Textbook of
Advanced Cardiac Life Support

Second Edition

 American Heart Association

Authors

Ramiro Albarran-Sotelo, MD
Youngstown, Ohio

Matt Anderson, NREMT-P
Juneau, Alaska

James M. Atkins, MD
Dallas, Texas

Doug Austin, EMT-P
Seattle, Washington

John E. Billi, MD
Ann Arbor, Michigan

Ronald S. Bloom, MD
Los Angeles, California

Frederick Campbell, MD
Philadelphia, Pennsylvania

Stephen W. Carveth, MD
Lincoln, Nebraska

Daniel L. Cavallaro, NREMT
Tampa, Florida

Leon Chameides, MD
Hartford, Connecticut

Jere D. Creed, MD
Plantation, Florida

Richard O. Cummins, MD,
    MPH, MSc
Seattle, Washington

James E. Dalen, MD
Worcester, Massachusetts

Judith Donegan, MD, PhD
San Francisco, California

Howard G. Dubin, MD
Providence, Rhode Island

Mickey Eisenberg, MD, PhD
Seattle, Washington

David Eitel, MD
York, Pennsylvania

Gordon A. Ewy, MD
Tucson, Arizona

Jane Freeman, RN
Gainesville, Florida

Randall Genton, MD
St. Louis, Missouri

Alan H. Goldberg, MD, PhD
Boston, Massachusetts

Edgar R. Gonzalez, PharmD
Richmond, Virginia

Joel M. Gore, MD
Worcester, Massachusetts

Ken Grauer, MD
Gainesville, Florida

Judy Graves, RN, MS
Seattle, Washington

Charles W. Guildner, MD
Everett, Washington

Cindy Hambly, EMT
Seattle, Washington

Mary T. Ho, MD, MPH
Seattle, Washington

NancySue Hudson, RN
Washington, DC

Allan S. Jaffe, MD
St. Louis, Missouri

Holly Jensen, RN
Gainesville, Florida

William Kaye, MD
Providence, Rhode Island

Costas T. Lambrew, MD
Portland, Maine

A. James Lewis, MD
Torrance, California

Robert C. Luten, MD
Jacksonville, Florida

Mary E. Mancini, RN, MSN
Dallas, Texas

James McCrory, MD
Jacksonville, Florida

Kevin M. McIntyre, MD, JD
Boston, Massachusetts

Richard Melker, MD, PhD
Gainesville, Florida

William H. Montgomery, MD
Honolulu, Hawaii

Mary M. Newman, BS
Carmel, Indiana

Joseph P. Ornato, MD
Richmond, Virginia

John M. Packard, MD
Birmingham, Alabama

John A. Paraskos, MD
Worcester, Massachusetts

Malcolm R. Parker, MD
Los Gatos, California

George J. Peckham, MD
Philadelphia, Pennsylvania

John R. Raye, MD
Farmington, Connecticut

Art Sanders, MD
Tucson, Arizona

Suzanne Sawtelle, RN
Providence, Rhode Island

Earl Schwartz, MD
Winston-Salem, North Carolina

James Seidel, MD, PhD
Torrance, California

Arnold Sladen, MD
Pittsburgh, Pennsylvania

Kenneth R. Stults, MS, PAC
Dallas, Texas

William H. Thies, PhD
Dallas, Texas

I. David Todres, MD
Boston, Massachusetts

Peter H. Viles, MD
Worcester, Massachusetts

W. Douglas Weaver, MD
Seattle, Washington

Roger D. White, MD
Rochester, Minnesota

Edward B.J. Winslow, MD
Chicago, Illinois

Arno Zaritzky, MD
Chapel Hill, North Carolina

ISBN 0-87493-603-9

Preface

The purpose of the *Textbook of Advanced Cardiac Life Support* is to serve as a reference source and as a course text for the training of advanced cardiac life support providers. With this edition the textbook has been revised to incorporate the suggestions of a large number of people who use the textbook, to accommodate anticipated changes in the ACLS course itself, and to incorporate the recommendations of the 1985 National Conference on Cardiopulmonary Resuscitation (CPR) and Emergency Cardiac Care (ECC).

The scope and content of the text was determined by the deliberations of the National Conference as published in the *Journal of the American Medical Association* in June 1986 and in a special supplement of *Circulation* in December 1986. As such, the text materials support the conjoint opinions of the National Conference itself rather than the views of the authors or the ACLS Working Group, which coordinated its production.

The present text provides more detailed background material that elucidates the rationale for the decisions of the National Conference along with illustrations and updated references that should enable those involved in ACLS to understand more fully the basis for and importance of these decisions.

This process represents a continuation of the efforts of many individuals since 1966 when the National Academy of Sciences and the National Research Council Conference on CPR recommended that external chest compressions according to the standards of the American Heart Association be taught to all medical professionals. In 1973, and again in 1980, a national conference on CPR and ECC standards was held and revised guidelines for ACLS were developed. Subsequently, educational materials such as the ACLS textbook were developed by the American Heart Association to teach the principles of ACLS and their practical implementation. These courses have provided the educational substrate for the training of large numbers of health professionals in this country and abroad.

Each national conference has developed a predominant theme. In 1980 the National Conference sought to expand the scope of the effort in ACLS by emphasizing the applicability of these guidelines to the out-patient setting by making the community part of the "cardiac care unit". The 1985 guidelines have built on this principle and present a strong advocacy for the rapid and widespread application of early and definitive care (most often defibrillation) in both the in-patient and the out-patient settings because of data that such a strategy will save lives.

The basic format of the textbook has not been altered substantially because, in general, there has been widespread satisfaction with it (over 900,000 copies distributed). Changes that have been made are largely in response to requests from those who use the textbook. The "Sudden Death" chapter, which was originally intended to present the rationale for the algorithms that had been developed, has been omitted, but the epidemiological material originally included is now part of Chapter 1 and the material relevant to postresuscitation is in Chapter 14. A new "Putting It All Together" chapter has been developed; it is hoped that this chapter can serve, published separately, as a pocket guide to resuscitation. In addition, a new chapter on "Special Resuscitation Situations" has been developed to guide resuscitation efforts when trauma, hypothermia, electrocution, near drowning, or pregnancy is present.

As in the past, the textbook has been planned to accompany a redeveloped ACLS course. The course will include a lecture and slides based on the information in the textbook. As part of this effort, core material and supplemental material will need to be designated, and a distinction between the two will be made in subsequent printings of the textbook.

It is important to remember that this textbook focuses on the end stage of the process that leads to cardiovascular disease by describing the management of "sudden death" and cardiac emergencies. At present, we can save individual lives if we are proficient. This is an important goal. However, we must also continue our efforts to better understand the processes that lead to cardiovascular disease and how to prevent them, the pathogenesis of cardiac arrest, and the physiology of cardiopulmonary resuscitation; and we must begin to develop improved techniques for prevention and for resuscitation and postresuscitation management because, in the long view, this is the way to save thousands.

Allan S. Jaffe, M.D.

Table of Contents

12. Invasive Monitoring Techniques

13. Invasive Therapeutic Techniques

14. Postresuscitation Management

15. Special Resuscitation Situations

Advanced Cardiac Life Support in Perspective

Chapter 1

The modern concept and practice of cardiopulmonary resuscitation (CPR) and emergency cardiac care (ECC) have been in evolution since 1960. This chapter is intended to put the development of CPR and ECC into perspective in terms of current practice and prospects for the future.

An Historical Perspective

Twenty-seven years have passed since the development of modern CPR began with the introduction of external chest compressions.[1] Modern CPR offers hope that the nearly 1,000 prehospital sudden deaths per day in the United States can be substantially reduced. In 1966, a National Academy of Sciences–National Research Council (NAS–NRC) Conference on CPR recommended the training of healthcare providers in the technique of external chest compressions according to the standards of the American Heart Association (AHA).[2] Widespread acceptance of CPR in this group ensued. Nevertheless, training, particularly of physicians, was not prevalent in many parts of the country; moreover, it was recommended that only on a supervised trial basis should CPR be taught to and administered by laypersons. From 1966 to 1973, contributions toward more widespread implementation were made by the AHA, the NAS–NRC, and the Inter-Society Commission on Heart Disease Resources, and by the recommendations and evaluations of governmental agencies, professional medical societies, and private groups.

In 1973, a National Conference on Standards for CPR and ECC, cosponsored by the AHA and the NAS–NRC, recommended that 1) the CPR training programs be extended to the general public, 2) training in CPR and ECC be in accordance with the standards of the AHA, 3) the association continue to review scientific data and clinical experience and revise and update the standards on those bases, 4) certification of competence at various levels of life support be based on nationally standardized curricula that include written and performance tests, 5) delivery of basic and advanced life support by highly trained personnel be required for all life support units and hospitals on an integrated, stratified, community-wide basis, 6) these goals be implemented by legislation and medicolegal action, where needed, to ensure the availability of prompt and effective CPR and ECC to the entire population, and 7) recognition of the early warning signs of heart attack and emphasis on access to the emergency medical services system be included in the definition of ECC. In addition, the 1973 National Conference described 1) the role of the American Red Cross and other agencies in training the lay public, 2) the role

of emergency care units in stratified systems providing ECC, and 3) the medicolegal problem areas of CPR and ECC, with possible approaches to solutions.

The recommendations and specific standards for both basic life support and advanced cardiac life support were published as a supplement to *The Journal of the American Medical Association*[3] in 1974. More than 5 million copies, in several different languages, were distributed worldwide. Materials for teaching CPR to laypersons and medical professionals, developed primarily by the AHA and the American Red Cross, were widely distributed.

In response to the recommendations of the 1973 National Conference, an advanced cardiac life support (ACLS) package of didactic and practical teaching and testing materials was produced by the AHA, based on a model developed by the Nebraska Affiliate;[4] and national and affiliate faculties in ACLS were organized to oversee and assist in implementation. Since 1975, many ACLS courses have been provided across the country; and the value of ACLS training is recognized by all professional medical organizations regularly involved in ECC.

Another national conference was convened in 1979. No major changes were made, but the standards and guidelines were revised in some areas.[5] In addition to those in CPR techniques, the revisions encompassed 1) a renewed, strong emphasis on community responsibility for coronary heart disease morbidity and mortality and for organized implementation of primary and secondary prevention programs in parallel with ECC efforts, 2) definition of the role of ECC units in stratified systems of emergency care, 3) a clearer definition of responsibility in life support for infants and children, 4) principles, techniques, and standards for the performance of basic life support (BLS), including CPR, in infants and children, and 5) principles, techniques, and guidelines for the performance of ACLS in neonates.

Each of the national conferences stimulated renewed interest and research. This activity necessitated another conference to update the standards and guidelines. The Fourth National Conference was convened in July 1985, and the most recent research and field experiences were incorporated.[6]

Since the 1973 National Conference, over 40 million people have been trained to perform CPR and tens of thousands of healthcare providers have completed the ACLS course. A number of factors have contributed to the success of this program; these include the development of emergency medical services systems nationwide, an increasing interest by laypersons in BLS–CPR, and the enthusiasm of healthcare providers for BLS–CPR and ACLS education. A major impetus has been an increased public awareness of the prevalence, morbidity, and mortality due to cardiovascular disease, plus new information provided through a resurgence of research.

Death From Cardiovascular Disease: The Magnitude of the Problem

The death rate due to cardiovascular disease increased each decade in the United States until the 1970's. Since then, there has been a dramatic decline in the death rates from myocardial ischemia and its complications (Figure 1). Although the reasons for this are not well understood, they are likely due, in part, to improved detection and treatment of hypertension, a reduction in cigarette use by middle-aged men, a change toward a more prudent diet, and improvements in the medical and surgical care for cardiovascular disease.[7,8] There is a general overall increase in health awareness in our society, more emphasis on disease prevention, and a growing interest in exercise, or "fitness". Despite these advances, the problem of premature death due to cardiovascular disease is formidable — more Americans die of cardiovascular disease than from any other cause (Table 1). In 1984 there were an estimated 2,047,000 deaths in the United States. Just under half (48%) of these were cardiovascular disease deaths, two-thirds of which were caused by underlying coronary and ischemic heart disease.

It is estimated that in 1987 approximately 1.5 million people in the United States will sustain a myocardial infarction, and roughly 540,000 (36%) of them will die (Table 2), 350,000 of those before they reach a hospital. Thus, more than half of the deaths due to ischemic heart disease will occur outside the hospital, most within two hours of the onset of symptoms.[10-15]

The need for educating the public to recognize life-threatening emergencies promptly and for developing rapid emergency response systems is clear.

For patients with acute myocardial infarction who reach the hospital, mortality from coronary disease has also substantially declined. This is due, in part, to the immediate resuscitation efforts possible in coronary care areas of hospitals and a reduction in the incidence of ventricular fibrillation by early antiarrhythmic drug therapy.[16,17] The recent results of clinical trials employing thrombolytic therapy and/or percutaneous transluminal angioplasty hold promise for further reducing mortality from acute ischemic heart disease.[18-22]

Table 1. Estimated Leading Causes of Death in the United States, 1985.

Cause	Number
Diseases of the heart and blood vessels	991,332
Cancer	457,670
Accidents	92,070
Chronic obstructive pulmonary disease	74,420
Pneumonia and influenza	66,630
All other causes	401,878

Source: National Center for Health Statistics, U.S. Public Health Service, DHHS

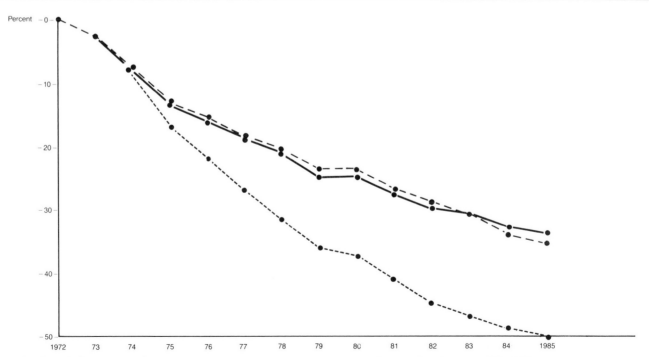

Figure 1. Cumulative percent change in age-adjusted death rates for major cardiovascular diseases, 1972-1985.

‐ ‐ ‐ CHD   ——— Total CVD   ••••• Stroke

Table 2. Estimated Deaths in the United States Due to Cardiovascular Diseases, 1984

CVD Type	No. of Deaths	Percent
Heart attack	540,400	54.8
Stroke	155,000	15.7
High blood pressure	30,000	3.1
Rheumatic fever and rheumatic heart disease	6,900	0.7
Other CVD	253,500	25.7

Source: National Center for Health Statistics, U.S. Public Health Service, DHHS.

Sudden Cardiac Death

There are two major clinical syndromes that result in death from ischemic heart disease: 1) sudden arrhythmic death due to cardiac arrest and 2) death due to myocardial failure. Although sudden arrhythmic death occurs most often in patients with previously recognized ischemic heart disease, unexpected cardiac arrest is the first manifestation of underlying heart disease in up to 20% of patients. The majority of patients who suffer sudden death have no premonitory symptoms immediately prior to collapse.[23-25] Thus, effective treatment for this condition cannot be symptom-initiated but is, instead, aimed at either preventing ventricular fibrillation or treating cardiac arrest itself.

Definition of Sudden Arrhythmic Death

Analyses to determine the etiology and exact incidence of sudden cardiac death have been hindered by variability in the definitions of the syndrome. Most definitions have been based on the apparent cause of death and duration of the final illness.[26] The World Health Organization classification (perhaps the most widely used) has defined sudden cardiac death as death occurring within 24 hours of the onset of illness or injury.[27]

A classification based solely on symptom duration is neither sensitive nor specific in determining the cause of death. Recently, a classification proposed by Hinkle and Thaler[28] has been used to determine the cause of cardiac death (Table 3). This classification has been validated in a multi-center prospective evaluation of mortality after acute myocardial infarction.[29] The findings of this study clearly show that although death within 1 hour of the onset of symptoms was specific for arrhythmic deaths, neither 1- nor 24-hour periods were useful in identifying the mechanism of death. For this reason, it seems prudent to modify the way in which we classify the deaths and to use the terms "sudden arrhythmic death" or "death due to myocardial failure". It is worthwhile to point out that the presence of ischemia or acute infarction is not accounted for in the classification, mainly because chest pain may be both absent and an imperfect indicator of ischemia.

Causes of Sudden Arrhythmic Death

Most episodes of sudden arrhythmic death occur outside the hospital.[24,26,30] It has been estimated that up to 1,000 cardiac arrests occur every day in the United States alone. In the overwhelming majority of patients, either coronary artery or ischemic heart disease is the underlying abnormality; valvular heart disease, congestive cardiomyopathy, or hypertensive heart disease is the underlying pathology in most of the remainder of cases.[31-35] Other, uncommon, conditions associated with cardiac arrest include preexcitation syndromes, hereditary or acquired prolonged QT disorders, metabolic abnormalities, and adverse reactions to drugs. In 1 or 2% of patients surviving cardiac arrest, no identifiable cardiac disorder can be found. The exact immediate cause of sudden arrhythmic death in all these conditions has been elusive. However, there are three conditions that are strongly associated with the development of ventricular fibrillation. They include 1) acute myocardial infarction in about 25% of patients, 2) transient myocardial ischemia in 25–30%, and 3) underlying structural myocardial abnormalities, usually caused by previous myocardial infarction, i.e., fibrosis or hypertrophy, in up to 50% of cases.

Identifying the High-Risk Patient

The major factors that increase the risk for sudden arrhythmic death are the same as those associated with the development of coronary heart disease: male sex, older age, elevated blood cholesterol, hypertension, diabetes mellitus, cigarette smoking, and a history of premature atherosclerosis.[36-41] Psychological and social factors such as a low level of education or a relatively high alcohol consumption appear also to be risk factors.[42-44] Although regular strenuous physical activity reduces the possibility of sudden death,[45,46] patients at risk for sudden arrhythmic death are more likely to collapse during or just following exercise than during sedentary activities.[47,48] Hypokalemia, hypomagnesemia, and prolongation of the QT interval also increase the risk for an arrhythmic death. In multivariant analysis of risk factors, age, left ventricular ejection

Table 3. Classification of Cardiac Deaths

Arrhythmic Death (abrupt loss of consciousness and disappearance of pulse without prior collapse of the circulation):

1. Not preceded by impairment of circulation
2. Preceded by chronic congestive heart failure, not disabling
3. Preceded by chronic congestive heart failure, disabling

Death Due to Myocardial Failure (gradual circulatory failure and collapse of circulation before disappearance of pulse):

1. Primarily caused by failure of peripheral circulation; e.g., due to hemorrhage, trauma, infarction, stroke, or respiratory failure
2. Primarily caused by failure of the myocardium

Modified from Hinkle and Thaler.[28]

fraction, and the presence of complex ventricular ectopy (greater than or equal to 10 PVC's/hour or three or more repetitive ectopic beats) were each independent predictors for a subsequent episode of cardiac arrest.[49-51] Unfortunately, neither the presence or absence of these factors is sufficiently specific or sensitive to be useful in accurately characterizing individual patients.

Prospects for the Future: Success and Potential of CPR and ACLS

Mortality from cardiovascular disease will be reduced when a significant decrease in the incidence and severity of coronary artery disease has occurred. However this long-term objective will not obviate the immediate problem of death from acute myocardial infarction and unheralded "sudden death". The approach to preventing cardiac arrest and resuscitating a cardiac arrest victim must involve a team effort that begins outside the hospital with the patient, bystanders trained in CPR, and the prompt and appropriate response of trained rescue personnel. It must be continued in the emergency department and hospital setting. An effective resuscitation commonly occurs through a coordinated team effort in which each member of the team anticipates the next step in the procedure and complements the efforts of the others.

The standards and guidelines for CPR and ECC have served as the framework for a coordinated approach that reflects extensive consideration of clinical and laboratory studies, education precepts, and the practicality of procedures advocated.[2,3,5,6] All were developed by consensus of an interdisciplinary group of experts to provide a reasoned and uniform approach to preventing and treating cardiac arrest. They represent the work of many distinguished clinicians and investigators — from the pioneers in resuscitation to those who have followed and have contributed by implementing, complementing, and broadening earlier achievements.

Reports from communities that have both large numbers of laypersons trained in BLS–CPR and an emergency medical services (EMS) system with a rapid response time have demonstrated that up to 30–40% of patients who receive bystander-initiated CPR and prompt defibrillation (ACLS) can survive an episode of cardiac arrest due to ventricular fibrillation.[52-59] When bystander-initiated CPR is delivered in a situation in which defibrillation is not immediately available, resuscitation and survival rates are still higher than when there is no bystander CPR. (Only one of the many studies in this area has failed to demonstrate improved survival or better neurological outcome in patients after bystander-initiated CPR.[60]) Thus, teaching citizens to recognize cardiac emergencies quickly, to provide CPR promptly and appropriately, and to know how to access the EMS system are uncontroversial benefits of community CPR programs. To maximize chances of survival, the delay

Table 4. Survival (%) Related to Response Times

Time to CPR (min)	Time to ACLS (min)		
	< 8	8-16	> 16
0-4	43%	19%	10%
4-8	26%	19%	5%
8-12	—	6%	0%

Adapted from Eisenberg.[70]

from onset of cardiac arrest until CPR and definitive care should be kept as short as possible, ideally to less than 4 and 8 minutes, respectively (Table 4).

Based on these types of data, it has been estimated that full implementation of these potentially lifesaving resources in the community may save between 100,000 and 200,000 lives per year in the United States.

There are several additional benefits associated with public enthusiasm for CPR. BLS–CPR programs incorporate education in both primary and secondary prevention of coronary heart disease, which results in a heightened awareness of coronary heart disease prevention, recognition, and early treatment.[61-65] Signals and action for survival are taught, which prompts lay rescuers to recognize the early warning signs of a cardiac emergency and tells them how to gain quick access into the EMS system. Given the increasing aggressive management of acute coronary emergencies, an even greater emphasis by physicians to patients and their families on how and when to seek emergency help is clearly mandated. Most studies show that patients with recognized heart disease delay longer before seeking emergency care than those who are not aware of their heart disease.[66,67]

There are three areas that deserve special attention during the next five years. The first is in targeting future layperson CPR efforts; the second, the need for early definitive care — specifically defibrillation; the third, changes in out-of-hospital care and the management of acute myocardial infarction (MI).

Targeting CPR Trainees

In surveys evaluating the demographics of laypersons taking CPR training in self-solicited community programs, trainees tended to be younger, more often male, and less often from a family with a known coronary heart disease victim than did persons who did not receive the training.[68,69] However, 70% of the time, cardiac arrest occurs at home; and most often, an older male is the victim. To take full advantage of community educational programs, family members of persons at risk for cardiac arrest need to be targeted to receive CPR training. This could be achieved by a greater involvement of healthcare providers in identifying and teaching the families of patients. Organized community efforts should try to attract older women to sign up for CPR courses, and CPR should be made a part of school curricula.

Early Defibrillation

Even in the best of EMS systems there is an inherent delay until the delivery of ACLS. The outcome for cardiac arrest, whether or not bystander CPR has been applied, is dismal if ACLS (defibrillation) is delayed beyond 8 minutes (Figure 2).[70,71] In the last decade, we have under-emphasized the role of prompt defibrillation. CPR should be initiated only when a defibrillator is not immediately at hand or after initial shocks have failed to restore spontaneous circulation. CPR should never be used as a substitute for definitive care. Efforts to provide a cadre of lesser-trained first responders with the training and equipment to administer early defibrillation have been initiated and should be aggressively supported.[72-74] In the future this trend of training first-arriving rescuers in defibrillation should include the training of fire, ambulance, and police personnel in tiered EMS systems — as well as, possibly, security and building attendants in public places and, finally, even family members of patients at risk for cardiac arrest.[75,76] Devices that will facilitate this effort of "early defibrillation" are known as "automatic (or semi-automatic) external defibrillators". Unlike conventional defibrillator-monitors, the automatic external defibrillator requires no rhythm recognition skills, is simpler to operate, and can be used by those less sophisticated in ACLS after only five hours of training. (The training required for first responders to use conventional defibrillators is two- to threefold greater, initially, and requires more extensive continuing education efforts to maintain satisfactory skill levels.[77-79]) Automatic devices should permit most small communities with volunteer emergency care providers, as well as most of all other first responding emergency care providers, to have enhanced lifesaving potential. Second, it may be a more fiscally responsible way to improve outcome after cardiac arrest in areas where the costs of paramedic services are prohibitive.

Changes in Out-of-Hospital Care and the Management of Acute MI

Emergency medical services systems have to deal with the problem of providing the best and most rapid care possible for patients with chest pain and acute coronary thrombosis. The evidence to date clearly shows that the greatest benefits of measures aimed at restoring blood flow to an acutely thrombosed coronary artery are realized when the delay from onset of chest pain to delivery of therapy is brief, suggesting that our pre-hospital care system should consider a return to the former "scoop and run" procedures in which only essential efforts were made in the field. This might shorten the delay until hospital arrival.

On the other hand, it is recognized that to prevent cardiac arrest, patients with chest pain, especially those with concomitant pulmonary congestion and/or shock,

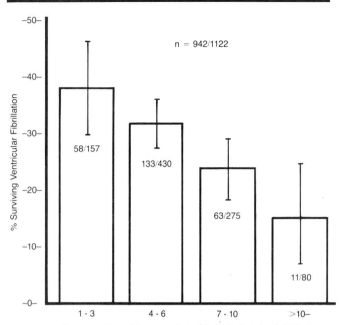

Figure 2. Survival rates for all patients (witnessed and unwitnessed) initially discovered in cardiac arrest. The response time was known in 942 of 1,122 consecutive cases. (From Weaver WD, Cobb LA, Hallstrom AP, Fahrenbruch C, Copass MK, Ray R: Factors influencing survival after out-of-hospital cardiac arrest. *J Am Coll Cardiol* 7:754, 1986.)

should be stabilized at the scene of the incident prior to transport. Pain relief needs to be initiated, an intravenous line started, and the cardiac rhythm stabilized. If necessary, blood pressure and ventilatory support should be ensured prior to initiating and during transport.[80-82] Because the anxiety induced by excessively rapid transportation may contribute to arrhythmias and in order to ensure the safety of the providers, the decision to provide high-speed transportation using a siren must be considered carefully. Substantial additional research is necessary to optimize care during helicopter transport. The feasibility of having EMT's and/or paramedics deliver thrombolytic therapy in the field must also be considered. The ability of the out-of-hospital team to make the diagnosis of acute myocardial infarction properly and to exclude patients with other emergencies that could be complicated or exacerbated by thrombolytic treatment is uncertain. However, EMS systems will be increasingly under pressure to rethink their organizations to minimize the delay in delivering definitive care to patients with chest pain and acute coronary thrombosis.

There are several obvious partial solutions to this delay. The patient must more promptly recognize the problem and seek help, transportation to the hospital must be facilitated, and the time from hospital admission until treatment must be reduced. Transport time is, in most cases, only a minor proportion of the total delay from initial symptoms to treatment. The delays encountered after the patient arrives at the hospital more often are far longer. The hospital emergency department should be prepared, using standing orders and guidelines, to quickly mobilize the personnel and resources needed to provide rapid pharmacological and/or invasive coronary reperfusion during the early hours of myocardial infarction.

A Systems Approach to Emergency Cardiac Care

Systems Conceptualization

Sudden arrhythmic death is the first manifestation of underlying coronary heart disease in approximately 15–25% of patients.[83] The majority will develop cardiac arrest outside the hospital without any, or with insignificant, premonitory symptoms.[84] Accordingly, the effective treatment of cardiac emergencies in the community requires a stratified or "systems" approach. This should begin with the instruction of the public in recognizing the manifestations of ischemic heart disease and an appropriate approach, by laypersons, to emergencies such as chest pain and cardiac arrest. Initial efforts need to be followed by a rapidly responding emergency medical services system with ACLS capability. In 1986, in Belfast, Ireland, the 20th year of out-of-hospital coronary care was celebrated. It was here that the concept of mobile coronary care was pioneered.[85] Now, every major city in the United States has paramedic level care, and almost all communities have some form of organized system for responding to emergencies.

In addition to the obvious benefit of these systems in the management of patients with cardiac arrest,[70,71] patients with acute myocardial infarction also benefit from organized systems.[86,87] Early prophylactic antiarrhythmia therapy is safe and results in a 50% reduction in the incidence of ventricular fibrillation en route to the hospital.[17]

In the setting of cardiac arrest, provision for defibrillation must be made for all prehospital emergency systems. When only CPR can be delivered initially and definitive therapy occurs only after arrival at the hospital, survival rates of 5% or less are usual. On the other hand, when prehospital defibrillation is available, survival rates for patients discovered in ventricular fibrillation range from 15 to 30%. The high rates of success in some communities are due in large part to widespread recognition of the problem, delivery of BLS–CPR by laypersons, plus a well-organized, rapidly responding EMS system (3–8 minutes) that provides ACLS (predominantly defibrillation).

ACLS will not be fully effective unless it is delivered almost immediately and is complemented by the prompt initiation of CPR. CPR is only a holding action to maintain the viability of the patient for a limited time until ACLS with "early defibrillation" is implemented.

An EMS system reflects coordination of the resources necessary to optimize the care required by an acutely ill or injured patient from the time the problem is recognized to the time he or she is discharged from the hospital and rehabilitation has been completed. Although this text deals primarily with advanced *cardiac* life support, the benefit of the EMS system to the victim of any kind of physical trauma is indisputable.

Dispatch of emergency care teams must be efficient and timely. Rapid response is facilitated through a widely publicized telephone number; all communities should adopt the 911 number for emergency assistance. It offers the advantage of ensuring prompt access to the system not only for the person familiar with the area but for transient populations as well. In some areas, advanced computerized systems now automatically provide the location of the caller, further facilitating the arrival of life support units.

The Emergency Care System

The EMS system should consist of primary response vehicles that are equipped and staffed to render both BLS and ACLS and to transport stabilized patients to better equipped facilities. In some areas, a tiered emergency response vehicle may be equipped and staffed to render only first aid and defibrillation. A limited number of secondary response vehicles may be simultaneously dispatched or summoned, with staff who are trained to provide full emergency care. The configuration of the specific emergency care system may vary from region to region since the best system will reflect the effective use and coordination of available resources.

Standing orders or protocols for ACLS providers are mandatory in order to minimize the delay until delivery of initial definitive care (ACLS). The initial management of cardiac arrest is straightforward and patients and conditions change so rapidly that efforts to communicate these changes to the hospital frequently only interfere with the delivery of lifesaving care. Therefore, initial procedures need to be defined and implemented by first-responding providers in order to maximize success rates. These initial steps must be defined by standing orders of the supervising physician; subsequent efforts not defined by standing orders must be supervised by the physician.

Medical Control of Prehospital Activity

Prehospital care is a logical extension of the hospital into the community. In this country rescue vehicles are rarely staffed by physicians. In most communities, nurses, emergency medical technicians (EMT's), and paramedics are trained to act as agents of the physician in the field. Every prehospital program must be supervised closely by a physician who provides direction and

Table 5. Medical Directors' Authorities, Responsibilities, and Roles

1. The adequate training and continuing education of providers of all care beyond first aid.
2. Criteria and policies for the certification and recertification of providers.
3. Guidelines for the management of all patients cared for by these providers.
4. Medically related dispatch procedures and transportation policies.
5. Criteria for patient disposition.
6. Quality assurance, including systematic audits.
7. A mechanism to allow supervision of all medical care delivered.

leadership and assumes responsibility for the emergency care team (Table 5). The physician must be thoroughly familiar with the local and regional EMS system and with the principles of advanced cardiac care as defined in the "Standards and Guidelines for Cardiopulmonary Resuscitation (CPR) and Emergency Cardiac Care (ECC)".[6] The system's medical director must ensure that both the on-site provider and the immediate medical supervisor are proficient in ACLS, and the medical director is ultimately responsible and should review the care given within the system.[88]

Direct involvement of the physician in virtually all aspects of care is mandatory. With the widespread provision of early defibrillation by first providers, there will be even more of a need to review the care delivered by these providers. It cannot be over-emphasized that out-of-hospital systems can be neither self-sustaining nor self-accountable. The use of a device or a drug is but a small portion of total patient care, and it is the evaluation of this total system of health care for which the medical director must be accountable. In addition, the physician should provide innovation and translate newly acquired medical knowledge into prehospital care. The director should set the expectations and criteria for performance of the providers. The most successful community emergency medical systems are in many ways a tribute to the extent of physician involvement, training, and supervision.

Voice communication from providers at the scene and to the supervising physician is mandatory and should be provided in every system. The need for telemetry of the electrocardiogram (ECG) will vary depending on the degree of training of the field personnel. It should be noted that the telephone is an inexpensive and readily accessible instrument that can be used to transmit the ECG.

Protocols and Standing Orders

All systems must have protocols for handling the most common emergencies.[56] These protocols are also essential for training prehospital personnel. In the cardiac arrest protocol, it is the option of the medical director to determine how much protocol should be followed before communication with the physician becomes obligatory. The use of standing orders is appropriate for only a few well-defined conditions, such as cardiac arrest.

For most other cardiac emergencies, the physician should be contacted prior to the initiation of invasive treatment by field personnel. The physician should be given a description of the patient's problem, the vital signs, and other information obtained during a brief physical assessment of the patient. Field personnel may suggest a plan for treatment that should be approved or modified by the consulting physician. Patient management protocols are predicated on a precise knowledge of the individual patient's condition as well as a clear recognition of what can and should be accomplished by treatment.[89] Therefore, the use of standard written orders for use by nonphysicians is appropriate for only a few well-defined conditions where therapeutic strategy is narrow and straightforward. The broad range of complex medical issues encountered by an EMS system does not lend itself to interventions based on an array of written standing orders. In addition, the communication process itself between physician and paramedic serves as a stimulus for careful thought and assessment of the patient's condition.

Issues relevant to urban-based EMS systems are, in principle, no different for rural areas; however, there are certain important modifiers. They include distances, resources available, economic/political aspects of hospital destination, the complexity and expectations of people living in the community, and the likelihood that multiple hospitals and multiple physicians will be involved.

If a physician is on the scene and willing to help and supervise, he or she should assume responsibility for the management of the patient by providing his/her identity and accompanying the patient to the receiving facility. If a physician has not been responsible, a retrospective review of each treatment record and other documents (voice or ECG tape recordings) is a means of quality assurance. In addition, personal observation of paramedic performance by the supervising physicians or their delegates should be accomplished periodically. Tabulations of procedures and performance carried out by each individual need to be made in order to establish constructive recommendations for continuing education.

Patient Disposition

The physician directing an emergency call must decide, based on the condition and medical needs of the patient, when and where the patient should be transported. The medical director should provide guidelines that consider the patient's prior medical care, the problem at hand, and the resources available in the community. Patients with suspected acute myocardial infarction, as well as other acute life-threatening cardiac conditions, should be closely monitored in a coronary care unit or its equivalent. Acutely ill or unstable cardiac patients should not be transported to a facility without this capability. If the need for an emergency cardiac catheterization or cardiopulmonary bypass is anticipated, the patient should be brought directly to a facility with such capability if feasible. Patients who develop, or who are at high risk to develop, life-threatening complications of extensive acute myocardial infarction are often managed best at specialized treatment facilities. The EMS system should make provisions for secondary ACLS transport of patients from primary care treatment centers to regional tertiary care institutions.

At times, it may be better for the patient to bypass the emergency department and go directly to the coronary care unit or to the cardiac catheterization laboratory.[90] Communication prior to transportation or while en route allows hospital personnel to properly prepare for the patient's arrival. All hospital medical personnel assigned to critical care areas, including the emergency department, the coronary care unit, and other intensive care units, should be trained in BLS–CPR and ACLS. Each hospital should have a committee that is responsible for assuring that such training is acquired and maintained.

Objectives of the American Heart Association: BLS and ACLS Support Programs

It is recognized that graduation from a health professional school and state licensure do not necessarily guarantee proficiency in performing BLS–CPR and ACLS. The CPR and ACLS training programs of the American Heart Association (AHA) were therefore developed to disseminate the AHA standards and guidelines for emergency cardiac care as broadly as possible by imparting knowledge and by providing an opportunity to develop and test the practical skills necessary to apply this knowledge. Laboratory simultations that promote effective learning of these skills through supervised practice have caused the ACLS program to become widely accepted.

The AHA training network pyramid allows for the maintenance of instructional quality and for adherence to the AHA standards and guidelines. The Subcommittee on Emergency Cardiac Care created the National Faculty Group. Representatives are appointed by each state affiliate and have the objective of providing a liaison with the Affiliate Faculty of each state, who are responsible ultimately for the teaching and supervision of ACLS programs in each state.

The ACLS training program has been a focus for interdisciplinary teaching. Physicians, nurses, and other healthcare providers have taught and learned together, promoting a climate of cooperation and teamwork in the acute care setting. The AHA standards and guidelines and the ACLS training package also have facilitated substantially the development of prehospital ACLS programs.

The AHA is charged with the responsibility for maintaining these standards. "Successful completion" of an ACLS course means in accordance with the cognitive

and performance standards of the American Heart Association. It does not warrant performance, nor does it, per se, qualify or authorize a person to perform any procedure. It is in no way related to licensure, which is a function of the appropriate legislative, health, or educational authority.[91] The primary objectives of ACLS courses are totally educational. They are not designated to regulate healthcare practices. Though ACLS courses may provide guidelines for medical and nursing personnel in the performance of certain jobs, the ACLS program should be considered to be only one component of the continuing in-service education in institutions responsible for the treatment of cardiac emergencies. It is not a substitute for either coronary care unit nursing educational programs or advanced cardiac training programs.

The schema and recommendations provided in this text are guidelines that represent a consensus. Future research may alter these guidelines considerably. The AHA standards and guidelines provide a stimulus to many investigators to reexamine the steps in resuscitation. Such research will likely lead to even further modifications. Although it is often difficult for students to practice or learn skills in an area where controversy exists, it is the reexamination of old and new "facts" that ultimately leads to even further improvements in resuscitation techniques. The American Heart Association supports new research in these areas and is aware of the continuous need to reassess the recommendations in this text.

References

1. Kouwenhoven WB, Jude JR, Knickerbocker GG: Closed-chest cardiac massage. *JAMA* 173:1064-1067, 1960.
2. *Cardiopulmonary Resuscitation Conference Proceedings,* May 23, 1966. Washington, National Academy of Sciences-National Research Council, 1967.
3. Standards for cardiopulmonary resuscitation (CPR) and emergency cardiac care (ECC). *JAMA* 227 (suppl):833-868, 1974.
4. Carveth SW, Burnap TK, Bechtel J, et al: Training in advanced cardiac life support. *JAMA* 235:2311-2315, 1976.
5. Standards and guidelines for cardiopulmonary resuscitation (CPR) and emergency cardiac care (ECC). *JAMA* 244:453-509, 1980.
6. Standards and guidelines for cardiopulmonary resuscitation (CPR) and emergency cardiac care (ECC). *JAMA* 255:2905-2989, 1986.
7. Kannel WB, Thom TJ: Implication of the recent decline in cardiovascular mortality. *Cardiovasc Med* 4:983, 1979.
8. Goldman L, Cook EF: The decline in ischemic heart disease mortality rates. An analysis of the comparative effects of medical interventions and changes in lifestyle. *Ann Intern Med* 101: 825-836, 1984.
9. Ornato JP, Garen EJ, Nelson N, et al: The impact of emergency cardiac care on the reduction of mortality from myocardial infarction. *J Cardiac Rehab* 3:863-866, 1983.
10. Bainton CR, Peterson DR: Deaths from coronary heart disease in persons fifty years of age or younger. A community-wide study. *N Engl J Med* 268:569-575, 1963.
11. McNeilly RH, Pemberton J: Duration of last attack in 988 fatal cases of coronary artery disease and its relation to possible cardiac resuscitation. *Br Med J* 3:139-142, 1968.
12. Kuller LH: Sudden death — definition and epidemiologic considerations. *Prog Cardiovasc Dis* 23:1-12, 1980.
13. Gordon T, Kannel WB: Premature mortality from coronary heart disease: The Framingham study. *JAMA* 215:1617-1625, 1971.

14. Kuller L, Cooper M, Perper J: Epidemiology of sudden death. *Arch Intern Med* 129:714-719, 1972.
15. Kuller L, Lilienfeld A, Fisher R: Sudden and unexpected deaths in young adults. An epidemiological study. *JAMA* 198:248-252, 1966.
16. Lie KI, Wellens HJ, Van Capelle FJ, Durrer D: Lidocaine in the prevention of primary ventricular fibrillation. A double-blind, randomized study of 212 consecutive patients. *N Engl J Med* 291(25):1324-1326, 1974.
17. Koster RW, Dunning AJ: Intramuscular lidocaine for prevention of lethal arrhythmias in the prehospitalization phase of acute myocardial infarction. *N Engl J Med* 313:1105-1110, 1985.
18. Simoons ML, Serruys PW, v d Brand M, Bars F, de Zwaan C, Res J, Verheugt FWA, Krauss XH, Remme WJ, Vermeer F, Lubsen J: Improved survival after early thrombolysis in acute myocardial infarction: A randomized trial conducted by the Inter-University Cardiology Institute in the Netherlands. *Lancet* 1:578-582, 1985.
19. Kennedy JW, Richey JL, Davis KB, Fritz JK: Western Washington randomized trial of intracoronary streptokinase in acute myocardial infarction. *N Engl J Med* 309:1477-1482, 1983.
20. Gruppo Ittalino per lo studio della streptochinasi nell'infarto miocardico (GISSI). Effectiveness of intravenous thrombolytic treatment in acute myocardial infarction. *Lancet* 1:397-401, 1986.
21. TIMI Study Group: The thrombolysis in myocardial infarction (TIMI) trial. Phase I findings. *N Engl J Med* 312:932-936, 1985.
22. O'Neill W, Timmis GC, Bourdellon PD, Lai P, Ganghadarhan V, Walton J Jr, Ramos R, Laufer N, Gordon S, Shork MA, Pitt B: A prospective randomized clinical trial of intracoronary steptokinase vs coronary angioplasty for acute myocardial infarction. *N Engl J Med* 314:812-818, 1986.
23. Schaffer WA, Cobb LA. Recurrent ventricular fibrillation and modes of death in survivors of out-of-hospital ventricular fibrillation. *N Engl J Med* 293:259-262, 1975.
24. Baum RS, Alvarez H 3rd, Cobb LA. Survival after resuscitation from out-of-hospital ventricular fibrillation. *Circulation* 50:1231-1235, 1974.
25. Eisenberg MS, Cummins RO, Litwin PE, Hallstrom AP. Out-of-Hospital cardiac arrest: Significance of symptoms in patients collapsing before and after arrival of paramedics. *Am J Emerg Med* 4:116-120, 1986.
26. Kuller LH. Sudden death — definition and epidemiologic considerations. *Prog Cardiovasc Dis* 23:1-12, 1980.
27. World Health Organization: *Manual of the International Statistical Classification of Diseases, Injuries, and Causes of Death,* based on the Recommendations of the Ninth Revision Conference, 1975, and adopted by the 29th World Health Assembly. 1975 revision. Geneva, World Health Organization, 1977, p 470.
28. Hinkle LE Jr, Thaler HT: Clinical classification of cardiac deaths. *Circulation* 65:457-464, 1982.
29. Marcus FI, Cobb LA, Edwards J, Kuller L, Serokman R: Multicenter post infarction research group. Mortality after acute myocardial infarction in the multi-center post infarction program. *J Am Col Cardiol* 7:67A, 1986.
30. Gordon T, Kannel WB. Premature mortality from coronary heart disease: The Framingham Study. *JAMA* 215:1617-1625, 1971.
31. Kuller L: Sudden and unexpected non-traumatic deaths in adults: A review of epidemiological and clinical studies. *J Chronic Dis* 19:1165-1192, 1966.
32. Schwartz CJ, Walsh WJ. The pathologic basis of sudden death. *Prog Cardiovasc Dis* 13:465-481, 1971.
33. Kehoe RF, Talano JV. Sudden death — a challenge for the 80's, in Moran JM, Michaelis LL (eds): *Surgery for the Complications of Myocardial Infarction.* New York, Grune & Stratton, 1980, pp 337-368.
34. Cobb LA, Hallstrom AP, Weaver WD, Copass MK, Hedgecock M, Haynes RE: Prognostic factors in patients resuscitated from sudden cardiac death, in Wilhelmsen L, Hjalmarson A(eds): *Acute and Long-Term Management of Myocardial Ischemia.* Mondak, Sweden, Lindgren and Soner AB, 1978, pp 106-113.
35. Cobb LA, Werner JA: Predictors and prevention of sudden cardiac death, in Hurst JW (ed): *The Heart.* New York, McGraw-Hill, 1982, pp 599-610.
36. Corday E: Symposium on identification and management of the candidate for sudden cardiac death: Introduction. *Am J Cardiol* 39(6):813-815, 1977.
37. Chiang BN, Perlman LV, Fulton M, et al: Predisposing factors in sudden cardiac death in Tecumseh, Michigan. A prospective study. *Circulation* 41:31-37, 1970.
38. Friedman GD, Dales LG, Ury HK: Mortality in middle-aged smokers and nonsmokers. *N Engl J Med* 300:213-217, 1979.
39. Moss AJ: Prediction and prevention of sudden cardiac death. *Ann Rev Med* 31:1-14, 1980.
40. Kannel WB, Doyle JT, McNamara PM, Quickenton P, Gordon T: Precursors of sudden coronary death. Factors related to the incidence of sudden death. *Circulation* 41:606-613, 1975.
41. Hallstrom AP, Cobb LA, Ray R: Smoking as a risk factor for recurrence of sudden cardiac arrest. *N Engl J Med* 314:271-275, 1986.
42. Weinblatt E, Ruberman W, Goldberg JD, et al: Relation of education to sudden death after myocardial infarction. *N Engl J Med* 299(2):60-65, 1978.
43. Jenkins CD: Low education: A risk factor for death (editorial). *N Engl J Med* 299(2):95-97, 1978.
44. Talbott E, Kuller LH, Detre K, Perper J: Biologic and psychosocial risk factors of sudden death from coronary disease in white women. *Am J Cardiol* 39(6):858-864, 1977.
45. Paffenbarger RS, Hale WE: Work activity and coronary heart mortality. *N Engl J Med* 292(11):545-550, 1975.
46. Siscovick DS, Weiss NS, Hallstrom AP, Inui TS, Peterson DR: Physical activity and primary cardiac arrest. *JAMA* 248:3113-3117, 1982.
47. Siscovick DS, Weiss NS, Fletcher RH, Laskey T: The incidence of primary cardiac arrest during vigorous exercise. *N Engl J Med* 311(14):874-877, 1974.
48. Cobb LA, Weaver WD: Exercise: a risk for sudden death in patients with coronary heart disease. *J Am Col Cardiol* 7(1):215-219, 1986.
49. Ritchie JL, Hallstrom AP, Trobaugh GB, Cobb LA: Out-of-hospital sudden coronary death: rest and exercise radionuclide left ventricular function in survivors. *Am J Cardiol* 55(6):645-651, 1985.
50. Bigger JT, Heller CA, Wenger TL, Weld FM: Risk stratification after acute myocardial infarction. *Am J Cardiol* 42(2):202-210, 1978.
51. The Multicenter Postinfarction Research Group: Risk stratification and survival after myocardial infarction. *N Engl J Med* 309:331-336, 1983.
52. Thompson RG, Hallstrom AP, Cobb LA: Bystander-initiated cardiopulmonary resuscitation in the management of ventricular fibrillation. *Ann Int Med* 90:737-740, 1979.
53. Cummins RO, Eisenberg MS: Prehosiptal cardiopulmonary resuscitation: Is it effective? *JAMA* 253:2408-2412, 1985.
54. Lund I, Skulberg A: Cardiopulmonary resuscitation by lay people. *Lancet* 2:702-704, 1976.
55. Vertesi L, Wilson L, Glick N: Cardiac arrest: Comparison of paramedic and conventional ambulance services. *Can Med Assoc J* 128:809-812, 1983.
56. Guzy PM, Pearce ML, Greenfield S: The survival benefit of bystander cardiopulmonary resuscitation in a paramedic-served metropolitan area. *Am J Public Health* 73:766-769, 1983.
57. Roth R, Stewart RD, Rogers K, Cannon GM: Out-of-hospital cardiac arrest: Factors associated with survival. *Ann Emerg Med* 13:237-243, 1984.
58. Copley DP, Mantle JA, Rogers WJ, Russell RO Jr, Rackley C: Improved outcome from prehospital cardiopulmonary collapse with resuscitation by bystander. *Circulation* 56:901-905, 1977.
59. Tweed WA, Bristow G, Donen N: Resuscitation from cardiac arrest: Assessment of a system providing only basic life support outside of hospital. *Can Med Assoc J* 122:297-300, 1980.
60. Kowalski R, Thompson BM, Horwitz L, Stueven H, Aprahamin C, Darin JC: Bystander CPR in prehospital coarse ventricular fibrillation. *Ann Emerg Med* 13:1016-1020, 1984.
61. Gordon T, Kannel WB, McGee D, et al: Death and coronary attacks in men after giving up cigarette smoking: A report from the Framingham study. *Lancet* 2:1345-1348, 1974.
62. Wilhelmsson C, Vedin JA, Elmfeldt D, et al: Smoking and myocardial infarction. *Lancet* 1:415-420, 1975.
63. Five-year findings of the hypertension detection and follow-up program. I. Reduction in mortality of persons with high blood pressure, including mild hypertension. *JAMA* 242:2562-2571, 1979.
64. The Lipid Research Clinics Coronary Primary Prevention Trial Results. I. Reduction in incidence of coronary heart arrest. *JAMA* 251:351-364, 1984.
65. Hallstrom AP, Cobb LA, Ray R: Smoking as a risk factor for recurrence of sudden cardiac death. *N Engl J Med* 314:271-275, 1986.

66. Goldstein S, Moss AJ, Greene W: Sudden death in acute myocardial infarction. Relationship to factors affecting delay in hospitalization. *Arch Intern Med* 129:720-724, 1972.

67. Moss AJ, Goldstein S: The pre-hospital phase of acute myocardial infarction. *Circulation* 41:737-742, 1970.

68. Mandel LP, Cobb LA: CPR training in the community. *Ann Emerg Med* 14:669-671, 1985.

69. Goldberg RJ, Gore JM, Love DG, Ockene JK, Dalen JE: Layperson CPR — Are we training the right people? *Ann Emerg Med* 13:701-704, 1984.

70. Eisenberg MS, Bergner L, Hallstrom A: Cardiac resuscitation in the community. Importance of rapid provision and implications for program planning. *JAMA* 241:1905-1907, 1979.

71. Weaver WD, Cobb LA, Hallstrom AP, Fahrenbruch C, Copass MK, Ray R: Factors influencing survival after out-of-hospital cardiac arrest. *J Am Coll Cardiol* 7:752-757, 1986.

72. Cummins RO, Eisenberg MS, Moore JE, Hearn TR, Anderson E, Wendt R, Litwin PE, Graves JR, Hallstrom AP, Pierce J: Automatic external defibrillators: Clinical, training, psychological, and public health issues. *Ann Emerg Med* 14:755-760, 1985.

73. Stults KR, Brown DD, Kerber RE: Efficacy of an automated external defibrillator in the management of out-of-hospital cardiac arrest: Validation of the diagnostic algorithm and initial clinical experience in a rural environment. *Circulation* 73:701-709, 1986.

74. Weaver WD, Copass MK, Hill DL, Fahrenbruch C, Hallstrom AP, Cobb LA: Cardiac arrest treated with a new automatic external defibrillator by out-of-hospital first responders. *Am J Cardiol* 57:1017-1021, 1986.

75. Weaver WD, Hill DL, Bolles J, Hallstrom AP, Cobb LA: Training families of victims at risk for cardiac arrest in the use of an automatic external defibrillator (abstracted). *Circulation* 72:III-9, 1985.

76. Moore JE, Eisenberg MS, Andresen E, Cummins RD, Hallstrom AP, Litwin P: Home placement of automatic external defibrillators among survivors of ventricular fibrillation. *Ann Emerg Med* 15:811-812, 1986.

77. Eisenberg MS, Hallstrom AP, Copass MK, Bergner L, Short F, Pierce J: Treatment of ventricular fibrillation. Emergency medical technician defibrillation and paramedic services. *JAMA* 251:1723-1726, 1984.

78. Stultz KR, Brown DD, Schug VL, Bean JA: Prehospital defibrillation performed by emergency medical technicians in rural communities. *N Engl J Med* 310:219-223, 1984.

79. Weaver WD, Copass MK, Bufi D, Ray R, Hallstrom AP, Cobb LA: Improved neurologic recovery and survival after early defibrillation. *Circulation* 69:943-948, 1984.

80. Lambrew CT: The experience in telemetry of the electrocardiogram to a base hospital. *Heart Lung* 3:756-764, 1974.

81. Pantridge JF: The effect of early therapy on the hospital mortality from acute myocardial infarction. *Quart J Med* 39:621-622, 1970.

82. Grace WJ, Chadbourn JA: The first hour in acute myocardial infarction. *Heart Lung* 3:736-741, 1974.

83. Cobb LA, Werner JA, Trobaugh GB: Sudden cardiac death. I. A decade's experience of out-of-hospital resuscitation. *Mod Con Cardiovasc Dis* 49:31-36, 1980.

84. Lown B, Klein MD, Hershberg PI: Coronary and precoronary care. *Am J Med* 46:705-724, 1970.

85. Pantridge JF, Geddes JS: Cardiac arrest after myocardial infarction. *Lancet* 1:807-808, 1966.

86. Lewis RP, Lanese RR, Stang JM, Chirikos TN, Keller MD, Warren JV: Reduction in mortality from prehospital myocardial infarction by prudent patient activation of mobile coronary care system. *Am Heart J* 103:123-127, 1982.

87. Cobb LA: Prehospital cardiac care: Does it make a difference? *Am Heart J* 103:316-318, 1982.

88. Thirteenth Bethesda Conference. Emergency Cardiac Care. *Am J Cardiol* 50:365-420, 1982.

89. Moloney TW, Rogers DE: Medical technology — A different view of the contentious debate over costs. *N Engl J Med* 301:1413-1419, 1979.

90. Standards for Emergency Cardiac Care in Advanced Life Support Units (including Hospital Emergency Departments). Dallas, American Heart Association, 1976.

91. Carveth SW, Burnap TK, Bechtel J, et al: Training in advanced cardiac life support. *JAMA* 235:2311-2315, 1976.

Myocardial Infarction Chapter 2

Myocardial infarction is the term used to refer to necrosis of heart muscle caused by an inadequate blood supply. In the majority of cases, it is the result of severe atherosclerotic narrowing of one or more of the coronary arteries. However, in individual patients, the extent and distribution of arterial narrowing is only a weak predictor of the likelihood that infarction will occur.[1,2] Factors that have been implicated in the pathogenesis of myocardial infarction include atherosclerotic plaque rupture (fissuring or hemorrhage)[3-5] and spasm.[6,7] During the early hours of an acute transmural (Q wave) myocardial infarction, one or more of these factors are usually associated with thrombosis of the involved coronary artery.[8] Nontransmural (non-Q wave) infarction may be less frequently associated with thrombosis.[9] A common pathogenetic sequence may be rupture of a plaque with extrusion of the atheromatous contents into the lumen and subsequent thrombosis. Coronary spasm and coronary embolism are uncommon causes of myocardial infarction. Rarely, myocardial infarction can occur in the absence of coronary artery narrowing if there is a marked disparity between myocardial oxygen supply and demand. Cocaine abuse has been implicated as a possible cause of such a disparity.[10]

The prompt recognition that infarction is occurring is critical since most deaths associated with acute infarction are due to electrical instability and occur suddenly, prior to presentation to hospital.[11] As such, they are potentially preventable.[12]

This chapter will review the principles of early management of the patient with acute myocardial infarction, the management of the more common life-threatening complications of myocardial infarction, and approaches designed to reduce long-term mortality after infarction.

Clinical Presentation

Precipitating Events

Despite a bias to the contrary, most patients suffer the onset of infarction at rest or with moderate activity. In one study, 59% were either at rest or asleep. Forty-one percent were involved in some activity, mostly requiring mild-to-moderate or usual exertion.[13] Other data also fail to support a cause-and-effect relation between vigorous exertion and myocardial infarction,[14] but some conflicting evidence also has been offered.[15-19] The recent description of a marked daily pattern (circadian rhythm) in the frequency of the time of the onset of acute infarction, which peaks from 6 AM to noon, also suggests that factors other than activity may be critical.[22] Nonetheless, the combination of severe exertion and excessive fatigue

or unusual emotional stress has been indicated as more likely to precipitate myocardial infarction.[15] Emotional stress and life events with powerful impact on the individual, e.g., death of a significant other person, divorce, or loss of job, are common prior to myocardial infarction and, in the long run, may prove to have an etiological relation with the event.[20,21]

Symptom Recognition and Response

All of the following symptoms may be due to acute myocardial infarction. As such they carry a risk of sudden death and must be recognized and acted on promptly:

1. New onset of chest pain suspicious for myocardial ischemia (see below) either at rest or with ordinary or usual activity.
2. A change in a previously stable pattern of anginal pain, i.e., either an increase in frequency or severity or the occurrence of rest angina for the first time.
3. Chest pain suspicious for myocardial ischemia, in a patient with known coronary heart disease, that is unrelieved by rest and/or nitroglycerin.

Chest pain or discomfort due to myocardial ischemia may be central (substernal) or more diffuse.[23] The pain is variably described as crushing, pressing ("like a vise"), constricting, oppressive, or heavy ("like an elephant on my chest") and tends to increase in intensity over a period of minutes. There may be radiation of the pain to one (more often the left) or both shoulders and arms, or to the neck, lower jaw, or back. Less commonly, high epigastric discomfort may be a manifestation of myocardial ischemia and may be dismissed as "indigestion". Any unusual or prolonged "indigestion" should raise suspicion, particularly in a high-risk individual. Discomfort in the arms, shoulders, neck, jaw, epigastrium, or back may be due to myocardial ischemia or infarction, even in the absence of substernal chest discomfort.

New discomfort in the chest or in the other areas described above, that is not otherwise explained and that persists more than a few minutes (especially in a patient known to be at high risk), should be evaluated. The American Heart Association recommends that a patient with known angina pectoris seek emergency medical care if chest pain is not relieved by three nitroglycerin tablets over a 10-minute period. In a person with previously unrecognized coronary disease, the persistence of suspicious chest pain for 2 minutes or longer is an indication for emergency medical assistance.[24]

The importance of a prompt response to symptoms suspicious for myocardial ischemia is emphasized by observations that ventricular fibrillation is 15 times more frequent during the first hour after symptoms than during the subsequent 12 hours.[12] In one study, ventricular fibrillation was found in 36% of patients with acute myocardial infarction within the first hour of symptoms.[25] Despite these facts, the average delay between the onset of symptoms of acute myocardial infarction and the decision to call for medical assistance is 3 hours,[26] and those who are aware of their illness and on cardiac medications are even less prompt in calling for medical assistance.[27] This unnecessary delay not only places the patient at higher risk of death from ventricular fibrillation but also diminishes the effectiveness of interventions designed to limit the size of the infarction. It is imperative, therefore, that patients, families, and communities be educated in the need for prompt response. Training in cardiopulmonary resuscitation for the patient's family and the community in general continues to be a critical link in efforts to reduce prehospital death from coronary artery disease.

General Management Approaches

Suspicion of acute myocardial infarction is based on the patient's symptoms. If the history is consistent with the diagnosis, the patient must be treated accordingly. Although the electrocardiogram often confirms the diagnosis, it also may be entirely normal. Therefore, a single normal electrocardiogram cannot be relied upon to exclude the diagnosis.

Electrocardiographic Monitoring

Because of the high incidence of ventricular fibrillation and other serious arrhythmias during the first hour of acute infarction,[11,25] electrocardiographic monitoring (with an oscilloscope) should be initiated immediately upon suspicion of the diagnosis.

Establishing Intravenous Access

Since pharmacological therapy may be needed rapidly, the placement of secure intravenous access is essential. A large-bore intravenous line should be placed in an arm vein. The percutaneous puncture of veins that are non-compressible should be discouraged since they will present a contraindication to the use of thrombolytic agents for several days.[28]

Oxygen in Myocardial Infarction

Hypoxemia in patients with uncomplicated acute infarction is usually caused by ventilation-perfusion abnormalities[29,30] and is exacerbated by left ventricular failure. Because significant hypoxemia may occur even in patients with uncomplicated infarction, therapy with supplemental oxygen is recommended until and unless a normal arterial oxygen tension (PaO_2) is documented. There is some evidence that an elevation of PaO_2 may reduce the size of the infarction.[31,32] However, super-physiological levels of oxygen may increase systemic vascular resistance and arterial pressure, lowering cardiac output and possibly compromising peripheral oxygen delivery.[33-35] Even at high concentrations, this concern is hypothetical and should not discourage the administration of oxygen to all patients with myocardial infarction. When oxygen is used, it should be administered by mask or nasal cannula at a flow rate of 1–10 L/min, or as described in Chapters 3 and 7. Further increase in the concentration of delivered oxygen is necessary only if serious left ventricular failure or pulmonary complications develop. Arterial blood gas determinations should be discouraged during the early stages of an acute myocardial infarction since they are associated with morbidity after the administration of thrombolytic agents.[36]

Relief of Pain

Relief of pain should have a high priority. Sublingual nitroglycerin usually is tried first unless the patient is hypotensive because in some patients severe ischemia may be difficult to distinguish from infarction. If chest pain and ECG changes resolve promptly, infarction is less likely. When infarction is present, nitroglycerin alone may not be adequate.[37] Nitroglycerin may reduce the mean arterial blood pressure (with a resultant fall in coronary perfusion pressure) and cause a reflex tachycardia (with a possible increase in myocardial oxygen demand).[33] Hence, blood pressure must be monitored closely. Even if blood pressure is normal when the patient is supine, there is a danger of orthostatic hypotension. If hypotension occurs, the patient should be placed in the supine position or with legs raised. Intravenous fluids may also be required. Pressor agents should be avoided if possible. If bradycardia occurs with hypotension, atropine should be administered.[39]

Among the potential additional beneficial effects of nitroglycerin may be a reduction in myocardial oxygen demand, a possible increase in collateral flow to the ischemic myocardium,[38] and a reduction of coronary artery spasm[40] with subsequent reduction in the extent of infarction if carefully titrated.[37,41,42] It has also been suggested that nitroglycerin decreases the susceptibility of the ischemic myocardium to ventricular fibrillation.[43] However, there is insufficient data at this time to recommend the continued use of nitroglycerin (after its original use to distinguish ischemia from infarction) in the routine patient with infarction. Its use may induce detrimental effects on coronary blood flow and significant arrhythmias if hypotension is induced.

Morphine sulfate is the drug of choice for the pain associated with acute infarction. Morphine is administered in small (2–5 mg) intravenous doses (see Chapter 7) and may be repeated at 5-minute intervals. In addition to its analgesic properties, morphine exerts favorable, though mild, hemodynamic effects by increasing venous capacitance (thereby reducing venous return and preload) and by reducing systemic vascular resistance (thereby reducing the impedance to left ventricular emptying or afterload). The result of both effects is a reduction in myocardial oxygen demand. Additionally, relief of pain alleviates anxiety and, thus, excretion of catecholamines.[44] Hypotension may occur after the administration of morphine, occasionally with an inappropriate heart rate response.[45] This is even more likely to occur if the patient has also been given nitroglycerin or a diuretic, and it usually resolves with fluid (with or without positioning the patient with head down and legs elevated). It is rarely necessary to employ a pressor agent. If bradycardia and hypotension occur, atropine should be given.[45]

Management of Arrhythmias and Heart Rate

Premature Ventricular Complexes and Ventricular Rhythms

Treatment with antiarrhythmic agents should be instituted in patients with acute myocardial infarction whenever "warning arrhythmias" occur. These arrhythmias include 1) six or more premature ventricular complexes (PVC's) per minute, 2) PVC's that are closely coupled (QR/QT <0.85), 3) PVC's that fall on the T wave of the preceding beat (R on T phenomenon), 4) PVC's that occur in pairs (couplets), plus in runs (i.e., ventricular tachycardia), or 5) PVC's that are multiformed.[46,47] However, ventricular fibrillation is infrequently preceded by such warning arrhythmias,[48] and ventricular fibrillation may occur in their absence.[49,50] The early use of lidocaine can significantly reduce the incidence of primary ventricular fibrillation (ventricular fibrillation without pump failure or hypotension), despite the absence of warning arrhythmias.[51,52] Therefore, even in the absence of PVC's, prophylactic therapy with lidocaine should be started as early as possible following the onset of symptoms and continued for at least 24 hours.[53]

There is a lower incidence of PVC's and ventricular tachycardia during the first several hours of acute infarction[54] but a higher incidence of ventricular fibrillation.[55] Thus, factors other than warning arrhythmias must play an important role in the genesis of ventricular fibrillation during the initial hours of acute infarction. There are several possibilities. The autonomic nervous system is abnormal during these early hours.[56] It is possible that the pharmacological inhibition of adrenergic

influences on the acutely ischemic myocardium may explain the apparent efficacy of beta-adrenergic blockade in improving survival after myocardial infarction.[56-58] Furthermore, if tachycardia is induced, it will lower the threshold for ventricular fibrillation in the ischemic left ventricle. Thus, the importance of the immediate correction of significant tachycardia whenever possible in patients with acute myocardial infarction should be clear.[59] Hypokalemia also is associated with ventricular arrhythmias during the early stage of myocardial infarction.[60] Prior diuretic therapy or elevated levels of circulating catecholamines may contribute to hypokalemia and may provide an explanation for the beneficial effects of beta-adrenergic blocking agents on potentially lethal arrythmias.[61,62] Hypomagnesemia may also occur, and the administration of magnesium has been reported to decrease the occurrence of ventricular arrhythmias in acute myocardial infarction.[63] The doses of lidocaine for the treatment of ventricular arrhythmias and for prophylactic use are delineated in Chapter 7.

Bradycardias

Controversy exists regarding the management of bradycardia during the course of acute myocardial infarction.[47,59,64,65] Early studies of nonischemic hearts emphasized the fact that bradycardia favored the development of ventricular fibrillation.[66] Investigations of ischemic myocardium, however, indicated that slow heart rates exert a protective effect.[64] These concepts are not mutually exclusive, and both must be considered when treating patients with myocardial infarction.

Bradycardia is particularly prevalent during the first hour after the onset of symptoms likely due to autonomic dysfunction.[21,25,55] Commonly encountered mechanisms for bradycardia are sinus bradycardia, junctional escape rhythm, and second- or third-degree atrioventricular block.[47] These rhythms usually are the result of increased parasympathetic tone and are particularly likely to be associated with inferior and posterior myocardial infarction. If the ventricular rate falls below 60 beats/min and is associated with symptoms, hypotension, or ventricular ectopy, treatment with atropine is indicated.[59] In the absence of symptoms, hypotension, or ventricular ectopy, no therapy is required. The increased vagal tone actually may contribute to improved electrical stability as long as blood pressure and coronary perfusion are maintained.[67-70] As the rate falls below 50 beats/min, more intense observation is necessary since an adequate cardiac output may not be maintained at such low rates in patients with compromised cardiac function.[71,72]

Ventricular escape rhythms ("idioventricular rhythms") with low rates often can be effectively treated with atropine by stimulating supraventricular pacemakers or by increasing the rate of the ventricular pacemaker.[73,74] Accelerated idioventricular rhythm (AIVR) is often seen with rates well above 40 beats/min but less than 100. Ventricular escape rhythms do not require treatment unless they are associated with symptoms. Occasionally, AIVR is suddenly observed to increase its rate with the same QRS morphology. Such a rhythm is presumed to represent ventricular tachycardia with varying exit block and should be treated as ventricular tachycardia.[75] In many cases, however, AIVR represents an escape ventricular rhythm that develops when the sinus rhythm is too slow. Under these circumstances, atropine or atrial pacing may be needed if hemodynamic consequences occur.

During the prehospital phase, bradycardia requiring therapy that is refractory to atropine may be managed with an external pacemaker, if available.[76] Alternatively, low doses of intravenous isoproterenol may be used although isoproterenol may worsen myocardial ischemia and provoke ventricular ectopy. Therefore, when iso-proterenol is needed to treat refractory symptomatic bradycardia, the lowest dose that results in an effective rate must be used. A constant infusion of 2–10 μg/min can be titrated to achieve an adequate heart rate until a transvenous pacemaker can be inserted.

Sinus Tachycardia

Sinus tachycardia is a physiological response to stress. In the patient with acute myocardial infarction it should alert the clinician to the likelihood of heart failure or hypovolemia, but other causes (e.g., anemia, infec-tion, etc.) must be excluded. Appropriate therapeutic decisions may require hemodynamic monitoring to guide proper therapy. In a small but significant number of cases, pain or anxiety or both may be responsible for sinus tachycardia. If so, analgesia and sedation may be the only therapy required. Young patients with their first anterior myocardial infarction may have sinus tachy-cardia along with a hyperdynamic state, including hypertension, associated with an increase in circulating catecholamines as well as local increases in catecholamines in injured areas of the heart.[77] Once definitively diagnosed (this often may require hemodynamic monitor-ing), the use of beta-adrenergic-receptor blocking agents may be useful, particularly in view of the potential negative impact of excessive catecholamines on myocar-dial ischemia, automaticity, cardiac work, and the threshold for ventricular fibrillation. However, in most instances, tachycardia is due to massive myocardial damage or hypovolemia. In both these circumstances beta-adrenergic-receptor blockade is contraindicated.

Supraventricular Arrythmias

Premature atrial complexes do not require therapy *per se* but may be manifestations of occult heart failure or excessive adrenergic tone, for which treatment, i.e., diuretics, analgesia, sedation, or beta-blockade, may be appropriate. Atrial tachycardia, flutter, and/or fibrillation may be due to atrial ischemia[78] but most often are associated with left ventricular failure due to increases in left atrial pressure (and pulmonary artery occlusive pressure).[79] Because of this association, these rhythms are seen more often after anterior wall infarction and are associated with increased mortality.[80] The success of therapy frequently depends on correction of the underly-ing abnormality.

When hemodynamic compromise occurs as a result of supraventricular arrhythmias, the prompt restoration of normal sinus rhythm and rate must be the immediate goal of therapy, even if the increased rate seems relatively modest (i.e., 100–120 beats/min). Synchronized cardioversion is the treatment of choice. Intravenous verapamil may be effective in terminating paroxysmal supraventricular tachycardias or in slowing the ven-tricular response in atrial flutter or fibrillation in asympto-matic patients. However, if the ventricular response is greater than 100–120 beats/min and verapamil is not immediately successful, cardioversion should be under-taken. If cardioversion is successful but supraventricular tachycardia recurs, cardioversion should not be repeated until underlying abnormalities that are inducing the arrythmia are corrected and/or pharmacological therapy to prevent recurrence (e.g., procainamide) has been instituted. Verapamil should not be used if hypotension or left ventricular failure is present.

Atrioventricular Junctional Rhythms

Atrioventricular junctional rhythms may compromise ventricular function by reducing ventricular filling due to the loss of atrial contraction. This is particularly likely when left ventricular failure or right ventricular infarction is present. Sequential atrioventricular pacing may help restore the contribution of atrial contraction in this setting. Unless the rate is slow and symptoms and/or signs of hemodynamic compromise are present, a junctional rhythm with a narrow QRS complex does not mandate pacemaker placement.

Ventricular Tachycardia

Ventricular tachycardia must be treated promptly. If the patient is hemodynamically stable and asymptomatic, lidocaine may be tried first. When ventricular tachycardia is rapid (i.e., greater than 150 beats/min) or when symptoms or signs of hemodynamic compromise are present, one sharp blow to the sternum with the fist from a position 12 inches above the chest (a "precordial thump") *may* be used first. Because this maneuver may cause the rhythm to degenerate to ventricular fibrillation, a defibrillator should be immediately accessible. Car-dioversion (Chapter 6) should be employed without delay if these approaches are unsuccessful or if the patient is unstable in any way.

Atrioventricular Block

First-degree atrioventricular (AV) block alone does not require treatment. The possibility of progression to higher degrees of block is always present and should be the primary concern. Careful monitoring is essential.[81,82]

Similarly, second-degree AV block of the Mobitz Type I (Wenckebach) variety does not require therapy in the absence of hemodynamically significant slowing of the ventricular rate. If treatment is required, atropine (0.5 mg IV) should be tried first. A temporary pacemaker may be necessary if atropine is not effective or if hemodynamically significant slowing is recurrent.

When second-degree AV block of the Mobitz Type II variety is associated with infarction, it carries a significant risk of progression to complete heart block. Therefore, its presence is an indication for the placement of a transvenous pacemaker.[82,83] The prognosis for patients who develop complete heart block (infranodal) is poor because of its usual association with extensive myocardial injury; there is little to suggest that pacing will markedly change outcome. The reestablishment of sequential atrioventricular contraction may be of some value in these patients.

Intraventricular Block

Serious forms of intraventricular block, including right bundle branch block and left anterior or posterior fascicular block, or any of the various forms of trifascicular block[84] are more likely to occur with anterior myocardial infarction and are an adverse prognostic sign. The prognostic significance of new isolated right bundle or left bundle branch block is less adverse.[85,86] Prognosis associated with intraventricular conduction disturbances is determined predominantly by the extent of myocardial damage rather than by the conduction disturbance *per se*.[83] There is no evidence that prophylactic pacing reduces mortality, but it and aggressive management of hemodynamic abnormalities remain the only therapeutic alternatives. Pacing should be employed in all patients with right bundle branch block unless it is clear that the right bundle branch block is old. The need for pacing is less clear with left bundle branch block.[87]

Ventricular Fibrillation

Although the risk of ventricular fibrillation is highest during the first few hours of infarction, it continues to be high for the first 48 hours and even after discharge from the coronary care unit. Lidocaine administered prophylactically reduces the incidence of primary ventricular fibrillation (unassociated with pump failure or hypotension) but may not reduce mortality.[51] When primary ventricular fibrillation in the setting of acute infarction is treated promptly with defibrillation, the event may not affect prognosis adversely. Nevertheless, since resuscitation is not uniformly successful after primary ventricular fibrillation, prevention seems unquestionably preferable.

Dosages of lidocaine for prophylaxis against ventricular fibrillation are detailed in Chapter 7.

Secondary ventricular fibrillation (ventricular fibrillation preceded and apparently provoked by pump failure or hypotension) is associated with high mortality; only 20–25% of patients survive hospitalization.[88,89] The likelihood of successful restoration of an effective cardiac rhythm declines rapidly with time. Thus, electrical countershock should be performed at the earliest possible instant.

Hemodynamic Patterns After Myocardial Infarction

Hemodynamic patterns after myocardial infarction are usually defined based on a determination of the pulmonary artery occlusive pressure (PAOP, or pulmonary capillary wedge pressure), cardiac output, heart rate, and systemic arterial pressure (see Chapter 12). When the systemic arterial pressure falls in association with pulmonary congestion because of the extensive myocardial damage, cardiogenic shock is said to be present. If hypotension is caused by a relative or absolute deficiency of circulating blood volume, the clinical syndrome is described as "hypovolemic". A clinical classification of hemodynamic patterns associated with myocardial infarction is outlined below, along with recommended therapeutic approaches.

Normal and Hyperdynamic States

For the patient with an acute myocardial infarction who is clinically stable and has neither symptoms nor signs suggesting hemodynamic compromise or other complications, ongoing electrocardiographic monitoring, oxygen therapy, symptomatic treatment, and reassurance are usually sufficient therapy. When there are signs of a hyperdynamic circulatory status, including tachycardia, hypertension (in a usually normotensive individual), bounding pulses, and other manifestations of a high-output state (elevated cardiac output), myocardial oxygen consumption (MVO_2) is usually significantly increased. Furthermore, the influence of catecholamines on the electrical, mechanical, and metabolic activity of the heart may be deleterious. Once the diagnosis of a hyperdynamic state is confirmed (this usually requires hemodynamic monitoring), beta-receptor blockade is recommended, presuming no contraindications are present. The dose should be titrated to decrease the heart rate, blood pressure, and cardiac output into the normal range.

Abnormal Blood Pressure Responses in Myocardial Infarction

Hypotension

During acute infarction, hypotension may occur for several reasons. Cardiac output may be decreased (because of low stroke volume or because the heart rate is too slow or too fast), or intravascular volume depletion (hypovolemia) may be present. On occasion, systemic vascular resistance (SVR) may be low transiently due to enhanced vagal tone in association with bradycardia. When hypotension is associated with pulmonary congestion (cardiogenic shock), usually 35% of the left ventricular myocardium has been destroyed. Right ventricular damage may also cause hypotension acutely (see below).

Hypertension

Patients who have been previously normotensive or mildly hypertensive may be significantly hypertensive during the evolution of acute infarction. This response may be transient and self-limited, but persistent elevations of systolic blood pressure above 140 mmHg is particularly undesirable since it results in increased myocardial oxygen demand and is associated with mechanical complications such as myocardial rupture.[90]

Initial therapy consists of the relief of pain and anxiety and the administration of oxygen. These measures may be sufficient to control mild hypertension. For more severe hypertension, sodium nitroprusside may be necessary.[87] If concomitant heart failure is present, diuretics and/or intravenous nitroglycerin may also be of benefit (see below). Beta-receptor blockade is indicated if a hyperdynamic state is present. During the first few hours of infarction, blood pressure control with a short-acting intravenous agent is preferred; after initial management, it is usually possible to substitute an oral antihypertensive drug.

Left Ventricular Pump Failure

Myocardial infarction may affect the pumping function of the heart in a generalized or a more localized manner. When the left ventricle is affected more diffusely, there is a decrease in wall motion with a proportionate fall in the amount of blood pumped with each heart beat (stroke volume). When localized areas are involved, the areas may fail to move (akinesis) or may bulge with each systole (dyskinesis).[91,92] With such localized areas of hypocontractility, other areas usually become hypercontractile in an attempt to compensate. The result may be a movement of blood into the bulging (dyskinetic) area during systole, thus decreasing the amount of blood ejected into the aorta. As the stroke volume falls, due to either diffuse or local compromise, the left ventricular volume and pressure increase. This increases the myocardial oxygen requirements (MVO_2) and the wall stress and reduces subendocardial perfusion — at a time when blood pressure and coronary perfusion have fallen. These changes adversely affect the relation of myocardial oxygen supply to demand, aggravate myocardial ischemia, extend infarction, and begin a pernicious cycle that may end with myocardial necrosis so extensive that the pumping mechanism of the heart is compromised (pump failure). When a critical amount of left ventricular myocardium is destroyed, pump failure may be recognized clinically as pulmonary congestion, or by systemic hypotension, or both. In its extreme form, pulmonary edema may occur. These syndromes, from mild to severe, are the major determinants of survival in hospitalized patients.[93,94] Thus, an aggressive approach to management is recommended.[95] The combination of hypotension with pump failure and pulmonary edema is known as "cardiogenic shock".

Hemodynamic Monitoring in the Management of Congestive Heart Failure

Until fairly recently, myocardial function was assessed from the patient's symptoms, evidence of tissue perfusion, including urine output and mental status, physical examination, and chest x-ray. Conclusions based on these clinical findings may be substantially different from those based on direct measurement of hemodynamic status.[96-98] Accordingly, hemodynamic monitoring should be employed when myocardial infarction is complicated by shock, hypotension unresponsive to simple measures such as control of bradycardia or volume challenge, significant pulmonary congestion, persistent chest pain despite analgesics, or other conditions such as unexplained hypoxemia, cyanosis, or acidosis. The proper use of parenteral inotropic drugs and vasodilators requires invasive hemodynamic monitoring. However, for the patient with uncomplicated infarction, invasive monitoring is unnecessary. The decision to proceed with invasive monitoring should not be used as an excuse to delay the institution of needed therapy.

The technique for placing a pulmonary artery catheter and an arterial line are described in Chapter 12. Right heart catheterization permits indirect assessment of left ventricular filling pressure, direct measurement of right ventricular and pulmonary pressures, and the determination of cardiac output. From these determinations and blood pressure, other hemodynamic measurements, such as systemic vascular resistance (SVR), can be calculated.

Clinical Classification

A useful classification to guide the clinical management of patients with acute myocardial infarction was developed by Killip and Kimball: Class I refers to patients with uncomplicated infarction without evidence of heart failure as judged by the absence of râles and a ventricular filling sound (third heart sound). Class II refers to patients with mild-to-moderate heart failure as evidenced by pulmonary râles in the lower half of the lung field and a ventricular filling sound. Class III refers to patients with severe left ventricular failure or pulmonary edema. Class IV refers to patients with cardiogenic shock, defined as systolic blood pressure less than 90 mmHg (in previously normotensive patients) with oliguria and other evidence of poor peripheral perfusion, such as mental obtundation.[99] Although this classification is a relatively poor predictor of exact hemodynamic status, it continues to be useful in determining which patients are likely to need therapeutic decisions that require hemodynamic monitoring.

Mortality in acute myocardial infarction is obviously greater for the more severe clinical and hemodynamic classes. While classification criteria have differed among investigators, four-level hemodynamic classification systems generally paralleling that of Killip and Kimball have provided comparable mortality figures. Among patients comparable to those in Killip's Class I, Resnekov observed a 5% mortality (Class A); in Class B (Killip's Class II) 7%; in Class C (Killip's Class III), 25%; and in Class D (Killip's Class IV), 85%. Forrester, et al., using a subset classification based on hemodynamic measurements, observed a mortality of 97% in patients with pulmonary congestion and peripheral hypoperfusion.[100]

Acute Pulmonary Edema

Pulmonary edema is an acute severe form of pulmonary congestion. It is characterized by extreme respiratory distress. Signs of adrenergic stimulation are usually present (e.g., tachycardia, diphoresis). Hyper- or hypotension may be present. In many patients, a pink frothy material is exuded from the mouth and/or nose. Generally, either pulmonary edema improves markedly or the patient dies.

Initial measures in the management of patients with pulmonary edema include placing the patient in a sitting or semisitting position and providing supplementary oxygen. Lasix is the drug of choice. In patients with pulmonary edema, its primary effects are to increase venous capacitance. Pulmonary edema usually has resolved prior to the induction of diuresis.[101] Morphine in a dose of 2–5 mg has also been used to increase venous capacitance and to relieve anxiety. Nitroglycerin may be useful to obviate ischemia.[102] Rotating tourniquets and phlebotomy are rarely used but are effective temporizing measures.

If the patient is normotensive or hypertensive, intravenous nitroprusside or nitroglycerin can be used to reduce the blood pressure and, thereby, improve heart failure due to impedance (afterload) reduction.[103] Proper titration is important to avoid hypotension and impaired coronary perfusion, especially if interventions that reduce preload (lasix and morphine) have been undertaken as well.[95] If the patient is hypotensive, dobutamine frequently is helpful.

In the absence of hypotension, parenteral vasodilators and/or inotropes are the drugs of choice. When congestive heart failure is present, intravenous nitroglycerin and nitroprusside have similar hemodynamic effects.[104] Since nitroglycerin benefits ischemia and may reduce infarct size[37,41,42] and there is controversy concerning beneficial versus detrimental effects with nitroprusside,[90,105] nitroglycerin is preferred. If the arterial pressure is inadequate to permit therapy with vasodilators, dobutamine may be used. In general, dobutamine improves contractility, resulting in increases in stroke volume and reflex decreases in systemic vascular resistance. At doses that do not increase heart rate by more than 10%, dobutamine appears unlikely to exacerbate myocardial ischemia.[106,107] Amrinone, another synthetic inotropic agent, may also be used and has hemodynamic properties similar to those of dobutamine.[108] However, there is concern that amrinone may exacerbate myocardial ischemia.[109]

Other Forms of Heart Failure

Patients with only mild heart failure require only hemodynamic monitoring if heart failure does not resolve in response to judicious doses of diuretics.

For more severe failure, hemodynamic monitoring is desirable because it permits an immediate determination of the patient's physiological status as well as a rapid titration and assessment of therapy. Rapid titration of intravenous drug therapy cannot be safely accomplished without such intervention. Nitroglycerin, dobutamine, and lasix are the mainstays of therapy. A PAOP of 15–18 mmHg will optimize cardiac output in patients with acute myocardial infarction.[110,111] This is also the level at which pulmonary congestion begins to develop.[112] Although each patient's hemodynamics are unique, in the hemodynamically decompensated patient, this level can be used as an initial goal. Efforts should be made to reduce the left ventricular filling pressure to this approximate range. Excessive diuresis and reduction of filling pressures below this range should be avoided in general.

The end points for therapy are clinical. Attempts to improve hemodynamic measurements in well-compensated patients are unlikely to induce any benefit and may induce morbidity.

Cardiogenic Shock

The hemodynamic diagnosis of cardiogenic shock is based on a depression of blood pressure (usually systolic pressure below 80–90 mmHg or a reduction of 70 mmHg or more), cardiac index of less than 1.8 L/min/m^2 with elevation of left ventricular filling pressure (PAOP above 16–18 mmHg), and clinical signs of hypoperfusion (e.g., oliguria, mental obtundation, pallor, sweating, and tachycardia).[113]

Cardiogenic shock is associated with a death rate in excess of 80%. Hemodynamic monitoring and diagnostic tests such as echocardiograms, radionuclide ventriculograms, and cardiac angiograms may aid in identifying reversible processes such as hypovolemia, vagally induced hypotension, right ventricular infarction, pericardial tamponade, ventricular septal rupture, papillary muscle rupture, and discrete left ventricular aneurysm which may be surgically treatable. These patients have a substantially better prognosis than patients without such correctable processes.[114] When cardiogenic shock is due to loss of a large area (greater than 35%) of the left ventricle (myocardiogenic shock), survival is not expected. Other causes of shock, such as aortic dissection, massive pulmonary embolism, and septic shock, also should be considered in the differential diagnosis.

If hypovolemia is found, volume expansion with dextran, blood, or saline may be beneficial. If a mechanical abnormality is identified, balloon counterpulsation, cardiac catheterization, and surgery are a reasonable approach.[114]

For myocardiogenic shock, there is little that can be done. Dobutamine can be tried, if severe hypotension is not present, in an attempt to improve cardiac output. For severe hypotension, dopamine is recommended.

Dopamine (see Chapter 8) should be titrated to maintain a systolic pressure of 80–100 mmHg. The lowest dose consistent with the desired result should be used. Careful monitoring of cardiac rhythm is essential because of the risk of serious ventricular arrhythmias with greater doses of dopamine. If all else fails, norepinephrine may be added.

Right Ventricular Infarction

Shock may occur in the course of myocardial infarction when the right ventricle is damaged to such an extent that it is unable to pump blood through the pulmonary circulation into the left ventricle. This syndrome occurs predominantly in patients with inferior infarction. Noninvasive studies have suggested that as many as 30% of patients with acute inferior infarction have associated right ventricular infarction.[115] Hemodynamically significant right ventricular infarction occurs in only about one half of these patients. Right ventricular infarction should be suspected in patients with inferior infarction, hypotension, and distended neck veins. Right-sided precordial leads often will demonstrate ST segment elevation,[116,117] and right atrial pressure (CVP) and right ventricular diastolic pressure are disproportionately high compared to PAOP.[118,119]

Treatment requires judicious fluid therapy to raise the left ventricular filling pressure (PAOP) and dobutamine.[120] Vasodilator drugs should be avoided.

Acute Mitral Regurgitation

Hemodynamic compromise may occur because of severe damage to the mitral valve apparatus in the course of an acute myocardial infarction. This is caused by involvement of the chordae or papillary muscles, which become damaged and dysfunctional, resulting in sudden severe mitral regurgitation. The patient may be hypotensive and have severe pulmonary congestion as well.[121] This syndrome may be suspected when shock is associated with a holosystolic murmur at the apex with a large systolic "regurgitant" or "V" wave observed on the PAOP pressure tracing. The murmur may be loud or soft and unimpressive. Furthermore, the absence of a large systolic "V" wave does not exclude the diagnosis, nor does its presence confirm it. Vasodilator drugs, which reduce left ventricular outflow impedance (afterload), result in a decrease in mitral regurgitation and may stabilize the patient long enough for mitral valve replacement to be considered. If vasodilator drugs are ineffective or inadequate in reversing the shock syndrome, intraaortic balloon pumping is warranted with early angiography and consideration of mitral valve replacement.[122]

Ventricular Septal Rupture

Ventricular septal rupture (VSR) occurs during the course of a myocardial infarction when a necrotic intraventricular septum ruptures. A shock syndrome develops that is easily confused with acute mitral regurgitation (described above) because of common clinical findings, i.e., shock often associated with pulmonary congestion, large systolic "V" waves on PAOP pressure tracing, and a holosystolic murmur. In a VSR, however, the murmur is more likely to be loudest at the lower left sternal edge, and the right ventricular and pulmonary artery oxygen content will be at least 1 vol% greater than the highest oxygen content to be found in the right atrium. Alternatively, the average oxygen saturation of several pulmonary artery samples will be at least 5% greater than the average saturation of samples taken from various locations in the right atrium.[123] Initial treatment of this complication is similar to that of acute mitral regurgitation. Vasodilator drugs or intraaortic balloon pumping will reduce impedance to left ventricular outflow and thereby reduce the amount of blood flowing across the VSR into the right ventricle and increase the cardiac output. Prompt cardiac angiography is warranted to assess the patient's ability to survive an attempt at repairing the VSR.[124-126] Recent data suggest that the presence of significant right ventricular dysfunction with VSR has a significant negative impact on surgical prognosis.[124,126]

Other Etiologies of Hemodynamic Collapse That Need to Be Distinguished From Acute Infarction

Massive Pulmonary Embolism

Massive pulmonary embolism may result in shock and cardiovascular collapse. The precipitating event is critical obstruction of the pulmonary arterial system, resulting in hypoxemia, pulmonary hypertension, and acute right ventricular failure, i.e., acute *cor pulmonale*.[127,128] Patients with pulmonary embolism may present with ischemic-type chest pain and electrocardiographic abnormalities consistent with myocardial ischemia and, more rarely, psuedo infarction. The hemodynamic hallmarks of acute *cor pulmonale* — i.e., depression of cardiac output, systemic hypotension, and increased SVR — may be thought secondary to cardiogenic shock or right ventricular infarction. However, the left ventricular filling pressure (PAOP) is usually normal while the pulmonary artery systolic and diastolic pressures are elevated, as is the right ventricular filling pressure (CVP).[129,130] Abnormal nuclear perfusion lung scans and evidence for deep venous thrombosis in the legs favors the diagnosis of pulmonary embolism. It must also be remembered that pulmonary embolism is not an infrequent complication of myocardial infarction although the routine use of low-dose subcutaneous heparin in the early stages of myocardial infarction has dramatically decreased the likelihood of this complication.[131]

Hypovolemic and Septic Shock

Hypovolemic shock may be associated with the clinical indices of hypoperfusion and hypotension. In contrast to cardiogenic shock, however, the left ventricular filling pressure (PAOP) is normal or low. The explanation for the low cardiac output, therefore, is inadequate left ventricular filling. This syndrome is very important to recognize because it is readily treatable, but hypotension may lead to changes on the electrocardiogram and, hence, diagnostic confusion. Unless the (PAOP) is 15–18 mmHg or higher, shock should first be treated with an attempt at volume replacement. When the hematocrit is normal, crystalloid or colloid solution should be used to correct hypovolemia. If the hematocrit is low, whole blood is usually preferable. The PAOP should not be raised above 15–18 mmHg since this is the filling pressure most

likely to be associated with an optimal cardiac output if myocardial infarction is the underlying process.[110,111] However, if the cardiac output, blood pressure, and urine flow are all adequate, a PAOP less than 18 mmHg is acceptable.

In septic shock, hypotension is due to a marked reduction in systemic vascular resistance (SVR), and the cardiac output is characteristically increased. Similar findings are frequently found in anaphylactic and neurogenic shock. In circumstances when a decreased SVR causes shock, dopamine or norepinephine may be helpful. Definitive therapy is the correction of the underlying cause.

Cardiac Tamponade

Acute pericarditis can mimic acute myocardial infarction. Its detection, especially if treatment with thrombolytic agents is considered, is essential.

Hemodynamic compromise associated with pericarditis usually occurs only when tamponade is present.

The presence of *pulsus paradoxus* (an inspiratory drop in systolic blood pressure of greater than 10–12 mmHg), if associated with distended neck veins and an enlarging heart shadow on x-ray, should lead to a strong suspicion of cardiac tamponade. An echocardiogram will help to make this diagnosis.[132,133] If the patient is in shock, augmentation of circulatory blood volume will improve the cardiac output. Emergency pericardiocentesis is warranted if the patient is deteriorating and a definitive surgical procedure cannot be accomplished immediately.[134]

Cardiac rupture after acute infarction can cause tamponade. Patients who sustain cardiac rupture are characteristically 60 years of age and older, with hypertension during the acute phase of their infarction. They frequently have no prior history of cardiac disease and are progressing to an uncomplicated recovery after their first infarction.[135] Pericardiocentesis may allow them to survive long enough to undergo emergency surgical repair.

Aortic Dissection

Acute aortic dissection may cause pain similar to that of acute myocardial infarction. It can cause infarction, acute cardiac tamponade, shock due to acute aortic rupture, or left ventricular failure due to sudden aortic valve regurgitation.

Aortic dissection occurs when a sudden tear of the aortic intima allows a column of blood to enter the aortic wall and strip the intima away from the outer wall of the aorta, driven by the force of the aortic blood pressure. When dissection occurs in the ascending aorta, it may occlude a coronary artery and cause a myocardial infarction. Occlusion of other vessels is apt to cause neurological abnormalities and pulse deficits. Dissection may involve the aortic valve itself and provoke severe regurgitation of the aortic valve. It may dissect into the pericardial space and cause cardiac tamponade. Rupture of the dissection into the pleural space, mediastinum, or retroperitoneal space will cause hypovolemia and shock.[136]

Without recognition and proper therapy, aortic dissection is almost universally fatal. Inappropriate treatment with thrombolytic therapy, under the mistaken opinion that one is treating an acute myocardial infarction, is likely to cause prompt exsanguination. Therefore, it is incumbent on the physician to exclude aortic dissection early with a patient suspected of or diagnosed as having an acute myocardial infarction. The history, physical examination, and chest x-ray may alert the clinician to the possibility of aortic dissection.

The pain of the dissection is usually very severe and may be found in the same area and with the same radiation patterns as that of a myocardial infarction. Dissection of the descending aorta is more likely to cause intrascapular pain or pain radiating to the abdomen. Most commonly, the pain of dissection is as severe at its onset as it ever becomes. In contrast, the pain at the beginning of a myocardial infarction usually increases progressively (crescendo pattern). In addition the clinician is alerted to the possibility of dissection by a history of hypertension or by congenital lesions, such as Marfan's syndrome, that weaken the aortic wall. The physical examination in dissection may reveal pulse deficits, neurological deficits, aortic regurgitation, pericardial rubs, or tamponade. The chest x-ray usually demonstrates a widened mediastinum.[137] Echocardiography may confirm the diagnosis of ascending aortic dissection.[138] When the clinical representation is suspicious of dissection, aortography or computerized tomography (CT scan) with contrast is needed for confirmation or exclusion of the diagnosis.[139]

If the patient is hypertensive or normotensive, the initial therapy of dissection is to lower the blood pressure and the contractile force of the left ventricle in order to stop progressive dissection by the column of aortic blood. This is best done with intravenous antihypertensive agents and beta blockers. Ascending aortic dissections are best treated with early surgical repair. Descending aortic dissections need not be operated upon unless 1) pain continues in spite of medical therapy, 2) there is a threat of infarction of bowel, kidney, or extremities, or 3) rupture occurs.[140,141]

Special Therapeutic Considerations

Beta-Receptor Blockers

Beta-adrenergic-blocking agents have been used in the setting of acute myocardial infarction to decrease myocardial oxygen demands and thus attempt to limit myocardial damage.[142-144] Beta-receptor blockers have been shown to improve long-term survival when used prophylactically,[57,58,145,146] and recent results with metoprolol[147,148] and atenolol[63] have shown that early institution of intravenous beta-receptor blockade in a subgroup of patients with high sympathetic tone has a significantly beneficial effect on mortality.[147,148] In the first day of acute myocardial infarction, beta-receptor blockers also have been shown to decrease the incidence and mortality from ventricular fibrillation.[149,61,63] Nonetheless, the use of beta blockers in patients with acute infarction cannot be routinely recommended.

Thrombolytic Therapy

Studies by Dewood, et al,[8] have shown that 87% of patients undergoing coronary arteriography within 4 hours of the onset of symptoms of transmural (Q wave) myocardial infarction have evidence of total coronary occlusion from coronary thrombi. The incidence of coronary thrombosis was found to decrease with the passage of hours following the onset of symptoms. After the role of thrombosis in the pathogenesis of myocardial infarction was demonstrated, interest quickly developed in the potential use of pharmacologic agents to dissolve the thrombus. Thrombolytic (or fibrinolytic) therapy involves the dissolution of thrombi or thromboemboli by digesting their fibrin supporting network. Thrombolytic agents have been used in the treatment of pulmonary and arterial thromboemboli, as well as deep venous thrombosis.

Several thrombolytic agents are currently being widely studied in acute myocardial infarction: streptokinase, acetylated streptokinase-plasminogen complexes, urokinase, prourokinase, and single- and double-stranded tissue plasminogen activator (tPA). Although effective thrombolytic agents are available, several critical questions remain regarding their use: overall efficacy, proper timing for optimal results, and safety. At the time of the 1985 National Conference on Cardiopulmonary Resuscitation and Emergency Cardiac Care, it was acknowledged that recent studies of thrombolytic agents have "yielded promising results", but it was felt that there was not "sufficient data to support the use of any of these attempts at infarct limitation for the routine patient with acute myocardial infarction".[150] At present, however, there are three published reports that mortality is reduced by thrombolytic agents at least for some patients with acute myocardial infarction (predominantly those with anterior infarction who can be treated early).[151-154] In addition, there is information that the size of the infarction[155,156] and, therefore, myocardial function are improved by the timely administration of thrombolytic agents.[156,157] The intravenous administration of newer clot-selective thrombolytic agents (r-tPA) induces coronary patency at rates similar to the intracoronary administration of other activators, is potentially safer, and is more expeditious.[158-160] Therefore, the efficacy and safety of thrombolytic therapy is likely to be enhanced by the more widespread availability of these agents. Based on a synthesis of the available data, it appears that patients with anterior myocardial infarction who can receive activator within 3 hours of the onset of symptoms and have no contraindications[161] are benefitted by thrombolytic therapy. The data for other subgroups of patients is not yet sufficient to sustain a similar conclusion at this time. If this early, optimistic view of thrombolytic therapy is supported by further studies, the patient with an acute myocardial infarction will need to be treated as an acute emergency requiring aggressive intervention comparable to the patient with acute hemorrhagic shock. Ongoing trials will determine further the role of thrombolytic therapy in clinical practice for all subgroups of patients with myocardial infarction. Several recent reviews are available that detail the approach necessary for safe and effective therapy.[36,162]

Percutaneous Transluminal Coronary Angioplasty

Percutaneous transluminal coronary angioplasty (PTCA) has recently been applied successfully in patients with acute myocardial infarction.[163-167] PTCA is considered to be potentially advantageous because it is often effective in reducing the degree of residual stenosis in the infarct-related artery and because it may open stenotic vessels when other therapies have failed. However, PTCA cannot be done in all patients with acute myocardial infarction. In some individuals, the coronary anatomy may not be suitable for PTCA or there may be a significant risk of dissection of the artery. There has also been a relatively high incidence of restenosis or reocclusion after acute PTCA. Finally, centers performing PTCA should have cardiac surgical back-up. Therefore, this mode of therapy has more limited general applicability than intravenous thrombolytic therapy.

Current interest has focused on the early use of thrombolytic therapy in community hospitals, with transfer of a patient within 10–48 hours to an institution that performs PTCA so that urgent angioplasty could be performed. A multicenter NHLBI-sponsored randomized trial (TIMI phase II) will assess the role of sequential thrombolytic therapy and PTCA (as well as the optimal timing for PTCA) in acute myocardial infarction.

Coronary Artery Bypass Grafting

The reestablishment of coronary artery flow with early coronary artery bypass grafting (CABG) has been attempted in acute myocardial infarction. Myocardial salvage has been demonstrated with significant improvement in left ventricular function after CABG in acute myocardial infarction.[168,169] Although acute revascularization by surgery may be efficacious, early acute bypass surgery is impractical for widespread use.

It is also unclear which patients, if any, would be benefitted by such surgery and which would be harmed.

Indications for Permanent Pacemakers After Myocardial Infarction

Survivors of myocardial infarction who have incurred bundle branch block and subsequent complete infranodal heart block (even transiently during the acute phase) have a higher frequency, subsequently, of progression to high-degree heart block than other patients with new bundle branch block. The use of a temporary pacemaker followed by the installation of a permanent pacemaker may reduce subsequent mortality.[84,170]

Late In-Hospital Post-Myocardial-Infarction Mortality: The Role of the Intermediate Coronary Care Unit

While the risk of sudden death is very high in the first hours after myocardial infarction, it is now clear that there is a significant risk of mortality and sudden death between the time the patient leaves the coronary care unit and final discharge from the hospital. As much as 20–30% of hospital deaths due to acute myocardial infarction may take place in this period.[171-173] Patients with complicated myocardial infarction are at a particularly high risk for sudden death in the late hospitalization phase. Included in the high-risk group are those patients who suffered extensive anterior myocardial infarction, those who experienced early rhythm abnormalities ranging from atrial fibrillation to ventricular tachycardia and fibrillation, and those with serious intraventricular conduction abnormalities.[172-174] It may be that monitoring the post-myocardial-infarction patient for a total of 3–5 days, either in the coronary care unit or an intermediate care unit, will have a positive effect on mortality, while continuous monitoring beyond that time will contribute little to further reduction of mortality.[175,176] In addition, patients with nontransmural (non-Q-wave) infarction seem to be at particular risk for extension of infarction.[177] The proper management of these patients is controversial, with some studies suggesting benefit from calcium channel blockers[178] and some not.[179]

Management After Hospital Discharge

Patients who are discharged from the hospital after an acute myocardial infarction have a mortality rate of 6–10% in the first year. Most of the deaths take place in the first 3 months. The major risk factors for late death following myocardial infarction are the severity of left ventricular damage,[180-186] the potential for continued ischemia,[181-185,187] and the predisposition to ventricular arrhythmias.[180,188-192]

Left ventricular damage may be detected by symptoms of heart failure or x-ray evidence of cardiac enlargement. Echocardiography or radionuclide angiography may demonstrate a depressed ejection fraction, diffuse wall motion abnormalities, or an aneurysm. Late mortality is greatest for those with an ejection fraction of less than 30%.

Evidence for ischemia at a site distant from the infarction may be detected by an exercise electrocardiogram with or without the use of Thallium 201 scintigraphy or radionuclide angiography. Coronary arteriography may demonstrate severely diseased vessels other than that precipitating the infarction. Modified treadmill exercise testing in the second or third week after myocardial infarction may be useful in certain uncomplicated cases.[193] There are conflicting reports on the ability of abnormal exercise results to predict mortality in the first year after myocardial infarction.[194-198] However, ischemic changes may help to identify those patients who are likely to experience angina and who are more likely to benefit from revascularization procedures.

Frequent or complex ventricular ectopy seen late after myocardial infarction correlates with an increased risk of sudden death,[189] as does the ability to induce ventricular tachycardias during electrophysiologic study.[199,200] It is not clear whether antiarrhythmic therapy decreases the risk of death in these patients.

Several studies have demonstrated a favorable effect of beta-receptor blockers in reducing mortality during the first several years following myocardial infarction. These results have been demonstrated for propranolol,[57] metoprolol,[201] and timolol.[58] The value of beta-receptor blockers, however, may be limited to high-risk patients.[202]

In addition to possible pharmacologic and invasive interventions, reduction of risk factors for coronary disease must be strongly advised.[203] Cessation of smoking may be the most important preventive measure. Also, hypertension, hyperlipidemia, and diabetes must be adequately managed.

Most patients who survive a myocardial infarction can be returned to normal activities within 6–8 weeks. Psychological and physical healing are often facilitated by a cardiac rehabilitation and education program. The patient's spouse and other close family members should be encouraged to participate in the education program; training in CPR and modification of their own life-style should favorably affect not only the patient's risk but also that of the whole family.

References

1. CASS Study: Myocardial infarction and mortality in the Coronary Artery Surgery Study randomized trial. *N Engl J Med* 310:750, 1984.
2. Califf RM, Tomabechi Y, Lee KL, et al: Outcome of one-vessel coronary artery disease. *Circulation* 67:283, 1983.
3. Chapman I: Morphogenesis of occluding coronary artery thrombosis. *Arch Pathol* 80:256, 1965.
4. Ambrose JA, Winters SL, Stern A, et al: Angiographic morphology and the pathogenesis of unstable angina pectoris. *J Am Coll Cardiol* 5:609, 1985.
5. Wilson RF, Holida MD, White CW: Quantitative angiographic morphology of coronary stenosis leading to myocardial infarction or unstable angina. *Circulation* 73:286, 1986.
6. Maseri A, L'Abbate A, Baroldi G, et al: Coronary vasospasm as a possible cause of myocardial infarction. A conclusion derived from the study of 'preinfarction' angina. *N Engl J Med* 299:1271, 1978.
7. Oliva PB, Breckinridge JC: Arteriographic evidence of coronary arterial spasm in acute myocardial infarction. *Circulation* 56:366, 1977.
8. DeWood MA, Spores J, Notske R, et al: Prevalence of total coronary occlusion during the early hours of transmural myocardial infarction. *N Engl J Med* 303:897, 1980.
9. DeWood MA, Stifter WF, Simpson CS, Spores J, Eugster GS, Judge TP, Hinnen ML: Coronary Arteriographic Findings Soon After Non-Q-Wave Myocardial Infarction. *N Engl J Med* 315:417-423, 1986.
10. Howard RE, Hueter DC, Davis GJ: Acute myocardial infarction following cocaine abuse in a young woman with normal coronary arteries. *JAMA* 254;95, 1985.
11. Kuller LH: Sudden death — Definition and epidemiologic considerations. *Prog Cardiovasc Dis* 23:1-12, 1980
12. Pantridge JF, Geddes JS: A mobile intensive care unit in the management of myocardial infarction. *Lancet* 2:271, 1967.
13. Phipps C: Contributory causes of coronary thrombosis. *JAMA* 106:761, 1936.
14. Master AM, Dack S, Jaffe HL: Factors and events associated with onset of coronary artery thrombosis. *JAMA* 109:546, 1937.
15. Fitzhugh G, Hamilton BE: Coronary occlusion and fatal angina pectoris: Study of the immediate causes and their prevention. *JAMA* 100:475, 1933.
16. Smith C, Sauls HC, Ballew J: Coronary occlusion: Clinical study of 100 patients. *Ann Intern Med* 17:681, 1942.
17. French AJ, Dock W: Fatal coronary arteriosclerosis in young soldiers. *JAMA* 124:1233, 1944.
18. Boas EP: Some immediate causes of cardiac infarction. *Am Heart J* 23:1, 1942.
19. Levine HD: Acute myocardial infarction following wasp sting. Report of two cases and critical survey of the literature. *Am Heart J* 91:365, 1976.
20. Jenkins CD: Recent evidence supporting psychologic and social risk factors for coronary disease. *N Engl J Med* 294:1033, 1976.
21. Rahe RH, Romo M, Bennett L, et al: Recent life changes, myocardial infarction, and abrupt coronary death. Studies in Helsinki. *Arch Intern Med* 133:221, 1974.
22. Muller JE, Stone PH, Turi ZG, et al: Circadian variation in the frequency of onset of acute myocardial infarction. *N Engl J Med* 313:1315, 1985.
23. Paraskos JA: Approach to the patient with chest pain, in Rippe JM, Irwin RS, Alpert JS, Dalen JE (eds): *Intensive Care Medicine*. Boston, Little Brown, 1985.
24. Heart Attack: *Signals and Actions for Survival*. Dallas, American Heart Association, 1976.
25. Rose RM, Lewis AJ, Fewkes J, et al: Occurrence of arrhythmias during the first hour in acute myocardial infarction, abstracted. *Circulation* 50 (suppl 3):III-121, 1974.
26. Moss AJ, Goldstein S: The prehospital phase of acute myocardial infarction. *Circulation* 41:737, 1970.
27. Turi ZG, Stone PH, Muller JE, et al: Implications for acute intervention related to time of hospital arrival in acute myocardial infarction. *Am J Cardiol* 58:203, 1986.
28. Standards and Guidelines for Cardiopulmonary Resuscitation (CPR) and Emergency Cardiac Care (ECC). *JAMA* 255:2905-2984, 1986.

29. Valentine PA, Fluck DC, Mounsey JP, et al: Blood-gas changes after acute myocardial infarction. *Lancet* 2:837, 1966.

30. Fillmore SJ, Shapiro M, Killip T: Arterial oxygen tension in acute myocardial infarction. Serial analysis of clinical state and blood gas changes. *Am Heart J* 79:620, 1970.

31. Maroko PR, Radvany P, Braunwald E, et al: Reduction of infarct size by oxygen inhalation following acute coronary occlusion. *Circulation* 52:360, 1975.

32. Madias JE, Hood WB Jr: Reduction of precordial ST-segment elevation in patients with anterior myocardial infarction by oxygen breathing. *Circulation* 53 (suppl I):I-198, 1976.

33. Thomas M, Malmcrona R, Shillingford J: Haemodynamic effects of oxygen in patients with acute myocardial infarction. *Br Heart J* 27:401, 1965.

34. Sukumalchantra Y, Levy S, Danzig R, et al: Correcting arterial hypoxemia by oxygen therapy in patients with acute myocardial infarction. Effect on ventilation and hemodynamics. *Am J Cardiol* 24:838, 1969.

35. Ganz W, Donoso R, Marcus H, et al: Coronary hemodynamics and myocardial oxygen metabolism during oxygen breathing in patients with and without coronary artery disease. *Circulation* 45:763, 1972.

36. Eisenberg PR, Jaffe AS: Coronary thrombolysis: Practical Considerations. *Cardiol Clin* 5:129-141,1987

37. Jaffe AS, Geltman EM, Tiefenbrunn AJ, et al: Reduction of infarct size in patients with inferior infarction with intravenous glylceryl trinitrate. *Br Heart J* 49:452-460, 1983.

38. Epstein SE, Borer JS, Kent KM, et al: Protection of ischemic myocardium by nitroglycerin: Experimental and clinical results. *Circulation* 53:(suppl I):I-191, 1976.

39. Come PC, Pitt B: Nitroglycerin-induced severe hypotension and bradycardia in patients with acute myocardial infarction. *Circulation* 54:624-628, 1976.

40. Dalen JE, Ockene IS, Alpert JS: Coronary spasm, coronary thrombosis, and myocardial infarction. A hypothesis concerning the pathophysiology of acute myocardial infarction. *Am Heart J* 104:1119, 1982.

41. Bussmann WD, Passek D, Seidel W, Kalterbach M: Reduction of CK and CK-MB indexes of infarct size by intravenous nitroglycerine. *Circulation* 63:615-622, 1981.

42. Flaherty JT, Becker LC, Bulkley BH, et al: A randomized prospective trial of intravenous nitroglycerin in patients with acute myocardial infarction. *Circulation* 68, 576-588, 1983.

43. Stockman MB, Verrier RL, Lown B: Effect of nitroglycerin on vulnerability to ventricular fibrillation during myocardial ischemia and reperfusion. *Am J Cardiol* 43:233, 1979.

44. Zelis R, Mansour EJ, Capone RJ, Mason DT: The cardiovascular effects of morphine: The peripheral capacitance and resistance vessels in human subjects. *J Clin Invest* 54:1247-1258, 1974.

45. Semenkovich CF and Jaffe AS: Adverse effects due to morphine sulfate — challenge to previous clinical doctrine. *Am J Med* 79:325-330, 1985.

46. DeSanctis RW, Block P, Hutter AM Jr: Tachyarrhythmias in myocardial infarction. *Circulation* 45:681, 1972.

47. Kimball JT, Killip T: Aggressive treatment of arrhythmias in acute myocardial infarction: Procedures and results. *Prog Cardiovasc Dis* 10:483, 1968.

48. Lawrie DM: Ventricular fibrillation in acute myocardial infarction. *Am Heart J* 78:424, 1969.

49. Lie KI, Wellens HJ, Downar E, et al: Observations on patients with primary ventricular fibrillation complicating acute myocardial infarction. *Circulation* 52:755, 1975.

50. Dhurandhar RW, MacMillan RL, Brown KW: Primary ventricular fibrillation complicating acute myocardial infarction. *Am J Cardiol* 27:347, 1971.

51. Lie KI, Wellens HJ, van Capelle FJ, et al: Lidocaine in the prevention of primary ventricular fibrillation: A double-blind, randomized study of 212 consecutive patients. *N Engl J Med* 291:1324, 1974.

52. Wyman MG, Hammersmith L: Comprehensive treatment plan for the prevention of primary ventricular fibrillation in acute myocardial infarction. *Am J Cardiol* 33:661, 1974.

53. Koster RW, Dunning AJ: Intramuscular lidocaine for the prevention of lethal arrhythmias in the prehospitalization phase of acute myocardial infarction. *N Eng J Med* 313:1105, 1985.

54. Oliver MF: Significance of ventricular arrhythmias during myocardial ischemia. *Circulation* 53 (suppl I):I-155, 1976.

55. Adgey AA, Allen JD, Geddes JS, et al: Acute phase of myocardial infarction. *Lancet* 2:501, 1971.

56. Lucchesi BR, Kniffen FJ: Pharmacological modification of arrhythmias after experimentally induced acute myocardial infarction. Drugs acting on the nervous system. *Circulation* 52 (suppl III): III-241, 1975.

57. β-Blocker Heart Attack Trial Research Group: A randomized trial of propranolol in patients with acute myocardial infarction. I. Mortality results. *JAMA* 247:1707, 1982.

58. Pedersen TR: Six-year follow-up of the Norwegian Multicenter Study on Timolol after Acute Myocardial Infarction. *N Engl J Med* 313:1055, 1985.

59. Rotman M, Wagner GS, Wallace AG: Bradyarrhythmias in acute myocardial infarction. *Circulation* 45:703, 1972.

60. Nordrehaug JE, Johannessen K, von der Lippe G: Serum potassium concentration as a risk factor of ventricular arrhythmias early in acute myocardial infarction. *Circulation* 71:645, 1985.

61. Norris RM, Brown MA, Clarke ED, et al: Prevention of ventricular fibrillation during acute myocardial infarction by intravenous propranolol. *Lancet* 2:883, 1984.

62. First International Study of Infarct Survival Collaborative Group. Randomized Trial of Intravenous atenolol among 16,027 cases of suspected acute myocardial infarction: ISIS-1. *Lancet* 2:56-66, 1986.

63. Smith LF, Heagerty AM, Bing RF, et al: Intravenous infusion of magnesium sulphate after acute myocardial infarction: Effects on arrhythmias and mortality. *Intern J Cardiol* 12:175, 1986.

64. Epstein SE, Goldstein RE, Redwood RD, et al: The early phase of acute myocardial infarction: Pharmacological aspects of therapy. *Ann Intern Med* 78:918, 1973.

65. Grauer LE, Gershen BJ, Orlando MM, et al: Bradycardia and its complications in the prehospital phase of acute myocardial infarction. *Am J Cardiol* 32:607, 1973.

66. Han J, Millet D, Chizzonitti B, et al: Temporal dispersion of recovery of excitability in atrium and ventricle as a function of heart rate. *Am Heart J* 71:481, 1966.

67. Corr PB, Gillis RA: Effect of autonomic neural influences on the cardiovascular changes induced by coronary occlusion. *Am Heart J* 89:766, 1975.

68. Goldstein RE, Karsh RB, Smith ER, et al: Influence of atropine and of vagally mediated bradycardia on the occurrence of ventricular arrhythmias following acute coronary occlusion in closed-chested dogs. *Circulation* 47:1180, 1973.

69. Scherlag BJ, Helfant RH, Haft JI, et al: Electrophysiology underlying ventricular arrhythmias due to coronary ligation. *Am J Physiol* 219:1665, 1970.

70. Kent KM, Smith ER, Redwood DR, et al: Electrical stability of acutely ischemic myocardium. Influences of heart rate and vagal stimulations. *Circulation* 47:291, 1973.

71. James TN: The coronary circulation and conduction system in acute myocardial infarction. *Prog Cardiovasc Dis* 10:410, 1968.

72. Gregory JJ, Grace WJ: The management of sinus bradycardia, nodal rhythm and heart block for the prevention of cardiac arrest in acute myocardial infarction. *Prog Cardiovasc Dis* 10:505, 1968.

73. Massumi RA, Mason DT, Amsterdam EA, et al: Ventricular fibrillation and tachycardia after intravenous atropine for treatment of bradycardias. *N Engl J Med* 287:336, 1972.

74. Higgins CB, Vatner SF, Braunwald E: Parasympathetic control of the heart. *Pharmacol Rev* 25:119, 1973.

75. de Soyza N, Bissett JK, Kane JJ, et al: Association of accelerated idioventricular rhythm and paroxysmal ventricular tachycardia in acute myocardial infarction. *Am J Cardiol* 34:667, 1974.

76. Zoll PM, Zoll RH, Falk RH, Clinton JE, Eitel DR, Antman EM: External noninvasive temporary cardiac pacing: Clinical trials. *Circulation* 71:937-944, 1985.

77. Corr PB, Gillis RA: Autonomic neural influences of the dysrhythmias resulting from myocardial infarction. *Circ Res* 43:1, 1978.

78. Hod H, Lew AS, Keltai M, et al: Early atrial fibrillation during evolving myocardial infarction: A consequence of impaired left atrial perfusion. *Circulation* 75:146, 1987.

79. Sugiura T, Iwasaka T, Ogawa A, et al: Atrial fibrillation in acute myocardial infarction. *Am J Cardiol* 56:27, 1985.

80. Cristal N, Szwarcberg J, Gueron M: Supraventricular arrhythmias in acute myocardial infarction: Prognostic importance of clinical setting; mechanism of production. *Ann Intern Med* 82:35, 1975.

81. Kitchen MG III, Kastor JA: Pacing in acute myocardial infarction: Indications, methods, hazards and results, in Brest AN, Wiener L, Chung EK, et al (eds): *Innovations in the Diagnosis and Management of Acute Myocardial Infarction.* Cardiovascular Clinics Series, vol 7, no 1. Philadelphia, FA Davis, 1975, p 219.

82. Norris RM, Mercer CJ: Significance of idioventricular rhythms in acute myocardial infarction. *Prog Cardiovasc Dis* 16:455, 1974.

83. Haft J: I. Clinical implications of atrioventricular and intra-ventricular conduction abnormalities. II. Acute myocardial infarction, in Rios JC (ed): *Clinical Electrocardiographic Correlations.* Cardiovascular Clinics Series, vol 8, no 3. Philadelphia, FA Davis, 1977, p. 65.

84. Hindman MC, Wagner GS, Jaro M, et al: The clinical significance of bundle branch block complicating acute myocardial infarction: II Indications for temporary and permanent pacemaker insertion. *Circulation* 58:689, 1978.

85. Hollander G, Nadiminti V, Lichstein E, et al: Bundle branch block in acute myocardial infarction. *Am Heart J* 105:738, 1983.

86. Klein RC, Vera Z, Mason DT: Intraventricular conduction defects in acute myocardial infarction: Incidence, prognosis, and therapy. *Am Heart J* 108:1007, 1984.

87. Jaffe AS: Complications of acute myocardial infarction. *Cardiol Clin* 2:79-94, 1984.

88. Bigger JT Jr, Dresdale FJ, Heissenbuttel RH, et al: Ventricular arrhythmias in ischemic heart disease: Mechanism, prevalence, significance, and management. *Prog Cardiovasc Dis* 19:255, 1977.

89. Goldberg RJ, Gore JM, Haffajee CI, et al: Outcome after cardiac arrest during acute myocardial infarction. *Am J Cardiol* 59:251, 1987.

90. Durrer JD, Lie K, vanCapelle F, et al: Effect of sodium nitro-prusside on mortality in acute myocardial infarction. *N Engl J Med* 306:1121, 1982.

91. Herman MV, Heinle RA, Klein MD, et al: Localized disorders in myocardial contraction: Asynergy and its role in congestive heart failure. *N Engl J Med* 277:222, 1967.

92. Herman MV, Gorlin R: Implications of left ventricular asynergy. *Am J Cardiol* 23:538, 1969.

93. Resnekov L: Management of acute myocardial infarction. *Cardiovasc Med* 2:949, 1977.

94. Hamosh P, Cohn JN: Left ventricular function in acute myocardial infarction. *J Clin Invest* 50:523, 1971.

95. Genton R, Jaffe AS: Management of congestive heart failure in patients with acute myocardial infarction. *JAMA* 256:2556-2560, 1986.

96. Constantin L: Extracardiac factors contributing to hypotension during coronary occlusion. *Am J Cardiol* 11:205, 1963.

97. Wolk MJ, Scheidt S, Killip T: Heart failure complicating myocardial infarction. *Circulation* 45:1125, 1972.

98. Weber KT, Ratshin RA, Janiki JS, et al: Left ventricular dysfunction following acute myocardial infarction: A clinicopathological and hemodynamic profile of shock and failure. *Am J Med* 54:697, 1973.

99. Killip T, Kimball JT: Treatment of myocardial infarction in a coronary care unit: A two-year experience with 250 patients. *Am J Cardiol* 20:457, 1967.

100. Forrester JS, Diamond G, Chatterjee K, et al: Medical therapy of acute myocardial infarction by application of hemodynamic subsets. *N Engl J Med* 295:1356, 1976.

101. Dikshit K, Vyden JK, Forrester JS, et al: Renal and extra-renal hemodynamic effects of furosemide in congestive heart failure after acute myocardial infarction. *N Engl J Med* 288:1087-1090, 1973.

102. Gold HK, Leinbach RC, Sanders CA: Use of sublingual nitro-glycerin in congestive failure following acute myocardial infarction. *Circulation* 46:839, 1972.

103. Cohn JN, Franciosa JA: Vasodilator therapy of cardiac failure (second of two parts). *N Engl J Med* 297:254, 1977.

104. Leier CV, Bambach D, Thompson MJ, et al: Central and regional hemodynamic effects of intravenous isosorbide dinitrate, nitro-glycerin and nitroprusside in patients with congestive heart failure. *Am J Cardiol* 48:1115-1123, 1981.

105. Cohn JN, Franciosa JA, Francis GS, et al: Effect of short-term infusion of sodium nitroprusside on mortality rates in acute myocardial infarction complicated by left ventricular failure. *N Engl J Med* 306:1129, 1982.

106. Gillespie TA, Ambos HD, Sobel BE, et al: Effects of dobutamine in patients with acute myocardial infarction. *Am J Cardiol* 39:588-594, 1977.

107. Rude RE, Izquierdo C, Buja LM, et al: Effects of inotropic and chronotropic stimuli on acute myocardial ischemic injury: I. Studies with dobutamine in the anesthetized dog. *Circulation* 65:1321-1328, 1982.

108. Taylor SH, Verma SP, Hussain M, et al: Intravenous amrinone in left ventricular failure complicated by acute myocardial infarction. *Am J Cardiol* 56:29B-32B, 1985.

109. Rude RE, Kloner RA, Maroko PR, et al: Effects of amrinone on experimental acute myocardial ischemic injury. *Cardiovasc Res* 14:419-427, 1980.

110. Crexells C, Chatterjee K, Forrester JS, et al: Optimum level of filling pressure in the left side of the heart in acute myocardial infarction. *N Engl J Med* 289:1263, 1973.

111. Russell RO Jr, Rackley CE, Pombo J, et al: Effects of increasing left ventricular filling pressure in patients with acute myocardial infarction. *J Clin Invest* 49:1539, 1970.

112. McHugh TJ, Forrester JS, Adler L, et al: Pulmonary vascular congestion with acute myocardial infarction: Hemodynamic and radiologic correlations. *Ann Intern Med* 76:29-33, 1972.

113. Rackley CE, Russell RO, Mantla JA, et al: Cardiogenic shock: Recognition and management. *Cardiovasc Clin* 7:251, 1975.

114. Jaffe AS: Who is likely to survive cardiogenic shock? *Clin Management* 7:699-713,1982.

115. Dell'Italia LJ, Starling MR, Crawford MH, et al: Right ventricular infarction: identification by hemodynamic measurements before and after volume loading and correlation with non-invasive techniques. *JACC* 4:931, 1984.

116. Lopez-Sendon J, Coma-Canella I, Alcasena S, et al: Electrocardiographic findings in acute right ventricular infarction: sensitivity and specificity of electrocardiographic alternations in right precordial leads V_4R, V_3R, V_1, V_2 and V_3. *J Am Coll Cardiol* 6:1273, 1985.

117. Reddy GV, Schamroth L: The electrocardiology of right ventricular myocardial infarction. *Chest* 90:756, 1986.

118. Lorell B, Leinbach RC, Pohost GM, et al: Right ventricular infarction. Clinical diagnosis and differentiation from cardiac tamponade and pericardial constriction. *Am J Cardiol* 43:465, 1979.

119. Cohn JN: Right ventricular infarction revisited (editorial). *Am J Cardiol* 43:666, 1979.

120. Dell'Italia LJ, Starling MR, Blumhardt R, et al: Comparative effects of volume loading, dobutamine, and nitroprusside in patients with predominant right ventricular infarction. *Circulation* 72:1327, 1985.

121. Meister SG, Helfant RH: Rapid bedside differentiation of ruptured interventricular septum from acute mitral insufficiency. *N Engl J Med* 287:1024, 1972.

122. Austen WG, Sokol DM, DeSanctis RW, et al: Surgical treatment of papillary muscle rupture complicating myocardial infarction. *N Engl J Med* 278:1137, 1968.

123. Antman EM, Marsh JD, Green LH, et al: Blood oxygen measurements in the assessment of intracardiac left to right shunts: A critical appraisal of methodology. *Am J Cardiol* 46:265, 1980.

124. Graham AF, Stinson EB, Daily PO, et al: Ventricular septal defects after myocardial infarction. Early operative treatment. *JAMA* 225:708, 1973.

125. Radford MJ, Johnson RA, Daggett WM Jr, et al: Ventricular septal rupture: A review of clinical and physiologic features and an analysis of survival. *Circulation* 64:545, 1981.

126. Moore CA, Nygaard TW, Kaiser DL, et al: Post-infarction ventricular septal rupture: the importance of location of infarction and right ventricular function in determining survival. *Circulation* 74:45, 1986.

127. McIntyre KM, Sasahara AA: Hemodynamic response to pulmonary embolism in patients without prior cardiopulmonary disease. *Am J Cardiol* 28:288, 1971.

128. Paraskos JA: Pulmonary heart disease including pulmonary embolism, in Parmley WW, Chatterjee K (eds): *Cardiology.* Philadelphia, Lippincott, 1987.

129. Dalen JE: Hemodynamic profile: Acute pulmonary embolism, in Grossman W (ed): *Cardiac Catheterization and Angiography.* Philadelphia, Lea & Febiger, 1974.

130. McIntyre KM, Sasahara AA: Pathophysiology of *cor pulmonale,* in Levine HJ (ed): *Cardiovascular Physiology,* chap 19. New York, Grune & Stratton, 1976.

131. Warlow C, Beattie AG, Terry G, et al: A double blind trial of low dose of subcutaneous heparin in the prevention of deep vein thrombosis after myocardial infarction. *Lancet* 2:934, 1973.

132. Feigenbaum H: Echocardiographic diagnosis of pericardial effusion. *Am J Cardiol* 26:475, 1970.

133. D'Cruz IA, Cohen HC, Prabha R, et al: Diagnosis of cardiac tamponade by echocardiography: Changes in mitral valve motion and ventricular dimensions, with special reference to paradoxical pulse. *Circulation* 52:460, 1975.

134. Spodick DH: Acute cardiac tamponade: Pathologic physiology, diagnosis and management. *Prog Cardiovasc Dis* 10:64, 1967.

135. Bates RJ, Beutler S, Resnekov L, et al: Cardiac rupture — challenge in diagnosis and management. *Am J Cardiol* 40:429, 1977.

136. Roberts WC: Aortic dissection: Anatomy, consequences, and causes. *Am Heart J* 101:195, 1981.

137. Slater EE, DeSanctis RW: The clinical recognition of dissecting aortic aneurysm. *Am J Med* 60:625, 1976.

138. Victor MF, Mintz GS, Kotler MN, et al: Two-dimensional echocardiographic diagnosis of aortic dissection. *Am J Cardiol* 48:1155, 1981.

139. Larde D, Belloir C, Vasile N, et al: Computed tomography of aortic dissection. *Radiology* 136:147, 1980.

140. Dalen JE, Alpert JS, Cohn LH, et al: Dissection of the thoracic aorta: Medical or surgical therapy? *Am J Cardiol* 34:803, 1974.

141. Doroghazi RM, Slater EE, DeSanctis RW, et al: Long-term survival of patients with treated aortic dissection. *J Am Coll Cardiol* 3:1026, 1984.

142. Maroko PR, Kjekshus JK, Sobel BE, et al: Factors influencing infarct size following experimental coronary artery occlusions. *Circulation* 43:67,1971.

143. International Collaborative Study Group. Reduction of infarct size with the early use of timolol in acute myocardial infarction. *N Engl J Med* 310:9, 1984.

144. Rude RE, Muller JE, Braunwald E: Efforts to limit size of myocardial infarcts. *Ann Intern Med* 95:736, 1981.

145. The Norwegian Multicenter Study Group: Timolol induced reduction in mortality and re-infarction in patients surviving acute myocardial infarction. *N Engl J Med* 304:801, 1981.

146. Herlitz J, et al: Göteborg Metoprolol Trial: Mortality and causes of death. *Am J Cardiol* 52:9D, 1984.

147. The MIAMI Trial Research Group: Metoprolol in acute myocardial infarction. Development of myocardial infarction. *Am J Cardiol* 56:23G, 1985.

148. The MIAMI Trial Research Group: Metoprolol in acute myocardial infarction. Enzymatic estimation of infarct size. *Am J Cardiol* 56:27G, 1985.

149. Hjalmarson Å, Herlitz J, Malek, I, et al: Effect on mortality of metoprolol in acute myocardial infarction: A double blind randomized trial. *Lancet* 2:823, 1981.

150. Standards and guidelines for cardiopulmonary resuscitation and emergency cardiac care. *JAMA* 255:2944, 1986.

151. Kennedy JW, Ritchie JL, Davis KB, et al: Western Washington randomized trial of intracoronary streptokinase in acute myocardial infarction. *N Engl J Med* 309:1477, 1983.

152. Kennedy JW, Ritchie JL, Davis KB, et al: The Western Washington randomized trial of intracoronary streptokinase in acute myocardial infarction: a 12-month follow-up report. *N Engl J Med* 312:1073, 1985.

153. Simoons ML, Serruys PW, v. d. Brand M, de Zwaan C, et al: Improved survival after early thrombolysis in acute myocardial infarction: A randomized trial by the Interuniversity Cardiology Institute in the Netherlands. *Lancet* 2:578, 1985.

154. Gruppo Italiano per lo Studio della Streptochinasi nell'Infarcto Miocardico (GISSI): Effectiveness of intravenous thrombolytic treatment in acute myocardial infarction. *Lancet* 1:397, 1986.

155. Sobel BE, Geltman EM, Tiefenbrunn AJ, et al: Improvement of regional myocardial metabolism after coronary thrombolysis with tissue-type plasminogen activator or streptokinase. *Circulation* 69:983, 1984.

156. Simoons ML, Serrruys PW, van den Brand M, et al: Early thrombolysis in acute myocardial infarction: Limitation of infarct size and improved survival. *J Am Coll Cardiol* 7:717, 1986.

157. Sheehan FH, Mathey DG, Schofer J, et al: Factors that determine recovery of left ventricular function after thrombolysis in patients with acute myocardial infarction. *Circulation* 71:1121, 1985.

158. TIMI Study Group: The thrombolysis in myocardial infarction (TIMI) trial: Phase I findings. *N Engl J Med* 312:932, 1985.

159. Verstraete M, Bory M, Collen D, et al: Randomized trial of intravenous recombinant tissue-type plasminogen activator versus intravenous streptokinase in acute myocardial infarction: Report from the European Cooperative Study Group for recombinant tissue-type plasminogen activator. *Lancet* 1:842, 1985.

160. van de Werf F, Nobuhara M, Collen D: Coronary thrombolysis with human single-chain urokinase type plasminogen activator (pro-urokinase) in patients with acute myocardial infarction. *Ann Intern Med* 104:345, 1986.

161. Thrombolytic Therapy in Thrombosis: A National Institutes of Heath consensus development conference. *Ann Intern Med* 93:141, 1980.

162. Smith B, Kennedy JW: Thrombolysis in the treatment of acute transmural myocardial infarction. *Ann Intern Med* 106:414-420, 1987.

163. Gold HK, Cowley MJ, Palacios IF, et al: Combined intracoronary streptokinase infusion and coronary angioplasty during acute myocardial infarction. *Am J Cardiol* 53:122c, 1984.

164. Hartzler GO, Rutherford, BD, McConahay DR: Percutaneous transluminal coronary angioplasty: Application for acute myocardial infarction. *Am J Cardiol* 53:117c, 1984.

165. Meyer J, Merx W, Schmitz H, et al: Percutaneous transluminal coronary angioplasty immediately after intracoronary streptolysis of transmural myocardial infarction. *Circulation* 66:905, 1982.

166. Papapietro SE, MacLean WA, Stanley AW Jr, et al: Percutaneous transluminal coronary angioplasty after intracoronary streptokinase in evolving myocardial infarction. *Am J Cardiol* 55:48, 1985.

167. Holmes DR Jr, Smith HC, Vliestra RE, et al: Percutaneous transluminal coronary angioplasty. Alone or in combination with streptokinase therapy, during acute myocardial infarction. *Mayo Clin Proc* 60:4498, 1985.

168. Phillips SJ, Kongtahworn C, Zeff RH: Emergency coronary artery revascularization: A possible therapy for acute myocardial infarction. *Circulation* 60:241, 1979.

169. Cohn LH, Gorlin R, Herman MV: Aortocoronary bypass for acute coronary occlusion. *J Thorac Cardiovasc Surg* 64:503, 1972.

170. Hindman MC, Wagner GS, JaRo M, et al: The clinical significance of bundle branch block complicating acute myocardial infarction: I Clinical characteristics, hospital mortality, and one-year follow-up. *Circulation* 58:679, 1978.

171. Roberts R, Ambos HD, Loh CW, et al: Initiation of repetitive ventricular depolarizations by relatively late premature complexes in patients with acute myocardial infarction. *Am J Cardiol* 41:678, 1978.

172. Wilson C, Adgey AA: Survival of patients with late ventricular fibrillation after myocardial infarction. *Lancet* 2:124, 1974.

173. Thompson P, Sloman G: Sudden death in hospital after discharge from coronary care unit. *Br Med J* 4:136, 1971.

174. Graboys TB: In-hospital sudden death after coronary care unit discharge: A high-risk profile. *Arch Intern Med* 135:512, 1975.

175. Lie KI, Liem KL, Schuilenburg RM, et al: Early identification of patients developing late in-hospital ventricular fibrillation after discharge from the coronary care unit. A 5½ year retrospective and prospective study of 1,897 patients. *Am J Cardiol* 41:674, 1978.

176. Resnekov L: Intermediate coronary care units. *JAMA* 237:1697, 1977

177. Marmor A, Sobel BE, Roberts R: Factors presaging early recurrent myocardial infarction (extension). *Am J Cardiol* 48:603-610, 1981.

178. Gibson RS, Boden WE, Theroux P, et al: Diltiazem and reinfarction in patients with non-Q-wave myocardial infarction. Results of a double-blind randomized, multicenter trial. *N Engl J Med* 315:423-429, 1986.

179. Eisenberg PR, Lee RG, Biello DR, Geltman EM, Jaffe AS: Chest pain after nontransmural infarction: The absence of remediable coronary vasospasm. *Am Heart J* 110:515-521,1985.

180. Schulze RA Jr, Strauss HW, Pitt B: Sudden death in the year following myocardial infarction. Relation to ventricular premature contractions in the late hospital phase and left ventricular ejection fraction. *Am J Med* 62:192, 1977.

181. Harris PJ, Harrell FE Jr, Lee KL, et al: Survival in medically treated coronary artery disease. *Circulation* 60:1259, 1979.

182. Davis HT, deCamilla J, Bayer LW, et al: Survivorship patterns in the posthospital phase of myocardial infarction. *Circulation* 60:1252, 1979.

183. Taylor GJ, Humphries JO, Mellits ED, et al: Predictors of clinical course, coronary anatomy and left ventricular function after recovery from acute myocardial infarction. *Circulation* 62:960, 1980.

184. DeFeyter PJ, Van Eenige MJ, Dighton DH, et al: Prognostic value of exercise testing, coronary angiography and left ventriculography 6-8 weeks after myocardial infarction. *Circulation* 66:527, 1982.

185. Norris RM, Barnaby PF, Brandt PWT, et al: Prognosis after recovery from first acute myocardial infarction: determinants of reinfarction and sudden death. *Am J Cardiol* 53:408, 1984.

186. Ahnve S, Gilpin E. Henning H, et al: Limitations and advantages of the ejection fraction for defining high risk after acute myocardial infarction. *Am J Cardiol* 58:872, 1986.

187. European Coronary Surgery Study Group. Prospective randomized study of coronary artery bypass surgery in stable angina pectoris: a progressive report on survival. *Circulation* 65:II 67, 1982.

188. Vismara LA, Amsterdam EA, Mason DT: Relation of ventricular arrhythmias in the late phase of acute myocardial infarction to sudden death after hospital discharge. *Am J Med* 59:6, 1975.

189. Ruberman W, Weinblatt E, Goldberg JD, et al: Ventricular premature beats and mortality after myocardial infarction. *N Engl J Med* 297:750, 1977.

190. Moss AJ, Davis HT, DeCamilla J, et al: Ventricular ectopic beats and their relation to sudden and non-sudden cardiac death after myocardial infarction. *Circulation* 60:998, 1979.

191. Bigger JT Jr, Weld FM, Rolnitzky LM: Prevalence, characteristics and significance of ventricular tachycardia (three or more complexes) detected with ambulatory electrocardiographic recording in the late hospital phase of acute myocardial infarction. *Am J Cardiol* 48:815, 1981.

192. Taylor GJ Jr, Humphries JO, Pitt B, et al: Complex ventricular arrhythmias after myocardial infarction during convalescence and follow-up: a harbinger of multivessel coronary disease, left ventricular dysfunction and sudden death. *Johns Hopkins Med J*: 149:1, 1981.

193. Fein SA, Klein NA, Frishman WH: Exercise testing soon after uncomplicated myocardial infarction: prognostic value and safety. *JAMA* 245:1863, 1981.

194. DeBusk RF, Blomqvist CG, Kouchoukos NT, et al: Identification and treatment of low-risk patients after acute myocardial infarction and coronary artery bypass graft surgery. *N Engl J Med* 314:161, 1986.

195. Williams WL, Nair RC Higginson LAJ, et al: Comparison of clinical and treadmill variables for the prediction of outcome after myocardial infarction. *J Am Coll Cardiol* 4:477, 1984.

196. Krone RJ, Gillespie JA, Weld FM, et al: Low-level exercise testing after myocardial infarction: usefulness in enhancing clinical risk stratification. *Circulation* 71:80, 1985.

197. Fioretti P, Brower RW, Simoons ML, et al: Prediction of mortality during the first year after acute myocardial infarction from clinical variables and stress test at hospital discharge. *Am J Cardiol* 55:1313, 1985.

198. Bigger JT Jr, Fleiss JL, Kleiger R, et al: The relationships among ventricular arrhythmias, left ventricular dysfunction, and mortality in the two years after myocardial infarction. *Circulation* 69:250, 1984.

199. Richards DA, Cody DV, Denniss AR, et al: Ventricular electrical instability: a predictor of death after myocardial infarction. *Am J Cardiol* 51:75, 1983.

200. Hamer A, Vohra J, Hunt D, et al: Prediction of sudden death by electrophysiologic studies in high risk patients surviving acute myocardial infarction. *Am J Cardiol* 50:223, 1982

201. Olsson G, Rehnqvist N, Sjogren A, et al: Long-term treatment witih metoprolol after myocardial infarction: effect on three year mortality and morbidity. *J Am Coll Cardiol* 5:1428, 1985.

202. Ahumada GG: Identification of patients who do not require beta antagonists after myocardial infarction. *Am J Med* 76:900, 1984.

203. American Heart Association: Special report: Secondary prevention in myocardial infarction survivors. *Circulation* 65:216A, 1982.

Adjuncts for Airway Control, Ventilation, and Supplemental Oxygen

Several special devices can be of help in controlling the airway, supplementing oxygen, and ventilating the patient. These devices and the techniques for their use are described in this chapter.

Overview

Anyone in respiratory distress or cardiovascular crisis (myocardial infarction, shock, etc.) — that is, anyone with decreased blood oxygen content or compromised oxygen transport to the cells — should receive supplemental oxygen. Supplemental oxygen in the patient who is breathing spontaneously may prevent a cardiac or respiratory arrest.

The patient may be making spontaneous respiratory efforts but not achieving alveolar ventilation because of upper airway obstruction from foreign material such as food or blood clots or from the posterior displacement of the tongue and/or epiglottis, occluding the pharynx and larynx. Severe upper airway obstruction is recognized when the patient becomes cyanotic and has noisy airflow during inspiration (stridor, or "crowing"). The contractions of the accessory muscles of respiration cause retractions of the suprasternal, supraclavicular, and intercostal spaces. This condition should be treated as if the airway were completely obstructed. The management of foreign body airway obstruction (FBAO) may include basic techniques such as subdiaphragmatic abdominal thrusts (the Heimlich maneuver) or advanced techniques such as direct laryngoscopy and removal of the foreign body with forceps and/or suctioning. For airway obstruction produced by the tongue and epiglottis, head-tilt with anterior displacement of the mandibular (chin-lift or jaw-thrust) is indicated. If this is not sufficient, an oropharyngeal or nasopharyngeal airway should be inserted.

If spontaneous ventilation is present after cleaning the airway, the patient should receive supplemental oxygen. If spontaneous breathing is absent, positive-pressure ventilations must be started. The preferred technique depends on circumstances, but that providing the best oxygenation should be used. These techniques include mouth-to-mouth and mouth-to-mask rescue breathing or the use of bag–valve–mask or oxygen-powered breathing devices.

Tracheal intubation is preferred for airway control and should therefore be attempted — by the most experienced person on the scene after ventilation and oxygenation have been established. An alternative, but less desirable, method of airway control is the esophageal obturator airway (EOA). After intubation by either technique, positive-pressure ventilation should be continued with a bag–valve unit or an oxygen-powered breathing device.

Once the airway is protected by an endotracheal tube, ventilations need not be synchronized with chest compressions.[1] The recommended rate for ventilation during CPR in the adult is 12–15 per minute.

Airway Control

Head and Jaw Position[2-6]

During acute airway obstruction of any etiology, attempts to open the airway have the highest priority. Upper airway obstruction in the unconscious person is the result of the loss of tonicity of the submandilar muscles, which provide direct support of the tongue and indirect support to the epiglottis. Posterior displacement of the tongue occludes the airway at the level of the pharynx, and the epiglottis may occlude the airway at the level of the larynx. The basic technique for opening the airway is head-tilt with anterior displacement of the mandible (chin-lift and, if necessary, jaw-thrust). In the trauma victim with suspected neck injury, the initial step for opening the airway is the chin-lift or jaw-thrust without head-tilt. If the airway remains obstructed, then head-tilt is added slowly and gently until the airway is open (see Figure 1).

These maneuvers should be attempted before any airway adjunct is used, and if the patient is capable of spontaneous respiration, proper airway positioning may

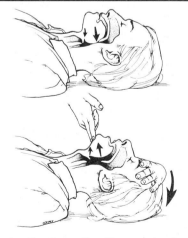

Figure 1. Opening the airway. Top: Airway obstruction produced by tongue and epiglottis. Bottom: Relief by head-tilt/chin-lift.

be all that is required. In some instances, an oropharyngeal or nasopharyngeal airway may be needed to maintain airway patency.

Oropharyngeal Airways

The oropharyngeal airway is a semicircular-shaped device that when in proper position will hold the tongue away from the posterior wall of the pharynx. Oropharyngeal airways facilitate suctioning of the pharynx and prevent the patient from biting and occluding an endotracheal tube. Those most frequently used are made of plastic and are disposable. There are two types, Guedel and Berman, the distinguishing differences being the tubular design of the Guedel and the airway channels along the sides of the Berman[7] (see Figure 2).

Sizes for Adults

The size is based on the distance, in millimeters, from the flange to the distal tip. The following sizes are recommended:

Large adult: 100 mm (Guedel size 5)
Medium adult: 90 mm (Guedel size 4)
Small adult: 80 mm (Guedel size 3)

Techniques of Insertion

If needed, the mouth and pharynx should be cleared of secretions, blood, or vomit, using a rigid pharyngeal suction tip (Yankauer). An easy way to place the airway is to turn it so that it is inserted backward as it enters the mouth, as the airway transverses the oral cavity and approaches the posterior wall of the pharynx, the operator rotates the airway into proper position. Another method is to move the tongue out of the way with a tongue blade depressor before the airway is inserted. The indication that the airway is in the proper position and of proper size is the presence of clear breath sounds on auscultation of the lungs during ventilation. It should be remembered that, even with the use of this airway, proper head position must be maintained.

Complications

If the airway is too long, it may press the epiglottis against the entrance of the larynx, producing complete airway obstruction.[8] If the airway is not inserted properly, it is possible to push the tongue posteriorly, aggravating the problem of upper airway obstruction. To prevent trauma, the operator should make sure that the lips and the tongue are not between the teeth and the airway. The insertion of the airway in the conscious or semiconscious patient may stimulate vomiting and laryngospasm and should therefore be performed only in the unconscious patient.

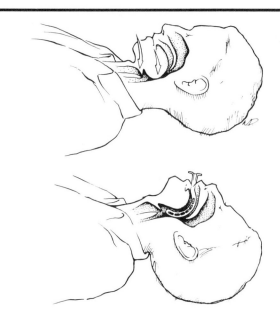

Figure 2. Placement of correctly inserted oropharyngeal airway. Top: Before insertion, incorrect head position. Bottom: After insertion, showing head tilted and oropharyngeal airway in place.

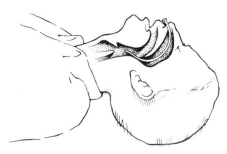

Figure 3. Nasopharyngeal airway in place. Note head tilted back for proper insertion.

Nasopharyngeal Airways

These are uncuffed tubes made of soft rubber or plastic material. Their use is indicated when the insertion of an oropharyngeal airway is technically difficult or impossible (trismus, massive trauma around the mouth, mandibulo-maxillary wiring, etc.) (see Figure 3).

Sizes for Adults

The sizes for this type of airway are indicated in millimeters for the internal diameter (i.d.). The length of the tubes varies with the internal diameter. Recommended sizes are as follows:

Large adult: 8.0–9.0 i.d.
Medium adult: 7.0–8.0 i.d.
Small adult: 6.0–7.0 i.d.

Technique of Insertion

The proper sized airway is lubricated with a water-soluble lubricant and gently inserted close to the midline along the floor of the nostril into the posterior pharynx behind the tongue. If resistance is encountered, slight rotation of the tube may facilitate the passage at the angle of the nasal passage and the nasopharynx.

Complications

If the tube is too long, it may enter the esophagus, causing gastric distention and hypoventilation during artificial ventilation. This type of airway is better tolerated by the semiconscious patient. However, its use may also precipitate laryngospasm and vomiting in these patients. The insertion of the airway may injure the nasal mucosa with bleeding and possible aspiration of clots into the trachea. Suction may be needed to remove secretions or blood. It is important to maintain head-tilt with anterior displacement of the mandible by chin-lift and, if necessary, jaw-thrust when using this airway.

Immediately after insertion of the pharyngeal airway (oral or nasal), check for respirations. If absent or inadequate, artificial positive-pressure ventilation should be initiated with a mouth-to-mask technique, bag–valve–mask, or the oxygen-powered breathing device. If adjuncts are not available, mouth-to-mouth ventilation should be used.

Esophageal Obturator Airway

The esophageal obturator airway (EOA)[9-13] is a large-bore tube, 37 cm in length, with a high-volume cuff close to the distal end that, when inflated in the lower part of the esophagus, prevents regurgitation and gastric insufflation during positive-pressure ventilation. The tube is mounted through a clear face mask. It has multiple openings at the level of the pharynx through which air or oxygen is delivered by artificial ventilation into the lungs via the larynx and trachea. The mask, when properly applied to the victim's face, prevents leaks around and through the nose.

The EOA is an alternative to tracheal intubation in situations where the rescuer cannot, or is not permitted to, intubate the trachea, when equipment for endotracheal intubation is not available or is not working properly, and in patients in whom tracheal intubation is not technically possible or desirable.

The potential advantage of the EOA is that since visualization is not required for insertion it can be introduced more easily and quickly than can an endotracheal tube. Because there is no need for hyperextension of the head and flexion of the neck during insertion, the EOA is an attractive technique for trauma victims with suspected neck injury. However, it is often difficult to maintain an adequate seal between the mask and the face, so ventilatory volumes can be inadequate. In this respect the disadvantage of the EOA is similar to that of the bag–valve–mask devices. Thus, esophageal airways must be used only by persons who are properly trained and proficient in their use. Practice and retraining are mandatory if proficiency is to be maintained.

Technique of Insertion (Figure 4)

Before insertion, the tube should be attached to the mask and the cuff tested for leaks. The cuff is then deflated before insertion and the tube lubricated.

With the head in mid-position or slight flexion, the rescuer elevates the tongue and jaw with one hand and with the other inserts the tube through the mouth and into the esophagus; the tube is advanced until the mask is seated on the face. When this is accomplished, the cuff will lie below the level of the carina (see Figure 5).

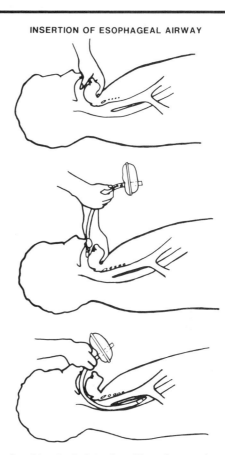

INSERTION OF ESOPHAGEAL AIRWAY

Figure 4. An obturator is introduced into the esophagus by elevating the tongue and jaw from the corner of the mouth with one hand, with head and neck flexed forward.

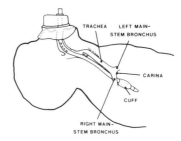

FINAL POSITION OF ESOPHAGEAL AIRWAY AND MASK

Figure 5. Properly positioned obturator airway. The rim of the face mask must be sealed tightly against the face to effect an airtight seal.

If the cuff is above the carina, it may, when inflated, compress the posterior membranous portion of the trachea and cause tracheal obstruction. Because of the possibility that the tube may enter the trachea, the rescuer should deliver positive-pressure ventilation before inflating the cuff. If the chest rises, indicating that the tube is in the esophagus, the cuff is inflated with 35 mL of air. After inflation of the cuff, breath sounds are listened for bilaterally in the midaxillary line. The epigastrium is also auscultated, and if the tube is improperly placed in the trachea, gurgling sounds will be heard. If there is difficulty in advancing the tube during insertion, it should be withdrawn slightly, the tongue-jaw lift should be improved, and the tube should be readvanced.

If the patient remains unconscious 2 hours after the insertion of the EOA, the trachea should be intubated with a cuffed endotracheal tube and the EOA removed. This will reduce the incidence of necrosis of the esophageal mucosa secondary to ischemia in the area of the cuff. Before removal the patient should be turned onto his or her side and suction provided, as regurgitation frequently follows removal.

Complications[14-16]

A number of studies have demonstrated that ventilation and oxygenation with the EOA may be inferior to that following tracheal intubation. Esophageal injuries, including rupture, have been reported. In the semiconscious victim, the insertion of the EOA could produce laryngospasm, vomiting, and aspiration. There is no protection by the EOA against aspiration into the trachea and bronchi of foreign material present in the mouth and pharynx.

In order to minimize complications the following observations are important:

1. The EOA should be used only by trained individuals.
2. It should not be used in individuals with esophageal disease or who have swallowed caustic material.
3. It is not for use in victims younger than 16 years of age.
4. It should not be used in conscious victims or those who are breathing spontaneously.
5. It should not be left in place for longer than 2 hours.
6. Force should not be used during insertion.
7. Suction should be immediately available during insertion and removal.

Esophageal Gastric Tube Airway[17]

A modification of the EOA is the EGTA (Figure 6). This tube is open throughout its entire length, providing for passage of a gastric tube for decompression of the stomach; because of this added advantage, it may be preferred over the EOA. Ventilation is carried out by way of an additional port in the mask. The technique of

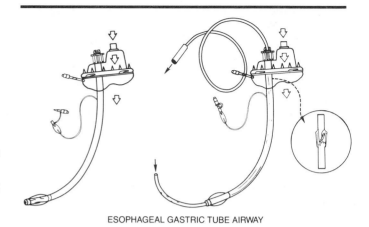

ESOPHAGEAL GASTRIC TUBE AIRWAY

Figure 6. Esophageal gastric tube airway (EGTA). The gastric tube can be passed through the lumen of the airway. Ventilation is carried out by standard mask technique, with the mask held securely against the face.

insertion and complications are the same as those for the EOA.

Several other devices have been reported that are similar to the EOA:

Esophageal Pharyngeal Airway (EPA)[18]
Pharyngeo–Tracheal Lumen Airway (PTLA)[19]
Laryngeal Mask Airway (LMA)[20]
Tracheal–Esophageal Airway (TEA)[21]
Berman Intubating-Pharyngeal Airway (BIPA)[22]

More clinical experience is needed before any of these devices can be recommended for use during CPR.

Tracheal Intubation

This technique consists of the passage of a tube directly into the trachea. The following advantages make tracheal intubation the preferred technique for airway control during CPR:

1. Isolates the airway, preventing aspiration of material into the lower airway.
2. Facilitates ventilation and oxygenation.
3. Facilitates suctioning of the trachea and bronchi.
4. Prevents wasted ventilation and gastric insufflation during positive-pressure ventilation.
5. Provides a route for the administration of some drugs (epinephrine, atropine, and lidocaine) during CPR.

This technique for airway control should be restricted to medical personnel and other healthcare personnel who are highly trained and who use it frequently or are retrained frequently. It is recommended that all medical[23] and paramedical personnel working in critical care areas in the hospital or providing ACLS in prehospital care should have adequate training in this technique and be able to place the tracheal tube properly in a high percent of those patients who require intubation.[24]

Indications

Indications for tracheal intubation include:

— The inability of the rescuer to ventilate the unconscious patient with conventional methods (mouth-to-mouth, mouth-to-mask, bag–valve–mask),
— The inability of the patient to protect her or his own airway (coma, areflexia, or cardiac arrest), and
— The need for prolonged artificial ventilation.

Because of the many advantages of tracheal intubation during cardiac or respiratory arrest, it should be performed as soon as possible by trained personnel. However, adequate ventilation and oxygenation should be provided before and between attempts to intubate. Because there is no ventilation and oxygenation during attempts to intubate, the maximum time allowed to complete the maneuver is 30 seconds.

Equipment

All equipment should be checked before attempting to intubate:

Laryngoscope (Figure 7): This device is used for exposure of the glottis. It has two parts: The handle that contains the batteries for the light source and the blade with a bulb placed in the distal third. The connection point between the blade and the handle is called the fitting, where electrical contact is made. In order to check for adequate light, the indentation of the blade is attached to the bar of the handle. When the blade is elevated to the point of making a right angle to the blade, the light should go on. If it does not, the fault may lie with the bulb or the batteries contained in the handle. There are two types of blades, 1) a curved blade (MacIntosh) and 2) a straight blade (Miller, Wisconsin, Flagg, etc.); it is a matter of personal preference as to which one is used.

Endotracheal Tube: The tube is open in both ends. The proximal end has a standard 15-mm connector that will fit the devices for positive-pressure ventilation. The distal end of the tube has a cuff that is attached by the inflating tube to a one-way inflating valve that is designed to accept a syringe for inflation. There is a pilot balloon between the one-way valve and the inflating tube that indicates whether the cuff is inflated. The cuff must always be tested for integrity prior to insertion. The markings indicate the size of the tube internal diameter (ID) in millimeters. The marking "IT" or Z-79 indicates that the tube has met certain tests or standards. The length of the tube from the distal end is indicated at several levels in centimeters.

Stylet: A malleable stylet, preferably plastic coated, may be inserted through the tube. It will conform to any desired configuration, thus facilitating the insertion of the tube into the larynx and trachea. The end of the stylet must always be recessed at least one-half inch from the distal end of the tube, and the stylet must be lubricated with a water-soluble lubricant prior to insertion into the endotracheal tube.

Additional Equipment:
— 10-mL syringe for cuff inflation
— Magill forceps, for removal of foreign material or to facilitate directing the tip of the tube into the larynx
— Water-soluble lubricant
— Suction unit should be functional and with one pharyngeal rigid suction tip (Yankauer) and tracheal suction catheter.

Technique

After checking all the equipment, the appropriate size tube is selected. Endotracheal tube sizes for females are 7.0–8.0 i.d.; and for males, 8.0–8.5 i.d. However, in an emergency a good standard size tube is 7.5 i.d., for both females and males.

Lubricate the tube with a water-soluble lubricant.

The next step is to obtain the proper head position (Figure 8). Three axes, those of the mouth, the pharynx, and the trachea, must be aligned in order to achieve

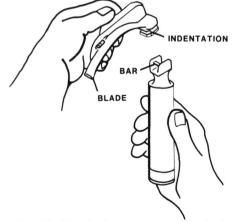

Figure 7. Attaching the laryngoscope blade to the handle. The blade locks into place when it is properly engaged.

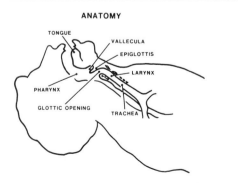

Figure 8. Essential anatomical landmarks in direct laryngoscopy.

direct visualization of the larynx. To accomplish this the head is extended and the neck flexed (i.e., the "sniffing position"). The head must not be allowed to hang over the end of the bed or table. In many cases it is helpful to place several layers of toweling under the patient's occiput in order to elevate it a few inches above the level of the bed. This provides proper flexion of the neck; extension of the head is effected by the individual performing the intubations.

It may be necessary to suction the mouth and pharynx prior to attempting intubation.

The mouth is opened with the fingers of the right hand. The laryngoscope is held in the left hand and the blade inserted in the right side of the mouth displacing the tongue to the left. Then the blade is moved slightly towards the midline and advanced to the base of the tongue. Simultaneously, the lower lip is moved away from the blade using the right index finger. Gentleness and the avoidance of pressure on the lips and teeth are essential. When the curved blade is used (Figure 9), the tip of the blade is advanced into the vallecula (i.e., the space between the base of the tongue and the pharyngeal surface of the epiglottis). The tip of the straight blade (Figure 10) is inserted under the epiglottis. The exposure of the glottic opening (Figure 11) is accomplished by exerting upward traction on the handle. The handle must not be used with a prying motion, and the upper teeth must not be used as a fulcrum.

An assistant, if available, may retract the right corner of the mouth. The tube is advanced through the right corner of the mouth and, under direct vision, through the vocal cords. If a stylet has been employed, it should be removed from the tube at this time. The intubator should view the proximal end of the cuff at the level of the vocal cords and advance the tube about 1–2.5 cm (0.5–1 inch) further into the trachea; this will place the tip of the tube about halfway between the vocal cords and the carina. This position will allow for some displacement of the tip of the tube during flexion or extension of the neck without extubation or movement of the tip into a main stem bronchus. Endotracheal intubation should take no longer than 30 seconds.

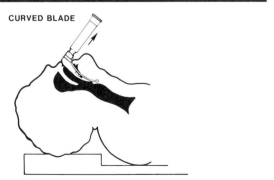

Figure 9. When a curved blade is used, the epiglottis is displaced anteriorly by upward traction, with the tip of the blade in the vallecula.

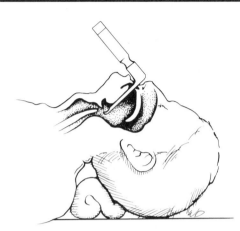

Figure 10. Laryngoscopic technique with a straight blade; the epiglottis is elevated anteriorly to expose the glottic aperture.

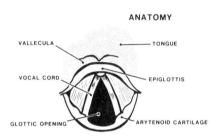

Figure 11. Anatomical structures to be seen during direct laryngoscopy.

Following inflation of the cuff, the patient is ventilated and oxygenated. During ventilation, the lateral aspect of the chest at the midaxillary line is auscultated for breath sounds on both sides. Auscultation is also performed over the epigastric area for gurgling sounds, which indicate esophageal intubation. If this problem is present, the endotracheal tube is removed immediately and the patient is ventilated and oxygenated prior to another attempt at endotracheal intubation.

Complications[25-27]

Trauma during intubation is a frequent complication. Lips or tongue compressed between the blade of the laryngoscope and the teeth may be lacerated. The tip of the tube or stylet may lacerate the pharyngeal or tracheal mucosa, resulting in bleeding, hematoma, or abscess formation. Rupture of the trachea has been reported.[28] Avulsion of an arytenoid cartilage and injury to the vocal cords is also possible. Other complications include pharyngeal–esophageal perforation[29] and intubation of the pyriform sinus.[30] In the semiconscious patient, vomiting and aspiration of gastric contents into the lower airway may occur. In the nonarrest patient the stimulation of endotracheal intubation produces significant release of epinephrine and norepinephrine, which may be manifested by hypertension, tachycardia, and/or arrhythmias.[31]

Insertion of the endotracheal tube into a mainstem bronchus is a frequent complication. Auscultation of the chest should be done to check for the presence of bilateral breath sounds and the chest examined to check for equal expansion of both sides during ventilation. Endobronchial intubation of a bronchus will result in hypoxemia due to one-lung ventilation. Accidental insertion of the endotracheal tube into the esophagus will result in no ventilation or oxygenation.[32]

In order to minimize complications the following observations are important:

1. Ventilation and oxygenation should be performed prior to intubation attempts, which should not be protracted or persisted with if unsuccessful.
2. Tracheal intubation should be performed only by trained personnel.
3. Cricoid pressure may decrease the incidence of gastric distention and pulmonary aspiration during positive-pressure ventilation.[33-35] This should be done if an assistant is available and familiar with the technique. To find the cricoid cartilage, the depression below the thyroid cartilage (Adam's apple) is palpated (Figure 12). This corresponds to the cricothyroid membrane. The prominence inferior to that is the cricoid cartilage. Firm backward pressure is applied with the thumb and index finger to the anterolateral aspects of the cricoid. The pressure is released when the cuff has been inflated and proper tube position verified.
4. Because of the possible need for prolonged intubation in the postresuscitation period, the recommended tube for use during CPR is one with a high-volume/low-pressure cuff. The intracuff pressure is measured and adjusted to 25–35 cmH$_2$O. The minimal intracuff

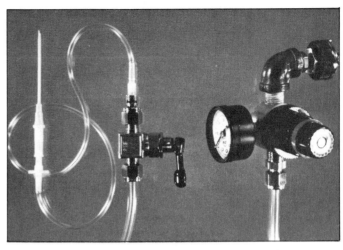

Figure 13. Equipment used in transtracheal catheter ventilation.

pressure to prevent aspiration appears to be 25 cmH$_2$O,[36] and the pressure that produces a decrease in capillary mucosal blood flow (ischemia) is higher than 40 cmH$_2$O.[37]

Transtracheal Catheter Ventilation[38-42]

Transtracheal catheter ventilation is a temporary procedure to provide oxygenation when airway obstruction has not been relieved by other methods until tracheal intubation or tracheostomy is accomplished. The technique consists of the insertion of an over-the-needle catheter through the cricothyroid membrane and intermittent jet ventilation.

Equipment (Figure 13)

— Over-the-needle catheter with a 5- or 10-mL syringe
— A pressure-regulating valve and a pressure gauge attached to a high-pressure (30–60 psi) oxygen supply
— A high-pressure tubing connects the pressure-regulating valve to a hand-operated release valve
— The relief valve connects by tubing to the catheter.

Technique

The small depression below the thyroid cartilage (Adam's apple) corresponds to the cricothyroid membrane (Figure 12). The catheter–needle combination attached to the syringe is directed in the midline downward and caudally at the angle of 45°. Negative pressure is applied to the syringe during insertion.

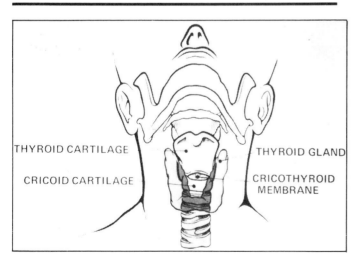

THYROID CARTILAGE

CRICOID CARTILAGE

THYROID GLAND

CRICOTHYRIOD MEMBRANE

Figure 12. Landmarks for locating the cricothyroid membrane.

Entrance of air into the syringe indicates that the needle is in the trachea (Figure 14).

The catheter is advanced over the needle; the needle and syringe are withdrawn; and the distal end of the tubing is attached to the catheter (Figure 15). An assistant holds the hub of the catheter to prevent accidental removal during the period of time required for tracheostomy or endotracheal intubation. The release valve is opened, and oxygen under pressure is introduced into the trachea. The pressure is adjusted to levels that allow adequate lung expansion. The chest must be observed carefully and the release valve turned off as soon as the chest rises. Exhalation then occurs passively.

The chest is observed during exhalation for deflation. If the chest remains inflated, a proximal complete airway obstruction may be present. In this case a second large-bore catheter is inserted next to the first catheter. If the chest continues to remain distended, cricothyrotomy should be done.

Complications[43]

High pressure during ventilation and air entrapment may produce pneumothorax. Hemorrhage may be produced at the site of the needle insertion, especially if the thyroid is perforated; and if the needle is advanced too far, the esophagus may be perforated. This technique does not allow direct suctioning of secretions — some secretions are expelled by the retrograde flow during jet ventilation into the pharynx. Subcutaneous or mediastinal emphysema may occur. A disadvantage of the technique is that while it can provide oxygenation, it does not allow for the efficient elimination of carbon dioxide.

Cricothyrotomy[44-47] (Figure 16)

This is another technique that allows rapid entrance to the airway for temporary ventilation and oxygenation in those patients in whom airway control is not possible by other methods. It consists of an opening in the cricothyroid membrane made with a knife.

Technique

— If possible the area is cleaned with alcohol or other antiseptic solution.
— A horizontal incision is made with a knife at the level of the cricothyroid membrane.
— The handle is inserted through the incision and rotated 90°.
— A pediatric tube, the largest possible, is inserted through this opening.
— Ventilation is done with a bag–valve unit, and the highest available oxygen concentration is provided.

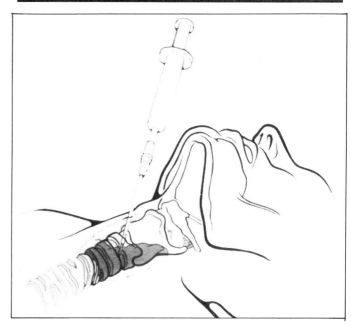

Figure 14. Insertion of a catheter with an attached syringe into the trachea across the cricothyroid membrane.

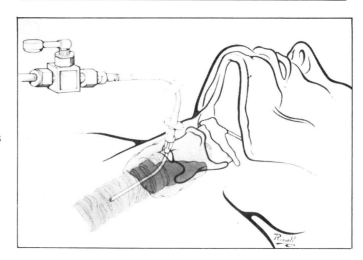

Figure 15. Attachment of a transtracheal ventilation system to an intratracheal catheter.

Complications

Hemorrhage, false passage, perforation of the esophagus, and subcutaneous or mediastinal emphysema are possible complications.

Tracheostomy

The surgical opening of the trachea and the insertion of the tracheostomy tube should ideally be performed under controlled conditions in the operating room by a skilled individual after the airway has first been secured by an endotracheal tube, translaryngeal catheter, or cricothyrotomy.

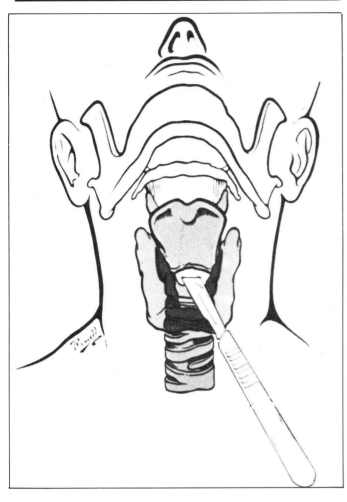

Figure 16. Cricothyrotomy performed with a scalpel.

Patients With Severe Trauma

The trauma victim poses particular problems in regard to airway control. If there is a known or suspected cervical spine injury, excessive movement of the spine, which may produce or exacerbate spinal cord injury, must be avoided. All patients with multiple trauma, head injury, and/or facial trauma should be presumed to have a cervical spine injury until this is definitely ruled out. In other instances a high index of suspicion for spinal injury may be triggered by the type of accident (e.g., motor vehicle accident, fall from a height).

The initial step in airway control in the victim with a suspected neck injury is chin-lift or jaw-thrust, without head-tilt. If the airway remains obstructed, head-tilt is added slowly and carefully until the airway is open. A trained rescuer should maintain the head in traction during airway manipulation to provide a check on any excessive flexion, extension, or lateral movement of the head during airway control. In order to avoid the necessity for manipulation of the head and neck during

intubation, the technique of "blind" nasal intubation may be preferred; however, this technique should be performed only by an experienced person. Nasal intubation is contraindicated in a patient with fractures in the base of the skull. In this instance, oral intubation in the usual manner should be attempted after suctioning the upper airway and ventilating the patient. If endotracheal intubation cannot be performed, a cricothyrotomy or tracheotomy may be necessary.

Administering Supplemental Oxygen

Because oxygen content and oxygen delivery are compromised during cardiac arrest, a system that provides a high inspired oxygen concentration (preferably 100%) should be selected for use during artificial ventilation. If a patient is breathing spontaneously, the administration of oxygen should be titrated according to the PaO_2, or oxygen saturation value.

The person taking care of a patient who is in need of supplemental oxygen should have a clear understanding of the oxygen delivery system, which consists of

— Oxygen supply (cylinder or piped wall oxygen),
— Valve handles to open the cylinder, pressure gauge, and flow meter,
— Connecting tubing from oxygen supply to the patient's oxygen administration unit, and
— Humidifier.

There are four commonly used devices for administering supplemental oxygen.[48]

Nasal Cannula

This is a low-flow system that does not provide sufficient gas to supply the entire inspired volume; therefore, part of the tidal volume must be supplied by room air. The inspired oxygen concentration depends on the flow of oxygen in the unit and the tidal volume of the patient. For every increase from 1 L/min flow, the inspired oxygen concentration will be increased by approximately 4%. The oxygen concentration supplied to a patient with a normal tidal volume by the nasal cannula with a flow of 1–6 L per minute is 24–44%.

Face Mask

This unit is well tolerated by the adult patient. In order to avoid accumulation of exhaled air in the mask reservoir that might be rebreathed, the oxygen flow should be higher than 5 L/min; the recommended flow is 8–10 L/min. Like the nasal cannula, there is dilution of the inspired oxygen by room air. This system provides concentrations of oxygen of 40–60%.

Face Mask With Oxygen Reservoir

This system, in which there is a constant flow of oxygen into the reservoir, will provide oxygen concentrations higher than 60%. A flow of 6 L/min will provide approximately 60% oxygen concentration, and each increase in flow of 1 L/min increases the inspired oxygen concentration by 10%. At 10 L/min the oxygen concentration is almost 100%.

Venturi Mask

The venturi mask provides a high gas flow with a fixed oxygen concentration. Oxygen under pressure is passed through a narrow orifice and, after leaving the orifice, provides a subatmospheric pressure that entrains room air into the system. By changing the orifice size and oxygen flow, the oxygen concentration is changed. This type of oxygen delivery is frequently used in patients with chronic hypercarbia (COPD) for the treatment of moderate-to-severe hypoxemia. The administration of high oxygen concentrations may produce respiratory depression in this type of patient by a sudden increase in PaO_2 which blocks the stimulant effect of hypoxemia on the respiratory centers. Oxygen concentrations available are 24%, 28%, 35%, and 40%. The oxygen flow rates to be used for these concentrations are 4, 4, 8, and 8 L/min, respectively. The mask with 24% oxygen concentration is used initially. The patient is observed for respiratory depression, and PaO_2 is evaluated. The oxygen concentration is then titrated to the desired level of PaO_2.

Oxygenation and Ventilation

Mouth-to-Mouth[49] and Mouth-to-Nose[50]

The basic technique of expired air ventilation provides adequate volumes of air to the victim. The only limitation is the vital capacity of the rescuer. However, the oxygen concentration is low since the concentration of oxygen in exhaled air is approximately 17%.

Mouth-to-Mask[51-53] (Figure 17)

This technique has many advantages: 1) it eliminates direct contact with the victim's mouth and nose; 2) administration of supplemental oxygen is possible; 3) it eliminates exposure to exhaled gas, if the unit has a one-way valve; 4) it is easy to teach and learn; 5) it provides effective ventilation and oxygenation; and 6) it is aesthetically more acceptable than mouth-to-mouth. With an oxygen flow rate of 10 L/min, combined with mouth-to-mask ventilation, an inspired oxygen concentration of about 50% can be achieved. The oxygen mixture delivered to a spontaneously breathing patient may also be enriched with this device. An oxygen flow rate of 15 L/min will provide an inspired oxygen concentration of approximately 80%.

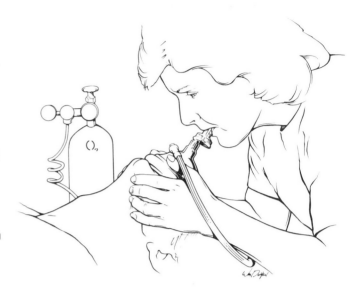

Figure 17.   Mouth-to-mask ventilation with a one-way valve.

The one-way valve should be connected to the mask and oxygen tubing connected to the inlet with an O_2 flow rate of 10 L/min. An oropharyngeal airway is inserted if needed. Head-tilt is applied, and the mask is placed on the face of the victim. With the thumb side (thenar) of the palm of both hands, pressure is applied to the sides of the mask; upward pressure is applied to the mandible just in front of the ear lobes using the index, middle, and ring fingers of both hands while maintaining head-tilt. If no oropharyngeal airway is in place, the rescuer should keep the mouth open. The operator should then blow in through the opening of the mask, observing the rise and fall of the chest.

If a trained assistant is available, cricoid pressure should be applied to avoid gastric inflation ventilation into the stomach during positive-pressure ventilation and to reduce the possibility of regurgitation and aspiration.

Bag–Valve Devices[54-56]

Bag–valve devices consist of a self-inflating bag and a non-rebreathing valve. They may be used with a mask, an endotracheal tube, or an esophageal obturator airway. It is recommended that these devices fulfill the following criteria:

1. A self-inflating bag that is easily cleaned and sterilized.
2. A non-jam valve system at 15 L/min of oxygen inlet flow.

3. No pressure-release valve ("pop-off valve"). If one is present, the valve should be manually bypassed to permit the higher pressure needed to ventilate a patient with high airway resistance and low lung compliance.
4. Standard 15 mm/22 mm fittings.
5. A system for delivery of high concentrations of oxygen through an ancillary oxygen inlet at the back of the bag or an oxygen reservoir.
6. A true non-rebreathing valve.
7. Satisfactory performance under extremes of environmental temperatures.
8. Suitability for manikin practice.
9. Should be available in adult and pediatric sizes.

Technique

The rescuer is positioned at the top of the victim's head. The victim's head is tilted back and, if victim is unconscious, an oropharyngeal airway is inserted. The victim's mouth should remain open under the mask.

The mask is applied to the face with the rescuer's left hand. The last two or three fingers are placed on the mandible while the remaining fingers are placed on the mask. The rescuer must maintain the head-tilt, keeping the anterior displacement of the mandible, while finding the optimum mask fit.

The bag is then compressed with the right hand and the chest observed to make certain that ventilation of the lungs is occurring.

Cricoid pressure should be applied while the airway is unprotected, if a trained assistant is available.

Complications

The most frequent problem with this type of device is the inability to provide adequate ventilatory volumes to a patient who is not intubated. This results from the difficulty of providing a leakproof seal to the face while maintaining an open airway. For this reason the BVM unit should be used only by well-trained and experienced personnel. Better BVM ventilation may be achieved with two persons, one holding the mask to the face and maintaining an open airway, the other compressing the bag with 2 hands; but this is an awkward procedure.[57]

Manually Triggered Oxygen-Powered Breathing Devices[58]

These devices allow for positive-pressure ventilation with 100% oxygen. They can be attached to a face mask, endotracheal tube, EOA, or tracheostomy tube. The system consists of a high-pressure tubing connecting the oxygen supply (under pressure, 50 psi) and a valve that is activated by a lever or push button. When the valve is in the open position, oxygen flows into the patient. The following characteristics are recommended in these devices:

1. Standard 15 mm/22 mm coupling
2. Rugged, breakage-resistant design that is compact and easy to hold
3. A constant flow rate of 100% oxygen at 40 L/min
4. An inspiratory release valve that opens at approximately 60 cmH_2O and vents any remaining volume to the atmosphere
5. An audible alarm that sounds whenever the release valve pressure is exceeded, indicating that the victim needs high inspiratory pressures and may not be receiving adequate ventilatory volumes[1]
6. A trigger positioned so that both hands of the rescuer can remain on the mask to hold it in position while maintaining a patent airway

Technique

The unit is checked and an appropriate mask attached. The mask is applied to the face of the victim, using both hands to maintain a tight fit between the face and the mask and to keep the lower jaw elevated. The valve is opened by activating the level or pushing the button.

The chest is observed for proper expansion. The valve is deactivated as soon as the chest rises. The flow of oxygen then ceases, and the exhaled gases are vented via a one-way valve into the atmosphere.

This type of device can also be used in the patient breathing spontaneously. The valve is opened by the negative pressure generated by the inspiratory effort of the patient; flow ceases when the negative pressure ends.

Complications

In patients who are not intubated, opening the esophagus with gastric distention is a frequent complication. Barotrauma to the lungs manifested by pneumothorax or subcutaneous emphysema is also possible with the use of these devices. OXYGEN-POWERED BREATHING DEVICES ARE NOT FOR USE IN PEDIATRIC PATIENTS.

Suction Devices

The rigid pharyngeal catheter (Yankauer) is used to clear secretions, blood clots, and other foreign material from the mouth and pharynx. High suction pressure is needed for pharyngeal suction (higher than − 120 mmHg). The tracheobronchial suction catheter is used to clear secretion through the endotracheal tube or the nasopharynx. The tracheobronchial suction catheter should have a design that will 1) produce minimal trauma to the mucosa with molded ends and side holes, 2) be long enough to pass through the tip of the endotracheal tube, 3) have minimal frictional resistance during insertion through the endotracheal tube, and 4) be sterile and disposable.

Technique of Tracheobronchial Suctioning[48]

The equipment is checked, and the suction pressure is set between -80 and -120 mmHg. The patient is pre-oxygenated with 100% O_2 for 5 minutes.

Using sterile technique, the catheter is inserted without closing the side opening in the proximal end of the catheter. The catheter is advanced to the desired location, which is approximately at the level of the carina. Suction is applied intermittently by closing the side opening while the catheter is withdrawn with a rotating motion.

Suction should not be applied for more than 15 seconds. If arrhythmias are present, suctioning is immediately discontinued and the patient is manually ventilated and oxygenated.

Prior to repeating the procedure, the patient should be ventilated with 100% oxygen for about 30 seconds.

Complications[59,60]

The most serious complication of suctioning is the sudden onset of severe hypoxemia secondary to a decrease in lung volume (functional residual capacity) during the application of negative pressure in the trachea. If severe enough this may lead to cardiac arrest. Suctioning produces stimulation to the airway similar to that produced during endotracheal intubation, and may increase arterial pressure and tachycardia. Significant cardiac arrhythmias may occur during suctioning, and this may be due to the decrease in myocardial oxygen supply secondary to hypoxemia, or to an increase in oxygen demand due to the hypertension and increase in heart rate. Some patients may manifest bradycardia and hypotension due to vagal stimulation. The stimulation of the catheter in the mucosa may trigger coughing, resulting in increased intercranial pressure and reduced cerebral blood flow. The incidence of mucosal damage is high and includes edema, hemorrhage, and areas of ulceration and loss of integrity, which may result in tracheal infection.

References

1. Melker RJ: Asynchronous and other alternative methods of ventilation during CPR. *Ann Emerg Med.* 13:758-761, 1984.
2. Safar P, Escarraga L, Chang F: Upper airway obstruction in the unconscious patient. *J Appl Physiol* 14:760-764, 1959.
3. Morikawa S, Safar P, DeCarlo J: Influence of head position upon upper airway patency. *Anesthesiology* 22:265, 1961.
4. Ruben HM, Elam JO, Ruben AM, et al: Investigation of upper airway problems in resuscitation. *Anesthesiology* 22:271-279, 1961.
5. Guildner CW: Resuscitation — Opening the airway: A comparative study of techniques for opening an airway obstructed by the tongue. *JACEP* 5:588-590, 1976.
6. Boidin MP: Airway patency in the unconscious patient. *Br J Anaesth* 57:306-310, 1985.
7. Berman RA, Lilienfield SM: Correspondence. *Anesthesiology* 11:136-137, 1950.
8. Spoerel WE: The unprotected airway, in Spoerel WE (ed): *Problems of the Upper Airway* (Int Anesthesiol Clin., Vol 10, No 3). Boston, Little, Brown and Company, 1972, pp 1-36.
9. Don Michael TA: Lamber EH, Mehran A: "Mouth-to-lung airway" for cardiac resuscitation. *Lancet* 2:1339, 1968.
10. Don Michael TA: The esophageal obturator airway. A critique. *JAMA* 246:1098-1101, 1981.
11. Smith JP, Bodai BI, Seifkin A, et al. The esophageal obturator airway. A review *JAMA* 250:1081-1084, 1983.
12. Donen N, Tweed WA, Dashfsky S, et al: The esophageal obturator airway: an appraisal. *Can Anaesth Soc J* 30:194-200, 1983.
13. Bryson TK, Benumof JL, Ward CF: The esophageal obturator airway: A clinical comparison to ventilation with a mask and oropharyngeal airway. *Chest* 74:537-539, 1978.
14. Pilcher DB, DeMeules JE: Esophageal perforation following use of esophageal airway. *Chest* 69:377-380, 1976.
15. Yancey W, Wears R, Kamajian G, et al: Unrecognized tracheal intubation: A complication of the esophageal obturator airway. *Ann Emerg Med.* 9:31-33, 1980.
16. Auerbach PS, Geehr EC: Inadequate oxygenation and ventilation using the esophageal gastric tube airway in the pre-hospital setting. *JAMA* 250:3067-3071, 1983.
17. Gordon AS: Improved esophageal obturator airway (EOA) and new esophageal gastric tube airway (EGTA), in Safar P, Elam JO (eds): *Advances in cardiopulmonary resuscitation.* The Wolf Creek Conference on CPR. New York, Springer-Verlag, 1977, pp 58-64.
18. Elam JO, Lim-Tan P, Shafieha M, et al: Airway management with the esophageal pharyngeal airway, in Safar P, Elam JO (eds): *Advances in cardiopulmonary resuscitation.* The Wolf Creek conferences on CPR. New York, Springer-Verlag, 1977, pp. 65-72.
19. Niemann JT, Rosborough JP, Myers R, et al: The pharyngeo-tracheal lumen airway: Preliminary investigation of a new adjunct. *Ann Emerg Med* 13:591-596, 1984.
20. Brain AI, McGhee TD, McAteer EJ, et al: The laryngeal mask airway. Development and preliminary trials of a new type of airway. *Anaesthesia* 40:356-361, 1985.
21. Eisenberg RS: A new airway for tracheal or esophageal insertion: Description and field experience. *Ann Emerg Med.* 9:270-272, 1980.
22. Berman RA: A method for blind oral intubation of the trachea or esophagus. *Anesth Analg* 56:866-867, 1977.
23. Natanson C, Shelhamer JH, Parrillo JE: Intubation of the trachea in the critical care setting. *JAMA* 253:1160-1165, 1985.
24. Sladen A: Emergency endotracheal intubation: Who can — who should?, editorial. *Chest* 75:535-536, 1979.
25. Blanc VF, Tremblay NAG: The complications of tracheal intubation. *Anesth Analg* 52:202-213, 1974.
26. Jones GOM, Hale DE, Wasmuth CE, et al: A survey of acute complications associated with endotracheal intubation. *Cleveland Clin Quart* 35:23-31, 1968.
27. Taryl DA, Chandler JE, Good JT Jr, et al: Emergency room intubations — complications and survival. *Chest* 75:541-543, 1979.
28. Thompson DS, Read RC: Rupture of the trachea following endotracheal intubation. *JAMA* 204:995-997, 1968.
29. Wolff AP, Kuhn FA, Oqura JH: Pharyngeal-esophageal perforations associated with rapid oral endotracheal intubation. *Ann Otol Rhinol Laryngol* 82:258-261, 1972.
30. Stauffer JL, Petty TL: Accidental intubation of the pyriform sinus: A complication of "roadside" resuscitation. *JAMA* 237:2324-2325, 1977.
31. Derbyshire DR, Chmielewski A, Fell D, et al: Plasma catecholamine responses to tracheal intubation. *Br J Anaesth* 55:855-859, 1983.
32. Pollard BJ, Junius F: Accidental intubation of the oesophagus. *Anaesth Intense Care* 8:183-186, 1980.
33. Keith A: Mechanism underlying various methods of artificial respiration. *Lancet* March 13,1909, p 747.
34. Sellick BA: Cricoid pressure to control regurgitation of stomach contents during induction of anaesthesia. *Lancet* 2:404-408, 1961.
35. Salem MR, Wong AY, Mani M, et al: Efficacy of cricoid pressure in preventing gastric insufflation during bag-mask ventilation in pediatric patients. *Anesthesiology* 40:96-98, 1974.
36. Bernhard WN, Cottrell JE, Sivakumaran C, et al: Adjustment of intracuff pressure to prevent aspiration. *Anesthesiology* 50:363-366, 1979.

37. Nordin U: The trachea and cuff-induced trachea injury. An experimental study on causative factors and prevention. *Acta Otolaryngl* 345 (suppl):1-71, 1977.

38. Jacoby JJ, Hamelberg W, Ziegler CH, et al: Transtracheal resuscitation. *JAMA* 162:625-628, 1956.

39. Sanders RD: Two ventilating attachments for bronchoscopes. *Del Med J* 39:170-175, 1967.

40. Spoerel WE, Narayanan PS, Singh NP: Transtracheal ventilation. *Brit J Anaesth* 43:932-939, 1971.

41. Jacobs HB. Emergency percutaneous transtracheal catheter and ventilator. *J Trauma* 12:50-55, 1972.

42. Smith RB, Babinksi M, Klain M, et al: Percutaneous transtracheal ventilation. *JACEP;* 5:765-770, 1976.

43. Poon YK: A life-threatening complication of cricothyroid membrane puncture. *Anesth Analg* 55:298-301, 1976.

44. Brantigan CO, Grow JB: Cricothyroidotomy: Elective use in respiratory problems requiring tracheotomy. *J Thorac Cardiovasc Surg* 71:72-81, 1976.

45. McGill J, Clinton JE, Ruiz E: Cricothyrotomy in the emergency department. *Ann Emerg Med* 11:361-364, 1982.

46. Simon RR, Brenner BE: Emergency cricothyroidotomy in the patient with massive neck swelling: Part 1; Anatomical aspects. *Crit Care Med* 111:114-118, 1983.

47. Simon RR, Brenner BE, Rosen MA: Emergency cricothyroidotomy in the patient with massive neck swelling: Part 2: Clinical Aspects. *Crit Care Med* 11:119-123, 1983.

48. Shapiro BA, Harrison RA, Trout CA: *Clinical Application of Respiratory Care.* Chicago, Year Book Medical Publishers, Inc., 1975, pp 130-137.

49. Elam JO, Greene DG: Mission accomplished. Successful mouth-to-mouth resuscitation. *Anesth Analg* 40:440-442, 578-580, 672-676, 1961.

50. Ruben H: The immediate treatment of respiratory failure. *Brit J Anaesth* 36:542-549, 1964.

51. Safar P: Pocket mask for emergency ventilation and oxygen inhalation. *Crit Care Med* 2:273-276, 1974.

52. Harrison RR, Maull KI, Keenan RL, et al: Mouth-to-mask ventilation: A superior method of rescue breathing. *Ann Emerg Med* 11:74-76, 1982.

53. Lawrences PJ, Sivaneswaran N: Ventilation during cardiopulmonary resuscitation: Which method? *Med J Austral* 143:443-446, 1985.

54. Ruben H: A new non-rebreathing valve. *Anesthesiology* 16:643, 1955.

55. Carden E, Hughes T: An evaluation of manually operated self inflating bags. *Anesth Analg* 54:133-138, 1975.

56. Elam JO: Bag-valve-mask O_2 ventilation, in Safar P, Elam JO (eds): *Advances in Cardiopulmonary Resuscitation.* The Wolf Creek Conference on CPR. New York, Springer-Verlag, 1977, pp 73-79.

57. Jesudian MCS, Harrison RR, Keenan RL, et al: Bag-valve-mask ventilation: Two rescuers are better than one. Preliminary report. *Crit Care Med* 13:122-123, 1985.

58. Pearson JW, Redding JS: Evaluation of the elder demand valve resuscitator for use by first-aid personnel. *Anesthesiology* 28:623-624, 1967.

59. Marx GF, Steen SN, Arkins RE, et al: Endotracheal suction and death. *New York J Med* 68:565-566, 1968.

60. Shim C, Fine N, Fernandez R, et al: Cardiac arrhythmias resulting from tracheal suctioning. *Ann Intern Med* 71:1149-1153, 1969.

Adjuncts for Artificial Circulation

Chapter 4

Mechanical devices are available that can be used as substitutes for manual external chest compression. Some also can provide a source of ventilation that is synchronized with chest compressions. The advantages of such devices are that they can 1) standardize the technique of CPR, 2) eliminate rescuer fatigue, 3) free trained persons to participate in the delivery of ACLS when there is a limited number of rescuers, and 4) assure adequacy of compression when a patient requires continued resuscitation during transportation. Mechanical CPR that is carefully and properly administered can be as effective as carefully administered manual CPR in adults.[1-3] In certain circumstances (such as during transportation or when CPR must be provided for prolonged periods), it may even be advantageous. Mechanically performed CPR should be used only for adults; its efficacy and safety have not been demonstrated in infants and children.

Manual Chest Compressors and CPR Devices

Cardiac Press

The simplest and least expensive adjunct is the cardiac press. This hinged, manually operated device gives the rescuer a mechanical advantage in performing chest compressions. The downstroke of the cardiac press can be adjusted to provide a stroke of 1½–2 inches (3.9–5.0 cm). It can be applied with only a brief interruption in manual CPR. Advantages include its relatively modest cost, its ease of storage, transportation, and assembly, its lightweight construction, and its simplicity, which reduces the possibilities of mechanical breakdown. Problems related to its use include the tendency for the compressor head to shift position and for the tightening device to become loosened so that the plunger does not compress the chest adequately. Therefore, constant monitoring of the position of the press and the adequacy of compression is necessary.

Automatic Resuscitators

A mechanical resuscitator can provide chest compressions and/or ventilations during CPR. Devices currently available consist of a compressed-gas powered plunger mounted on a backboard and a time-pressure cycled ventilator. The devices are programmed to deliver standard AHA-recommended CPR in a 5:1 compression-to-ventilation ratio using a compression duration that is 50% of the cycle length.

This type of device does not require electrical power since it is usually powered by 100% oxygen gas. The depth of plunger compression can be adjusted by the rescuer to compress the sternum 1½–2 inches with each cycle or 20–25% of the patient's anterior-posterior diameter (for patients with a large anterior-posterior diameter). When used properly, this device causes less injury to the chest wall and internal organs during patient transport (as in the back of a moving ambulance) than manually performed CPR because the patient can be "harnessed" to the device's backboard, fixing the position of the plunger on the sternum. An acceptable ECG can often be recorded with the compressor in operation, and the patient can be defibrillated or transported without interrupting CPR. Defibrillation is timed to occur during the downstroke of a chest compression when the lungs are relatively empty, which will result in more energy being delivered to the heart and, perhaps, more successful defibrillations since chest impedance is lower when the lungs are deflated.[4]

The principle disadvantage of the automatic resuscitator is its cost. Its disadvantage in size and weight is balanced by its ability to permit rescuers to perform other tasks and by providing better access to the patient for procedures by reducing the number of rescuers at the patient's side.

Pneumatic Antishock Garment

The pneumatic antishock garment (PASG) raises mean arterial pressure by selectively increasing peripheral vascular resistance in the lower half of the body. Other names for this device include medical antishock trousers, military antishock trousers, antishock garments, G suits, antishock air pants, external counterpressure devices, pneumatic trousers, circumferential pneumatic compression devices, and MAST suits.

The PASG consists of a one-piece double-layered fabric with inflatable bladder(s) capable of maintaining high internal pressure. Most suits have three separate compartments that can be inflated individually to compress each lower extremity and the abdomen. The PASG is usually inflated with a foot pump; pressure gauges or pop-off valves are used to regulate the internal pressure.[5]

Physiological Effects

Mean arterial pressure generally increases when the PASG is inflated. Initially, this effect on the blood pressure was thought to be due to autotransfusion of blood from the lower half of the body into the central circulation (producing a reversible increase in preload).[6] More recent studies have shown that the preload effect from the PASG is minimal. The dominant hemodynamic effect of PASG inflation is an increase in arterial impedance.[7-10] When circumferential pneumatic counterpressure is applied to the lower half of the body, blood vessels under the suit constrict.[11] This decreases blood flow to the lower half of the body and increases peripheral vascular resistance. A second important feature of pneumatic counterpressure is that the circumferential tension improves hemostasis and decreases blood flow to torn vessels under the garment.[12-14] The PASG also may be useful as an air splint or a compression bandage for traumatic injuries to the lower half of the body.

Clinical Effects

The most common clinical indication for PASG application is hypovolemic shock due to traumatic injury to the lower half of the body. Patients who have pelvic and/or lower extremity long bone fractures may benefit from the splinting, hemostatic, and pressor effects. The antishock garment is useful only as a temporary measure. Because it compromises blood flow and tissue perfusion to the lower half of the body, more definitive treatment (fluids, blood tranfusions, fracture reduction, surgical repair, etc.) must be instituted as soon as possible.

Although use of the PASG increases mean arterial pressure, it is not indicated for use during cardiac resuscitation because it raises central venous pressure as well and, therefore, does not increase coronary blood flow. Survival is not improved either.[15] Liver laceration has been noted in animals when CPR was performed with the abdominal binding inflated.[16] Thus, there is concern that if CPR is done in patients with the abdominal portion of the antishock garment inflated, it also may lead to abdominal injury.

The PASG has been advocated as an adjunct in the treatment of hypotensive patients with paroxysmal supraventricular tachycardia.[17] In general, these patients should be cardioverted instead.

Complications

Potential complications associated with the use of PASG include

1. lower extremity compartment syndromes,
2. metabolic acidosis after prolonged use due to decreased lower extremity tissue perfusion,
3. decreased renal function, and
4. decreased diaphragmatic excursion and reduced vital capacity when the abdominal section is inflated.

Inflation of the abdominal section is discouraged in pregnant women because of the potential decrease in blood flow to the fetus. Its use also should be discouraged in patients with a foreign body impaled in the abdomen, evisceration of abdominal contents, tension pneumothorax, cardiac tamponade, pulmonary edema, and cardiogenic shock.[5]

Whenever the device is removed from a patient, it should be deflated gradually over a period of several minutes during which vital signs should be monitored closely. Sudden deflation in a patient who still has a marginal blood volume can cause sudden reappearance of shock.

Direct Cardiac Massage

Before the introduction in 1960 of closed chest massage, i.e., external compressions, direct cardiac massage was used frequently to treat patients with in-hospital cardiac arrest. Studies from the 1950's show survival rates ranging from 16 to 37%.[18,19] A large percent of these arrests, however, occurred in the operating room. Following the introduction of closed-chest CPR, no studies were done comparing survival with both techniques. Closed-chest CPR seemed to be effective, was considerably less invasive, and quickly became the standard method for resuscitation.

It is now clear that properly performed direct cardiac massage provides better hemodynamics than closed-chest compression.[20-26] Cardiac index and coronary perfusion pressure often are improved by switching from closed- to open-chest CPR.[25,26] There are several case reports of patients who have been resuscitated after direct cardiac massage when attempts during closed-chest CPR have been unsuccessful.[26-28] Studies in animal models also support the notion that survival is improved when open-chest CPR is used soon after the onset of cardiac arrest (15 minutes or less).[22-24] When open-chest CPR is initiated after cardiac arrest has been managed with closed-chest CPR for 20–25 minutes or more, there is no improvement in outcome despite a significant improvement in hemodynamics.[23] In one of the few outcome studies on humans, open-chest CPR did not improve survival for patients with out-of-hospital arrest when applied after 30 minutes of arrest time.[29]

Few physicians today are skilled in the technique of direct cardiac massage. Since most cardiac arrests occur outside of the hospital and since most patients cannot be brought to a facility where a thoracotomy and direct cardiac massage can be performed in less than 15 minutes of total arrest time, the applicability of direct cardiac massage is limited. The risks and benefits of open-chest cardiac massage used early (within the first 15 minutes of cardiac arrest) in humans have not yet been adequately studied. Thoracotomy and direct cardiac massage cannot be recommended for the routine patients with cardiac arrest.

An exception is the victim with cardiac trauma due to penetrating chest trauma. Most studies indicate clear benefit from thoracotomy for victims of penetrating chest trauma who develop cardiac arrest.[30-33] A thoracotomy potentially allows for 1) relief of pericardial tamponade and 2) identification and control of severe intrathoracic hemorrhage (or adjunctive treatment of concomitant abdominal hemorrhage by aortic cross-clamping).

Emergency thoracotomy is practical as a resuscitation technique in well equipped trauma treatment centers. A multi-disciplinary team should be present that can provide definitive surgical treatment in the operating room as soon as possible. If direct cardiac massage is used at all, it should be applied early. Opening the chest as a "last ditch effort" to resuscitate a patient in cardiac arrest is of little or no value.

Though penetrating chest trauma is the only clear indication for a thoracotomy and open-chest CPR, there are other specific instances in which open-chest CPR may be considered:

1. Cardiac arrest due to hypothermia, pulmonary embolism, pericardial tamponade, or abdominal hemorrhage.
2. Chest deformity where closed-chest CPR is not effective.
3. Penetrating abdominal trauma with deterioration and cardiac arrest.
4. Blunt trauma with cardiac arrest.

Emergency Cardiopulmonary Bypass

Cardiopulmonary bypass (CPB) is an important adjunct for patients undergoing cardiac surgery. CPB has been applied experimentally in the treatment of selected patients with cardiac arrest[34,35] without thoracotomy, using the femoral artery and vein for access to the circulation. Animal models of cardiac arrest show improved hemodynamics and survival when CPB is used soon after the onset of cardiac arrest.[34,35] Further study in humans will be necessary before CPB can be recommended for general use in treating patients with cardiac arrest. It is useful as a method for rapidly rewarming patients with severe hypothermia who develop cardiac arrest.

Mechanical Assistance to the Failing Circulation

Intraaortic Balloon Counterpulsation

Patients in cardiogenic shock who are unresponsive to pharmacologic treatment may require mechanical assistance using CPB or intraaortic balloon counterpulsation. The latter technique involves placing a catheter encircled by a balloon percutaneously or via a femoral artery cutdown into the descending aorta under fluoroscopic guidance.[36] The balloon can be rapidly inflated and deflated by an external pump synchronized with the cardiac rhythm (either the ECG signal or the arterial waveform).

Counterpulsation consists of two hemodynamic phases, systolic unloading and diastolic augmentation. Rapid deflation of the balloon at the onset of systole causes a fall in intraaortic pressure and afterload (systolic unloading). Rapid inflation of the balloon early in diastole propels blood distal and proximal to the balloon, increasing forward cardiac output and augmenting coronary and cerebral perfusion (diastolic augmentation). The net effects are a decrease in systolic pressure, an increase in diastolic pressure at the aortic root, improved coronary and cerebral blood flow, and decreased myocardial oxygen consumption and work.[37-40]

External counterpulsation devices produce external pressure on the patient's leg and abdomen by filling a suit with water during the diastolic cycle. They are less effective than the intraaortic balloon device in improving coronary blood flow or oxygen consumption.[41,42]

Indications for Use

The major indication for intraaortic balloon counterpulsation is cardiogenic shock. The prognosis for patients in cardiogenic shock is very poor. Counterpulsation will not improve the long-term prognosis for patients whose shock is based on the excessive loss of myocardium (myocardiogenic shock). However, it can improve hemodynamics sufficiently to permit assessment of possible mechanical interventions (e.g., coronary artery angioplasty and/or coronary artery bypass surgery, ventricular septal defect repair, mitral valve replacement) which can in some circumstances improve outcome.[37,43-48] Other indications for intraaortic counterpulsation include 1) treatment of patients with unstable angina who are unresponsive to pharmacological intervention until mechanical interventions can be instituted[37-49] and 2) postsurgical patients who are difficult to wean from cardiopulmonary bypass.[37-49]

Complications from intraaortic counterpulsation occur frequently,[36,50,51] especially in patients with preexisting atherosclerotic vascular disease involving the aorta, the iliofemoral system, and the lower extremities. Among the more frequent complications are intravascular thrombosis and/or emboli and lower extremity vascular insufficiency. Anticoagulation with heparin is generally maintained throughout the duration of counterpulsation. Other complications include aortic dissection, false aneurysm at the catheterization site, balloon rupture, intimal perforation, and sepsis.

References

1. Taylor GJ, Rubin R, Tucker M, Greene HL, Rudikoff MT, Weisfeldt ML: External cardiac compression — A randomized comparison of mechanical and manual techniques. *JAMA* 240:644-646, 1978.

2. McDonald JL: Systolic and mean arterial pressures during manual and mechanical CPR in humans. *Ann Emer Med* 11:292-295, 1982.

3. Barkalow CB: Mechanized cardiopulmonary resuscitation: Past, present and future. *Am J Emerg Med* 2:262-269, 1984.

4. Ewy GA, Hellman DA, McClung S, et al: Influence of ventilation phase on transthoracic impedance and defibrillation effectiveness. *Crit Care Med* 8:164-166, 1980.

5. Kaback KR, Sanders AB, Meislin HW: MAST suit update. *JAMA* 252:2598-2603, 1984.

6. McSwain NE: Pneumatic trousers and the management of shock. *J Trauma* 77:719-724, 1977.

7. Gaffney FA, Thal ER, Taylor WF, et al: Hemodynamic effects of medical antishock trousers (MAST garment). *J Trauma* 21:931-935, 1981.

8. Goldsmith SR: Comparative hemodynamic effects of antishock suits and volume expansion in normal human beings. *Ann Emerg Med* 12:348-350, 1983.

9. Bivins HG, Knopp R, Tiernan C, et al: Blood volume displacement with inflation of anti-shock trousers. *Ann Emerg Med* 11:409-411, 1982.

10. Niemann JT, Stapczynski JS, Rosborough JP, et al: Hemodynamic effects of pneumatic external counterpressure in canine hemorrhagic shock. *Ann Emerg Med* 12:661-667, 1983.

11. Wangensteen SL, Ludewig RM, Eddy DM: The effect of external counterpressure on the intact circulation. *Surg Gynecol Obstet* 127:252-258, 1968.

12. Wangensteen SL, Ludewig RM, Cox JM, et al: The effect of external counterpressure on arterial bleeding. *Surgery* 64:922- 927, 1968.

13. Ludewig RM, Wangensteen SL: Effect of external counterpressure on venous bleeding. *Surgery* 66:515-520, 1969.

14. Ludewig RM, Wangensteen SL: Aortic bleeding and the effect of external counterpressure. *Surg Gynecol Obstet* 128:252-258, 1969.

15. Mahoney BD, Mirick MJ: Efficacy of pneumatic trousers in refractory prehospital cardiopulmonary arrest. *Ann Emerg Med* 12:8-12, 1983.

16. Harris LC Jr, Kirimli B, Safar P: Augmentation of artificial circulation during cardiopulmonary resuscitation. *Anesthesiology* 28:730-734, 1967.

17. Tandberg D, Rusnak R, Sklar D, et al: Successful treatment of paroxysmal supraventricular tachycardia with MAST. *Ann Emerg Med*.13:1068-1070, 1984.

18. Stephenson HE Jr, Reid C, Hinton JW: Some common denominators in 1200 cases of cardiac arrest. *Ann Surg* 137:731-744, 1953.

19. Turk LN, Glenn WW: Cardiac arrest — results of attempted resuscitation in 42 cases. *N Engl J Med* 251:795-803, 1954.

20. Weiser FM, Adler LN, Kuhn LA: Hemodynamic effects of closed and open chest cardiac resuscitation in normal dogs and those with acute myocardial infarction. *Am J Cardiol* 10:555-61, 1962.

21. Bircher N, Safar P: Comparison of standard and "new" closed-chest CPR and open-chest CPR in dogs. *Crit Care Med* 9:384-385, 1981.

22. Sanders AB, Kern KB, Ewy GA, et al: Improved resuscitation from cardiac arrest with open-chest massage. *Ann Emerg Med* 13:672-5, 1984.

23. Sanders AB, Kern KB, Atlas M, et al: Importance of the duration of inadequate coronary perfusion pressure in resuscitation from cardiac arrest. *J Am Coll Cardiol* 6:113-118, 1985.

24. Bircher NG, Safar P: Cerebral preservation during cardiopulmonary resuscitation. *Crit Care Med* 13:185-190, 1985.

25. Howard MA, Labadie LL, Martin GB, et al: Improvement in coronary perfusion pressures after open-chest cardiac massage in humans: Preliminary report (abstract). *Ann Emerg Med* 15:664-5, 1986.

26. Del Guercio LRM, Feins NR, Cohn JD, Coomarswamly RP, et al: Comparison to blood flow during external and internal cardiac massage in man. *Circulation* 31(suppl 1):171-180, 1965.

27. Shockett E, Rosenblum R: Successful open cardiac massage after 75 minutes of closed chest massage. *JAMA* 200:157-159, 1967.

28. Sykes MK, Ahmed N: Emergency treatment of cardiac arrest. *Lancet* 2:347-349, 1963.

29. Geehr EC, Lewis FR, Auerbach PS: Failure of open-heart massage to improve survival after prehospital nontraumatic cardiac arrest (letter). *N Engl J Med* 314:1189-1190, 1986.

30. Bodai BI, Smith JP, Ward RE, et al: Emergency thoracotomy in the management of trauma — A review. *JAMA* 249:1891-1896, 1983.

31. Cogbill TH, Moore EE, Millikan JS, et al: Rationale for selective application of emergency department thoracotomy in trauma. *J Trauma* 23:453-460, 1983.

32. Danne PD, Finelli F, Champion HR: Emergency bay thoracotomy. *J Trauma* 24:796-802, 1984.

33. Roberge RJ, Invatury RR, Stahl W, et al: Emergency department thoracotomy for penetrating injuries: Predictive value of patient classification. *Am J Emerg Med* 4:129-135, 1986.

34. Martin GB, Nowak RM, Carden DL, et al: Cardiopulmonary bypass vs CPR as treatment for prolonged canine cardiopulmonary arrest. *Ann Emerg Med* 16:628-636, 1987.

35. Levine R, Gorayeb M, Safer P, et al: Emergency cardiopulmonary bypass after cardiac arrest and prolonged closed-chest CPR in dogs. *Ann Emerg Med* 16:620-627, 1987.

36. Gottleib SO, Brinker JA, Borkon AM, et al: Identification of patients at high risk for complications of intraaortic balloon counterpulsation: A multivariant risk factor analysis. *Am J Cardiol* 53:1135-1139, 1984.

37. Bolooki H: *Clinical Application of Intra-aortic Balloon Pump,* 2 ed. Mount Kisco, New York, Futura Publishing Co, 1984, pp 1-421.

38. Fuchs RM, Brin KP, Brinker JA, et al: Augmentation of regional coronary blood flow by intra-aortic balloon counterpulsation in patients with unstable angina. *Circulation* 68:117-123, 1983.

39. Williams DO, Korr KS, Gewirtz H, et al: The effect of intraaortic balloon counterpulsation on regional myocardial blood flow and oxygen consumption in the presence of coronary artery stenosis in patients with unstable angina. *Circulation* 66:593-597, 1982.

40. Gewirtz H, Ohley C, Williams DO, et al: Effect of intra-aortic balloon counterpulsation on regional myocardial blood flow and oxygen consumption in the presence of coronary artery stenosis: Observations in an awake animal model. *Am J Cardiol* 50:829-837, 1982.

41. Kern MJ, Henry RH, Lembo N, et al: Effects of pulsed external augmentation of diastolic pressure on coronary and systemic hemodynamics in patients with coronary artery disease. *Am Heart J* 110:727-735, 1985.

42. Heck HA, Doty DB: Assisted circulation by phasic external lower body compression. *Circulation* 64(suppl II):118-122, 1981.

43. Scheidt S, Wilner G, Mueller H, et al: Intra-aortic balloon counterpulsation in cardiogenic shock: Report of a co-operative clinical trial. *N Engl J Med* 288:979-984, 1973.

44. Weiss AT, Engel S, Gotsman CH, et al: Regional and global left ventricular function during intraaortic balloon counterpulsation in patients with acute myocardial infarction shock. *Am Heart J* 108:249-254, 1984.

45. Bregman D: Assessment of intra-aortic balloon counterpulsation in cardiogenic shock. *Crit Care Med* 3:90-93, 1975.

46. Dunkman WE, Leinbach RC, Buckley MJ, et al: Clinical and hemodynamic results of intraaortic balloon pumping and surgery for cardiogenic shock. *Circulation* 46:465-477, 1972.

47. O'Rourke MF, Norris RM, Campbell TJ, et al: Randomized controlled trial of intraaortic balloon counterpulsation in early myocardial infarction with acute heart failure. *Am J Cardiol* 47:815-820, 1981.

48. Flaherty JT, Becker LC, Weiss JL, et al: Results of a randomized prospective trial of intraaortic balloon counterpulsation and intravenous nitroglycerin in patients with acute myocardial infarction. *J Am Coll Cardiol* 6:434-446, 1985.

49. Downing TP, Miller DC, Stinson EB, et al: Therapeutic efficacy of intraaortic balloon pump counterpulsation. *Circulation* 64(suppl II):108-113, 1981.

50. Harvey JC, Goldstein JE, McCabe JC, et al: Complications of percutaneous intra-aortic balloon pumping. *Circulation* 64(suppl II):114-117, 1981.

51. Vignola PA, Swaye PS, Gosselin AJ: Guidelines for effective and safe percutaneous intraaortic balloon pump insertion and removal. *Am J Cardiol* 48:6 60-664, 1981.

Arrhythmias

The purpose of this chapter is to review the essential diagnostic features and significance of arrhythmias commonly encountered in emergency cardiac care. Part I contains background material on the electrical activity of the heart. Part II is an introduction, for the novice, to basic methods of determining rhythms. Part III contains brief descriptions of the characteristics of various rhythms; Part IV, information on the treatment of arrhythmias not discussed elsewhere in this text.

The terms "dysrhythmia" and "arrhythmia" are used interchangeably in the medical literature. "Dysrhythmia" is the more accurately descriptive term as it means *an abnormality in rhythm*, whereas "arrhythmia" means *an absence of rhythm*. However, most journal editors now prefer "arrhythmia"; hence, that term will be used herein.

Part I: Electrical Activity of the Heart

Myocardial Cell Types

There are two basic groups of cells within the myocardium that are important for cardiac function:

1. The Working Myocardial Cells

Such cells possess the property of contractility, or the ability to shorten and then return to their original length. In order for a working cell to contract, the cell membrane must be electrically discharged (a process called depolarization), causing a change in the electrical charge across the cell membrane resulting from the flux or movement of certain ions (especially sodium) across the cell membrane. The process of depolarization also allows the entry of calcium into the cell, where it activates the points of attraction between the actin and myosin filaments of the sarcomere (the basic contractile unit of the myocardial fiber), resulting in contraction.

2. The Electrical System

Cells belonging to the electrical system of the heart are responsible for the formation of an electrical current and for conduction of this impulse to the working cells of the myocardium where the depolarization activates contraction. Certain cells of the electrical system have the ability to generate an electrical impulse (a property referred to as automaticity or spontaneous depolarization). Cells possessing this property are known as "pacemaker cells." Such cells are found in the sinus (or sino-atrial, or SA) node, probably in the atrial conduction

pathways, in the area immediately above the AV node, in the lower portion of the AV node, in the bundle of His (the AV node, the bundle of His, and an area immediately above the AV node are called the "AV junction"), in the bundle branches, and in the ventricular Purkinje system.[1] The electrical impulse is conducted over specialized pathways to be described later in this section.

Basic Electrophysiology

In order to better understand disturbances in the electrical activity of the heart, it is important to have a basic knowledge of the electrical properties of the working myocardial cells and of the pacemaker cells (see Figure 1). With the use of a microelectrode, the electrical events (or action potential) in a single cell can be recorded.

In order for a cell either to do work by contracting or to conduct an impulse, it must be electrically charged. This charge occurs by the active transport of ions across the cell membrane. Hence, there are different concentrations of potassium, sodium, and calcium, among others, inside of the cell, as compared to the outside of the cell. This normal gradient causes a -80 to -90 mV electrical charge to occur across the membrane. When the cell is activated this charge heads toward 0 mV, causing either conduction or contraction to be initiated.

The process of depolarization results in a momentary change in the physical properties of the cell membrane. Positively charged ions can enter the cell causing the inside of the cell to become electrically positive. Two channels by which ions can enter the cell have been described.[2,3] The fast channel operates at membrane potentials that are more negative than -60 mV, permitting the rapid entry of sodium ions. This is the "normal channel" for nonpacemaker myocardial cells. The slow channel operates at membrane potentials that are less negative than -50 mV. This channel permits the entry of calcium ions (and possibly sodium ions). Slow-channel depolarization as well as potassium flux are responsible for the pacemaker activity of the sinus node and the AV junction. Slow-channel depolarization may also be responsible for abnormal types of depolarization such as might exist in an area of myocardium bordering an infarct. In this situation, local extracellular hyperkalemia may occur and result in a reduction in the resting membrane potential (e.g., from a normal of -90 mV to -40 mV).[2,3]

In recording the action potential of a typical ventricular myocardial (working) cell, it is found that the resting membrane potential (the electrical potential across the cell membrane before depolarization) is approximately -80 to -90 mV (Figure 1). In other words, the inside of the cell membrane is electrically negative compared to the outside of the cell membrane. This is due to the distribution of ions across the very complex cell membrane. During this resting phase of the action potential (Phase 4), sodium is found in high concentration outside the cell and in low concentration inside the cell. Because of this concentration gradient, there is a physical force attempting to cause sodium ions to enter the cell. Energy is expended in order to develop this gradient. However, during this phase of the action potential, the cell membrane is relatively impermeable to sodium. Potassium is found in high concentration inside the cell and in low concentration outside the cell. This ion, in small amounts, is able to cross the cell membrane. During Phase 4, therefore, potassium is able to traverse the cell membrane from inside to outside. Because of this direction of potassium flux or movement, the interior of the cell becomes electrically negative while the exterior is positive. The resting membrane potential, then, is primarily dependent on the potassium gradient across the cell membrane.[2-5]

At the onset of depolarization (Figure 1), a complex gating mechanism (the fast channel) in the cell membrane opens momentarily (the duration is approximately 1 msec), permitting the rapid entry of sodium into the cell with its concentration gradient. Since there is now a flow of positively charged ions from outside to inside the cell, the interior of the cell becomes electrically positive (about $+20$ mV) while the outside of the cell membrane is negative. This portion of the action potential is labelled Phase 0. When Phase 0 occurs in the ventricular muscle cells at the same time, the QRS complex of the electro-cardiogram is generated. The P wave is generated by Phase 0 in the atrial muscle mass. As the gating mechanism closes and the entry of sodium slows down, the electrical charge inside the cell becomes less

positive, initiating the process of repolarization (Phase 1). During Phase 2, the action potential is approximately isoelectric and the cell remains depolarized. Significant amounts of sodium are no longer entering the cell through the fast channel, whereas calcium and possibly sodium are entering the cell through the slow channel.[2] Phase 2 of the ventricular muscle occurs at the time of the ST segment of the electrocardiogram. Phase 3 represents rapid repolarization during which the inside of the cell again becomes negative. This is caused by an increased efflux or movement of potassium ions from inside to outside the cell. Phase 3 in the ventricular muscle occurs during the T wave.

Repolarization is completed at the end of Phase 3. The interior of the cell is again approximately -90 mV. However, the ionic distribution across the cell membrane is different from that immediately prior to the onset of depolarization. Because of the entry of sodium into the cell and the loss of potassium from the cell, there is a higher concentration of intracellular sodium and a lower concentration of intracellular potassium. This would not prevent the cell from being depolarized a second time, but repeated depolarizations without an appropriate redistribution of sodium and potassium ions would lead to a serious impairment of cell function. Hence, during Phase 4 a special pumping mechanism in the cell membrane is activated. It transports sodium ions from inside to outside the cell and brings potassium ions into the cell. This pumping mechanism is dependent on adenosine triphosphate (ATP) as its energy source. The level of resting membrane potential (Phase 4) at the onset of depolarization is an important determinant of the conductivity (the ability to cause an adjoining cell to depolarize and the speed by which the adjoining cell is depolarized) of that electrical impulse to other cells. The less negative the resting membrane potential at the onset of Phase 0 (e.g., -60 mV as opposed to -90 mV), the slower will be the rate of rise of Phase 0. Conductivity is directly related to the rate of rise of Phase 0 of the action potential. Among the factors that determine the rate of rise of Phase 0 (and hence conductivity) are the sodium gradient across the cell membrane at the onset of Phase 0 and potassium gradient during Phase 4. For example, an increase in extracellular potassium will result in a decrease in the potassium gradient and a decrease in the resting membrane potential.

The action potential of a pacemaker cell differs significantly from that of a working myocardial cell (Figure 2).[2-5] Pacemaker cells possess the property of automaticity — that is, they are able to depolarize spontaneously. An important feature of the pacemaker cell action potential is that Phase 4 does not remain at a constant level. During this phase there is a gradual

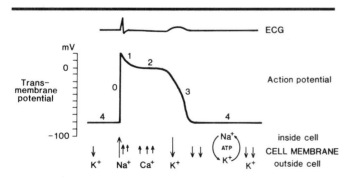

Figure 1. Schematic representation of ventricular myocardial working cell action potential. Arrows indicate times of major ionic movement across cell membrane.

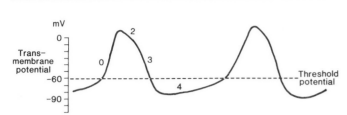

Figure 2. Schematic representation of pacemaker cell action potential.

lessening of the resting membrane potential. This occurs because of the entry of small amounts of calcium as well as sodium and a decrease in the outward flow of potassium ions during Phase 4. Hence, the resting membrane potential becomes less negative (a process called spontaneous diastolic depolarization). When the resting membrane potential reaches a certain critical voltage (threshold), Phase 0 begins. Since Phase 0 begins at a less negative resting membrane potential, the rate of rise of Phase 0 is slower than is seen in a normal myocardial working cell. The slow rate of rise of the action potential (Phase 0) in cells of the sinus node and AV junction is dependent on the accelerated entry of calcium and, possibly, sodium ions through the slow channel. The slope of Phase 4 will be an important factor in the rate of impulse formation. The steeper the slope, the more rapid will be the rate of the pacemaker cell; conversely, the more gradual the slope, the slower the rate. Activation of the sympathetic nervous system (or the administration of a catecholamine) will make the slope steeper and thereby enhance automaticity. Stimulation of the parasympathetic nervous system (i.e., vagal stimulation) will produce the opposite effect. Commonly used antiarrhythmic drugs (lidocaine, procainamide, quinidine, disopyramide, flecainide, amiodarone, tocainide, mexiletine, diphenylhydantoin) may decrease the rate of spontaneous depolarization (although this is not the only mechanism by which such drugs affect arrhythmias).[2]

Clinically, the most important groups of pacemaker cells are found in the sinus node, the AV junction, and the ventricular conduction system. The rate of spontaneous depolarization (the "firing rate") differs in these several locations. The sinus node is the primary pacemaker of the heart and has a firing rate of 60–100 per minute. The firing rate of the AV junction is 40–60 per minute and that of the ventricle (Purkinje fibers) is less than 40 per minute. This decrement in the firing rate has important physiologic implications. The lower pacemakers (AV junction and ventricle) fail to reach threshold potential (that is, they are prevented from spontaneously depolarizing) before being depolarized in Phase 4 by a sinus node impulse. Thus, the pacemakers in the AV junction and ventricle are "escape pacemakers"; that is, they do not spontaneously produce an electrical impulse unless the faster pacemaker (e.g., the

sinus node) fails. Hence, if the sinus rate falls significantly below 60 per minute, a junctional escape beat should occur. Likewise, if a supraventricular impulse does not reach the ventricles within approximately 1.5 seconds (equivalent to a rate of 40 per minute), a ventricular escape beat should occur. However, the rates of these escape pacemakers can be increased or decreased in various disease states, with drugs, or with sympathetic and/or parasympathetic stimulation.

Another important concept is that of the refractory period (Figure 3). The refractory period of the ventricle begins with the onset of Phase 0 (the onset of the QRS complex) and terminates at the end of Phase 3 (the end of the T wave). It can most conveniently be divided into two portions: 1) the absolute refractory period and 2) the relative refractory period. During the absolute refractory period, the cell cannot propagate or conduct an action potential. During the relative refractory period, a strong stimulus may result in a propagated but not necessarily normal action potential. The absolute refractory period begins with the onset of Phase 0 and ends midway through Phase 3 (at about the apex of the T wave); the relative refractory period extends through the remainder of Phase 3 (to the end of the T wave).

Mechanisms of Impulse Formation

There are two basic mechanisms whereby an electrical impulse may arise in the myocardium: 1) automaticity and 2) reentry.

Automaticity: An impulse may arise through the mechanism of automaticity described above. Other "abnormal" forms of automaticity may also be responsible for impulse formation and have been related to

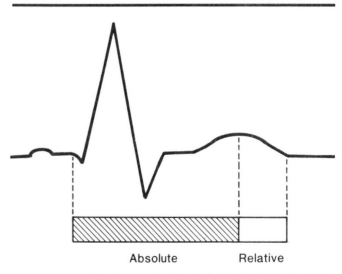

Figure 3. Relationship of refractory period to electrocardiogram.

abnormalities in slow channel activity.[2,3,5,6] 1) An after-potential is a transient decrease in the resting membrane potential following the action potential (i.e., during Phase 4.) If such an afterpotential is able to reach threshold, spontaneous depolarization will occur. 2) Multiple afterpotentials may occur (these are referred to as oscillations). 3) Differences in potential between nearby groups of cells may result when incomplete repolarization occurs in one group of cells (e.g., in cells adjacent to an infarct), whereas normal repolarization occurs elsewhere. Current may then flow between these groups of cells causing the normal cells to depolarize. 4) Triggered automaticity describes the induction of an automatic focus dependent on an initiating premature beat, which because of an abnormal repolarization causes a second depolarization or a series of depolarizations.

Reentry: The second mechanism for impulse formation is reentry.[2,5] This mechanism may occur in the sinus node, the atrium, the AV junction, or the ventricular conduction system. It may be responsible for isolated beats such as premature ventricular complexes (PVC) or abnormal rhythms such as ventricular tachycardia. As an example of this mechanism (Figure 4), consider an electrical impulse traveling down a ventricular Purkinje fiber that divides into two branches (A and B) and joins a muscle fiber. If conduction in both Purkinje branches is normal, the electrical impulse will travel down both branches to the muscle fiber. If, however, unidirectional (antegrade) block is present in one Purkinje branch (Branch A) and conduction down the other branch (Branch B) is slow, the electrical impulse will reach the muscle fiber though Branch B. It will then travel down the muscle fiber. When it reaches Branch A, the electrical impulse can be conducted back through A (since only antegrade block was present) to the original Purkinje fiber. From that point this electrical impulse can travel

though the remainder of the Purkinje system, giving rise to an ectopic impulse (e.g., a PVC). The same result would occur if the refractory period of Branch A was longer than that of Branch B. When an electrical impulse reached the point of division, it would find A refractory and would travel down B and then down the muscle fiber. It could then be conducted retrogradely through A if A had recovered from its refractory period. The basic components of the reentry mechanism include dual conduction pathways, one of which has unidirectional block (or a longer refractory period); the other has slow conduction so that transit time around the circuit is long enough that the refractory period of the Purkinje conduction tissue at the site of and proximal to the block is no longer absolute. Many of these changes from the normal pattern are caused by diseases such as coronary artery disease, cardiomyopathy, etc.

Conduction of the Cardiac Impulse[7-9]

The normal cardiac impulse originates in the sinus node, a structure located in the superior portion of the right atrium at its juncture with the superior vena cava (Figure 5). Conduction from the sinus node is thought to occur over internodal pathways. Three internodal pathways have been described. The anterior pathway arises at the cranial end of the sinus node. It divides into two branches, one to the left atrium (Bachmann's bundle) and the other along the right side of the interatrial septum to the AV node. The middle internodal pathway arises along the endocardial surface of the sinus node and descends through the interatrial septum to the AV node. The posterior pathway arises from the caudal end of the sinus node and approaches the AV node at its posterior aspect. The speed of conduction through the atria is approximately 1,000 mm/sec.

The AV node is located inferiorly in the right atrium, anterior to the ostium of the coronary sinus, and above the tricuspid valve. The speed of conduction is slowed (about 200 mm/sec) through the AV node. The AV node

RE–ENTRY

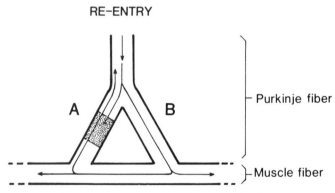

Figure 4. Diagrammatic representation of mechanism of reentry. Branches of Purkinje fiber which join muscle fiber are represented by A and B. Shaded area in A represents area of unidirectional block.

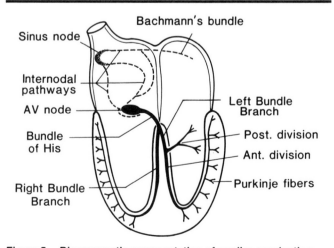

Figure 5. Diagrammatic representation of cardiac conduction system.

is anatomically a complicated network of fibers. These fibers converge at its lower margin to form a discrete bundle of fibers, the bundle of His (or AV bundle). This structure penetrates the annulus fibrosis and arrives at the upper margin of the muscular interventricular septum where it gives origin to the bundle branches.

The left bundle branch arises as a series of radiations at right angles to the bundle of His. Although the anatomy of these radiations is complex and variable, two groups can be considered. The superior, anterior radiation courses down the anterior aspect of the interventricular septum to the anterolateral papillary muscle where it breaks up into a Purkinje network. The inferior, posterior radiation is shorter and thicker, passing posteriorly to the base of the posteromedial papillary muscle where it branches into the Purkinje network. Purkinje fibers to the interventricular septum may arise as a separate radiation or as fibers from either the anterior or posterior radiation.

The right bundle branch courses down the interventricular septum on the right side. It contributes Purkinje fibers to the septum only near the apex of the right ventricle. At the lower end of the septum it passes into the right ventricular wall where it branches into a Purkinje network.

As the electrical impulse leaves the AV node, it passes into the bundle of His and then down both bundle branches simultaneously. The first section of the ventricle to begin depolarization is the midportion of the interventricular septum from the left side. The free walls of both ventricles are depolarized simultaneously. The speed of conduction through the ventricular Purkinje network is rapid, about 4,000 mm/sec.

Causes of Cardiac Arrhythmias[3-7,10]

Based on the above discussion, cardiac arrhythmias may result from the following mechanisms:

1. *Disturbances in Automaticity:* This may involve, for example, a speeding up or slowing down of the sinus node (sinus tachycardia or sinus bradycardia). Premature beats (more appropriately called "depolarizations" or "complexes" rather than "beats" or "contractions") may arise through this mechanism from the atria, the junction, or the ventricles. Abnormal rhythms, such as atrial or ventricular tachycardia, may also occur.
2. *Disturbances in Conductivity:* Conduction may be either too rapid (as in the Wolff-Parkinson-White syndrome) or too slow (as in atrioventricular block). The mechanism of reentry as described above is dependent on the presence of slowed conduction.
3. *Combinations of Altered Automaticity and Conductivity:* A simple example would be a premature atrial complex (PAC) with first-degree AV block or atrial flutter with 3:1 or higher grades of AV block.

The Electrocardiogram

The electrocardiogram (ECG) is a recording of the electrical forces produced by the heart. For the purposes of this discussion, an ECG machine or an oscilloscope may be used. The body itself acts as a giant conductor of electrical currents, and any two points on the body may be connected by electrical "leads" to register an ECG or to monitor the rhythm of the heart. The tracing recorded by the electrical activity of the heart forms a series of waves and complexes that have been arbitrarily labelled as the P wave, the QRS complex, the T wave, and U wave (Figure 6). The waves or deflections are separated by regularly occurring intervals.

Depolarization of the atria produces the P wave; the depolarization of the ventricles produces the QRS complex. Repolarization of the ventricles causes the T waves. The significance of the U wave is uncertain but may be due to repolarization of the Purkinje system. It appears at a time when many premature ventricular complexes occur and is affected by a variety of factors such as digitalis and electrolytes, as well as others.

In summary: The P wave represents depolarization of the atria (Figure 7). The PR interval extends from the beginning of the P wave (the beginning of atrial depolarization) to the onset of the QRS complex (the beginning of ventricular depolarization). It should not exceed 0.20 second as measured on ECG graph paper where each small square represents 0.04 second. The QRS complex represents the electrical depolarization of the ventricles. The upper limit of normal duration of the QRS is <0.12 second. A QRS duration of less than 0.12 second means that the impulse was initiated from the AV node or above (supraventricular). A wide QRS (≥0.12 sec) may signify conduction which either arises from the ventricle or comes from supraventricular tissue but has prolonged conduction through the ventricle and, thus, a widened QRS. The T wave is the ventricular recovery or repolarization of the ventricles.

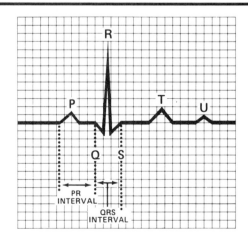

Figure 6.   The electrocardiogram.

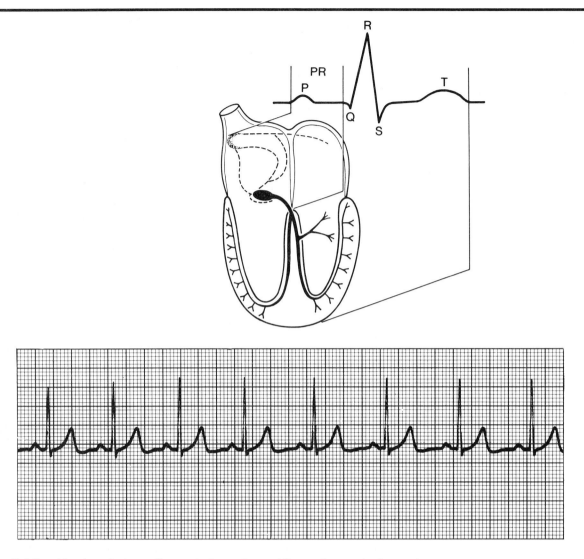

Figure 7. Relationship of an electrocardiogram to the anatomy of the cardiac conduction system.

The key to arrhythmia interpretation is the analysis of the interrelation of the P wave, the PR interval, and the QRS complex, including its width and configuration. The ECG should be analyzed with respect to its rate, rhythm, the site of the dominant pacemaker, and the configuration of the P and QRS waves. The relation of the ECG rhythm strip to cardiac anatomy is shown in Figure 7. The middle line in the diagram is at the bundle branches of the conduction system. Any malfunction above this point will largely affect the P wave and PR interval, while malfunction below this level will largely affect the QRS complex.

P Wave: If for some reason the sinus node fails to act as the normal cardiac pacemaker, other atrial foci may take over, and the P wave may have a different configuration. Alternatively, a secondary pacemaker, e.g., the AV junction, may provide an "escape rhythm."

PR Interval: When conduction though the atria, the AV node, or bundle of His is slowed, the PR interval becomes longer. Changes in conduction through the AV

node are the most common cause of changes in the PR interval.

QRS Complex: If there is a delay or interruption in conduction in either bundle branch, the QRS will widen in a manner typical for either right or left bundle branch block. An ectopic focus that initiates an impulse from the ventricle also can alter the shape of the QRS. When an ectopic beat arises above the bundle branches, the ventricles are activated in a normal fashion and the QRS complex will remain the same, assuming that there is no conduction delay in either bundle branch. If the beat occurs below the bundle branches, the QRS complex will be widened and notched or slurred because a different sequence of conduction will ensue.

The rate of any regular cardiac rhythm can be quickly determined from an ECG rhythm strip. Most ECG recorders in North America run ECG paper at 25 mm/sec. The ECG graph paper has heavy lines every 5 mm or 0.20 second (i.e., 300 heavy lines/min). The smaller

(1 mm) squares are 0.04 second apart. The markers at the top margin of the paper are 3 seconds apart. Thus, the heart (QRS) rate can be estimated at 10 times the number of complexes within three markers (6 seconds). Another method of establishing the rate is to divide the number 300 by the number of thick lines between complexes. For example, two thick lines between complexes represent a rate of 150 per minute, three thick lines a rate of 100 per minute, and four thick lines a rate of 75 per minute. The rates of irregular rhythms must be determined by counting the number of beats over a period of time and converting to beats per minute. For example, count the number of beats in 6 seconds and multiply by 10, or the number of beats in 12 seconds multiplied by 5, or the number of beats in 30 seconds multiplied by 2.

Monitoring Systems

Cardiac monitoring systems may be of many types, but they generally consist of a monitor screen (cathode ray oscilloscope) on which the ECG is visualized and a "write-out" system which directly transcribes the rhythm strip on paper. The write-out may be controlled by a switch or be automatic, and a ratemeter may be set to write out a rhythm strip should the rate go below a preset figure (for example, 50 beats/min) or above a certain rate (for example, 120 beats/min) for at least 6 seconds, sometimes as long as 30 seconds. A ratemeter is usually part of the system and is triggered by the QRS complex of the ECG. Lights and beepers may provide appropriate visual and audible signals of the heart rate.

Monitor leads or electrodes may be attached to the patient's chest or to his or her extremities. It is especially important that the chest leads be placed so as to show clearly the waves and complexes of the ECG strip and to leave the chest clear for treatment with a defibrillator if necessary.

Conventional locations for the chest electrodes are illustrated (Figure 8). The arrow indicates the direction of polarity from negative to positive. In Lead 1, the positive electrode is below the left clavicle and the negative below the right (Figure 8A). In Lead 2, the positive electrode is below the left pectoral muscle and the negative below the right clavicle (Figure 8B). Lead 3 is displayed by attaching the positive electrode beneath the left pectoral muscle and the negative below the left clavicle (Figure 8C). Another popular monitoring lead is that called MCL$_1$ (Figure 8D). To connect this lead the negative electrode is placed near the left shoulder, usually under the outer third of the left clavicle and the positive is placed to the right of the sternum in the fourth intercostal space. Representative samples of the resulting ECG are displayed beneath diagrams. The ground electrode in all four leads can usually be placed almost anywhere but is commonly located below the right pectoral muscle. The electrodes are often color-coded for ease of application, lessening confusion in their location.

It is especially significant to remember the following points when monitoring patients:

1. A prominent P wave should be displayed if organized atrial activity is present. Leads should be chosen which will show the P wave well.
2. The QRS amplitude should be sufficient to properly trigger the ratemeter.
3. The precordium of the patient must be left exposed so that defibrillation paddles can be readily employed if necessary.
4. It must be remembered that monitoring is for rhythm interpretation only. One should not try to read ST abnormalities or attempt more elaborate ECG interpretation.
5. Artifacts should be noted — a straight line will show if the electrode is loose, or a bizarre, wavy baseline resembling ventricular fibrillation may appear with patient movement. Sixty-cycle interference also may be present.

It is basic that any ECG findings should be correlated with clinical observation of the patient.

Different electrode placements may be used for telemetry or other special purposes. Unless the positive electrode is to the left or below the negative electrode, the deflections will all be reversed and the rhythm strips can be confusing.

Each rhythm strip must be analyzed in a systematic fashion. It is helpful to consider the following questions:

1. Is the rate fast or slow? Are the atrial and ventricular rates the same?
2. Are the P wave to P wave and R wave to R wave intervals regular or irregular? If the rhythm is irregular, is it consistent or is it an irregular irregularity?
3. Is there a P wave before each ventricular complex? Does a P wave follow the QRS complex? Are the P waves and the QRS complexes identical and normal in configuration?
4. Are the PR and QRS intervals within normal limits?
5. When correlated with clinical observation of the patient, what is the significance of the arrhythmia?

Part II: How to Identify Arrhythmias

Personnel providing ACLS must be able to recognize the following electrocardiographic arrhythmias:

1. Sinus tachycardia
2. Sinus bradycardia
3. Premature atrial complexes
4. Paroxysmal supraventricular tachycardia (atrial tachycardia)
5. Atrial flutter

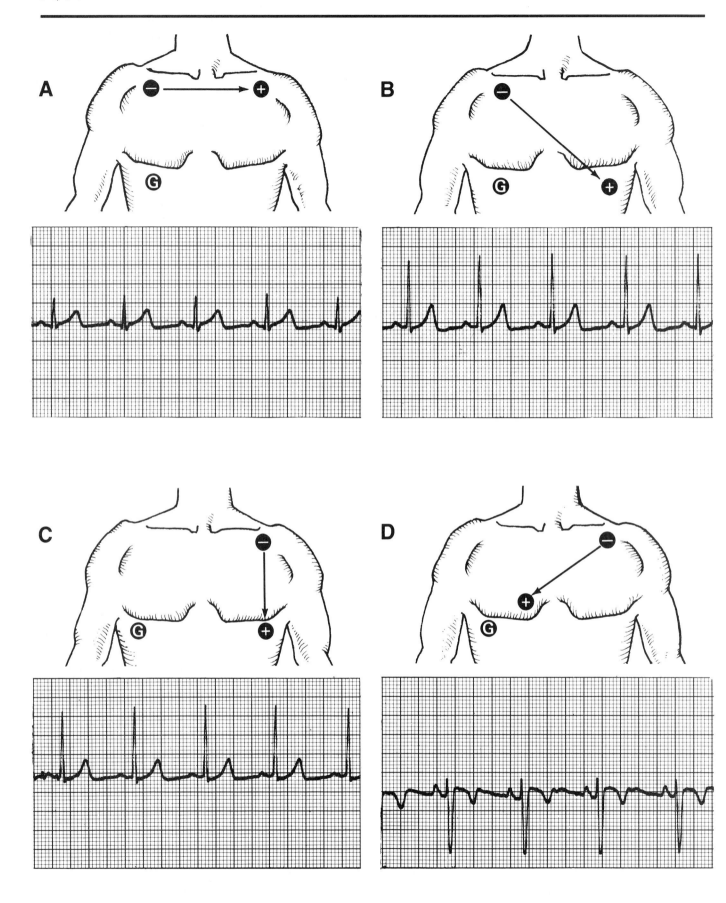

Figure 8. Location for chest electrodes. (A) Lead 1. (B) Lead 2. (C) Lead 3. (D) Lead MCL$_1$.

6. Atrial fibrillation
7. Junctional rhythms
8. Premature ventricular complexes (frequent, multi-formed, and R-on-T phenomenon)
9. Ventricular tachycardia (including the variant *torsade de pointes*
10. Ventricular fibrillation
11. Ventricular asystole (cardiac standstill)
12. AV block: first degree, second degree (Mobitz Types I and II), and third degree

In addition, ACLS personnel should be able to distinguish ventricular rhythms from supraventricular rhythms with ventricular aberrancy when such a distinction is possible.

The occurrence of these arrhythmias may be of significance clinically because of electrical and/or mechanical effects. For example, premature ventricular complexes may presage the sudden development of a life-threatening rhythm disturbance such as ventricular tachycardia or ventricular fibrillation. Alternatively, an increase in heart rate may lead to increases in cardiac work, resulting in a need for increased coronary blood flow. In the presence of significant coronary atherosclerosis, coronary flow may not be able to increase, and myocardial ischemia or infarction may be induced. Similarly, too slow a heart rate can also be problematic. If the heart rate decreases below 40 beats/min, cardiac output may fall.

Basic Information Needed for Identifying Arrhythmias

The identification of an arrhythmia or a cardiac rhythm, from either an ECG strip or a monitor, requires relatively simple logic. To begin the process, we must first learn how to determine the six basic blocks of information that are essential to understanding and recognizing an arrhythmia:

1. The rate of the arrhythmia
2. The pattern, or regularity, of the arrhythmia
3. Whether a QRS complex has normal or abnormal conduction
4. Whether atrial activity is present
5. What type of atrial activity is present
6. How the atrial activity is related to the ventricular activity

Determination of Rate (Figure 9)

Of the many ways that rate can be determined from an ECG, the most accurate is to count the number of complexes that occur in 1 minute. However, for an approximate rate there is a faster method: Many types of ECG paper have 3-second marks above or below the grid work of the ECG. A simple way of calculating the rate is to count the number of ventricular (QRS) complexes within two of these 3-second intervals. This gives you the number of ventricular complexes in 6 seconds, and by multiplying that times 10, you will have an approximate rate. The only problem with this method is that ECG's in books and on slides (and some ECG paper) may not have 3-second marks.

Another method is to determine the rate between two beats. If you can count the number of complete, large 5-mm boxes between two ventricular (QRS) complexes and divide 300 by the number of large boxes, you have an approximate rate per minute. An alternative is to count the number of small 1-mm boxes between two ventricular (QRS) complexes and divide 1500 by the number of small boxes to get an approximate rate.

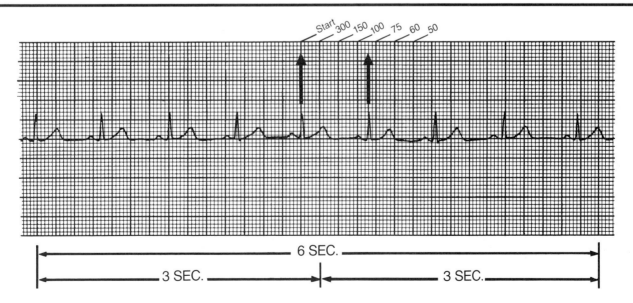

Figure 9. Determination of a rate.

Any of these methods may be used to determine an approximate rate, and they all assume that the paper is run at 25 mm/sec, which is the standard paper speed for an electrocardiogram. If the paper speed has been changed, then the method of calculation must be changed. For example, if the paper is run at 50 mm/sec, then the marks at the top and bottom of the paper are no longer 3-second marks but are 1.5-second marks and you must use four intervals between these marks to find 6 seconds. Rates of irregular rhythms need to be averaged over longer periods of time.

Is the heart rate fast, normal, or slow? If the rate is faster than 100 beats/min, it is faster than "normal," which is called tachycardia. If the rate is slower than 60 beats/min, the rate is slower than "normal" — bradycardia. If the rate is from 60 to 100, it is called a "normal" rate.

Hence, if the impulse begins in the sinus node and has a rate of 50, then it is a sinus bradycardia. If the impulse begins in the sinus node and is 70, it is a normal sinus rhythm. If the impulse begins in the sinus node and is 120, it is a sinus tachycardia. (See "Other Sites," below, for further discussion.)

Pattern Regularity (Figure 10)

The next step is to look at the pattern, or regularity, on the ECG. Are the ventricular complexes in a regular pattern, i.e., is the distance between any two QRS complexes, called the R–R interval, constant? If the interval between any two complexes is constant, the rhythm is regular. There are five abnormalities in rhythmicity or pattern:

1. The pattern may be abnormal because there is suddenly a beat earlier than you would have expected (a "premature beat").
2. There may be a periodic speeding up and/or slowing down of the rhythm that occurs with respiration. This periodic speeding up and slowing down should occur only with a sinus rhythm; this pattern is called sinus arrhythmia.
3. There may be a situation in which the rhythm is regular until a sudden, prolonged R–R interval occurs (a pause).
4. Another abnormal pattern is known as "group beating" in which a group of several beats are seen, followed by a pause, then another group of beats, then another pause. This sequence differs from pauses alone in that the groups of beats may be slightly irregular.
5. The rhythm may be totally irregular, or chaotic, so that it is impossible to define a pattern.

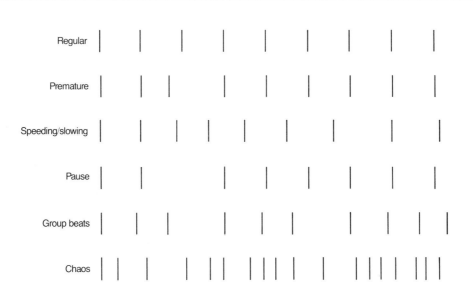

Figure 10. Patterns of rhythm disturbances.

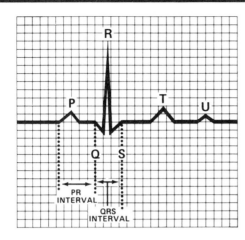

Figure 11. The electrocardiogram.

Width of Ventricular Complex (Figure 11)

If a ventricular complex arises in the ventricle, the QRS will be 0.12 second wide or wider (three of the 1-mm boxes at a 25 mm/sec paper speed). However, if the ventricular complex arises supraventricularly ("above the ventricles," i.e., sinus, atrial, or AV node), usually the QRS duration (or interval) will be less than 0.12 second wide (less than three of the 1-mm boxes at a paper speed of 25 mm/sec). There are times, however, when a supraventricular complex can be wide or abnormal. Hence, if a QRS complex is less than 0.12 second wide, it is supraventricular, i.e., it arose in the sinus node, the atrium, or the AV junction (node). If the QRS is 0.12 second wide or wider, there are two possibilities: 1) the impulse may have been initiated in the ventricle, or 2) the impulse began in the supraventricular area and was conducted abnormally (aberrantly, e.g., bundle branch block).

Recognizing Atrial Activity

To recognize atrial activity, you must carefully identify the various waves on the electrocardiogram. If the heart rate is fast or a premature beat occurs, the P wave may be superimposed on top of the previous T wave. One must be able to recognize normal T waves and, if a U wave is present, normal U waves. Then, if one is thorough, identification of changes in the T wave or U wave that could represent a P wave may be possible.

The T wave in any individual patient, in any lead may be upright, inverted, or biphasic (partially upright and partially inverted). Hence, you need to look at what the T wave and U wave for that particular person looks like in the lead you are using to determine if there is an extra notching (or P wave) that has been added.

In general, a P wave has relatively low amplitude but is relatively narrow. Most P waves are less than 0.08

second wide; occasionally, an abnormal P wave may be 0.12 second wide. T waves, on the other hand, are usually broader. The width of the T wave itself at the base is generally at least 0.20 second. When the heart rate gets faster than 150 beats/min, the T wave may encompass the entire interval between two QRS complexes. Hence, if the wave you are looking at is narrow (0.08–0.12 second), it is more likely to be a U wave or a P wave than a T wave. Remember, the U wave follows the T wave; thus, the interval from the QRS to the U wave should be constant even when the rate speeds up or slows. A P wave, on the other hand, may be on top of a T wave or buried in the upstroke or downstroke of the T wave. However, when the rate changes, the interval between the QRS and the next P wave may vary; search the T wave and U wave carefully in the intervals being analyzed for evidence of a P wave.

Definition of Atrial Activity

When using a Lead 2, use the positivity or negativity of the P wave for information about its origin. Lead 2 points from the right shoulder to the left leg at an angle about 60° below the horizontal in the same direction as normal depolarization from the sinus node toward the AV node. Since the sinus (SA) node causes a depolarization wave that sweeps from the top of the atrium toward the AV node in Lead 2, the P wave will be positive. A positive P wave in Lead 2 means that the impulse originated in either the sinus node or near the sinus node. If the P wave is negative, the impulse likely began in the AV node or near the AV node and was conducted retrograde (i.e., away from the region of the AV node toward the sinus node). In other leads the shape of the P wave may vary, in Lead V1 or MCL$_1$, a sinus P wave may be positive, negative, or biphasic. In Leads 2, 3, or aVF, atrial flutter will have a characteristic sawtooth appearance, like a positive P wave and a negative P wave hooked together with a little notch in between. In Lead V1 or MCL$_1$, atrial flutter usually looks like discrete positive P waves. Atrial flutter is not usually apparent in many other leads.

In atrial fibrillation, the atrial activity may have many different patterns. At times, atrial fibrillation may have a positive P wave, a negative P wave, a pattern similar to atrial flutter, or a flat line; the pattern is never consistent. The only consistent thing about atrial fibrillation is that nothing is consistent. The wavy baseline can mimic many other patterns. Therefore, inconsistency is the chief characteristic of the atrial activity in atrial fibrillation.

Relationship of P's to QRS's

Conduction of atrial impulses (P waves) to the ventricles results in QRS complexes that may have varying relationships: 1) There may be a fixed 1-to-1 relationship, in which each P wave is followed by a QRS after a constant PR interval and a duration ≤ 0.20 second. 2)

There may be a fixed 1-to-1 relationship in which each P is followed by a QRS after a constant PR interval that is longer than 0.20 second. 3) There are more P's than QRS's. Hence, when analyzing the basic rhythm on the ECG, there are only three ways in which P's can cause QRS's:

1. A normal, 1-to-1, fixed relationship.
2. A prolonged, 1-to-1, fixed relationship.
3. More P's than QRS's.

If none of these relationships is present, the P waves did not lead to all of the QRS complexes.

There are many reasons why P waves may not be associated with QRS complexes. The atrium may be generating the impulses, but not all of the impulses may be transmitted; this is known as block. P waves may not be associated with QRS complexes if the ventricle is inducing electrical activity faster than the atrium; hence, the QRS complexes are going at a faster rate than the P waves. The relation between the P waves and QRS complexes must follow one of the three patterns mentioned above if propagation of atrial activity causes the QRS complexes.

Sites of Origin for Impulses

There are four major sites within the heart from which an impulse or rhythm can be generated: the sinus node, the atrium, the AV node or junction, and the ventricle. Hence, one of the steps in identifying an arrhythmia is to decide which of the four sites could have originated the impulse.

The Sinus Node

The sinus node is acted on by the sympathetic and the parasympathetic (vagus) nervous systems. The sympathetic system speeds the sinus node up; the parasympathetic (or vagus nerve) slows the sinus node down. Changes in rate induced by sympathetic or parasympathetic systems resemble acceleration or braking. The sinus node does not change suddenly from one rate to a much faster or slower one. It speeds up over several beats or slows down over several beats. Thus, when a patient goes from a sinus rhythm of 70 to a sinus tachycardia of 120, there should be an acceleration over several beats from the slower to the faster rate. Likewise, if the sinus node slows from 70 to 40, there should be a deceleration (or braking) over several beats. Breathing in and out changes parasympathetic, or vagal, tone and causes a periodic speeding and slowing of the sinus node with respiration. This effect is accentuated in younger and physically fit individuals.

The Atrium

There are three rhythm disturbances that occur in the atrium. 1) The atrium can give rise to a premature atrial complex, which is a beat originating in the atrium that is earlier than expected. Unlike the acceleration or deceleration of the sinus node, it induces a sudden change in rhythm. 2) A second type of arrhythmia that begins in the atrium is atrial flutter. It has a characteristic sawtooth appearance in Leads 2, 3, and aVF. 3) The third type is atrial fibrillation, or a chaotic firing of the atrium.

The AV Junction

The third site at which a rhythm can originate is the AV junction. Impulse initiation at the AV node can also be responsible for arrhythmias. When the junction (or AV node) originates the arrhythmia, the arrhythmia is usually extremely regular (with a few rare exceptions).

The Ventricle

The fourth site at which the impulse can be initiated is the ventricle. When the ventricle originates an impulse, it is not caused by a P wave or atrial activity, and the QRS or ventricular complex is always wide and bizarre — generally 0.12 second wide or wider due to the different sequence of ventricular depolarization.

Naming the Arrhythmia

To name an arrhythmia, first look at the basic (or underlying) rhythm that is constant through the tracing. Identify this arrhythmia by 1) site of origin, 2) whether it is fast, slow, or normal in rate, and 3) what happens to it as it is conducted from its site of origin through the heart. After identifying the rhythm, then identify any other abnormalities that might be present on the ECG in the same manner — by identifying the site of origin of the abnormality and its relation to other electrical activity. To analyze the arrhythmia, use the six building blocks already described. First, determine its rate. Is it fast, normal, or slow? Second, look at the pattern. Third, look at the width of the QRS. Fourth, look for atrial activity. Fifth, define the atrial activity. Sixth, determine the relation of that atrial activity to the ventricular activity.

Identifying Specific Arrhythmias

The following section is a discussion of the differentiation of each arrhythmia in Lead 2. The minor changes encountered when using leads other than Lead 2 will be discussed later. Use the building blocks provided earlier to analyze these arrhythmias.

Sinus Rhythm

In Figure 12 the rate is four complete, large squares, or 20 mm. Three-hundred divided by 4 is 75 beats/min, so the rate on this ECG is 75 per minute or "normal," i.e., between 60 and 100. The pattern shown is very regular. The R–R intervals are equal and there is no variation in pattern or timing. The QRS's are two small squares wide, or approximately 0.08 second. These are normal, narrow QRS complexes. A distinct P can be identified and the P wave is positive. Since we are using Lead 2, the P wave came from the area of the sinus node and the impulse was propagated toward the AV node. Every P is followed by a QRS complex in a fixed relationship with a PR interval that is constant, with a duration of 0.16 second (normal). Therefore, there is a sinus rhythm — the impulse that began in the sinus node at a rate between 60 and 100 was conducted with a normal PR interval that resulted in a narrow QRS. Each P wave was followed by a QRS complex.

Sinus Bradycardia

An example of sinus bradycardia is shown in Figure 13. There are almost exactly six large boxes between two of the QRS's; 300 divided by 6 is 50; the rate is 50 beats/min. As this is less than 60, the heart rate is slow. Therefore, it is a bradycardia. The pattern of the electrical activity is consistent and regular. The duration of the QRS complex is two small squares, or 0.08 second wide, and has normal morphology. There is a P wave after each T wave and before each QRS. The P wave is positive; hence, it came from the area of the sinus node. Every P wave is followed by a QRS complex in a normal 1-to-1 relationship, with a PR interval of approximately 0.16 second, or four small squares. This rhythm started in the sinus node and is slow. Its conduction through the AV node and ventricle is normal. It is called a sinus bradycardia.

Sinus Tachycardia

There are approximately 2½ large squares between two of the QRS's in Figure 14; therefore, the rate is approximately 125. Again the pattern is very regular. The QRS's are narrow — two small squares — or 0.08 second wide. Each T wave is followed by a P wave. That P wave is positive in Lead 2. There is a fixed 1-to-1 relation between P waves and QRS complexes, and the PR interval is 3½ small squares, or approximately 0.14 second. This rhythm began in the sinus node, was faster than 100, and is therefore a sinus tachycardia.

Sinus Arrhythmia

On Figure 15 the rate is somewhat irregular. It varies from 47 to 95 beats/min. Average would be around 70 beats/min. The pattern too is irregular: The ECG starts out slow, speeds, and then slows again, but it does so slowly. The QRS complexes are of normal width (0.08

second). The P waves are positive in our Lead 2, and there is a constant 1-to-1 relation between the P's and the QRS's. The PR relationship is 4½ small squares, or 0.18 second. Hence, the QRS complexes speed up and slow down as the P waves speed up and slow down. This periodic speeding up and slowing is known as sinus arrhythmia. Sinus arrhythmia is a normal rhythm. The younger and more physically fit people are, the more sinus arrhythmia they tend to exhibit.

Other Sites

Rhythms can also begin in the AV junction. If it was slow, it would be a junctional bradycardia. If the rhythm began in the junction and had a normal rate, it would be a junctional rhythm. If it had a fast rate (> 100 beats/min), it would be a junctional tachycardia. The same principles apply when the impulses arise in the ventricle. If the impulse arises in the ventricle and is slow, it is a ventricular bradycardia. If the impulse arises in the ventricle and has a normal rate, then it is a ventricular rhythm. And if it arises in the ventricle and is fast, it is a ventricular tachycardia.

With junctional or ventricular rhythms, there is no respiratory variation. The periodic speeding up and slowing down with respiration only occurs in the sinus node. There is a problem with the nomenclature of junctional and ventricular rhythms. As herein, some authors use 60–100 as normal; therefore, a junctional or ventricular rhythm less than 60 is bradycardia and one greater than 100 is tachycardia. Other authors state that the normal escape rate of the AV junction is 40–60 per minute; and they therefore define rates of 40-60 as junctional rhythms, those less than 40 as junctional bradycardias, those of 60–100 as accelerated junctional rhythms, and those above 100 as junctional tachycardias. Since the normal ventricular escape rate is 30–40 per minute, some authors define ventricular rhythms with a rate of less than 30 as ventricular bradycardia or an idioventricular rhythm; 40–100 as accelerated ventricular or idioventricular rhythm or slow ventricular tachycardia, and those above 100 as ventricular tachycardia. It is thus best to state the rate after the name so that there is no confusion, i.e., a junctional rhythm of 65. For simplicity, we will herein consider rates less than 60 to be bradycardias, rates of 60-100 to be rhythms, and rates above 100 to be tachycardias.

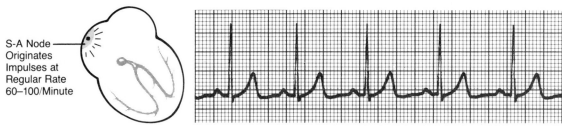

Figure 12. Normal sinus rhythm. S-A node originates impulses at regular rate 60–100 per minute. (Adapted with permission from THE CIBA COLLECTION OF MEDICAL ILLUSTRATIONS, Frank H. Netter, M.D., illustrator.)

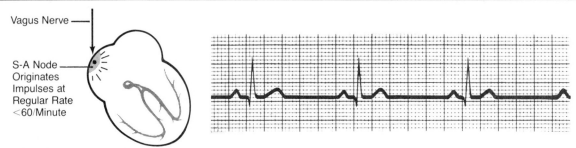

Figure 13. Sinus bradycardia. S-A node originates impulses at regular rate < 60 per minute. (Adapted with permission from THE CIBA COLLECTION OF MEDICAL ILLUSTRATIONS, Frank H. Netter, M.D., illustrator.)

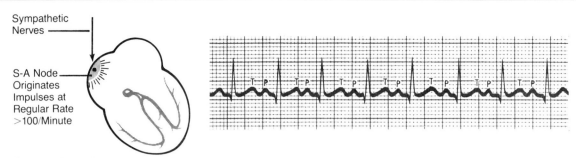

Figure 14. Sinus tachycardia. S-A node originates impulses at regular rate >100 per minute. (Adapted with permission from THE CIBA COLLECTION OF MEDICAL ILLUSTRATIONS, Frank H. Netter, M.D., illustrator.)

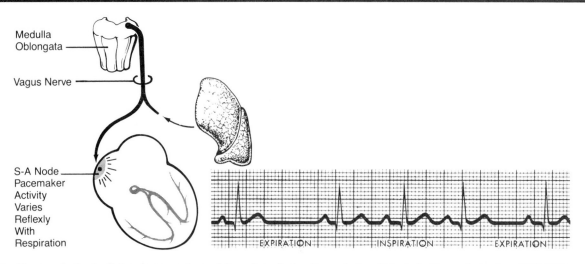

Figure 15. Sinus arrhythmia. S-A node pacemaker activity varies reflexly with respiration. (Adapted with permission from THE CIBA COLLECTION OF MEDICAL ILLUSTRATIONS, Frank H. Netter, M.D., illustrator.)

Premature Complexes

Premature complexes (Figure 16) are beats that occur earlier than expected. If a regular rhythm is present and suddenly a beat occurs earlier than the pattern would have predicted, it is a premature complex — also called premature beats or premature contractions. If there is a positive P wave before that premature complex, it is a premature atrial complex. If there is not a positive P wave before that premature complex, and if the QRS is narrow, less than 0.12 second (or three small squares wide), then the premature complex is junctional; and if that QRS complex is wide, then the premature complex is ventricular. Therefore, in Lead 2, a premature atrial complex has two characteristics: It is earlier than expected and it starts with a positive P wave. This is not called a premature sinus complex because the sinus node speeds up or slows down over several beats. Thus, the positive P wave did not come from the sinus node but, since it is positive, must have originated in the high, right atrium near the sinus node. Therefore, it is called a premature atrial complex.

A premature junctional complex has three characteristics in Lead 2: 1) It is early; 2) it is not preceded by a positive P wave; and 3) the QRS is of normal duration (less than 0.12 second width).

A premature ventricular complex also has three characteristics in Lead 2: 1) It is early; 2) it is not preceded by a positive P wave; and 3) the QRS complexes are wide (0.12 second wide or wider).

Premature Atrial Complexes (Figure 17A): The first three beats have normal QRS complexes, positive P waves, and normal PR intervals. Hence, we have a normal sinus rhythm. The sinus beats are followed by a premature complex. That premature complex has a positive P wave before it; therefore, it is a premature atrial complex. Premature atrial complexes may have normal, longer, or occasionally slightly shorter (0.01–0.03 second shorter) PR intervals than the underlying rhythm. Sometimes the premature atrial complex does not cause a QRS complex because it is so early that the AV junction is refractory to conduction. A premature atrial complex can be followed by either a normal (narrow) or wide QRS complex after a normal or prolonged PR interval.

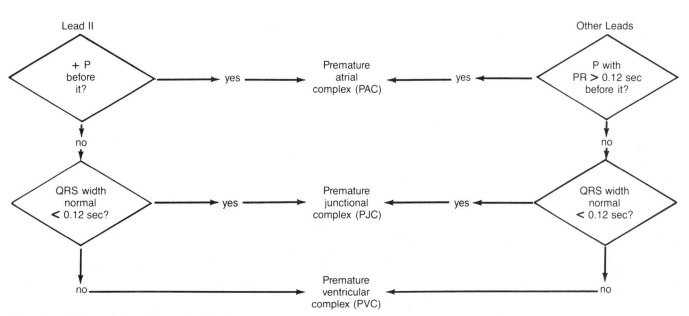

Figure 16. Differentiation of premature beats.

Premature Junctional Complexes (Figure 17B,C,D): The first three beats of these examples demonstrate a regular rhythm, normal QRS complexes, positive P waves, and normal PR intervals. Thus, it is a sinus rhythm. On all three strips the fourth beat is a premature complex. On the top strip the premature complex has a negative P wave before it, and the QRS complex is narrow and normal in configuration. Hence, this is a premature junctional complex. Premature junctional complexes frequently have negative P waves before QRS complexes in Lead 2. If the impulse arises high in the junction (on top of the zone where conduction is slowed or delayed), then it can cause a negative P wave followed by a QRS complex with a longer PR interval because the impulse has to go through the slow conduction zone of the AV node before initiating ventricular depolarization (a QRS complex). The junction actually depolarizes prior to the negative P wave (Figure 17C).

On the second strip the first three beats again are sinus beats. The premature complex (beat 4) does not have a positive P wave before the QRS complex, which is narrow and normal in appearance. Hence, again, it is a premature junctional complex. On occasion, a P wave may not be associated with the premature junctional complex for either of two reasons: 1) the impulse could have begun in the middle of the delay zone so that it was equidistant (or equal time) in transmission back up to the atrium and down to the ventricle, so that the P wave is buried in the higher frequency and amplitude QRS complex, or 2) the premature junctional beat may not have been conducted back (retrograde) into the atrium and a P wave is not present. In the second instance, no P wave may be seen or, on occasion, the sinus node may depolarize and cause a positive P wave that is unrelated to the QRS (Figure 17D).

On the third strip, again, the first three beats are sinus beats; the fourth is a premature complex. There is no positive P wave before the premature QRS complex in Lead 2, and the QRS is narrow. It is, then, a premature junctional complex. In this case there is a negative P wave after the QRS. When the impulse arises from the lower portions of the AV node, it may conduct more rapidly to the ventricle, causing a QRS complex but only slowly, retrograde through the slow conduction zone, causing a negative P wave after the QRS complex.

On occasion, a premature junctional complex might have a wide or abnormal QRS. In this circumstance it is difficult to properly interpret the rhythm from the surface ECG unless the abnormal QRS complex observed in the premature beat is identical in all leads to the QRS while in sinus rhythm. Frequently, it can be determined only in the electrophysiology lab. Fortunately, premature junctional complexes with aberrant QRS complexes are not common.

Premature Ventricular Complexes (Figure 17E,F): The first three beats of both examples have a regular rhythm with normal QRS complexes preceded by positive P's with a normal PR interval. Hence, the first three beats of each strip are sinus beats. The fourth beat is again early (premature). There are no P waves preceding the premature beats. The T wave preceding each of those QRS's is identical to the T waves of the beats prior to them, so there is no evidence that P waves are buried in the T waves. (This rule is not absolute; there can be late PVC's that occur right after the next sinus P wave. Usually, when a widened QRS complex follows a P wave, the PR interval is the same or longer than a normal PR interval. If the PR interval is suddenly shorter, the P wave probably did not cause the QRS complex and the beat is probably ventricular.) The QRS complexes are wide and aberrant appearing (0.12 second or wider). Hence, they are premature ventricular complexes. In the first example the premature ventricular complex induces a positive QRS complex; in the second, a negative QRS.

Several special terms are used to describe premature ventricular complexes. When all of the premature ventricular complexes on a single lead strip have exactly the same shape, they are called uniform (or unifocal) premature ventricular complexes. When the premature ventricular complexes have different shapes in the same lead, they are called multiformed (or multifocal) premature ventricular complexes.

Patterns of Premature Complexes: There are special names for different groupings of premature complexes. When two premature complexes occur in a row, they are called a "couplet." When three or more premature complexes occur in succession, it is called a "tachycardia," and if the tachycardia is recurrent, it is designated a "paroxysmal tachycardia." Three or more premature atrial complexes in a row is termed an atrial tachycardia, and three or more premature ventricular complexes, a ventricular tachycardia. When a normal beat alternates with a premature complex, it is called bigeminy. A normal sinus beat alternating with a premature atrial complex would be an atrial bigeminy and with a ventricular complex, it would be designated as ventricular bigeminy. When every third beat is a premature complex, it is

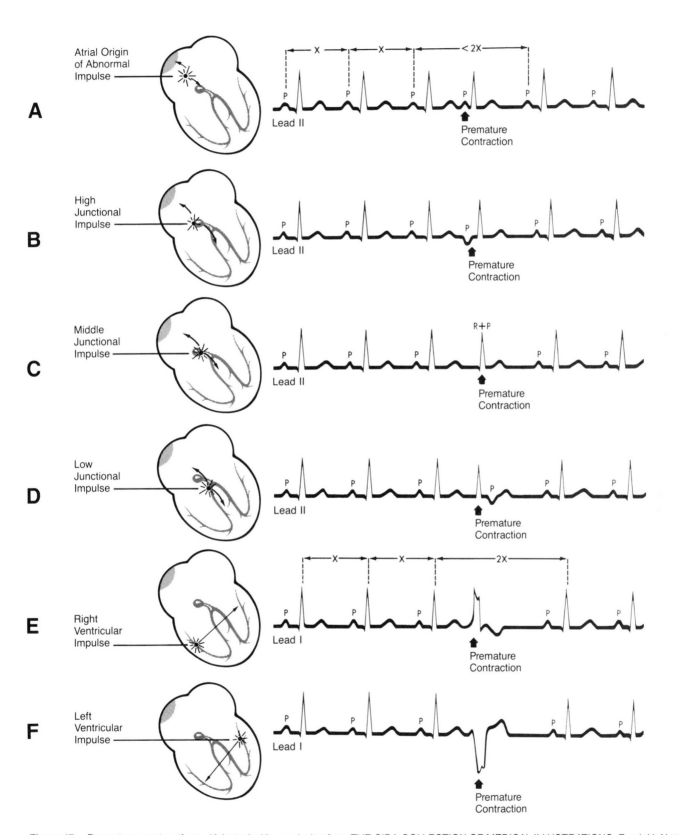

Figure 17. Premature contractions. (Adapted with permission from THE CIBA COLLECTION OF MEDICAL ILLUSTRATIONS, Frank H. Netter, M.D., illustrator.)

called a trigeminy; when every fourth beat is a premature complex, it is called a quadrageminy, and so forth.

Atrial Tachycardia (Figure 18A): On this strip the first two beats are normal. The rate is 75, the QRS complexes are normal, with a positive P wave before them and a normal PR interval. They are followed by three or more premature complexes in a row, which are preceded by positive P waves. They are premature atrial complexes, and with three or more in a row, this is an atrial tachycardia. If recurrent, it is known as paroxysmal atrial tachycardia (PAT).

Junctional Tachycardia (Figure 18B): On this strip, again, the first two beats have a rate of approximately 75 and normal QRS complexes preceded by positive P's with a normal PR interval. Thus, it is a sinus rhythm. However, the three or more premature complexes do not have positive P waves. The QRS complex is normal. The rhythm is a junctional tachycardia. In this case, there are negative P waves that precede the QRS complexes. The rhythm is regular. Junctional pacemakers tend to depolarize regularly. If recurrent, it is known as paroxysmal junctional tachycardia (PJT).

Paroxysmal Supraventricular Tachycardia: Paroxysmal atrial tachycardia and paroxysmal junctional tachycardia are two types of paroxysmal supraventricular tachycardia. Often it is difficult to define P waves clearly; hence, the use of the term "supraventricular" has become widespread to describe all narrow non-sinus tachycardias. It is also clear that there are many different locations and mechanisms for these rhythms and they are often subdivided into paroxysmal (usually due to a reentry mechanism) and nonparoxysmal (usually due to altered automaticity). (See Part IV for explanation.) Both PAT and PJT are usually due to reentry within the AV junction and/or atrium. Practically, it may be difficult to tell where the reentry circuit is located. In addition, therapy is similar for the majority of these arrhythmias though physiologically they use different pathways. As the majority of these arrhythmias have rates faster than 150 beats/min, it may be difficult to determine the atrial activity. Hence, if the rhythm is regular and faster than 150 beats/min and associated with narrow QRS complexes, it is called a paroxysmal supraventricular tachycardia or PSVT.

There are times when several PAC's are seen in succession but not in a regular pattern and have different P waves. If the rate of these premature beats is less than 100 beats/min then the term "wandering atrial pacemaker" (WAP) is sometimes used. If the rate of these irregular PAC's is faster than 100 beats/min, then the term "multifocal atrial tachycardia" (MAT) is sometimes used. Purists will often say that wandering atrial pacemakers or multifocal atrial tachycardias should have at least three different P wave morphologies or shapes and three different P-to-P intervals.

Supraventricular tachycardias, including junctional rhythms with rates between 60 and 150 beats/min, are usually not due to reentry but to enhanced automaticity.

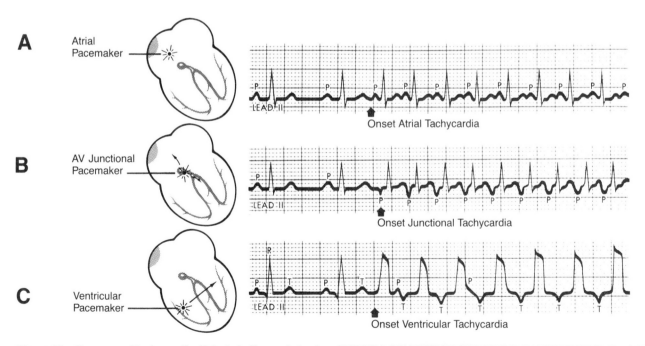

Figure 18. Paroxysmal tachycardia. (Adapted with permission from THE CIBA COLLECTION OF MEDICAL ILLUSTRATIONS, Frank H. Netter, M.D., illustrator.)

Accelerated junctional rhythms may be seen when exogenous catecholamines are being administered, in patients in the recovery room after open heart surgery (usually receiving some catecholamine), or in patients who are digitalis intoxicated.

When one has a regular, narrow QRS (QRS < 0.12 sec) tachycardia that is not sinus in mechanism and is faster than 150 beats/min, it is called a "paroxysmal supraventricular tachycardia." Care must be taken to make sure that it is not a sinus tachycardia or an atrial flutter with a 2:1 block, which also is regular and has a rate of about 150 beats/min. The importance of looking for P waves must be emphasized, particularly when the tachycardia has wide QRS's. A wide QRS tachycardia may be ventricular tachycardia or a supraventricular tachycardia with a bundle branch block or aberration. If atrial activity can be seen that is not associated with the QRS's, it is a ventricular tachycardia. If positive atrial activity is seen in a Lead 2 that is associated with the QRS's, it is a supraventricular tachycardia with a bundle branch block. If atrial activity cannot be defined, it is not certain whether a supraventricular or ventricular rhythm is present.

Ventricular Tachycardia (Figure 18C): On this strip the first two complexes have a rate of 75 with normal, narrow QRS complexes preceded by positive P waves with fixed, normal PR intervals. Hence, the first two complexes are sinus beats. They are followed by three or more premature complexes not preceded by positive P waves, and the QRS complexes are wide and abnormal. This is paroxysmal ventricular tachycardia. Please note that a couple of positive P waves are seen in the tracing and are labelled "P." However, there is no P wave before each QRS complex, so the P waves are dissociated from the QRS complexes. Thus, the origin of the QRS complexes is ventricular.

Atrial Flutter (Figure 19)

Atrial flutter is a rhythm that involves a circus movement (conduction around some loop) in the atrium. In atrial flutter the impulse is conducted around some area of the atrium in a circular motion, arriving back at the same point at a rapid interval. This rapid interval is generally around 300 per minute. Though the rate of atrial flutter can vary tremendously, commonly it is between 240 and 360 per minute. On rare occasions it can be slower than 240. Most frequently the atrial flutter circles the atrium in the atrioventricular groove. The atrial flutter conducts from the groove back up one side of the atrium, over the top of the atrium, and down the other side. This means that part of the time it is going from the AV groove towards the sinus node, and part of the time it is going from the sinus node toward the AV groove. In an inferior lead (2, 3, aVF), when the impulse is being

conducted from the AV groove toward the sinus node, a negative deflection of the base line will be present. However, when the impulse goes from the high right atrium back down toward the AV groove, here will be a positive deflection of the base line. This is like taking a positive P wave and following it by a negative P wave. There is also generally a slight pause between the two, and the resultant atrial activity looks much like a sawtooth or picket fence pattern. Atrial activity is very consistent and very regular in atrial flutter. The QRS complexes, however, may not be regular; because, as seen later, atrial flutter frequently is associated with some degree of AV block. Thus, there are more flutter waves than QRS's. Always suspect atrial flutter when the rate is about 150 beats/min.

Atrial Fibrillation (Figure 20)

Atrial fibrillation is a chaotic rhythm. The atrial muscle is firing in a random manner. These impulses are therefore being conducted to the AV node randomly. The atrium is frequently firing between 350 and 600 times per minute. This is so fast, and the muscle mass being depolarized is so small, that it may cause just a little bit of waviness of the base line. Since what is being conducted to the AV node is very irregular, what gets conducted through the AV node is going to be markedly irregular as well, and intervals between QRS complexes (known as R-R intervals) are constantly changing. Because they are totally erratic, the pulse or heart rate is totally erratic. Because the rhythm is erratic, it may be difficult to diagnose. In the examples provided, the QRS complexes are narrow. Thus, we have for the most part ruled out a ventricular rhythm. Since the QRS's are narrow, they must have originated in the sinus node, the atrium, or the junction. If the impulses began in the sinus node, they would be regular, with positive P waves before each one. Since this is not the case, it cannot be a sinus rhythm. If this had been junctional, the rhythm likely would have been regular; since this rhythm is irregular, it cannot be junctional. There is only one other site that is left, the atrium. Hence, by ruling out sinus, junctional, and ventricular, we know that this is an atrial rhythm.

There are three common types of rhythm disturbances in the atrium: 1) premature atrial complexes, which have positive P waves before them; 2) atrial flutter with the regular sawtooth appearance of the atrial activity; and 3) atrial fibrillation. Since there are no positive P waves before each of these QRS complexes and there is no sawtooth pattern, neither atrial tachycardia nor atrial flutter is present. The only possibility left is that this is atrial fibrillation. Atrial fibrillation may be diagnosed by exclusion, ruling out all potential sites and mechanisms other than atrial fibrillation.

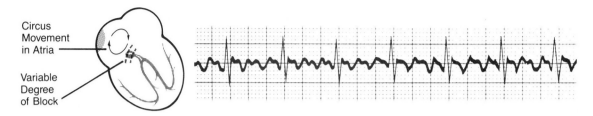

Figure 19. Atrial flutter. (Adapted with permission from THE CIBA COLLECTION OF MEDICAL ILLUSTRATIONS, Frank H. Netter, M.D., illustrator.)

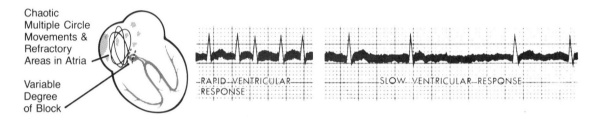

Figure 20. Atrial fibrillation. (Adapted with permission from THE CIBA COLLECTION OF MEDICAL ILLUSTRATIONS, Frank H. Netter, M.D., illustrator.)

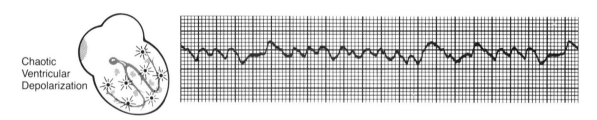

Figure 21. Ventricular fibrillation. (Adapted with permission from THE CIBA COLLECTION OF MEDICAL ILLUSTRATIONS, Frank H. Netter, M.D., illustrator.)

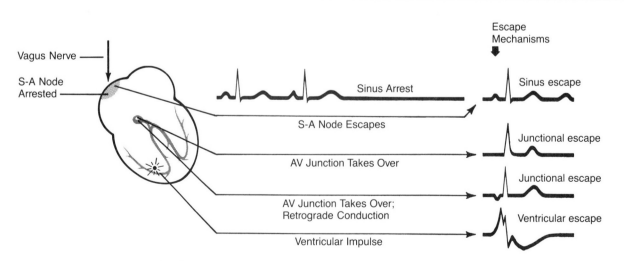

Figure 22. Escape mechanisms following sinus arrest. (Adapted with permission from THE CIBA COLLECTION OF MEDICAL ILLUSTRATIONS, Frank H. Netter, M.D., illustrator.)

Ventricular Fibrillation (Figure 21)

Ventricular fibrillation is the absence of any apparent organization of electrical activity. With ventricular fibrillation, an apparently chaotic pattern of electrical activity is present, and there is nothing identifiable on the tracing, not QRS complexes, T waves, or P waves. Ventricular fibrillation may appear to be "noise." Also, artifacts that represent electrical noise can mimic VF; for example, if an electrode pops off, a wire is broken, the electrode is dry, or during certain patient movements. The patient with ventricular fibrillation does not have a pulse and loses consciousness within 6–10 seconds. Thus, frequent assessment of the cardiac pulse is very helpful in determining when VF is present.

Escapes (Figure 22)

Occasionally, there may be pauses in electrical activity. The sinus node, for example, may suddenly stop and cause a pause. This is termed "sinus pause" or "sinus arrest." Whatever beat occurs after the pause is an escape beat. Escape beats can occur from three different sites. If the escape beat in Lead 2 has a positive P wave before it, we call it a "sinus escape," not an "atrial escape" — because we usually know that an escape with a positive P wave before it is a sinus escape. If the escape has no positive P wave before it in Lead 2 and has a normal, narrow QRS, then it is a junctional escape. If the escape beat has no positive P wave in front of it and has a wide, aberrant QRS, then it is a ventricular escape. If there is no escape, and you thus have no rhythm following a pause, it is called "asystole," or cardiac standstill.

Atrioventricular (AV) Block (Figure 23)

In the AV node, the impulse is normally delayed for no more than 0.20 second. Delays longer than 0.20 second or atrial activity that is not transmitted to the ventricles are termed "heart block." There are three grades of heart block: first-, second-, and third-degree (complete). With first-degree heart block, every P wave causes a QRS complex, but the PR interval is prolonged — longer than 0.20 second. With second-degree heart block, there are more P waves than QRS complexes. Thus, some P waves are associated with QRS complexes and some are not. There are multiple ways in which this can occur.

With third-degree (complete) heart block, there are more P waves than QRS complexes, and the P waves and QRS complexes are not associated. The QRS complexes occur due to junctional or ventricular escape rhythm.

It is sometimes very difficult to differentiate among second- and third-degree heart block on a monitor. One simple method is to determine whether the PR interval is constant or variable. If the PR is fixed or constant, a second-degree block is present. The fixed variety is

generally called a Mobitz II or Type II block. The Type II block may occur either in the AV node, in which case the QRS's are normal or narrow, or it may occur below the bundle of His (the so-called infra-His block), in which case the QRS complexes are ≥ 0.12 second in duration. (Rarely, the QRS may be normal due to simultaneous delays down all pathways. This situation can be diagnosed only in the electrophysiology lab.) Type II block with wide QRS complexes may lead to asystole. (Some authors reserve the designation Type II for infra-His blocks with wide QRS's; however, herein it will denote a pattern of block.) Always designate whether Type II block is infra-His or not. If the PR interval varies and the QRS complexes are all the same and are regular in pattern, third-degree heart block is present. If the QRS's that look alike are irregular in pattern, some degree of variable second-degree block, called Mobitz I, Wenckebach, or just Type I block, is present. In third-degree heart block, the rhythm may be irregular because there may be more than one escape mechanism and premature complexes may also be present. Thus, the similarity of the QRS complexes is important. A junctional escape mechanism will cause a narrow QRS at one regular rate, and a ventricular escape mechanism may cause regular wide QRS complexes at different rates. Hence, with third-degree heart block, comparing the QRS's that look alike and the intervals between them to determine the rhythm is recommended.

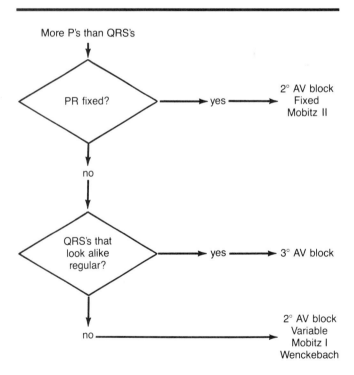

Figure 23. Differentiation of second- and third-degree blocks.

First-Degree AV Block (Figure 24A): In this example there is a regular rhythm with normal QRS complexes. A positive P wave precedes each QRS, but the PR interval is longer than 0.20 second and fixed or constant.

Second-Degree AV Block Type II (Figure 24B): In this example there are more P waves than QRS complexes. Looking at the P wave just before each QRS complex, the PR interval is fixed. Therefore, this is a second-degree block, Type II, or fixed.

Third-Degree (Complete) AV Block (Figure 24C,D): In these two examples there are more P waves than QRS complexes and the PR interval is varying. The QRS complexes are identical to one another and they are regular in pattern. Third-degree heart block is present. On the top tracing the QRS's are narrow since there is junctional escape rhythm. On the lower tracing the QRS's are wide because there is a ventricular escape rhythm.

Second-Degree AV Block Type I (Figure 24E): In this example the pattern of the QRS complexes is irregular and there are more P's than QRS's. Notice also that the PR is varying. The PR interval varies and the QRS

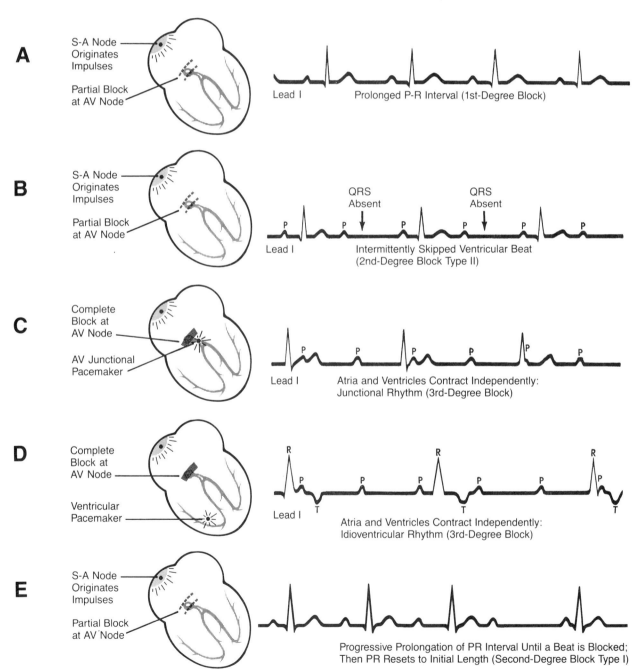

Figure 24. Atrioventricular block. (Adapted with permission from THE CIBA COLLECTION OF MEDICAL ILLUSTRATIONS, Frank H. Netter, M.D., illustrator.)

complexes that look alike have an irregular pattern. This is second-degree variable block. Most second-degree variable blocks are Wenckebach. But, some second-degree variable blocks may not meet criteria for Wenckebach (which see below).

Bundle Branch Block (Aberrant Conduction): If a supraventricular rhythm is present but the QRS is wide (0.12 second or wider), a conduction defect such as "bundle branch block" or "aberrant conduction" is present. To differentiate a bundle branch block or aberrantly conducted beats from ventricular complexes, one must determine whether there is atrial activity preceding the QRS complex. If there is a sinus P wave prior to the wide QRS complex, it is likely a complex with a bundle branch block or aberrant conduction. Atrial flutter or fibrillation also may be associated with aberrant conduction. With atrial flutter there should be a discernable though not necessarily constant relation between the atrial flutter waves and the wide QRS's. In atrial fibrillation, the wide QRS's will be irregular in pattern. When ventricular tachycardia is present, QRS complexes usually occur in a fairly regular pattern. If there is no atrial activity in front of a wide QRS, it is likely a ventricular complex.

Identifying Arrhythmias in Leads Other Than Lead 2

Criteria based on the positivity or negativity of the P wave to determine in which direction the atrium was depolarized apply predominantly to Lead 2. In Lead 2 positivity or negativity of the P wave definitively represents the direction in which the atrium has been depolarized. However, in other leads, such criteria are not as reliable!

In general, if the PR interval is longer than 0.12 second, then the P wave probably originated either in the sinus node or atrium. Hence, a premature complex with a P wave before it with a PR interval of 0.16 second is probably a premature atrial complex. A regular rhythm with a P wave before each QRS complex and a PR interval of 0.18 second probably is a sinus rhythm. On the other hand, impulses beginning in the junction usually have a PR interval of 0.12 second or less. Thus, a premature complex with a P wave in front of it but a PR interval of only 0.10 second, is probably a premature junctional complex. A regular rhythm with a P wave in front of each QRS complex with a PR interval of 0.10 second is probably a junctional rhythm. These guidelines describe probabilities; there can be errors.

Sometimes, it is very difficult to differentiate between atrial flutter and paroxysmal atrial tachycardia (or sinus tachycardia) in leads other than 2, 3, or aVF. In Lead 2 sinus tachycardia or PAT has discrete positive P waves whereas atrial flutter has a sawtooth appearance. But in other leads such as V1 or MCL$_1$, atrial flutter may also appear to have discrete P waves and it may be impossible to tell the difference between atrial flutter and PAT. That most PAT's have atrial rates less than 240 and most atrial flutters have atrial rates greater than 240 can

be used as a criterion to help differentiate atrial flutter from PAT (or sinus tachycardia) in Lead V1 or Lead MCL$_1$. However, some atrial flutters can be slower than 240, and occasionally a PAT can have a rate faster than 240 beats/min.

Part III: Definitions of Arrhythmias

The arrhythmias basic to a knowledge of ACLS are analyzed below. More detailed discussion of these rhythms may be found in standard textbooks on electrocardiography or cardiology.[5,7,11]

Normal Sinus Rhythm (NSR) (Figure 25)

Description

Normal sinus rhythm is characterized by a regular discharge of the sinus node leading to atrial depolarization at a rate of 60–100 beats/min. The rhythm is regular (or slightly irregular). The spread of atrial depolarization is inferior and leftward, resulting in positive P waves in Leads 1, 2, and aVF.

Summary of ECG Criteria

a. Rate: 60–100 per minute.
b. Rhythm: Regular.
c. P waves: Upright in Leads 1, 2, aVF.

Sinus Tachycardia (Figure 26)

Description

Sinus tachycardia is characterized by an increase in the rate of discharge of the sinus node. Perhaps secondary to multiple factors (e.g., exercise, fever, anxiety, hypovolemia, etc.), it is a physiologic response to a demand for a higher cardiac output.

Summary of ECG Criteria

a. Rate: Greater than 100 per minute.
b. Rhythm: Regular.
c. P waves: Upright in Leads 1, 2, aVF.

Sinus Bradycardia (Figure 27)

Description

Sinus bradycardia is characterized by a decrease in the rate of atrial depolarization due to slowing of the sinus node. It may be secondary to sinus node disease, increased parasympathetic tone, or drug effects (e.g., digitalis, propranolol, or verapamil).

Summary of ECG Criteria

a. Rate: Less than 60 per minute.
b. Rhythm: Regular.
c. P waves: Upright in leads 1, 2, aVF.

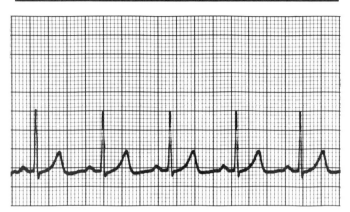

Figure 25. **Normal sinus rhythm.** Note regular rhythm at the rate of 81 beats/min. P waves are upright in Lead 2, consistent with sinus rhythm.

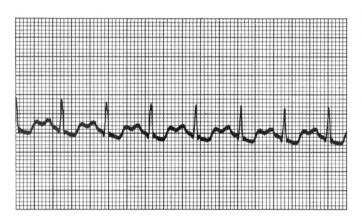

Figure 26. **Sinus tachycardia.** Note regular rhythm at the rate of 121 beats/min. Each QRS is preceded by upright P wave in Lead 2.

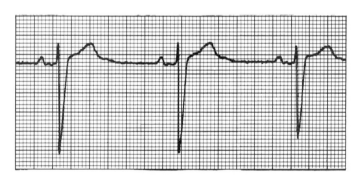

Figure 27. **Sinus bradycardia.** Sinus rate is 46 beats/min and rhythm is regular.

Premature Atrial Complexes (PAC's)
(Figure 28)

Description

A premature atrial complex is an electrical impulse that originates in the atria outside of the sinus node. It is premature, occurring before the next expected sinus beat. Since it arises in the atrium (hence, close to the sinus node), it usually causes depolarization of the sinus node. Therefore, the interval between the premature wave (P′) and the next sinus P wave is equal to (or slightly longer) than the usual P–P interval. It is for this reason that the interval between the sinus P waves preceding and following the PAC is usually less than twice the normal P–P interval (Figure 29). This phenomenon is referred to as a noncompensatory pause. However, on occasions the PAC may suppress the sinus node for a prolonged period, causing a pause that is longer; also, on occasions, the sinus node may not be reset, and a compensatory pause may occur. (The next P wave will occur on time as if unaffected by the premature beat.) A PAC normally may be conducted through the AV node and ventricles, or it may be conducted with partial or complete block at either level. This may give rise to a PAC with first-degree AV block, a blocked (or nonconducted) PAC, or a PAC with aberrant ventricular conduction (usually in the form of right bundle branch block) (Figure 30).

Premature atrial complexes often occur without apparent cause. Clinically, commonly recognized causes include the use of "stimulants" (caffeine, tobacco, alcohol) and sympathomimetic drugs, hypoxia, elevation of atrial pressure, and digitalis intoxication. Premature atrial complexes may initiate other atrial tachycardias (Figure 31).

Summary of ECG Criteria

a. Rhythm: Irregular.
b. P waves: A P′ wave, differing in morphology from that of sinus node origin, occurring before the next expected sinus beat, hence, the P–P′ interval is shorter than the P–P interval. Premature atrial complexes originating from the same focus have similar P′ waves and a similar coupling interval (the P–P′ interval). A noncompensatory pause is usually present.
c. PR interval: The PR interval may be normal or prolonged (i.e., PAC with first-degree AV block). Complete block may occur with no QRS complex following the P′ wave.
d. QRS interval: The QRS may be normal or widened (aberrant ventricular conduction). When aberrant, it usually takes the form of a right bundle branch block.

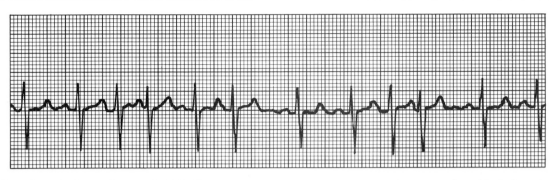

Figure 28. Premature atrial complexes. Multiple PAC's are present (the 3rd, 4th, 6th, 9th, and 10th complexes) resulting in irregular rhythm.

Figure 29. Premature atrial complex. Normal sinus rhythm at the rate of 75 beats/min (P–P interval is 0.80 second). The fourth P wave (indicated by arrow) is premature and differs morphologically from sinus P waves. The accompanying ladder diagram indicates a premature P wave arising in the atrium, outside the sinus node, and conducted normally through the AV node and ventricle. The sinus node was depolarized by PAC; hence, the distance between the normal sinus beat preceding and following PAC (1.32 seconds) is less than twice the P–P interval (0.80 × 2 = 1.60 seconds). A = atrium, AVN = atrioventricular node, V = ventricle.

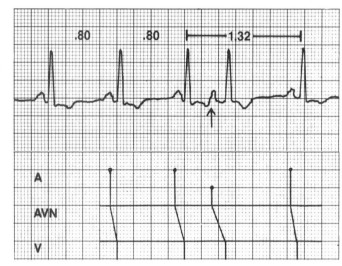

Figure 30. Premature atrial complex with first-degree AV block and aberrant ventricular conduction. The second and fourth P waves (indicated by dot) are PAC's. In both, the P wave falls on the T wave of the preceding beat. In both, the PR interval is prolonged (0.25 second); hence, first-degree AV block is present. The QRS complex of each PAC is prolonged (0.16 second) with morphologic features indicating right bundle branch block.

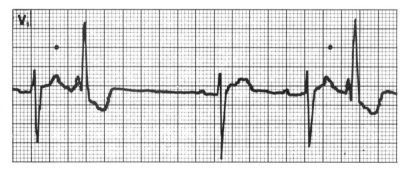

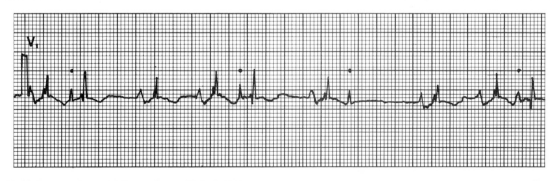

Figure 31. Multiple premature atrial complexes. Multiple PAC's are present and are indicated by the dot above the premature P wave. The third PAC was not conducted to ventricles.

Atrial Tachycardia (AT)

Description (Figures 32, 33)

Atrial tachycardia may be either uniform or multiform. Multiform AT is most often seen in patients with respiratory failure. This section will deal with only two of the multiple clinical forms of uniform AT.

Paroxysmal Supraventricular Tachycardia (PSVT):[5,12] This is a distinct clinical syndrome characterized by repeated episodes (i.e., paroxysms) of AT with an abrupt onset lasting from a few seconds to many hours. They usually end abruptly and often can be terminated by vagal maneuvers. Such paroxysms may recur for many years. An episode of AT is usually initiated by a closely coupled PAC with a prolonged AV node conduction time which is manifested on the surface electrocardiogram by a prolonged PR interval. Studies have indicated that this delayed AV conduction permits the impulse to be deflected back into the atrium, i.e., reentry either at AV node level or through a variety of concealed or apparent bypass tracts (Figure 32). This sequence of events is continuously repeated, resulting in a supraventricular tachycardia. This mechanism is the same as that which induces junctional tachycardia, hence the term "paroxysmal supraventricular tachycardia" employed for both by some authors. Episodes of PAT are usually well tolerated in the young in the absence of other coexistent forms of heart disease. In the elderly, and in those with other forms of heart disease (especially coronary atherosclerosis or stenosis of the mitral or aortic valves), serious problems such as myocardial ischemia, infarction, or pulmonary edema can be precipitated by the rapid heart rate.

Nonparoxysmal Atrial Tachycardia: This arrhythmia is secondary to some other primary event. The most common cause is digitalis intoxication. When the primary event is corrected, the AT may be terminated. Its mechanism of production involves the rapid firing of an automatic focus within either atrium due to enhanced automaticity. Although both the paroxysmal and non-paroxysmal forms of AT may be indistinguishable on the ECG (hence, the importance of an accurate history), certain important ECG clues may be present. In the undigitalized patient, PAT is usually associated with 1:1 AV conduction or 2:1 conduction when the atrial rate exceeds 240 beats/min though on occasion 2:1 block may be seen at slower rates. When nonparoxysmal AT is due to digitalis excess, it is characterized by atrioventricular block which occurs at lower atrial rates or is associated with higher grades of AV block (e.g., 3:1, 4:1, etc.) and more variable conduction (Figure 33). In the latter circumstances, the ventricular rate may be irregular.

Summary of ECG Criteria

a. Rate: The atrial rate is usually 160–240 beats/min.
b. Rhythm: The atrial rhythm is regular. The ventricular rhythm is most often regular with 1:1 AV conduction when the atrial rate is under 200. With atrial rates above 200, 2:1 AV block is common. Higher grades of block may also occur (e.g., with digitalis intoxication).
c. P waves: P waves may be difficult to identify because they can be buried in the preceding T wave. They differ morphologically from sinus P waves when the comparison can be made.
d. PR interval: This interval may be normal or prolonged.
e. QRS interval: The QRS may be normal or prolonged because of bundle branch block or aberrant conduction.

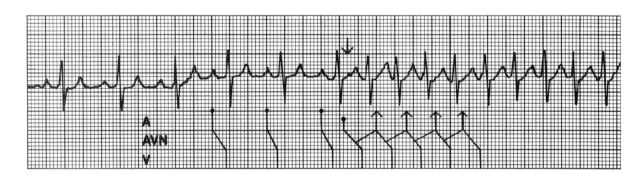

Figure 32. Atrial tachycardia. Initially, a normal sinus rhythm is present. This is interrupted by a PAC (arrow), which initiates an episode of atrial tachycardia with a rate of 185 beats/min. The proposed reentry mechanism at the AV node level is illustrated in the ladder diagram. A = atrium, AVN = AV node, V = ventricle.

Atrial Flutter (Figures 34–36)

Description

This arrhythmia probably is the result of a reentry circuit at the atrial level (Figure 34). Atrial depolarization occurs in a caudad-to-cephalad direction and, hence, is best observed in Leads 2, 3, and aVF. It is often described as resembling a "sawtooth" or "picket fence." Such a wave is called an F wave.

When slower atrial rates (e.g., 220 per minute) are present, it is possible to have 1:1 AV conduction: More commonly, however, there is a physiologic block at AV nodal level because the refractory period of the AV node results in 2:1 AV conduction.

Since the atrial rate is most commonly approximately 300 per minute, 2:1 AV block usually is present and the ventricular rate is usually 150 per minute. AV conduction ratio may be altered by AV nodal disease, increased vagal tone, and certain drugs (e.g., digitalis, propranolol, verapamil), which will induce a higher degree of AV block (3:1, 4:1, etc.) or at times a variable block (Figures 35, 36). Atrial flutter seldom occurs in the absence of organic heart disease. It is seen in association with mitral or tricuspid valvular heart disease, acute or chronic *cor pulmonale,* and coronary heart disease. It is rarely a manifestation of digitalis intoxication.

Summary of ECG Criteria

a. Rate: The atrial rate is usually 300 beats/min, ranging between 220 and 350 beats/min.
b. Rhythm: The atrial rhythm is regular. The ventricular rhythm may be regular if a constant degree of AV block is present (such as 2:1 or, less commonly, 1:1) but can be grossly irregular if variable block is present.
c. P waves: Flutter (F) waves resemble a "sawtooth" or "picket fence" and are best seen in Leads 2, 3, or aVF. In the presence of 2:1 or 1:1 conduction ratios, it may be difficult to identify the F waves. In this instance carotid sinus massage may produce a transient delay in AV node conduction resulting in a higher degree of AV block. This will "uncover" the F waves, permitting their identification.
d. PR interval: Usually the PR interval is regular, but it may vary.
e. QRS interval: This pattern is usually normal, but aberrant ventricular conduction, usually with right bundle branch block can occur.

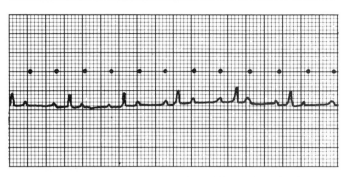

Figure 33. Atrial tachycardia with block. The atrial rate is 200 beats/min, and the rhythm is regular. Every other P wave is conducted to ventricles (2:1 conduction ratio). P waves are indicated by dots.

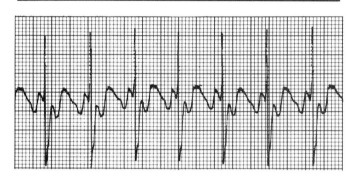

Figure 34. Atrial flutter. The atrial rate is 250 beats/min, and the rhythm is regular. Every other F wave is conducted to ventricles (2:1 block), resulting in regular ventricular rhythm at a rate of 125 beats/min.

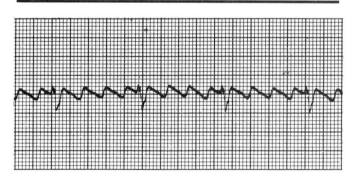

Figure 35. Atrial flutter with high-grade AV block. Atrial rhythm is regular (260 beats/min), but only every fourth F wave is followed by QRS (4:1 conduction).

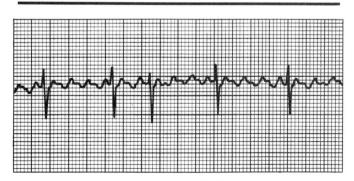

Figure 36. Atrial flutter with variable AV block. Atrial rhythm is regular, but there is variable AV block present (2:1, 4:1 conduction ratios), resulting in irregular ventricular rhythm.

Atrial Fibrillation (AF) (Figures 37–39)

Description

Atrial fibrillation may result from multiple areas of reentry within the atria or from multiple ectopic foci. The atrial electrical activity is very rapid (approximately 400–700 per minute), but each electrical impulse results in the depolarization of only a small islet of atrial myocardium rather than the whole atrium.

As a result, there is no contraction of the atria as a whole. Since there is no uniform atrial depolarization, there is no P wave. The chaotic electrical activity does produce a deflection on the ECG referred to as an "f wave" (Figure 37). Such f waves vary in size and shape and are irregular in rhythm. Transmission of these multiple atrial impulses through the AV node is thought to occur at random, resulting in an irregular rhythm. Some impulses are conducted into but not through the AV node; that is, they are blocked within the AV node. This is a form of "concealed conduction" and is important since such nonconducted impulses contribute to the overall refractoriness of the AV node (Figure 38). It is for this reason that the ventricular rate of AF is often slower (averaging 160–180 per minute) than that seen in AT or atrial flutter with 1:1 conduction. Atrial fibrillation is usually the result of some underlying form of heart disease (usually with congestive heart failure) and may occur intermittently or as a chronic rhythm. It may, however, be seen in a paroxysmal form in which there is no other evidence of heart disease (similar to PAT).

Summary of ECG Criteria

a. Rate: The atrial rate is usually from 400 to 700 per minute but as a rule cannot be counted. In the undigitalized patient the ventricular rate is usually between 160 and 180 per minute.
b. Rhythm: The ventricular rhythm is irregularly irregular except in the presence of digitalis intoxication.
c. P waves: Organized atrial electrical activity is absent, so there are no P waves. Chaotic electrical activity, or f waves, may be seen.
d. QRS interval: Ventricular depolarization is normal unless aberrant ventricular conduction occurs.

Premature Junctional (Nodal) Complexes (PJC's) (Figure 40)

Description

A premature junctional complex is an electrical impulse that originates in the AV junction and occurs before the next expected sinus impulse, usually resulting in retrograde atrial depolarization (hence, the P wave in Leads 2, 3, and aVF will be negative) (Figure 40). The P wave may precede, coincide with, or follow the QRS. The relation of P wave to QRS complex depends on the relative conduction times from the site of origin within the junction to the atria and ventricles. It is likely, therefore, that an impulse arising in the higher portion of the junction, above the AV node (i.e., bundle of His), would result in a P wave occurring before or during the QRS complex whereas one arising at a lower level will result in a P wave that occurs after the QRS complex. Conduction from the junction to the ventricles usually occurs along normal pathways. Thus, the QRS complex is usually normal although it can be wide due to either a bundle branch block or aberrant conduction. The pause following a PJC may be noncompensatory (if the sinus node is depolarized by the premature beat) or fully compensatory if the sinus node has discharged before it is reached by the premature beat. The causes of PJC's are similar to those described for PAC's.

Summary of ECG Criteria

a. Rhythm: Irregular.
b. P waves: Because atrial depolarization is usually retrograde, P waves are generally negative in Leads 2, 3, and aVF. P waves can precede, coincide with, or follow the QRS. Either a noncompensatory or a fully compensatory pause may occur.
c. PR interval: If the P wave precedes the QRS, the PR interval is usually less than 0.12 second. The PR interval may, however, be prolonged. Complete AV block may occur.
d. QRS interval: The QRS may be normal or, if widened, (aberrant ventricular conduction), it usually takes the form of a right bundle branch block.

Junctional Escape Complexes and Rhythms (Figure 41)

Description

The AV junction can function as a pacemaker. Under normal circumstances, because it initiates impulses at a rate of from 40 to 60 per minute (equivalent to an R–R interval between 1.5 and 1.0 seconds) the sinus node pacemaker, which is faster, predominates. If the AV node is not depolarized by the arrival of a sinus impulse within approximately 1.0–1.5 seconds, it will initiate an impulse. This is called a junctional escape complex. It occurs because of failure of the sinus node to initiate an

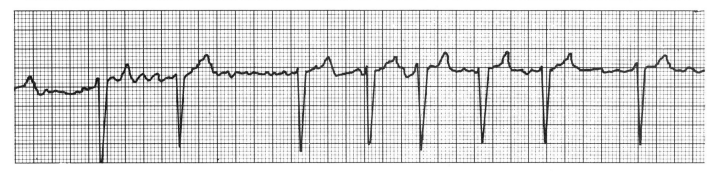

Figure 37.   Atrial fibrillation with controlled ventricular response. Note irregular undulations of baseline representing atrial electrical activity (f waves). The f waves vary in size and shape and are irregular in rhythm. Conduction through AV node occurs at random; hence, ventricular rhythm is irregular.

Figure 38.   Atrial fibrillation with rapid ventricular response.

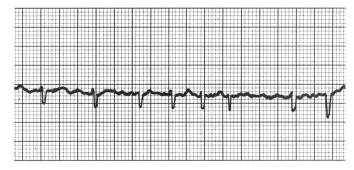

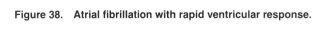

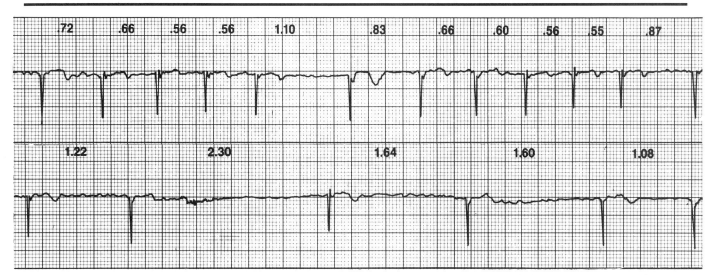

Figure 39.   Atrial fibrillation with Type I second-degree AV block and high-grade AV block. In upper tracing, note that R–R intervals (indicated by number above ECG) become progressively shorter prior to pause. Cycle is then repeated. The mechanism of this phenomenon may involve high-grade block in the AV node and the emergence of a junctional pacemaker with exit block. In lower tracing, note long R–R intervals indicative of high-grade AV block. Patient had digitalis intoxication (serum digoxin level was 3.0 ng/mL and serum potassium was 3.2 mEq/L). The time interval between upper and lower tracing was approximately 30 seconds.

Figure 40.   Premature junctional complexes. Third and fifth complexes occur early and are initiated by inverted P waves. In Lead 2 this is consistent with retrograde atrial depolarization.

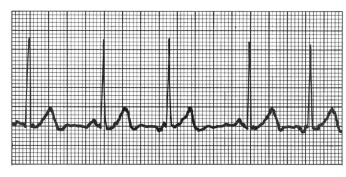

appropriately timed impulse or because of some problem with conduction between the sinus node and the AV junction (Figure 41). A series of such impulses in series is referred to as a junctional escape rhythm.

Summary of ECG Criteria

a. Rate: A junctional escape rhythm has a rate of between 40 and 60 per minute.
b. Rhythm: The presence of some junctional escape complexes may lead to an irregular rhythm. Junctional escape complexes occur approximately 1.0 second or more following the last depolarization. A junctional escape rhythm is usually regular.
c. P waves: Retrograde P waves (negative) may be seen in Leads 2, 3, and aVF. P waves may precede, coincide with, or follow the QRS. Sinus P waves, at a rate equal to or slower than the junctional rhythm, may occur. This may result in atrioventricular dissociation (discussed in more detail in "Ventricular Tachycardia").
d. PR interval: This interval is variable but is usually less than the PR interval of the normally conducted beat from the sinus node.
e. QRS interval: Ventricular conduction is usually normal unless a ventricular conduction problem is present or aberrant conduction occurs (see Part I).

Premature Ventricular Complex (PVC)
(Figures 42–50)

Description

A premature ventricular complex is a depolarization that arises in either ventricle prior to the next expected sinus beat, i.e., prematurely (Figure 42). It may result from the firing of an automatic focus or by reentry.

Since PVC's originate in the ventricle, the normal sequence of ventricular depolarization is altered — i.e., instead of the two ventricles depolarizing simultaneously, they depolarize sequentially (Figure 43). In addition, conduction occurs more slowly through myocardium than through specialized conduction pathways. This results in a wide (0.12 second or greater) and bizarre-appearing QRS. The sequence of repolarization is also altered, usually resulting in a ST segment and T wave in a direction opposite to the QRS complex.

The interval between the previous normal beat and the PVC (the coupling interval) usually remains constant when PVC's are due to reentry from the same focus (uniform PVC's). When the coupling interval and the QRS morphology vary, the PVC's may be arising from different areas within the ventricles; or if arising from a single focus, ventricular conduction may vary (Figure 44). Such PVC's are referred to as multifocal or, more appropriately, multiformed.

A PVC may occur nearly simultaneously with the firing of the sinus node. The antegrade impulse originating in the sinus node (resulting in normal atrial depolarization)

and the retrograde impulse traveling towards the atria from the ventricles may meet in the AV node. Then neither can spread further because of the refractory period of the other.

Since the rhythm of the sinus node is not disturbed, a fully compensatory pause usually results (i.e., the next P wave should occur at the proper time) (Figure 45). In this instance the interval between the normal beat preceding the PVC and the normal beat following the PVC are equal to twice the normal sinus (P–P) interval. However, on occasions retrograde conduction can spread to the atria and reset the SA node. Also, the sinus rate can be so slow that the PVC occurs long before the next sinus P; hence, the PVC occurs — between two sinus complexes — which is known as interpolation of the premature beat (Figure 46). In neither of these cases will a compensatory pause occur. The sinus impulse following an interpolated PVC may have a prolonged PR interval because of retrograde conduction from the ventricle into the AV node where it is blocked by the refractory period of the AV node. Since it is conducted into the AV node, however, it may further prolong the refractory period of the AV node (an example of the phenomenon of concealed conduction) and lead to a prolonged PR interval in the next sinus beat. Occasionally, a longer than fully compensatory pause may be seen. This may be due to the presence of sinoatrial block which delays atrial depolarization.

PVC's may occur as isolated complexes, or they may occur repetitively in succession in pairs (two PVC's in a row) (see Figure 47). When three or more PVC's occur in a row, ventricular tachycardia is present.

If every other beat is a PVC, ventricular bigeminy is present (Figure 48). If every third beat is a PVC, the term ventricular trigeminy is used; if every fourth beat is a PVC, ventricular quadrigeminy is present; and so forth.

A PVC that falls on the T wave (during the so-called vulnerable period of ventricular repolarization) may precipitate ventricular tachycardia or ventricular fibrillation (Figure 49). However, PVC's occurring after the T wave may also initiate such ventricular tachycardia.[15,16] (See Figure 50.)

Summary of ECG Criteria

a. Rhythm: Irregular.
b. P waves: The sinus P wave is usually obscured by the QRS, ST segment, or T wave of the PVC. It may, however, sometimes be recognized as a notching during the ST segment or T wave. Retrograde P waves may occur. The presence of a sinus P wave (when it cannot be seen) may be inferred by the presence of a fully compensatory pause.
c. QRS, ST segment, T wave: 1) The PVC is premature — i.e., it must occur before the next expected sinus beat unless atrial fibrillation is present since preactivity

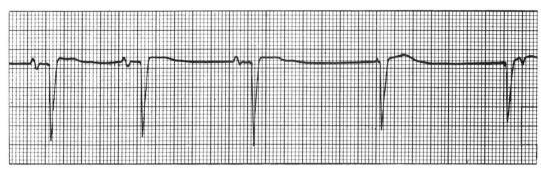

Figure 41. Junctional escape complexes. Sinus bradycardia with prolonging P–P interval (sinus arrhythmia) is present. Second P–P interval is 1.2 seconds. Third P–P interval is 1.5 seconds, but before it can be conducted to ventricles, QRS occurs. Morphology is similar to sinus beats, consistent with site of origin in AV junction. Fifth QRS also represents junctional escape complex.

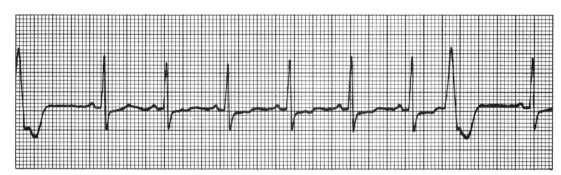

Figure 42. Premature ventricular complex.

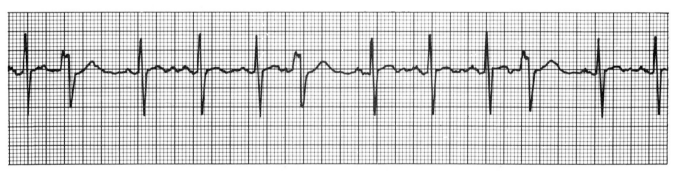

Figure 43. Unifocal premature ventricular complexes. Note occurrence of wide, premature QRS complexes with no preceding P wave. Interval between preceding normal QRS and PVC (coupling interval) remains constant and morphology remains the same.

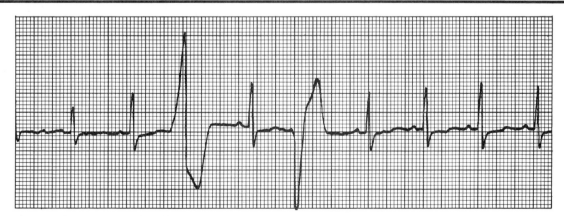

Figure 44. Multiformed premature ventricular complexes. Note variation in morphology and in coupling interval of PVC's.

cannot be assessed. 2) The width of the QRS is 0.12 second or greater. 3) The QRS morphology is often bizarre, with notching. 4) The ST segment and T wave are usually opposite in polarity to the QRS. 5) When multiformed (or multifocal), both the coupling interval and morphology of the QRS vary. 6) A fully compensatory pause is usually present.

Ventricular Tachycardia (VT) (Figure 51)

Description[17]

When three or more beats of ventricular origin occur in succession at a rate in excess of 100 per minute, ventricular tachycardia is present (Figure 51). The rhythm is usually regular, but on occasion it may be irregular. This arrhythmia may be well tolerated or associated with grave, life-threatening hemodynamic compromise. The hemodynamic consequences of VT depend largely on the presence or absence of myocardial dysfunction (such as might result from ischemia or infarction) and on the rate of the VT. Atrioventricular dissociation usually is present. This means that the sinus node is depolarizing the atria in a normal manner at a rate either equal to or slower than the ventricular rate. Thus, sinus P waves sometimes can be recognized between QRS complexes. They bear no fixed relationship to the QRS complexes

unless the atrial and ventricular rates happen to be equal. Conduction from atria to ventricles is usually prevented because the AV node and/or ventricular conduction system is refractory due to ventricular depolarizations. Sometimes retrograde conduction from ventricles to atria occurs. In this instance, there will be a relation between the QRS complex and the retrograde P wave. Thus, it may be very difficult to distinguish VT from a supraventricular tachycardia with aberrant ventricular conduction. This topic will be discussed below.

Occasionally, an atrial impulse arrives when the AV node and His–Purkinje system is not refractory and AV conduction can occur. This results in a "capture beat" in which ventricular conduction occurs over the normal pathways, resulting in a normal-appearing (narrow) QRS complex. A capture beat occurs at a shorter R–R interval than the R–R interval of the VT. Atrioventricular conduction also may occur simultaneously with depolarization of the ventricular focus. In this instance, the ventricle will be depolarized in part over the normal pathway and in part from the ventricular focus. The resulting QRS complex will be intermediate in morphology between a normal QRS and a QRS of ventricular origin. In this instance the R–R interval will not change. This is called a "fusion beat." Ventricular tachycardia may be monomorphic (all QRS's with the same shape) or polymorphic (varying QRS shapes during the tachycardia).

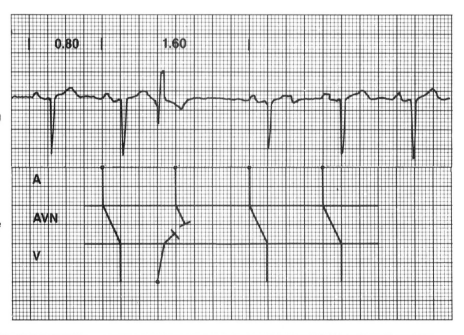

Figure 45. Premature ventricular complex with fully compensatory pause. Two normal sinus beats are followed by premature, wide QRS which is not preceded by P wave. As illustrated in accompanying ladder diagram, firing of sinus node was not disturbed; therefore, next sinus beat comes at expected time. Hence, interval between normal beat preceding and following PVC is twice normal sinus interval. This is a fully compensatory pause. Sinus impulse that occurs coincident with PVC depolarizes atria but cannot reach ventricles because it is blocked in AV node by refractory period of impulse that arose in ventricle and is attempting to reach atria retrogradely. Neither impulse can be conducted through AV node because it is blocked by refractory period of the other. A = atrium, AVN = AV node, V = ventricle.

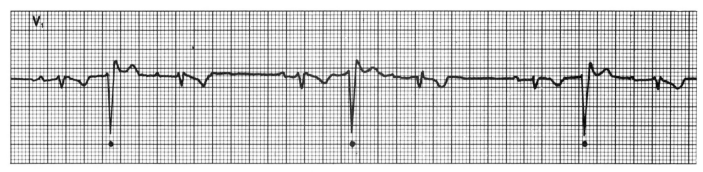

Figure 46.   Interpolated premature ventricular complexes. Second, fifth, and eighth QRS complexes (indicated by dot) are PVC's. Note that there is no pause, i.e., R–R interval of sinus beats remains unchanged. Note also that PR interval following PVC is longer than that preceding PVC. This indicates there was retrograde conduction from ventricles into, but not through, AV node (concealed conduction).

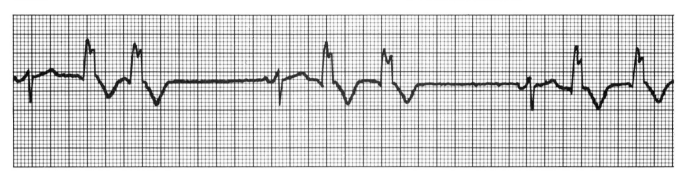

Figure 47.   Pairs of premature ventricular complexes.

Figure 48.   Ventricular bigeminy.
Note that every other beat is PVC. Both coupling interval and morphology remain constant; hence, they are unifocal.

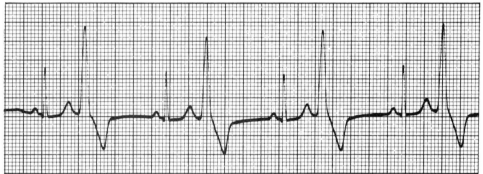

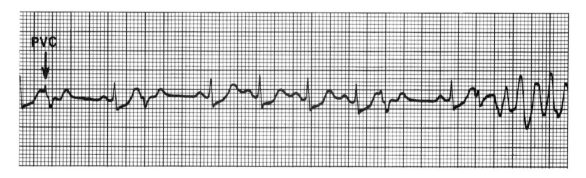

Figure 49.   R-on-T phenomenon. Multiple PVC's are present. On right side of illustration, a PVC falls on downslope of T wave, precipitating ventricular fibrillation.

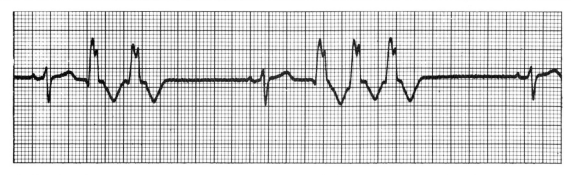

Figure 50.   Precipitation of ventricular tachycardia by late cycle PVC. Note brief salvo of ventricular tachycardia that is initiated by PVC occurring well beyond T wave.

Figure 51.   Ventricular tachycardia. The rhythm is regular at rate of 158 beats/min. The QRS is wide. No evidence of atrial depolarization is seen.

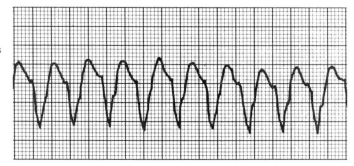

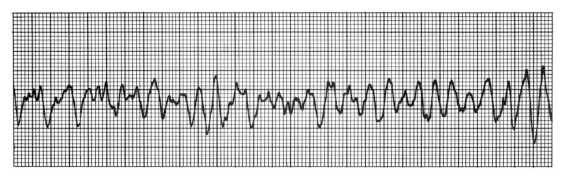

Figure 52.   Coarse ventricular fibrillation. Note high amplitude waveforms, which vary in size, shape, and rhythm representing chaotic ventricular electrical activity.

Figure 53.   Fine ventricular fibrillation. By comparison to Figure 52, amplitude of electrical activity is much reduced.

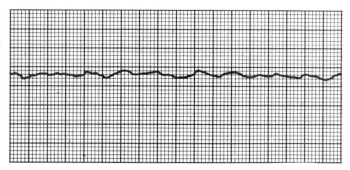

Summary of ECG Criteria

a. Rate: The rate is greater than 100 per minute and usually not faster than 220 per minute.
b. Rhythm: The rhythm of the VT is usually regular but may be irregular.
c. P waves: In rapid VT, the P waves are often not recognizable. At slower ventricular rates P waves may be recognized and may represent normal atrial depolarization from the sinus node at a rate slower than the VT (or occasionally at the same rate), but the electrical activities do not affect one another. This is known as atrioventricular dissociation. Since the atria and ventricles are usually beating at different rates, there is no fixed relation between the P wave and the QRS. In other instances retrograde ventriculo-atrial conduction may occur, resulting in a fixed QRS–P relationship.
d. QRS: The QRS, ST segment, and T wave were described in the section dealing with PVC's. Occasionally, a QRS complex that is narrow may occur after a short preceding R–R interval (capture beat), or a QRS complex may be seen with morphologic features intermediate between a beat of ventricular origin and one of supraventricular origin but with a constant R–R interval (fusion beat).

Torsade de Pointes

Torsade de pointes is an unusual form of ventricular tachycardia in which the QRS's appear to be constantly changing. It gets its name from the fact that it looks as if the electrical activity is twisted into a helix. This form of ventricular tachycardia is usually due to toxicity or an idiosyncratic reaction to Type IA antiarrhythmic agents such as quinidine, procainamide, or disopyramide or other agents that prolong the QT interval. This arrhythmia is usually accompanied by prolongation of the QT interval. The QT interval is measured from the onset of the Q wave to the end of the T wave. At most rates the QT interval is 0.40 second or less though it may be prolonged at slow rates. If the QT is abnormally prolonged in a patient receiving a Type IA antiarrhythmic agent, the possibility of inducing *torsade* should be considered.

Ventricular Fibrillation (VF)
(Figures 52, 53)

Description

Ventricular fibrillation is a ventricular rhythm in which there are multiple areas within the ventricles exhibiting varying degrees of depolarization and repolarization (Figure 52). Since there is no organized ventricular depolarization, the ventricles do not contract as a unit. When observed, the ventricular myocardium appears to be quivering.

There is no cardiac output. This is the most common mechanism of cardiac arrest resulting from myocardial ischemia or infarction. The terms "coarse" and "fine" have been used to describe the amplitude of these waveforms (see Figure 53). Coarse VF usually indicates the recent onset of VF, which can be readily corrected by prompt defibrillation. In the presence of fine VF, there has usually been a considerable delay since collapse, and successful resuscitation is unusual.

Summary of ECG Criteria

a. Rate: The rate of VF is very rapid but usually too disorganized to count.
b. Rhythm: The rhythm is irregular. The electrical waveforms vary in size and shape. There is no P wave, QRS, ST segment, or T wave. On occasion, VF may masquerade in one lead as asystole.

Ventricular Asystole (Cardiac Standstill) (Figure 54)

Description

Ventricular systole represents the total absence of ventricular electrical activity. Since depolarization does not occur, there is no ventricular contraction. This may occur as a primary event in cardiac arrest, or it may follow VF or electromechanical dissociation (EMD) (see Chapter 16).

Ventricular asystole can occur also in patients with

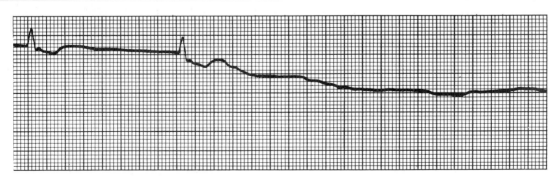

Figure 54. Ventricular asystole. Only two QRS complexes are seen, probably representing ventricular escape beats. This is followed by absence of electrical activity.

complete heart block in whom there is no escape pacemaker (see "Third-Degree Atrioventricular Block"). Ventricular fibrillation may masquerade as asystole; it is best always to check two leads perpendicular to each other to make sure that the rhythm is not ventricular fibrillation. If there is any question that it might be VF, it should be treated as VF.

Summary of ECG Criteria

There is a complete absence of any ventricular electrical activity. Sometimes, however, P waves may occur.

Atrioventricular Block (AV Block)

Description[18]

Atrioventricular block is defined as a delay or interruption in conduction between atria and ventricles. It may be due to 1) lesions along the conduction pathway (e.g., calcium, fibrosis, necrosis), 2) increases in the refractory period of some portion of the conduction pathway (such as may occur in the AV node when a digitalis preparation is administered), or 3) shortening of the supraventricular cycle length with encroachment on the normal refractory period (such as with atrial flutter in which 2:1 AV block at the level of the AV node occurs because the normal AV node refractory period will not allow conduction at a rate of 300 beats/min but will allow it at 150 beats/min).

AV block may be classified in two ways:

1. According to the degree of block:
   a. Partial
      (i) First-degree AV block
      (ii) Second-degree AV block, Type I and Type II
   b. Third-degree or complete AV block

2. According to the site of block:
   a. AV node
   b. Infranodal
      (i) Bundle of His
      (ii) Bundle branches

It must be recognized that each degree of block (first-degree, second-degree, third-degree) may occur either at the AV node level or below it. This distinction is not academic since the pathogenesis, treatment, and prognosis may differ.

First-Degree AV Block (Figure 55)

Description: First-degree AV block is simply a delay in passage of the impulse from atria to ventricles. This delay usually occurs at the level of the AV node but may be infranodal.

Summary of ECG Criteria:
a. Rhythm: Regular.
b. P waves: Each P wave is followed by a QRS complex.
c. PR interval: This interval is prolonged beyond 0.20 second. It usually remains constant but may vary.
d. QRS: The QRS morphology is unaffected.

Second-Degree AV Block (Figures 56-58)[18-20]

In second-degree AV block, some impulses are conducted while others are blocked. This type of block is divided into two additional types.

Type I Second-Degree AV Block (Wenckebach):
Description: This form of block almost always occurs at the level of the AV node (rarely at His bundle or bundle branch level) and is often due to increased parasympathetic tone or to drug effect (e.g., digitalis, propranolol, or verapamil). It is usually a transient phenomenon, and

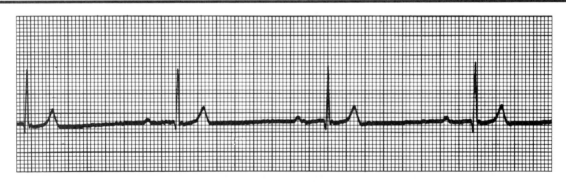

Figure 55. **First-degree AV block.** The PR interval is prolonged to 0.31 second.

short- and long-term prognosis is good. It is characterized by a progressive prolongation of the PR interval indicative of decreasing conduction velocity through the AV node before an impulse is completely blocked (see Figure 56). Usually, only a single impulse is blocked, then the pattern is repeated.

The repetition of this pattern results in "group beating" — e.g., three conducted sinus beats with progressively lengthening PR intervals and a fourth sinus beat that is not followed by a QRS. Such a "group" is referred to as "4:3 conduction." Although the conduction ratio may remain constant, it is not unusual for it to change — e.g., 4.3, 3:2, 2:1 (Figure 57). When the ratio is 2:1, obviously one cannot detect prolongation of the PR interval. In this case the diagnosis of Type I second-degree AV block is based on the presence of a normal QRS duration and more typical Wenckebach periods at other times. The ventricular rhythm is irregular except in the presence of 2:1 block.

In addition to a gradual prolongation of the PR interval, the typical Wenckebach is characterized by a decreasing R–R interval prior to the dropped beat (Figure 58). This is due to the fact that the increment of PR prolongation becomes progressively less. The recognition of a de-

creasing R–R interval prior to a pause is the only way that Type I second-degree AV block can be recognized in the presence of atrial fibrillation since P waves cannot be observed. This may be an important clue to the presence of digitalis intoxication (Figure 59). In atypical forms of Wenckebach block, however, the R–R interval may remain constant for variable periods of time or may lengthen prior to a nonconducted beat.

Summary of ECG Criteria:

a. Rate: The atrial rate is unaffected, but the ventricular rate will be less than the atrial rate because of the nonconducted beats.

b. Rhythm: The atrial rhythm is usually regular. The ventricular rhythm is usually irregular with progressive shortening of the R–R interval before the block impulse. The R–R interval that brackets the nonconducted P wave is less than twice the normal cycle length.

c. P waves: The P waves will appear normal, and each P wave will be followed by a QRS complex except for the blocked P wave.

d. PR interval: There is a progressive increase in PR interval until one P wave is blocked.

e. QRS: The QRS complex is unaffected.

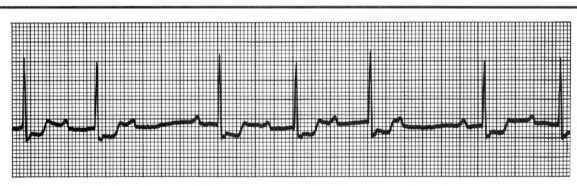

Figure 56. Second-degree AV block, Type I. Atrial rhythm is nearly regular, but there are pauses in ventricular rhythm because every fourth P wave does not conduct into ventricles. Note progressive prolongation of PR interval indicating increasing conduction delay in AV node prior to nonconducted beat. There are four P waves and three QRS complexes in this example representing a 4:3 cycle. The QRS complexes are normal.

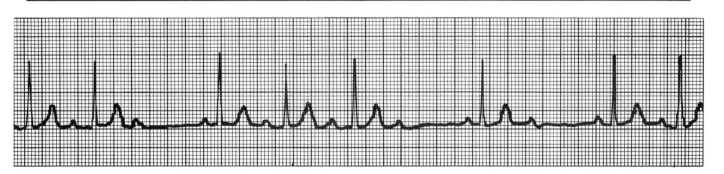

Figure 57. Second-degree AV block Type I, with variable conduction ratios. First cycle is 3:2, then 4:3, followed by 2:1 cycle.

Type II Second-Degree AV Block (Figure 59):

Description: This form of second-degree AV block occurs below the level of the AV node either at bundle of His (uncommon) or bundle branch level (more common). It is usually associated with an organic lesion in the conduction pathway, and unlike Type I second-degree AV block, it is rarely the result of increased parasympathetic tone or drug effect. It is thus associated with a poorer prognosis, and complete heart block may develop. A hallmark of this type second-degree AV block is that the PR interval does not lengthen prior to a dropped beat. It is not unusual for more than one nonconducted beat to occur in succession. This type of block most often occurs at the level of the bundle branches. In order for a dropped beat to occur, there must be complete block in one bundle branch (i.e., right or left bundle branch block) with intermittent interruption in conduction in the con-tralateral bundle as well. As such, Type II second-degree AV block is associated with a wide QRS complex (Figure 59). When block occurs at His bundle level, the QRS may be narrow since ventricular conduction is not disturbed in those beats that are not blocked. The rhythm may be irregular when block is intermittent or when the conduction ratio is variable. With a constant conduction ratio (e.g., 2:1) the ventricular rhythm is regular.

Summary of ECG Criteria:

a. Rate: The atrial rate is unaffected, but the ventricular rate will be less than the atrial rate.
b. Rhythm: The atrial rhythm is usually regular, whereas the ventricular rhythm may be regular or irregular, with pauses corresponding to the nonconducted beats.
c. P waves: The P waves will appear normal and each will be followed by a QRS except for the blocked P wave.
d. PR interval: This interval may be normal or prolonged in duration, but it will remain constant. There may be shortening of the PR interval following a pause.
e. QRS: This interval will be normal when the level of block is at the bundle of His. However, the QRS will be widened with the features of bundle branch block if the level of block is at the level of the bundle branches.

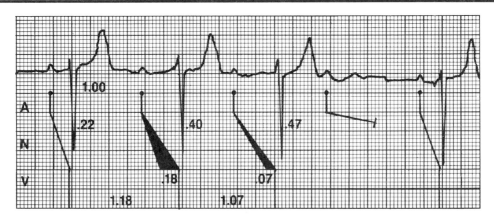

Figure 58. Second-degree AV block Type I, demonstrating progressive shortening of R–R interval. In ladder diagram, dot below each P wave represents firing of sinus node, and vertical line extending down from dot represents atrial depolarization. Slanted line represents conduction through AV node. Subsequent vertical line represents ventricular depolarization. Time is indicated on horizontal axis. A 4:3 Wenckebach cycle is shown. The P–P interval is 1.00 second (rate 60 beats/min). There is progressive prolongation of PR interval (0.22, 0.40, 0.47 second) before failure of conduction occurs. Despite progressive prolongation of PR interval, R–R interval becomes progressively shorter (1.18, 1.07 seconds). The reason is that increment of PR prolongation (indicated by shaded area) becomes progressively shorter. The R–R interval is obtained by adding increment of PR prolongation to P–P interval: 0.18 + 1.00 = 1.18; 0.07 + 1.00 = 1.07. A = atrium, N = AV node, V = ventricle.

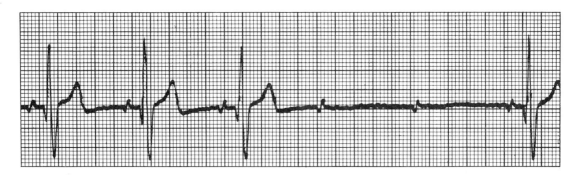

Figure 59. Second-degree AV block Type II. In this example there are three conducted sinus beats followed by two nonconducted P waves. The PR interval of conducted beats remains constant and QRS is wide.

Third-Degree AV Block (Figures 60–62)

Description: Third-degree AV block indicates complete absence of conduction between atria and ventricles. It may occur at AV node (see Figure 60), bundle of His, or bundle branch level. This distinction, as discussed for second-degree AV block, is not merely academic since the pathogenesis, treatment, and prognosis may vary considerably depending on the level of block. When third-degree AV block occurs at the level of the AV node, a junctional escape pacemaker frequently will initiate ventricular depolarization. This is usually a stable pacemaker with a rate between 40–60 per minute. Since it is located above the bifurcation of the bundle of His, the sequence of ventricular depolarization usually is normal, resulting in a normal QRS. This type of third-degree AV block can result from increased parasympathetic tone associated with inferior infarction from drug effect (e.g., digitalis, propranolol), or from damage to the AV node. Third-degree AV block with a junctional escape rhythm is usually transient and is associated with a favorable prognosis.

When third-degree AV block occurs at the infranodal level, it is most often due to block involving both bundle branches. This indicates the presence of extensive infranodal conduction system disease. When it results from coronary atherosclerosis, it is usually associated with extensive anterior myocardial infarction. It usually does not result from increases in parasympathetic tone or from drug effects. The only escape mechanism available is in the ventricle distal to the site of block. Such a ventricular escape pacemaker has an intrinsic rate that is slow, less than 40 beats/min. Like any depolarization originating in a ventricle, the QRS complex will be wide (Figure 61). It is not a stable pacemaker, and episodes of ventricular asystole are common (Figure 62).

Summary of ECG Criteria:

a. Rate: The atrial rate will be unaffected by third-degree AV block, and the ventricular rate will be slower than the atrial rate. With third-degree AV block, the ventricular rate is usually 40–60 per minute; with infranodal third-degree AV block, the ventricular rate is usually less than 40 per minute.

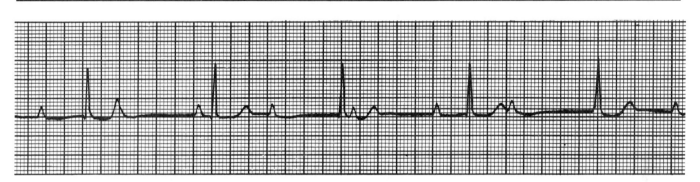

Figure 60. Third-degree AV block occurring at level of AV node. Atrial rhythm is slightly irregular due to presence of sinus arrhythmia. Ventricular rhythm is regular at slower rate (44 beats/min). There is no constant PR interval. The QRS complexes are narrow, indicating supraventricular origin below level of block.

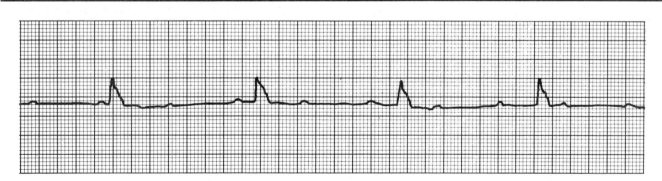

Figure 61. Third-degree AV block occurring at ventricular level. In this example, as in Figure 44, there is no relation between atrial and ventricular rhythm. Ventricular rhythm is regular at very slow rate (38 beats/min). The QRS is wide because block is at bundle branch level, and ventricular pacemaker is distal to that level.

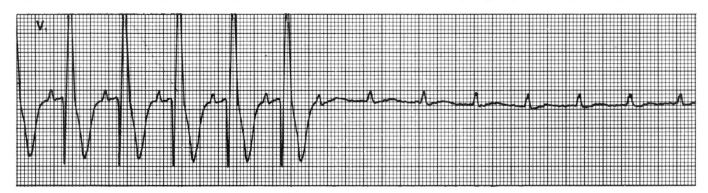

Figure 62.   Third-degree AV block with ventricular asystole. Rhythm strip is from patient with acute anterior myocardial infarction who developed right bundle branch block as indicated by wide QRS complex with terminal R wave (left half of rhythm strip). Complete heart block abruptly developed. On right side of rhythm strip only P waves are seen. There is absence of ventricular escape resulting in ventricular asystole.

b. Rhythm: The atrial rhythm is usually regular although sinus arrhythmia may be present. The ventricular rhythm will be regular.

c. P waves: Normal.

d. PR interval: Since the atria and ventricles are depolarized from different pacemakers, they are independent of each other and the PR interval will vary.

e. QRS: When block occurs at AV node or bundle of His level, the QRS complex will appear normal. When block occurs at bundle branch level, the QRS complex will be widened.

The major characteristics for heart blocks are summarized in Figure 63.

Supraventricular and Ventricular Complexes and Rhythm

It can, at times, be difficult to differentiate 1) ventricular ectopic beats or ventricular tachycardia from 2) supraventricular ectopic beats or supraventricular tachycardia with aberrant ventricular conduction.[17] The problem is very complex, and sometimes the differentiation is virtually impossible even by experienced electrocardiographers. The clinical significance of the distinction, however, may be considerable, since ventricular tachycardia is a potentially life-threatening arrhythmia, usually requiring more immediate treatment while supraventricular arrhythmias usually are less dangerous.

The most salient features used in the differentiation of isolated beats are as follows:

1. Premature atrial complexes with aberration are characterized by a wide QRS complex preceded by a premature P wave (Figure 64). The premature P wave may be difficult to identify since it may be buried in the preceding T wave. Often one can identify some distortion of the T wave. In the case of premature junctional complexes, a premature P wave may not be identifiable.

ECG FEATURE		FIRST-DEGREE	SECOND-DEGREE	THIRD-DEGREE (COMPLETE)
RATE	A	UNAFFECTED	UNAFFECTED	UNAFFECTED
	V	SAME AS A	SLOWER THAN A	SLOWER THAN A
VENTRICULAR RHYTHM		SAME AS A	TYPE I: IRREGULAR TYPE II: IRREGULAR OR REGULAR	REGULAR
P–QRS RELATIONSHIP		CONSISTENT 1:1	TYPE I: VARIABLE (RECURRING PATTERN) TYPE II: FIXED	ABSENT
QRS DURATION		UNAFFECTED	TYPE I: NARROW TYPE II: USUALLY WIDE	DEPENDS ON SITE OF ESCAPE RHYTHM
SITE OF BLOCK		ANYWHERE FROM AV NODE TO BUNDLE BRANCHES	TYPE I: AV NODE TYPE II: HIS OR BELOW	ANYWHERE FROM AV NODE TO BUNDLE BRANCHES

Figure 63.   Summary of ECG features of AV block.

2. Aberrant conduction may take the form of either right or left bundle branch block although the former is more common.

3. In the presence of atrial fibrillation, the occurrence of a wide QRS complex in V_1 (or other right precordial lead) with right bundle branch block morphology (RSR') following a normally conducted beat which is preceded by a relatively long R–R interval favors aberrant conduction (Ashman phenomenon); however, if the coupling between the normal beat and the following wide beat is repetitive and constant, they are probably PVC's (see Figure 65). When a wide QRS tachycardia develops, an irregularly irregular rhythm of the aberrantly conducted beats favors a supraventricular origin (Figure 66).

Wellens and associates have studied the distinction between a supraventricular or ventricular site of origin in patients with tachycardia and a wide QRS complex.[17] They found that the following features favor the presence of ventricular tachycardia:

1. Atrioventricular dissociation: As was pointed out previously, atrioventricular dissociation is not always present since ventriculo-atrial conduction can occur.

Figure 64. Premature atrial complex with aberrant ventricular conduction. Fourth QRS complex is wide, with RSR′ configuration indicating block of right bundle branch. It is preceded by a premature P wave that distorts the T wave of the previous beat.

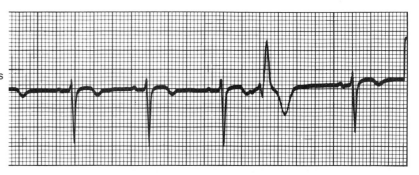

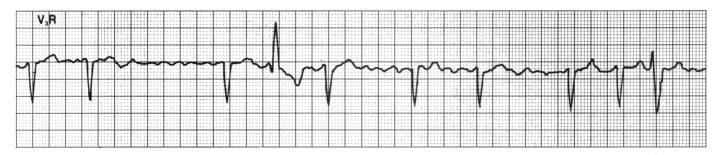

Figure 65. Atrial fibrillation with aberrant conduction. Fourth QRS complex is wide, with morphologic features of right bundle branch block (RSR′). It is preceded by a normally conducted QRS which follows a long R–R interval.

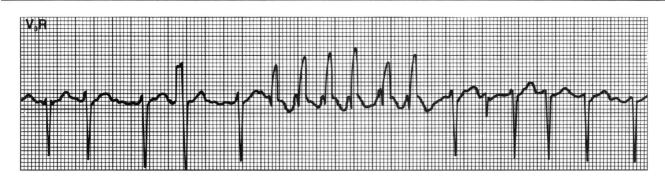

Figure 66. Atrial fibrillation with aberrant conduction simulating ventricular tachycardia. Sixth through eleventh QRS complexes are wide with features of right bundle branch block (RSR′). Rhythm remains irregular throughout. This is also an example of the Ashman phenomenon.

However, the presence of atrioventricular dissociation or the occurrence of fusion or capture beats (although rare) is diagnostic of ventricular tachycardia.

2. A QRS duration greater than 0.14 second.
3. A monophasic or biphasic "right bundle branch-like" QRS complex in V_1 (rather than the typical triphasic RSR′ of right bundle branch block).
4. Left axis deviation in the frontal plane during tachycardia which is not present in the absence of tachycardia.

In the final judgement, clinical observation of the patient should determine the gravity of the situation, recognizing that a ventricular arrhythmia is more likely to cause hemodynamic decompensation. Emergency therapy should be so directed by the hemodynamic consequences of the arrhythmia.

Conclusion

This section has provided a brief description of cardiac rhythm disturbances commonly encountered in the emergency cardiac care setting. It is important that both the individual arrhythmias and their significance be recognized promptly so that appropriate therapy can be instituted.

Part IV: Therapy

This section will only superficially cover arrhythmias that are not usually life threatening. Life threatening and potentially life threatening arrhythmias are covered in Chapter 16. Cardiac arrest is also covered in that chapter.

Atrial Arrhythmias

Premature Atrial Complexes (PAC's)[21-24]

Premature atrial complexes seldom require therapy. Though some physicians have advocated treating premature atrial complexes in order to prevent atrial flutter or atrial fibrillation, there is no data that supports this approach. Premature atrial complexes can occur in normal individuals. Few patients become symptomatic with premature atrial complexes. If the patient becomes symptomatic with PAC's, reassurance that this is not a serious problem frequently will relieve the symptoms. Removal of stimulants can also decrease the incidence of PAC's in some individuals. Cessation of smoking, reduction in the use of caffeine-based beverages and other stimulants (amphetamines, cocaine, etc.) should be attempted first. Encouraging the patient to obtain proper sleep and exercise also may be of benefit. The patient who remains symptomatic after these interventions may respond to one of several different therapies. Sedation or the use of tranquilizers may be of benefit. Specific drugs that can be tried include quinidine, procainamide, verapamil, beta-adrenergic blocking agents, and diltiazem. The drugs may be effective; however, suppression of PAC's can be difficult. Flecainide and amiodarone can also suppress PAC's, but their potentially serious side effects preclude their use for PAC's.

One special consideration is the patient having very frequent early PAC's that do not conduct and result in a slow underlying heart rate. For example, a patient with atrial bigeminy and an average heart rate of 80 per minute may have an effective rate of only 40 and be symptomatic. If the PAC's are contributing to an effective bradycardia, first look for a cause. Several drugs, including digitalis (toxicity), clonidine, methyldopa, guanethidine, beta-adrenergic blocking agents, verapamil, and diltiazem can be implicated. If one of these agents is present, discontinue it and observe to see if the symptoms abate. If bradycardia persists, then a pacemaker may be required.

Paroxysmal Atrial Tachycardia (PAT)

This is considered to be a form of PSVT and is discussed in Chapter 16.

Atrial Flutter[21-24]

Atrial flutter may be associated with sick sinus syndrome, hypoxia, pericarditis, valvular heart disease, and less commonly, acute myocardial infarction. This rhythm usually presents with 2:1 AV block and a ventricular rate of about 150 beats/min. If the patient is hypotensive, having ischemic pain, or in severe congestive heart failure, synchronized cardioversion is the treatment of choice. If the patient is only mildly symptomatic, then an attempt might be made to control the rate with pharmacological therapy first; however, some feel that atrial flutter should always be cardioverted initially if possible. The ventricular rate can be slowed with digitalis, verapamil or beta-blocking agents. Verapamil and beta blockers may exacerbate bradycardia and/or congestive heart failure. If digitalis is used to control the rate, care must be taken to keep from causing intoxication. Once the rate is controlled, the patient can be placed on a Type I antiarrhythmic agent, such as quinidine or procainamide to convert flutter. After a reasonable trial of pharmacological conversion, the patient should be electronically cardioverted.

Atrial Fibrillation[21-24]

Atrial fibrillation may be associated with sick sinus syndrome, hypoxia, increased atrial pressure, pericarditis, and many other conditions. In the setting of acute ischemic heart disease, increased left atrial pressure secondary to congestive heart failure is the most common cause. If the patient with atrial fibrillation and a rapid ventricular response presents *in extremis,* synchronized cardioversion is the treatment of choice. Hypotension induced by atrial fibrillation is usually seen only in patients with acute myocardial infarction or abnormalities of ventricular filling, e.g., IHSS or mitral stenosis; these patients should be immediately cardioverted. The vast majority of patients presenting with atrial fibrillation will have ventricular rates between 120 and 200 beats/min. If acute ischemic heart disease is present, cardioversion is recommended. Other asymptomatic patients, even those with a modest response (>120 beats/min), can be treated conservatively by controlling their rate initially with digitalis, verapamil, or beta-adrenergic blocking agents. Beta-adrenergic blocking agents and verapamil in the undigitalized patient may not cause sufficient slowing and may exacerbate bradycardia and/or congestive heart failure.

Once the heart rate is controlled, or if symptoms occur, a decision about cardioversion should be made. Success in cardioverting and maintaining a patient out of atrial fibrillation depends on atrial size and the length of time the patient has been in atrial fibrillation. The larger the atria and the longer the patient has been in atrial fibrillation, the lower the likelihood of successful maintenance of sinus rhythm. Before cardioversion is attempted either electrically or pharmacologically with an agent such as quinidine or procainamide, the need of anticoagulation should be investigated. Patients with mitral stenosis, cardiomyopathy, and large atria are more likely to have thrombus in the atrium and are thus at higher risk for emboli. A careful evaluation of the patient should be made prior to cardioversion to determine the relative risks of anticoagulation and cardioversion.

Junctional Arrhythmias

Premature Junctional Complexes (PJC's)

Premature junctional complexes are usually asymptomatic and rarely of any consequence. In the symptomatic patient they have the same significance as PAC's. If therapy is mandated due to severe symptoms, they can be treated similar to PAC's. When PJC's represent escape beats, they should not be suppressed.

Junctional Tachycardia[21-24]

Most commonly junctional tachycardia is simply a variant of PSVT. (See Chapter 16 for therapy guidelines for PSVT.) Junctional tachycardia may also be due to digitalis intoxication. In nonparoxysmal junctional tachycardia due to digitalis intoxication the digitalis should be withheld. The serum potassium should be checked, and if low, potassium should be given to raise the serum potassium to the normal range. If the patient is *in extremis*, antibodies to digitalis may be used.

Other Arrhythmias

Ventricular Arrhythmias

Ventricular arrhythmias are discussed in Chapter 16.

Heart Blocks

First-degree AV block does not require therapy. If it is associated with an acute cardiac problem, the patient should be observed for the development of second- or third-degree AV block. Second- and third-degree heart blocks are discussed in Chapter 16.

References

1. Rosen MR: Electrophysiology of the cardiac specialized conduction system, in Narula OS (ed): *His Bundle Electrocardiography and Clinical Electrophysiology.* Philadelphia, FA Davis Co, 1975.
2. Cranefield P: *Conduction of the Cardiac Impulse.* Mt Kisco, NY, Futura Publishing Co Inc, 1975.
3. Gettes LS: Electrophysiology of cardiac arrhythmias, in Eliot RS, Wolf GL, Forker AD (eds): *Cardiac Emergencies.* Mt Kisco, NY, Futura Publishing Co Inc, 1977.
4. Hoffman BF, Cranefield PF: *Electrophysiology of the Heart.* Mt Kisco, NY, Futura Publishing Co Inc, 1960.
5. Marriott HJ, Myerburg RJ: Recognition and treatment of cardiac arrhythmias and conduction disturbances, in Hurst JW (ed): *The Heart, Arteries, and Veins,* ed 6. New York, McGraw-Hill Book Co, 1985, pp 431-474.
6. Bigger JT Jr: Electrical properties of cardiac muscle and possible causes of cardiac arrhythmias, in Dreifus LS, Likoff W (eds): *Cardiac Arrhythmias.* New York, Grune & Stratton, 1973.
7. Schamroth L: *The Disorders of Cardiac Rhythm.* New York, JB Lippincott Co, 1971.
8. Lev M, Bharati S: Anatomic basis for impulse generation and atrioventricular transmission, in Narula OS (ed): *His Bundle Electrocardiography and Clinical Electrophysiology.* Philadelphia, FA Davis Co, 1975.
9. Truex RC: Anatomy of the specialized tissues of the heart, in Dreifus LS, Likoff W (eds): *Cardiac Arrhythmias.* New York, Grune & Stratton, 1973.
10. Myerburg RJ, Lazzara R: Electrophysiologic basis of cardiac arrhythmias and conduction disturbances, in Fisch C (ed): *Complex Electrocardiography I. Cardiovascular Clinics Series,* vol 5, no 3, Philadelphia, FA Davis Co, 1973.
11. Marriott HJ: *Practical Electrocardiography,* ed 5. Baltimore, Williams & Wilkins Co, 1972.
12. Goldreyer BN, Bigger JT Jr: Site of reentry in paroxysmal supraventricular tachycardia in man. *Circulation* 43:15-26, 1971.
13. Mason DT, Vera Z, Miller RR, et al: Treatment of tachyarrhythmias, in Mason DT (ed): *Cardiac Emergencies.* Baltimore, Williams & Wilkins Co, 1978.
14. Morgan JR, Dzindzio B, Starke H, et al: Management of tachyarrhythmias, in Eliot RS, Wolf GL, Forker AD (eds): *Cardiac Emergencies.* Mt Kisco, NY, Futura Publishing Co Inc, 1977.
15. Lie KI, Wellens HJJ, Downar E, et al: Observations on patients with primary ventricular fibrillation complicating acute myocardial infarction. *Circulation* 52:755-759, 1975.
16. Dhurandhar RW, MacMillan RL, Brown KW: Primary ventricular fibrillation complicating myocardial infarction. *Am J Cardiol* 27:347-351, 1971.
17. Wellens HJJ, Bar FW, Lie KI: The value of the electrocardiogram in the differential diagnosis of a tachycardia with a widened QRS complex. *Am J Med* 64:27-33, 1978.
18. Narula OS, Scherlag BJ, Samet P, et al: Atrioventricular block. Localization and classification by His bundle recordings. *Am J Med* 50:146-165, 1971.
19. Langendorf R, Cohen H, Gozo EG Jr: Observations on second degree atrioventricular block, including new criteria for the differential diagnosis between type I and type II block. *Am J Cardiol* 29:111-119, 1972.
20. Zipes DP: Second-degree atrioventricular block. *Circulation* 60:465-472, 1979.
21. Smith WM, Wallace AG: Management of arrhythmias and conduction abnormalities, in Hurst JW (ed): *The Heart, Arteries, and Veins,* ed 6. New York, McGraw-Hill, 1985, 475-485.
22. Zipes DP: Management of cardiac arrhythmias: Pharmacological, surgical, and electrical techniques, in Braunwald E (ed): *Heart Disease: A Textbook of Cardiovascular Medicine,* ed 2. Philadelphia, WB Saunders Co, 1984, pp 648-682.
23. Zipes DP: Specific arrhythmias: Diagnosis and treatment, in Braunwald E (ed): *Heart Disease: A Textbook of Cardiovascular Medicine,* ed 2. Philadelphia, WB Saunders Co, 1984, p 6.
24. Lindsay BD, Cain ME: Cardiac arrhythmias, in Orland MJ, Saltman RJ: *Manual of Medical Therapy.* Boston, Little, Brown and Company, 1986, pp 107-140.

Electrical Therapy in the Malignant Arrhythmias

Chapter 6

Electrical defibrillation is presently the most effective method of terminating ventricular fibrillation. The hemodynamic result of defibrillation depends on the metabolic state of the myocardium. The longer the duration of ventricular fibrillation, the greater the myocardial deterioration and the less likely defibrillation is to be successful. This is true in the experimental laboratory,[1,2] in the hospital, and in the community. Patients with primary ventricular fibrillation occurring in a coronary care unit or with a witnessed cardiac arrest occurring in a modern cardiac rehabilitation center can almost always be successfully resuscitated.[3] As documented by the out-of-hospital cardiac arrest experience, the success of resuscitation of patients with ventricular fibrillation relates to how soon electrical defibrillation can be applied.[4-7] Since a major determinant of survival from out-of-hospital cardiac arrest is the rapidity of defibrillation, recent efforts have been directed toward shortening the delays in treatment through training experienced first-aid providers to use defibrillators and by developing automatic and semi-automatic external defibrillators.[4,8-10]

Defibrillators

Defibrillators require a power source. Portable defibrillators contain their own power source, derived from a battery. A direct current defibrillator typically consists of a variable transformer, allowing the operator to select a high but variable voltage potential, an AC to DC converter that includes a capacitor to store the direct current, a charge switch that allows the capacitor to

charge, and discharge switches to complete the circuit from the capacitor to the electrodes (Figure 1). By placing an inductance coil in series with the capacitor (Figure 1), the resultant power waveforms are half sinusoidal in configuration (Figure 2). The output of most defibrillators is half sinusoidal. Some defibrillators are designed to deliver trapezoidal or near square waveforms. The optimal duration of defibrillation power waves is 4–12 msec.[11-14]

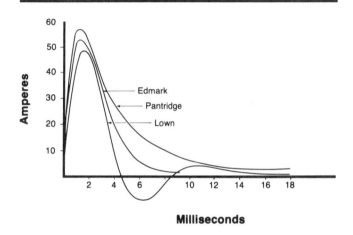

Milliseconds

Figure 2. **Graphic illustration of the waveforms of damped capacitor–inductor discharges.** The Lown waveform is non-critically damped and has a negative after-wave. The Edmark and Pantridge waveforms are critically damped.

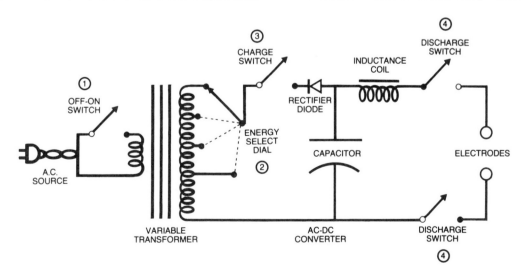

Figure 1. **Schematic of direct current defibrillator.**

Energy, Current, and Voltage

The output of defibrillators is quantified in joules (or watt-seconds), a measure of energy. The energy is the time integral of the power wave. Since power is measured in watts, integrating the area under the power wave over time in seconds gives watt-seconds. One watt-second equals one joule.

Formula 1

Energy(joules) = Power(watts) × Duration(seconds)

When a defibrillator discharges, the power output can be analyzed as potential (measured in volts) and current (measured in amperes). As shown in Formula 2, potential times current equals power.

Formula 2

Power(watts) = Potential(volts) × Current(amperes)

An analogy can be made with the cardiovascular system. When the heart ejects blood, the output can be measured as blood pressure and blood flow. The same is true of an electrical discharge. The potential is the "pressure" and current is the "flow".[14] If the potential in volts is multiplied by the current in amperes, the result is power in watts (Figure 3). If this is done at each point along the potential and current wave, a power wave can be constructed. When the area under the power wave is integrated over time, energy is derived (Figure 3).

Formula 3

Energy(joules) = Potential(volts) × Current(amperes)
              × Duration(seconds)

Although the defibrillator operator selects the shock energy (in joules), it is the current flow (in amperes) that actually defibrillates.[14,15] With a constant amount of energy stored in the defibrillator capacitor, the delivered current depends on the impedance present between the defibrillator electrodes. The transchest impedance is primarily resistive. Figure 4 illustrates the effect of increasing resistance on delivered current. The greater the resistance the less the delivered current.

Formula 4

$$\text{Current(amperes)} = \frac{\text{Potential(volts)}}{\text{Resistance(ohms)}}$$

Since the internal resistance of the defibrillator is small, the major determinants of the resistance to defibrillator discharge are operator and patient dependent.

Factors known to influence transthoracic resistance to direct current defibrillation include 1) delivered energy, 2) electrode size and composition, 3) interface between electrode and the skin, 4) the number of and time interval between previous discharges, 5) electrode pres-

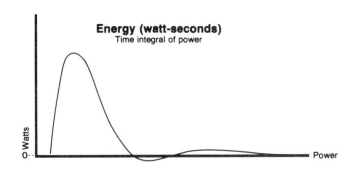

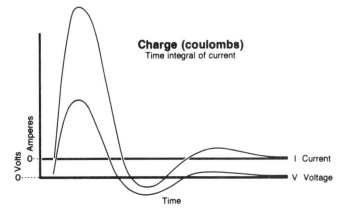

Figure 3. Graphic illustration of the current, voltage, and power waves of a defibrillator discharge delivering a damped half-sinusoidal waveform.

Defibrillator Dial Setting 400 Joules

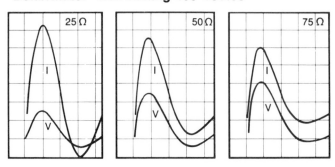

Figure 4. Simultaneous voltage (V) and current (I) waves from three separate defibrillator discharges (400 J stored energy) into 25, 50, and 75 ohms. Note that with increasing resistance, the delivered current decreases.

sure, 6) phase of the patient's ventilation, and 7) interelectrode distance.

Energy-dependent resistance[16] is not controllable by the operator. The electrode size and composition is seldom under control of the operator, but the importance of these factors must be clearly understood by those responsible for the purchase of defibrillators and for the selection of defibrillator electrodes.[17,18] The correct electrode size is unknown, but several studies suggest that electrodes with a circular diameter of 13 cm are near optimal for adults.[14,19,20] The interface between the chest wall and the electrode is important. Resistance is very high if metal electrodes are bare.[18,21,22] The lowest resistances are provided by electrodes covered with appropriate electrode paste.[18] Some electrode pads are also acceptable.[23,24]

Previous defibrillator shocks lower the transchest resistance.[25,26] In humans the transthoracic resistance declines by an average of 8% with the second shock.[27] Electrode–chest contact pressure influences transchest resistance when hand-held paddle electrodes are used.[27] It is recommended that firm pressure of about 11 kg (25 lbs) per paddle be used. The transchest resistance is also a function of the phase of ventilation and is minimum at full expiration.[28] Finally, the inter-electrode distance influences transchest resistance.[27] Therefore, forceful paddle electrode pressure not only assures good electrode skin contact and compresses the thorax but also often results in a smaller interelectrode distance, all of which decreases resistance to electrical defibrillation. If the resistance or impedance is high, it has been shown that low-energy shocks will fail to defibrillate.[19,29]

Electrode Placement

Defibrillation is accomplished by passage of an appropriate electrical current through the heart sufficient to depolarize a critical mass of the left ventricular myocardium.[30,31] One of the most important factors determining whether a critical mass of myocardium is depolarized is electrode placement.[14] Standard or anterolateral electrode placement calls for one electrode to be placed to the right of the upper sternum just below the right clavicle; the other, just to the left of nipple in the midaxillary line. With anterior posterior position, one paddle is positioned anteriorly over the precordium, just to the left of the lower sternal border and the other is positioned behind the heart. There is inadequate data to indicate that one position is superior to the other. To be effective, the current between the two electrodes must depolarize a critical mass of the left ventricle.[30,31]

Defibrillation

Energy Requirements for Defibrillation

Defibrillation is a probability function.[32] There are energies too low to defibrillate, energies that have a reasonable degree of defibrillation success with each shock, and energy levels that are clearly excessive and have a high probability of cardiac damage and/or death.[32-36] Another consideration is the dose–weight concept of defibrillation.[37-40] This concept is valid in humans as the energy necessary for defibrillation is less in children than in adults. Nevertheless, over the weight

range of most adults, body weight does not appear to be a major factor determining defibrillation energy requirements.[41-45]

Prospective studies of low (175–200 J) versus higher (300–400 J) energy for first shocks failed to show any benefit from initial shocks above 200 J.[46,47] Therefore, recommended strength for the initial shock is 200 J. If the first shock fails, the recommended strength of the second shock is 200–300 J. Those favoring a second shock strength of 200 J point to three observations: the study by Weaver and associates of out-of-hospital cardiac arrest where two low-energy shocks were as effective as two higher-energy shocks,[46] to the probability function of defibrillation,[32] and to the fact that the transchest resistance decreases with successive shock.[48,49] Those who favor 300 J energy levels for the second shock point to the observations of Kerber and associates who found the transthoracic impedance declined only 8% and peak current increased an average of only 4% with the second shock.[27] The fall in transthoracic impedance and rise in current is not uniform, and when it does occur is small.[27]

Since the probability of defibrillation increases with increasing energy, some argue for a second shock strength of 300 J. Because of this controversy, the recommended strength of the second shock is 200–300 J.

The patient with persistent ventricular fibrillation following the first two shocks should receive a third and subsequent shock of up to 360 J. If available, 360 J should be delivered. However, since the major determinant of successful resuscitation is the speed of defibrillation, the wording "up to 360 J" allows for use of automatic or semi-automatic units that deliver several shocks of energy levels lower than 360 J rather than performing BLS until the patient can be brought to the hospital for a 360 J shock.[50] If the initial or second shock is successful and the patient subsequently refibrillates, there is no reason to increase the energy for the subsequent shock.

Pediatric Defibrillation

A critical ventricular mass is necessary to sustain ventricular fibrillation.[30,31] For this reason, fibrillation is uncommon in children and rare in infants. Cardiac arrest in the pediatric age group is most often secondary to respiratory arrest. Therefore, when an infant or child is found to be without a pulse, therapy should first be directed toward adequate ventilation and oxygenation and to supporting the circulation by external chest compressions. The bradycardias secondary to respiratory arrest are most likely to respond to this approach. If ventricular fibrillation is present, a weight-related energy dose of 1 J/pound (2 J/kg) is recommended.[51] The electrode size should be appropriate to the chest size. If defibrillation is not successful the dose should be doubled and repeated twice. The presently available 4.5-

cm diameter electrodes are appropriate for infants, and 8.0-cm and 10.0-cm diameter electrodes are suitable for children.

Electrocardiographic Recognition

The disordered state of ventricular fibrillation has a characteristic electrocardiographic pattern, yet in some subjects, coarse ventricular fibrillation can be present in some leads while very small undulations or a straight line is present in others (Figure 5). Therefore, more than one lead needs to be monitored before one concludes that the patient should not be defibrillated because of very fine ventricular fibrillation or asystole.[52,53]

Procedure for Defibrillation

Once the decision is made to defibrillate, the following steps should be taken:

1. Apply conductive material to electrodes if necessary.
2. Turn on the defibrillator [Figure 1 (1)].
3. Select energy level [Figure 1 (2)].
4. Charge capacitors [Figure 1 (3)]. Note that this may take several seconds. Some units will not discharge until the capacitor is charged to the energy levels selected.
5. Assure proper placement of electrodes on the chest. If paddle electrodes are used, apply approximately 25 lb of pressure on each. (Do not lean on paddles as they may slip.)
6. Make sure no personnel are directly or indirectly in contact with the patient.
7. Deliver countershock by depressing both discharge buttons simultaneously [Figure 1 (4)].

For automatic and semi-automatic external defibrillators, some of these steps are automatic.

Urgent Synchronized Cardioversion

Electrical cardioversion is the therapy of choice for hemodynamically unstable ventricular or supraventricular tachyarrhythmias. Ventricular tachycardia often precedes ventricular fibrillation, and therefore, effective therapy of this arrhythmia may prevent potentially lethal ventricular fibrillation.

When a pulse is absent, the patient is treated like the patient with ventricular fibrillation. If the patient is severely unstable (in pulmonary edema, unconscious, or hypotensive), unsynchronized cardioversion is recommended. This strategy avoids delays inherent in synchronization, which can be substantial, and when ventricular tachycardia is rapid, may be safer.[54,55] Because at very rapid rates the T wave may not be easily distinguished from the QRS, it has been suggested that a non-synchronized shock may be less likely to fall on the T wave than a synchronized shock.[54]

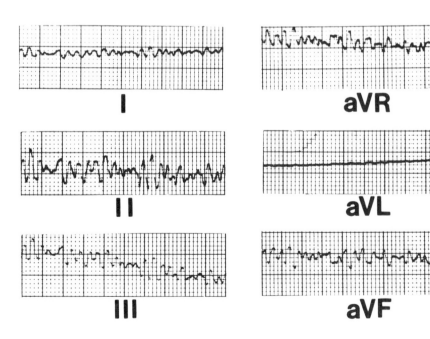

Figure 5. Simultaneous recordings of leads I, II, and III, and aVR, aVL, aVF from a subject with ventricular fibrillation. Note that the near flat line electrocardiogram recorded in aVL is the electrical sum of leads aVR and aVF. (From Ewy GA: Ventricular fibrillation masquerading as ventricular standstill. *Crit Care Med* 9:841, 1982, with permission.)

If the patient is hemodynamically stable, pacing or synchronized electrical cardioversion is indicated for ventricular tachycardia unresponsive to intravenous drugs as the probability of this arrhythmia deteriorating into ventricular fibrillation is great. If the patient is hemodynamically stable, a standard 12-lead electrocardiogram should be obtained prior to cardioversion as this might be useful if electrophysiologic testing becomes necessary. Maintenance of the patency of the airway and observation to prevent aspiration should vomiting occur are essential whenever a cardioversion is done. It is especially necessary when sedation with a short-acting sedative or hypnotic is used during less urgent procedures.

Some patients who are initially asymptomatic may become unstable while preparations (e.g., synchronization or sedation) for the procedure are being made. These patients may need to be cardioverted immediately.

Synchronized cardioversion also should be used urgently to convert hemodynamically unstable supraventricular arrhythmias and those unresponsive to drugs. Elective cardioversion is warranted only after the initiation mechanism of the arrhythmia is controlled.[56,57]

A synchronizing circuit allows the delivery of a countershock to be "programmed" to occur during the QRS complex of the electrocardiogram. Synchronized countershocks have been shown to reduce the energy requirements and complications.[56,57]

Technique: The procedure is the same as for defibrillation except as follows. Since the patient is conscious, anesthesia or analgesia is necessary, and the synchronizer circuit must be activated. The recommended energy for cardioversion of atrial fibrillation is 100 J for the first shock, 200 J for the second, and 360 J if a third shock is needed. The first shock probability of successful cardioversion of atrial fibrillation is only 50% with the capacitor charged to 100 J and is near 85% at 200 J, but there is less morbidity with lower energies.[56-61] If the patient is not cardioverted with 360 J, the likelihood of cardioversion with subsequent 360 J shocks is small. For paroxysmal supraventricular tachycardia, an initial energy of 75–100 J is recommended to accommodate the treatment of all of the various types of paroxysmal supraventricular tachycardia.[62,63] If conversion to normal sinus rhythm occurs, even transiently, prior to the redevelopment of supraventricular tachycardia, cardioversion should not be repeated until additional therapy has been initiated to maintain sinus rhythm after a second cardioversion.

Such rhythms as ventricular tachycardia or atrial flutter will revert with a dose as low as 10 J, yet in an urgent or emergency situation, an initial shock energy of 50 J for ventricular tachycardia and 25 J for atrial flutter is recommended in adults. For ventricular tachycardia, subsequent shocks of 100, 200, and up to 360 J are recommended. However, ventricular tachycardia is very responsive to electrical therapy, and it is rare for it to be resistant to cardioversion.[58] When ventricular tachycardia appears to persist, it is far more likely that it is actually recurrent.

A large number of arrhythmias can occur in response to cardioversion. In general, they are easily treated pharmacologically.[56-58] If ventricular fibrillation should occur during preparation or following emergency cardioversion, immediately:

1. Turn off the synchronizer circuit,
2. Charge the unit to 200 J, and
3. Defibrillate.

Routine Maintenance of Defibrillators

The amount of energy stored in the capacitor and that indicated on the energy select meter do not always coincide with the delivered energy into a standard 50-ohm load.[64] The energy doses recommended in the sections above are for delivered and not stored energy. All defibrillators should be checked at regular intervals with suitable testing equipment that can accurately determine the delivered energy of the defibrillator into a 50-ohm test load. The optimal frequency of testing is unknown. More frequent testing may be warranted if back-up defibrillators are not available. However, the clinicians should be aware that excessive testing may result in increased defibrillator failure. With a test every 8-hour shift, over 1,000 tests per year would be performed exclusive of defibrillation attempts. If frequent testing is required, it is recommended that the selected energy be limited to 50 J.[65]

The following protocols have been recommended for routine testing of line-powered and battery-powered defibrillation.[65]

Line-Powered Defibrillators: Engineering personnel should perform a maintenance check on the equipment every 3 months. Clinical personnel should perform a full energy charge–discharge test into an artificial load once a week and a visual inspection and charge–discharge test at 50 J into a test load each day.[65] With some of the newer defibrillators, it is probable that daily testing is not mandatory.

Battery-Powered Defibrillators: Engineering and clinical personnel should perform duties as described above. Battery inspection and/or maintenance should be performed as described in the operating instructions, service instructions, or labels on the unit or battery charger.

Special Situations

Resuscitation of Patients With Automatic Implantable Cardioverter-Defibrillators

Patients with automatic implantable cardioverter-defibrillators (AICD) are at high risk for ventricular fibrillation. When caring for a patient with an implanted defibrillator who has experienced cardiac arrest, the rescuer should know the following principles:

1. If the automatic implanted defibrillator discharges while the rescuer has his or her hands on the victim's chest, the shock from the automatic implanted defibrillator will be perceptible and possibly painful but almost certainly will not be dangerous to the rescuer.[66]
2. Automatic implantable defibrillators are protected against damage from conventional external transchest defibrillator shock.
3. If an unconscious patient with an AICD has muscle contractions with shocks, and then the contractions stop, the unit has gone into the disabled mode, as only a few shocks are applied by the unit for each episode of tachycardia or fibrillation. Under such conditions, if ventricular tachycardia or fibrillation is present, an external countershock should be applied as it is possible that the limited energy output of the AICD was insufficient to defibrillate the heart. The AICD will reactivate only if a period of nonfibrillatory rhythm occurs to reset the unit.[67,68]

Emergency Pacing During CPR

There are three basic approaches to pacing: external, transthoracic, and transvenous. External pacing is the oldest and simplest technique for temporarily stabilizing patients with profound bradycardia.[69] Early noninvasive pacing was limited by the large external currents necessary to excite the heart. The result was contractions of thoracic muscles and unacceptable pain in conscious patients. The large stimulus artifacts obscured the electrocardiographic response. The forceful muscle contractions were often confused with arterial pulsation.[70]

Placement of transthoracic electrodes via the precordium were limited by the possibility of injury to the coronaries, heart, or adjacent structure and by the unsuitability of this technqiue for prophylactic use in conscious patients.[71,72]

Transvenous pacing techniques, introduced in the late 1950's, soon became the preferred method for emergency as well as temporary and long-term pacing.[73]

However, in the emergency situation, effective placement of the transvenous pacing electrodes requires skill and time, and there is always the potential for complication.[74,75] Therefore, transvenous pacing is not always optimal for emergency pacing.

Recently developed external noninvasive temporary pacing techniques with specially designed direct current waveform combined with large high-impedance electrodes have significant promise.[72,76] The ease of application, effectiveness, safety, lack of significant pain, and significant skeletal muscle contraction on stimulation are definite advances.[70] Demand-mode pacing adds to noninvasive external pacing safety.[70]

The effectiveness of pacing depends on the condition of the myocardium. The patient with severe bradycardia, heart block, or idioventricular rhythm who can generate a pulse with each QRS complex has a cardiovascular system that will respond to pacing — all that is lacking is frequent enough electrical stimuli.[77] On the other hand, the majority of patients with cardiac arrest will not respond to pacing. Electrocardiographic activity without cardiac contraction and asystole is the electrocardiographic reaction of a heart that is metabolically compromised from inadequate myocardial perfusion, and electrical pacing will not be effective.[77]

In some circumstances, electrical pacing can be employed to suppress malignant ventricular arrythmias. Pacing (atrial pacing is preferable) is the treatment of choice for *torsade de pointes* until the stimulus to the arrythmia can be corrected.[78] In some emergency circumstances, ventricular pacing (generally at a rate of 90–110) can be used to "overdrive suppress" ventricular ectopy.[79] This is usually attempted only if other attempts to control the arrhythmia have been unsuccessful.

Rapid atrial pacing has been used to convert supraventricular tachycardias[79] but is rarely the treatment of choice in the emergent situation.

Electrical Defibrillation or Cardioversion in Patients with Permanent Pacemakers

Improvements in the internal protection circuits of the present generation of implanted pacemakers make loss of pacemaker function secondary to a transchest shock unlikely.[80] However, if one of the defibrillation electrodes is placed too close to the generator of an implanted unipolar pacemaker, the defibrillator shock may induce a significant increase in pacemaker stimulation thresholds.[80] This probably results from the shunting of current via the housing of the pulse generator down the pacemaker lead, concentrating energy at the electrode–myocardial interface. This can cause burns or local electrical trauma. Therefore, it is recommended that defibrillator paddles or self-adhesive electrodes be placed at least 5 inches (12.7 cm) from the pulse generator of permanent pacemakers.[80]

In some patients, the rise in pacemaker stimulation threshold is more gradual. Therefore, it is recommended that serial measurements of stimulation threshold be made on a frequent basis for the next 2 months to screen for a significant rise in stimulation threshold. This procedure is especially important in patients who are pacemaker dependent.[80]

Precordial Thump

Conversion of an abnormal rhythm following a precordial thump or cough has been well demonstrated in patients with ventricular tachycardia and complete heart block.[81] Recently, it has been demonstrated as well for ventricular fibrillation.[81] Because the speed of defibrillation is critical, a solitary precordial thump is recommended for all witnessed cardiac arrests when a defibrillator is unavailable. When a precordial thump is used in patients who have ventricular tachycardia and a pulse, a defibrillator should be available since ventricular fibrillation can be induced.[81]

A precordial thump is delivered to the center of the sternum with the hypothenar aspect of the fist and from a height of no more than 12 inches.

New Trends in Defibrillation

Advance Prediction of Transthoracic Resistance

Techniques developed at Purdue University[82] have been shown by Kerber and associates to accurately determine transthoracic impedance in advance of any defibrillator shocks.[29,83] Using a "test pulse" technqiue, a low-level current is passed between the electrode during the defibrillator charge cycle. A microprocessor monitored the predischarge current flow and determined the predischarge transthoracic resistance.[29,83]

Automatic External Defibrillators

Automatic and semi-automatic defibrillators have been developed to allow early defibrillation by a trained spouse or companion of high-risk patients. The semi-automatic units detect ventricular fibrillation but do not allow defibrillation unless there is also positive identification of ventricular fibrillation and absence of respiratory motion. Selected emergency medical technicians have been provided additional training in defibrillation using standard or semi-automatic defibrillators. This approach has allowed a markedly improved survival of out-of-hospital cardiac arrest victims in rural settings.[4,8,10]

References

1. Sanders AB, Kern KB, Atlas M, Bragg S, Ewy GA: Importance of the duration of inadequate coronary perfusion pressure on resuscitation from cardiac arrest. *JACC* 6:113, 1985.
2. Sanders AB, Kern KB, Ewy GA, Atlas M, Bailey L: Improved resuscitation from cardiac arrest with open-chest massage. *Ann Emerg Med* 13:672, 1984.
3. Hossack KF, Hartwig R: Cardiac arrest associated with supervised cardiac rehabilitation. *J Cardiac Rehab* 2:402, 1982.
4. Eisenberg MA, Bergner L, Hallstrom AP: Paramedic programs and out-of-hospital cardiac arrest: Factors associated with successful resuscitation. *Am J Public Health* 69:30, 1979.
5. Eisenberg MS, Copass MK, Hallstrom AP, et al: Treatment of out-of-hospital cardiac arrest with rapid defibrillation by emergency medical technicians. *N Engl J Med* 302:1379, 1980.
6. Cobb LA, Hallstrom AP: Community-based cardiopulmonary resuscitation: What have we learned? *Ann NY Acad Sci* 382:330, 1982.
7. Weaver WD, Copass MK, Buffi D, et al : Improved neurologic recovery and survival after early defibrillation. *Circulation* 69:943, 1984.
8. Stults KR, Brown DD, Schung V, et al: Prehospital defibrillation performed by emergency medical technicians in rural communities. *N Engl J Med* 310:219, 1984.
9. Cummins RO, Eisenberg MS, Bergner L, et al: Sensitivity, accuracy and safety of an automatic external defibrillator. *Lancet* 2:381, 1984.
10. Weaver WD, Copass MK, Cobb LA, Hill D, Newman BH: A new compact, automatic external defibrillator designed for lay person use (abstract). *J Am Coll Cardiol* 5:457, 1985.
11. Schuder JC, Stoeckle H, Dolan AM: Transthoracic ventricular defibrillation with square wave stimuli. *Circ Res* 15:258, 1964.
12. Schuder JC, Rahmoeller GA, Stoeckle H: Transthoracic ventricular defibrillation with triangular and trapezoidal waveforms. *Circ Res* 19:689, 1966.
13. Bourland JD, Tacker WA Jr, Geddes LA, et al: Comparative efficacy of damped sine wave and square wave current for transchest ventricular defibrillation in animals. *Med Instrum* 12:42, 1978.
14. Ewy GA: Cardiac arrest and resuscitation: Defibrillators and defibrillation. *Curr Probl Cardiol* 2:1, 1978.
15. Patton JN, Pantridge JF: Current required for ventricular fibrillation. *Br Med J* 1:513, 1979.
16. Ewy GA, Ewy MD, Nuttall AJ, Nuttall AW: Canine transthoracic resistance. *J Appl Physiol* 32:91, 1972.
17. Patel AS, Galysh FT: Experimental studies to design safe external pediatric paddles for a DC defibrillator. *IEEE Trans Biomed Eng* 19:228, 1972.
18. Connell PN, Ewy GA, Dahl CF, Ewy MD: Transthoracic impedance to defibrillation discharge. Effect of electrode size and electrode chest wall interface. *J Electrocardiol* 6:313, 1973.
19. Thomas ED, Ewy GA, Dahl CF, et al: Effectiveness of direct current defibrillation: Role of paddle electrode size. *Am Heart J* 93:463, 1977.
20. Kerber RE, Grayzel J, Hoyt R, et al: Transthoracic resistance in human defibrillation. Influence of body weight, chest size, serial shocks, paddle size, and paddle contact pressure. *Circulation* 63:676, 1981.
21. Ewy GA, Taren DT: Comparison of paddle electrode pastes used for defibrillation. *Heart Lung* 6:847, 1977.
22. Ewy GA, Taren DT: Impedance of transthoracic direct current discharge: A model for testing interface material. *Med Instrum* 12:47, 1978.
23. Tacker WA, Paris RL: Defibrillation effectiveness using disposable conductive gel pads, in *Proceedings of AAMI 16th Annual Meeting.* Washington D.C., Arlington VA Association for Advancement of Medical Instrumentation, May 1981, p.97.
24. Kerber RE, Martins JB, Kelly KJ, Ferguson DW, Kouba C, Jensen SR, Newman B, Parke JD, Kieso R, Melton J: Self-adhesive preapplied electrode pads for defibrillation and cardioversion. *J Am Coll Cardiol* 3:815, 1984.
25. Geddes LA, Tacker WA, Cabler DP, Chapman R, Rivera BS, and Kidder H: The decrease in transthoracic impedance during successive ventricular defibrillation trials. *Med Instrum* 9:179, 1975.

26. Dahl CR, Ewy GA, Ewy MD, Thomas ED: Transthoracic impedance to direct current discharge: Effect of repeated countershocks. *Med Instrum* 10:151, 1976.

27. Kerber RE, Grayzel J, Hoyt R, Marcus M, Kennedy J: Transthoracic resistance in human defibrillation. Influence of body weight, chest size, serial shocks, paddle size and paddle contact pressure. *Circulation* 63:676, 1981.

28. Ewy GA, Hellman DA, McClung S, et al: Influence of ventilation phase on transthoracic impedance and defibrillation effectiveness. *Crit Care Med* 8:164, 1980.

29. Kerber RE, Kouba C, Martins J, Kelly K, Low R, Hoyt R, Ferguson D, Bailey L, Bennett P, Charbonnier F: Advance prediction of transthoracic impedance in human defibrillation and cardioversion: Importance of impedance in determining the success of low energy shocks. *Circulation* 70:303, 1984.

30. Garrey WE: The nature of fibrillatory contraction of the heart — Its relation to tissue mass and form. *Am J Physiol* 33:397, 1914.

31. Zipes DP, Fisher J, King RM, Nicoll A deB, and Jolly W: Termination of ventricular fibrillation in dogs by depolarizing a critical amount of myocardium. *Am J Cardiol* 36:37, 1975.

32. Tacker WA, Geddes LA: *Electrical Defibrillation*. Boca Raton, CRC Press Inc., 1980, p. 141.

33. Dahl CF, Ewy GA, Warner ED, et al: Myocardial necrosis from direct current countershock. *Circulation* 50:956, 1974.

34. Warner ED, Dahl C, Ewy GA: Myocardial injury from transthoracic defibrillator countershock. *Arch Pathol* 99:55, 1975.

35. Ehsani A, Ewy GA, Sobel BE: Effects of electrical countershock on serum creatine phosphokinase (CPK) isoenzyme activity. *Am J Cardiol* 37:12, 1976.

36. Ewy GA, Taren D, Bangert J, McClung S, Hellman DA: Comparison of myocardial damage from defibrillator discharges at various dosages. *Med Instrum* 14:9, 1980.

37. Geddes LA, Tacker WA, Rosborough JP, et al: Electrical dose for ventricular defibrillation of large and small animals using precordial electrodes. *J Clin Invest* 53:310, 1974.

38. Collins RE, Giuliani ER, Tacker WA, et al: Transthoracic ventricular defibrillation: Success and body weight. *Med Instrum* 12:53, 1978.

39. Gold JH, Schuder JC, Stoeckle H, et al: Transthoracic ventricular defibrillation in the 100 kg calf with unidirectional rectangular pulses. *Circulation* 56:745, 1977.

40. Tacker WA Jr, Galioto FM Jr, Giuliani E, et al: Energy dosage for human transchest electrical ventricular defibrillation. *N Engl J Med* 290:214,1974.

41. Gascho JA, Crampton RS, Cherwek M, et al: Determinants of ventricular defibrillation in adults. *Circulation* 60:231, 1979.

42. Kerber RE, Sarnat W: Factors influencing the success of ventricular defibrillation in man. *Circulation* 60:226, 1979.

43. Pantridge JF, Adgey AA, Webb SW, et al: Electrical requirements for ventricular defibrillation. *Br Med J* 2:313, 1975.

44. Pantridge JF, Adgey AA, Geddes JS, et al: *The Acute Coronary Attack*. New York, Grune and Stratton, 1975, p. 71.

45. Campbell NP, Webb SW, Adgey AA, et al: Transthoracic ventricular defibrillation in adults. *Br Med J* 2:1379, 1977.

46. Weaver WD, Cobb LA, Copass MK, Holstrom AP: Ventricular defibrillation — A comparative trial using 175 J and 320 J shocks. *N Engl J Med* 307:1101, 1982.

47. Kerber RE, Jensen SR, Gascho JA, Grayzel J, Hoyt R, Kennedy J: Determinants of defibrillation: Prospective analysis of 183 patients. *Am J Cardiol* 52:739, 1983.

48. Geddes LA, Tacker WA, Cabler DP, Chapman K, Riveria BS, Idder H: The decrease in transthoracic impedance during successive ventricular defibrillation trials. *Med Instrum* 9:179, 1975.

49. Dahl CF, Ewy GA, Ewy MD, Thomas ED: Transthoracic impedance to direct current discharge: Effect of repeated countershocks. *Med Instrum* 10:151, 1976.

50. Standards and guidelines for cardiopulmonary resuscitation (CPR) and emergency cardiac care (ECC). *JAMA* 244:453, 1980.

51. Gutgesell HP, Tacker WA, Geddes LA, et al: Energy dose for defibrillation in children. *Pediatrics* 58:898, 1976.

52. Ewy GA, Dahl CF, Zimmerman M, et al: Ventricular fibrillation masquerading as ventricular standstill. *Crit Care Med* 12:41, 1981.

53. McDonald JL: Coarse ventricular fibrillation presenting as asystole or very low amplitude ventricular fibrillation. *Crit Care Med* 10:790, 1982.

54. Standards and guidelines for cardiopulmonary resuscitation (CPR) and emergency cardiac care (ECC). *JAMA* 255:2841-3044,1986.

55. Ewy G: Electrical therapy of cardiovascular emergencies. *Circulation* 74(suppl IV), IV-111, 1986.

56. Lown B, Amarasingham R, Neuman J: New methods for terminating cardiac arrhythmias: Use of synchronized capacitor discharge. *JAMA* 182:548, 1962.

57. Killip T: Synchronized DC precordial shock for arrhythmias. Safe new technique to establish normal rhythm may be utilized on an elective or emergency basis. *JAMA* 186:1, 1963.

58. Lown B: Electrical reversion of cardiac arrhythmias. *Br Heart J* 29:469, 1967.

59. DeSilva RA, Grayboys TB, Podrid PJ, et al: Cardioversion and defibrillation. *Am Heart J* 100:881, 1980.

60. Kerber RE, Jensen SR, Grayzel J, et al: Elective cardioversion: Influence of paddle-electrode location and size on success rates and energy requirements. *N Engl J Med* 305:658, 1981.

61. Ewy GA: Influence of paddle electrode location and size on success of cardioversion (letter). *N Engl J Med* 306:174, 1982.

62. Resnekov L and McDonald L: Appraisal of electroconversion in treatment of cardiac dysrhythmias. *Br Heart J* 30:786,1968.

63. Resnekov L: Drug therapy before and after electroversion of cardiac dysrhythmias. *Prog Cardiovasc Dis* XVI:531, 1974.

64. Ewy GA, Fletcher RD, Ewy MD: Comparative analysis of direct current defibrillators. *J Electrocardiol* 5:349, 1972.

65. Creed JD, Packard JM, Lambrew CT, Lewis AJ: Defibrillation and Synchronized Cardioversion, in McIntyre KM, Lewis AJ (eds): *Textbook of Advanced Cardiac Life Support*. Dallas, American Heart Association, 1981, pp. VII-I.

66. Tacker WA: Personal communication.

67. Mirowski M: Prevention of sudden arrhythmic death with implanted automatic defibrillators. *Ann Intern Med* 97:606, 1982.

68. Mirowski M, Reid PR, Mower MM, et al: Termination of malignant ventricular arrhythmias with an implanted automatic defibrillator in human beings. *N Engl J Med* 303:322, 1980.

69. Zoll PM: Resuscitation of the heart in ventricular standstill by external electrical stimulation. *N Engl J Med* 247:768, 1952.

70. Zoll PM, Zoll RH, Falk RH, Clinton JE, Eitel DP, Antman EM: External noninvasive temporary cardiac pacing: Clinical trials. *Circulation* 71:937, 1985.

71. Thevenet A, Hodges PC, Lillehei CW: The use of a myocardial electrode inserted percutaneously for control of complete atrioventricular block by an artificial pacemaker. *Dis Chest* 34:621, 1958.

72. Brown CG, Gurley HT, Hutchins GM, MacKenzie EJ, White JD: Injuries associated with percutaneous placement of transthoracic pacemakers. *Ann Emerg Med* 14:223, 1985.

73. Furman S, Robinson G: Use of an intracardiac pacemaker in the correction of total heart block. *Surg Forum* 9:245, 1958.

74. Austin JL, Preis LK, Crampton RS, Beller GA, Martin RP: Analysis of pacemaker malfunction and complications of temporary pacing in the coronary care unit. *Am J Cardiol* 49:301, 1982.

75. Hynes JK, Holmes DR Jr, Harrison CE: Five-year experience with temporary pacemaker therapy in the coronary care unit. *Mayo Clin Proc* 58:122, 1983.

76. Zoll RH, Zoll PM, Belgard AH: External noninvasive electric stimulation of the heart. *Crit Care Med* 9:393, 1981.

77. Ewy GA: Defining electromechanical dissociation. *Ann Emerg Med* 13:830, 1984.

78. Smith WM and Gallagher JJ: "Les Torsade de Pointes": An unusual ventricular arrhythmia. *Ann Intern Med* 93:578, 1980.

79. Waldo AL, Wells JL, Cooper TB, and MacLean WAH: Temporary cardiac pacing: applications and techniques in the treatment of cardiac arrhythmias. *Prog Cardiovasc Dis* 23:451, 1981.

80. Levine PA, Barvold SS, Fletcher RD, Talbot P: Adverse acute and chronic effect of electrical defibrillation and cardioversion on implanted unipolar cardiac pacing system. *JACC* 6:1413, 1983.

81. Standards and Guidelines for Cardiopulmonary Resuscitation (CPR) and Emergency Cardiac Care (ECC). *JAMA* 255:2953,2954, 1985.

82. Geddes LA, Tacker WA, Schoenlein W, Minton M, Grubbs S, Wilcox P: The prediction of the impedance of the thorax to defibrillating current. *Med Instrum* 10:159, 1976.

83. Kerber RE, McPherson D, Charbonnier F, Kleso R, Hite P: Automated impedance-based energy adjustment for defibrillation: Experimental studies. *Circulation* 71:136, 1985.

Cardiovascular Pharmacology I

Chapter 7

This chapter is a review of the pharmacology of drugs commonly used during ACLS, with an emphasis on the proper indications, contraindications, and doses for each agent. The pharmacotherapeutic objectives of advanced cardiac life support (ACLS) are:

1. To correct hypoxemia,
2. To reestablish spontaneous circulation,
3. To optimize cardiac function,
4. To suppress sustained ventricular arrhythmia,
5. To correct acidosis,
6. To relieve pain, and
7. To treat congestive heart failure.

Oxygen

Mechanisms of Action

Although many do not think of oxygen as a drug, all of the considerations pertinent to a pharmacological agent are appropriate for oxygen. It is an essential component of cardiac resuscitation and emergency cardiac care.

Numerous factors contribute to hypoxemia in the patient with cardiac arrest. Even under ideal conditions, expired air provides only 16–17% oxygen. Mouth-to-mouth resuscitation produces an alveolar oxygen tension of no more than 80 mmHg, which is inadequate to oxygenate mixed venous blood that is severely desaturated due to the low cardiac output (25–30% of normal), the ventilation-perfusion abnormalities, and right-to-left shunting that can occur in the cardiac arrest victim.[1] Similar abnormalities have been described in patients with pulmonary edema and gastric aspiration.[2] Accordingly, supplemental oxygen is obligatory during resuscitation.

Modest changes in oxygen tension will substantially affect hemoglobin saturation in patients who are functioning on the steep portion of the oxyhemoglobin saturation curve (Figure 1). In hypoxemic patients, oxygen administration elevates arterial oxygen tension and increases arterial oxygen content, thereby improving tissue oxygenation.[3]

Indications

Oxygen should be given to all patients with 1) acute chest pain that may be due to cardiac ischemia,[4] 2) suspected hypoxemia of any cause, and 3) cardiopulmonary arrest. Prompt treatment of hypoxemia may prevent cardiac arrest.

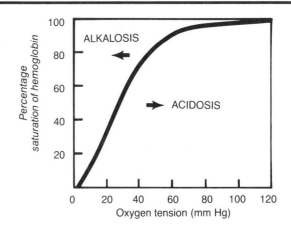

Figure 1. Oxyhemoglobin dissociation curve.

Dosage

Several different devices, including masks and nasal cannulae, can be used to administer oxygen to patients who are breathing spontaneously. Oxygen can also be delivered by positive-pressure ventilation devices, e.g., demand valve. Oxygen can be adequately delivered by volume-regulated ventilators even during resuscitation of intubated patients. For further details of oxygen administration, see Chapters 2 and 3.

Precautions

Oxygen toxicity may occur after prolonged ventilatory support with a high oxygen concentration. However, even 100% oxygen is not hazardous to the patient's lungs during the brief time required for clinical resuscitation. It should never be withheld or diluted during resuscitation because of the mistaken belief that it will be harmful. In patients with chronic pulmonary disease, e.g., pulmonary emphysema, it may be necessary to assist ventilation during the administration of oxygen if reversal of hypoxemia reduces respiratory drive in a patient with a chronically high $PaCO_2$. If clinically indicated, oxygen should never be withheld. Depression of the respiratory drive sufficient to necessitate ventilatory support is infrequent since the PO_2 need not be raised into the normal range. (See Chapter 3, "Venturi Mask".)

Epinephrine

Mechanisms of Action

Epinephrine is an endogenous catecholamine with both alpha- and beta-adrenergic activity. Its usefulness in cardiac arrest has been substantiated experimentally[5] and clinically. Epinephrine's pharmacologic actions are complex since they are modulated in part by reflex circulatory adjustments. In general, the following cardio-vascular responses can be expected from the dosages used during resuscitation:

1. Increased systemic vascular resistance.
2. Increased arterial blood pressure.
3. Increased heart rate.
4. Increased coronary and cerebral blood flow.
5. Increased myocardial contraction.
6. Increased myocardial oxygen requirements.
7. Increased automaticity.

Peripheral vasoconstriction, which improves coronary and cerebral perfusion pressure, is the primary beneficial effect of epinephrine in cardiac arrest (Figures 2 and 3).[6-8] Epinephrine's potent alpha-1 and alpha-2 post-synaptic adrenergic effects improve cerebral and coronary blood flow by preventing arterial collapse and increasing peripheral vasoconstriction.[6-8] Recent studies in animals indicate that epinephrine's alpha-adrenergic effect (not its beta-adrenergic effect) makes ventricular fibrillation (VF) more susceptible to direct current coun-tershock.[9] Pure alpha-adrenergic agonists appear to be as effective as epinephrine in restoring spontaneous circulation without producing beta-adrenergic mediated myocardial ischemia.[10-12] However, epinephrine may produce a greater improvement in cerebral blood flow than either phenylephrine or methoxamine,[13-17] possibly due to its combined alpha- and beta-adrenergic ac-tivity.[12] The role of pure alpha-adrenergic agonists in cardiac resuscitation needs further evaluation before they can be recommended as an alternative to epinephrine.

Indications

Epinephrine produces a favorable redistribution of blood flow during CPR. The elevation of coronary perfusion pressure following the administration of epi-nephrine is a potentially beneficial effect applicable to all forms of cardiorespiratory arrest.[6-8] Epinephrine may be a useful vasoactive, inotropic agent in rare selected refractory patients with circulatory shock, e.g., after cardiopulmonary bypass.[18,19]

Dosage

The optimal dose of epinephrine to augment aortic diastolic blood pressure in humans during resuscitation is unknown. However, most data suggest that higher rather than lower doses may be optimal.[8,20] Epinephrine produces a dose-dependent vasopressor effect in ani-mals and humans.[20] Kosnik and coworkers compared the effects of different doses of epinephrine on aortic diastolic blood pressure in dogs during cardiac arrest.[21] Epinephrine (15 μg/kg) did not affect aortic diastolic

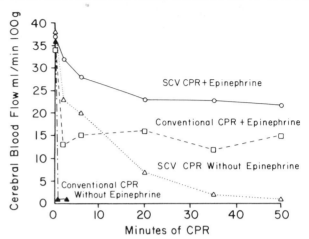

Figure 2. **Cerebral blood flow measurement by radiolabelled microsphere technique in dogs during conventional CPR with and without epinephrine.** Without epinephrine there is essentially no measurable flow, whereas flow is substantially increased by the drug, correlating with higher perfusion pressures. Modified from Michael JR, Guerci AD, Koehler RC, Shi AY, Tsitlik J, Chandra N, Niedermeyer E, Rogers MC, Traystman RJ, Weisfeldt ML: Mechanisms by which epinephrine augments cerebral and myocardial perfusion during cardiopulmonary resuscitation in dogs. *Circulation* 69:822-835, 1984.

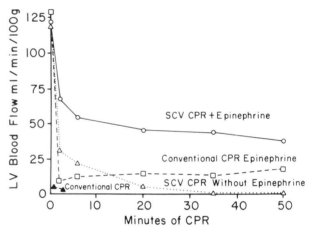

Figure 3. **Left ventricular blood flow in dogs with and without epinephrine.** As with cerebral blood flow, myocardial blood flow is increased by epinephrine as perfusion pressure is increased. Modified from Michael JR, Guerci AD, Koehler RC, Shi AY, Tsitlik J, Chandra N, Niedermeyer E, Rogers MC, Traystman RJ, Weisfeldt ML: Mechanisms by which epinephrine augments cerebral and myocardial perfusion during cardiopulmonary resuscitation in dogs. *Circulation* 69:822-835, 1984.

blood pressure; however, doses of 45, 75, and 150 μg/kg sustained a diastolic blood pressure of > 30 mmHg for up to 5 minutes. Since the recommended dose of epi-nephrine is 0.5–1.0 mg (7.5–15 μg/kg in a 70-kg male) given intravenously (IV) during the resuscitation, in general the higher range of doses should be used and should be repeated at least every 5 minutes.

If there is a delay in establishing an IV route, epinephrine can be instilled directly into the tracheobronchial tree via an endotracheal tube. Chest compression must be momentarily interrupted when epinephrine is introduced intratracheally. Positive-pressure ventilation is then applied and compression resumed. The rate of absorption of endotracheally administered epinephrine during CPR has been measured in dogs and in primates.[22-24] In dogs, following an initial peak concentration, endotracheal epinephrine results in a lower, but more sustained, plasma concentration of epinephrine due to continued absorption of the drug from the airway.[22,23] In primates, epinephrine is absorbed rapidly after intratracheal administration, has prompt vasopressor action,[24] and produces quantitatively similar effects on heart rate and blood pressure at comparable doses.[25]

In humans, endotracheal injection produces lower and slightly delayed peak plasma epinephrine concentrations.[26] A localized vasoconstricting effect may impede absorption from the lung, explaining the more sustained physiological response observed after endotracheal administration.[23,24] Drug dilution is an important factor in assuring a good pharmacologic response following endotracheal drug administration.[25,27] Epinephrine should be diluted with 10 mL of either normal saline or sterile water before administration to adults. In children, undiluted epinephrine has been used with good clinical results.[28]

Epinephrine should be injected directly into the heart only in rare circumstances when it cannot be given intravenously or intratracheally. The hazards of intracardiac administration include interruption of chest compression and ventilation, coronary artery laceration, cardiac tamponade, pneumothorax, and intramyocardial injection with intractable ventricular fibrillation.[26] For these reasons, it is the route of last resort.

Epinephrine also can be administered as a continuous infusion to increase and sustain the arterial pressure and/or the heart rate. An infusion can be prepared by adding 1 mg of epinephrine to 250 mL 5% dextrose in water, initiated at a rate of 2 μg/min, and titrated to effect. Epinephrine infused at a rate of 0.04 μg/kg/min (2.8 μg/min for a 70-kg person) usually increases cardiac index and arterial pressure in patients not receiving CPR.[29]

Precautions

Auto-oxidation of catecholamines and related sympathomimetic compounds is pH dependent. Although contact of epinephrine with other drugs that have an alkaline pH (such as sodium bicarbonate) can cause auto-oxidation, the rate of breakdown is too slow[30] to be clinically important when epinephrine is given by IV bolus or when it is infused rapidly IV. However, epinephrine or other related sympathomimetic drugs should not be mixed in the same infusion bag or bottle with alkaline solutions such as sodium bicarbonate. Epinephrine's positive inotropic and chronotropic effects can precipitate or exacerbate myocardial ischemia.[5] Doses in excess of 20 μg/min or 0.3 μg/kg/min frequently produce hypertension in patients who are not receiving CPR.[31] Epinephrine may induce or exacerbate ventricular ectopy, especially in patients who are receiving digitalis.[32]

Atropine

Mechanisms of Action

Atropine sulfate is a parasympatholytic drug that enhances both sinus node automaticity and atrioventricular (AV) conduction via its direct vagolytic action.

Indications

In diseased myocardium, heightened parasympathetic tone may precipitate conduction disturbances or asystole.[33] Atropine is indicated as initial therapy for patients with symptomatic bradycardia, including occasional patients who have a heart rate in the "physiological" range under circumstances in which a sinus tachycardia would be more appropriate (e.g., a patient who has acute myocardial infarction, symptomatic hypotension, and a heart rate of 70 beats/min). "Symptomatic" bradycardia includes conditions in which absolute or relative bradycardia are associated with hypotension, ventricular ectopy, or myocardial ischemia.[34] Atropine is not needed and may produce adverse consequences when the bradycardia is not accompanied by symptoms or signs of hemodynamic compromise, ischemia, or frequent ventricular ectopy.[35] Atropine may restore normal AV nodal conduction and initiate electrical activity during asystolic cardiac arrest.[33]

Atropine's beneficial effects in treating asystole or pulseless idioventricular rhythms is suspected but unproven in humans.[33,36-40] Brown and coworkers reported that 3 of 8 patients survived after the administration of atropine for asystole.[33] However, all survivors experienced cardiac arrest in the hospital (2 in the catheterization laboratory, 1 in intensive care) and had ACLS initiated within 2 minutes. Steuven and coworkers reported a significant ($P < 0.04$) increase in the number of patients who survived until arrival to the emergency room after out-of-hospital arrest with asystole in response to atropine (14% compared to 0% in those who received only epinephrine and bicarbonate), but none of the short-term survivors was discharged from the hospital. Iseri, et al., observed no response in 10 asystolic patients.[39] Coon and coworkers found that 10 of 11 patients who did not receive atropine and 8 of 10 who did receive atropine developed rhythms other than asystole, yet only 1 patient (who did not receive atropine) was discharged alive.[40] Unfortunately, asystolic cardiac arrest is nearly always fatal,[38] regardless of therapy. Although there is no unequivocal proof of its value, there is little evidence that atropine is harmful in this setting. A well-designed prospective, controlled trial to determine the utility of atropine in treating asystole would be helpful.

Dosage and Administration

For patients without cardiac arrest, atropine is given in 0.5-mg aliquots IV and may be repeated at 5-minute intervals until the desired response is achieved (i.e., an increased heart rate usually to 60 beats/min or greater or abatement of signs and symptoms). Two milligrams given intravenously is a fully vagolytic dose in most patients.[41] Doses smaller than 0.5 mg can produce a paradoxical bradycardia due to the central and/or peripheral para-sympathomimetic effects of low doses. This effect can precipitate ventricular fibrillation.[34,42] For patients with asystole, a dose of 1 mg (repeated once if necessary) is recommended.

Endotracheal administration of atropine can be used in patients without intravenous access (Figure 4).[26,43] Endotracheally administered atropine produces a rapid onset of action similar to that observed with intravenous injection.[43,44] The recommended adult dose of atropine for endotracheal administration is 1.0–2.0 mg diluted in 10 mL of sterile water or normal saline.[26,44]

Precautions

Atropine may induce tachycardia, which may be deleterious in patients with acute myocardial ischemia or infarction.[45] Atropine should be administered with caution in the setting of myocardial ischemia.[45,46] Ventricular fibrillation and tachycardia have occurred after IV administration of atropine.[47-49] Excessive doses of atropine can cause delirium, tachycardia, coma, flushed and hot skin, ataxia, and blurred vision.[50]

Figure 4. Changes in cardiac rate and rhythm following endotracheal administration of atropine. Measurement of atropine blood levels confirmed absorption of the drug. From Greenberg MI, Mayeda DV, Chrzanowski R, Brumwell D, Baskin SI, Roberts JR: Endotracheal administration of atropine sulfate. *Ann Emerg Med* 11:546-548, 1982. (1) Initial cardiac rhythm strip, supraventricular mechanism, 30–40 beats/min. (2) Cardiac rhythm strip 75 sec after endotracheal intubation. Atropine sulfate 1.0 mg, administered ET. (3) 30 sec after ET atropine. (4) 90 sec after ET atropine.

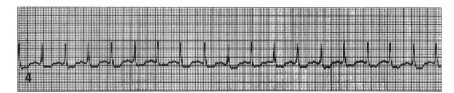
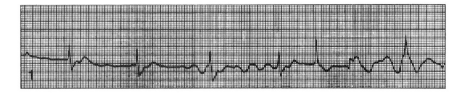
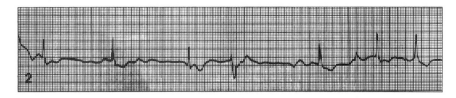
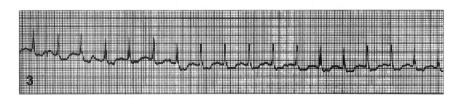

Antiarrhythmic Agents

Arrhythmias result from altered impulse formation (automaticity), abnormal impulse conduction (reentry), or a combination of both mechanisms. During myocardial ischemia, either or both mechanisms may exist. In addition, ischemia leads to a decrease in the threshold for ventricular fibrillation (the energy necessary to induce ventricular fibrillation). Antiarrhythmic drugs comprise a heterogenous group of agents. The Vaughn-Williams and Singh Classification system (Table 1) lists antiarrhythmic agents according to their predominant electrophysiologic effects.

Lidocaine

Mechanisms of Action

Lidocaine suppresses ventricular arrhythmias predominantly by decreasing automaticity by reducing the slope of Phase 4 diastolic depolarization (Figure 5).[51] Its local anesthetic properties may also help to suppress ventricular ectopy after acute myocardial infarction.[52] Lidocaine may terminate reentrant ventricular arrhythmias by further depressing conduction in reentrant pathways, thus converting unidirectional block to bidirectional block (Figure 6).[53] This prevents the emergence of wavefronts from zones of ischemic myocardium. Lidocaine has been shown also to reduce the disparity in action potential duration between ischemic and normal zones and to prolong conduction and refractoriness in ischemic tissue[54] (Figure 7).

Table 1. Vaughn-Williams and Singh Classification of Anti-arrhythmic Drugs

Class	Drugs
I	A. *Procainamide*
	Disopyramide
	Quinidine
	B. *Lidocaine*
	Tocainide
	Phenytoin
	Mexilitine
	C. Flecainide
	Encainide
	Lorcainide
II	Propranolol
	Acebutolol
	Atenolol
	Labetolol
	Metoprolol
	Nadolol
	Pindolol
	Timolol
III	*Bretylium*
	Amiodarone
	Sotalol
IV	*Verapamil*
	Diltiazem
	Nifedipine

During acute myocardial ischemia, the threshold for the induction of ventricular fibrillation is reduced (less energy is required and thus fibrillation is more likely to occur). In some studies lidocaine has been shown to elevate the fibrillation threshold.[55] Elevation of the fibrillation threshold correlates closely with blood levels of lidocaine.[55] However, in other studies, lidocaine either does not alter or may increase the ventricular defibrillation threshold, i.e., the energy needed to reverse ventricular fibrillation.[56,57] In a comparison study with bretylium, lidocaine and bretylium behaved similarly in this regard.[56] In man, clinical studies do not indicate that lidocaine has a major antifibrillatory effect in prehospital VF refractory to direct-current countershock.[58] Thus, its comparable efficacy with agents that do have "primary antifibrillatory effects" may be related to the fact that some apparently refractory episodes of ventricular fibrillation represent recurrent rather than resistant episodes and that lidocaine is capable of preventing recurrence.[59,60] Higher plasma lidocaine concentrations

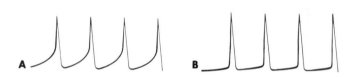

Figure 5. Effect of lidocaine on Phase 4 depolarization in canine Purkinje fiber action potentials. (A) Prior to lidocaine administration, there is spontaneous depolarization (automaticity). (B) After lidocaine, slope of Phase 4 depolarization has been depressed.

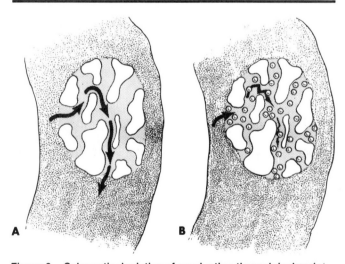

Figure 6. Schematic depiction of conduction through ischemic/ infarcted intramural zone of ventricular muscle. White areas are islands of inexcitable, severely depressed tissue. Dotted areas within ischemic zone are still excitable, though also depressed, and conduct wavefront at reduced conduction velocities. Ischemic zone is surrounded by normal muscle, indicated by wavy lines. (A) Wavefront propagates through depressed area at reduced conduction velocity, but is able to sustain itself and emerge to reenter surrounding normal myocardium. (B) After lidocaine administration, lidocaine-induced further depression of conduction velocity impairs advance of wavefront to extent that it is blocked, unable to reenter normal surrounding muscle. Reentrant arrhythmias sustained via such pathways of depressed conduction would then be terminated.

Control

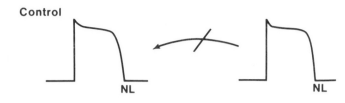

Acute Ischemia

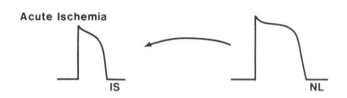

After Lidocaine

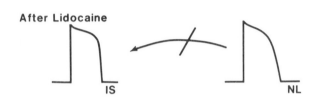

Figure 7. Boundary current in a canine model during acute ischemia and after lidocaine administration. Top: There is no boundary current flow between normal zones (NL) of heart because action potentials are of essentially equal duration. Middle: In acute ischemia of 15-minute duration, current flows from normal zone into acutely ischemic zone (IS). This is because acute ischemia shortens action potential duration in ischemic tissue, which therefore recovers excitability earlier than surrounding normal tissue. This current can pass through ischemic tissue slowly and emerge to reexcite heart as PVC. Bottom: Lidocaine acts on normal tissue to make action potentials more uniform, thus preventing current flow.

are required to achieve an antifibrillatory effect than to control ventricular ectopy.[61,62]

Lidocaine usually does not affect myocardial contractility, arterial blood pressure, atrial arrhythmogenesis, or intraventricular conduction. It can on occasion facilitate atrioventricular conduction.[51]

Indications

Lidocaine reduces the incidence of primary ventricular fibrillation in patients with acute myocardial infarction.[63-65] In a randomized controlled study of patients with suspected acute myocardial infarction, 400 mg of (prophylactic) lidocaine injected intramuscularly reduced the incidence of subsequent ventricular fibrillation.[65] Prophylactic lidocaine is recommended for patients strongly suspected of having acute myocardial infarction, though some have questioned both the safety and efficacy of this intervention.[66,67]

Lidocaine is the drug of choice for the supression of ventricular ectopy, including ventricular tachycardia and ventricular fibrillation, as well as ventricular premature complexes (PVC's) in critically ill patients, especially

those with acute ischemic heart disease. Traditional indications for treatment of PVC's include PVC's that are frequent (more than 6 per minute), close-coupled (R on T phenomenon), multiform, or occurring in short bursts of two or more PVC's or salvos.

Lidocaine is useful in the treatment of both ventricular tachycardia and fibrillation. In controlled studies, lidocaine is as effective as agents with "primary antifibrillatory effects".[59,60] In ventricular fibrillation that reverts after an initially successful conversion, lidocaine should be given and other causes of recurrent VF (e.g., persistent acidosis or hypoxemia) should be sought. To prevent recurrent VF, lidocaine should be continued for at least 24 hours after ventricular tachycardia or fibrillation has been terminated.

Dosage

There is an extensive literature on the proper way to load and to maintain blood levels of lidocaine in an effective suppressive range of 1.5–6.0 μg/ mL.[68-70] One reasonable approach consists of a bolus injection of 1 mg/kg, with additional bolus injections of 0.5 mg/kg every 2–10 minutes if needed to a total dose of 3 mg/kg.[69] Since the half-life of a bolus of lidocaine is short and the time for the drug to achieve reasonable levels with a continuous infusion is long,[69] only bolus therapy should be used in treating patients in cardiac arrest. After restoration of circulatory function, a continuous infusion should be started at 30–50 μg/kg/min (or approximately 2-4 mg/min).[69]

For primary prophylaxis against ventricular fibrillation, an initial bolus of 1.5 mg/kg is followed by a continuous infusion at 2–4 mg/min. To prevent subtherapeutic plasma lidocaine levels after the initial bolus, a second bolus of 0.5 mg/kg is administered after 10 minutes. The maintenance infusion can be titrated upward if ventricular ectopy is present, and additional 50-mg boluses may be given every 5 minutes up to a total dose of 2 mg/kg or 225 mg. The dose of lidocaine should be decreased by 50% in the presence of impaired hepatic blood flow (acute myocardial infarction, congestive heart failure, or shock) because total body clearance of lidocaine is reduced.[71,72] Above the age of 70 years, patients have a reduced volume of distribution; in such patients the dose should also be reduced by 50%.[69]

Precautions

Excessive doses of lidocaine are capable of producing myocardial and circulatory depression. Clinical indicators of lidocaine toxicity include drowsiness, disorientation, decreased hearing ability, paresthesias, and muscle twitching.[68] Some patients may become very agitated. More serious toxic effects include focal and grand mal seizures.[51] Treatment consists of withdrawal of lidocaine and, if necessary, administration of CNS depressants such as barbituates or diazepam to control seizures.

Lidocaine undergoes hepatic degradation. If hepatic function is impaired, the dose should be reduced. The dose should also be reduced in the presence of reductions in cardiac output associated with myocardial infarction, acute pulmonary edema, or shock[71-73] and in patients over 70 years of age.[74] Advanced heart failure may be associated with near-toxic plasma levels of lidocaine after relatively brief infusions (Figure 8). In one anecdote, only 2 hours of infusion produced plasma levels of 5 μg/mL.[72] If the infusion had been continued, toxic levels would have been reached shortly thereafter.

The pharmacokinetics of lidocaine in patients with cardiac arrest are not well-understood, but available experimental evidence in dogs indicates that disposition of the drug is greatly altered, most likely a consequence of the severe reduction of cardiac output and blood flow during CPR.[75] Consequently, high levels are achieved. This may be the reason why apparent beneficial effects are observed in humans (2 bretylium comparisons) when such effects are only seen at very high doses in experimental animals.[61,62] Additional data in humans receiving CPR is needed.

While neither volume of distribution nor clearance of lidocaine is abnormal in patients with renal disease, after prolonged infusions metabolites normally excreted in the urine may accumulate and may have pharmacologic activity.[71]

In therapeutic doses, lidocaine can be used safely in patients with conduction disturbances. Large doses may infrequently induce heart block, depress spontaneous discharge from the sinus node, or alter AV conduction.[51,76] However, in usual doses lidocaine does not change the AH and HV times measured by a bundle of His recording.[77] Nevertheless, caution should be observed in the use of lidocaine in a patient with documented conduction system disorder.

Procainamide

Mechanisms of Action

Procainamide effectively suppresses ventricular ectopy and may be effective when lidocaine has not achieved suppression of life-threatening ventricular arrhythmias.[78] In normal ventricular muscle and Purkinje fibers, procainamide suppresses Phase 4 diastolic depolarization reducing the automaticity of ectopic pacemakers. Procainamide also slows intraventricular conduction by reducing the slope of Phase 0 of the action potential. If conduction already is slowed, e.g., in ischemic tissue, further slowing may produce bidirectional block and may terminate reentrant arrhythmias.[79,80]

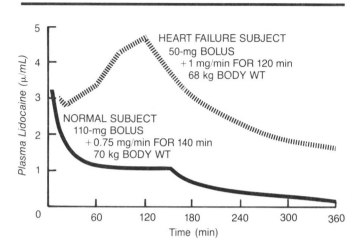

Figure 8. Illustration of difference in plasma level response to infused lidocaine in normal subject and heart failure subject of similar size. Within 2 hours, concentrations of lidocaine approached toxic levels in patient with advanced heart failure, even though infusion rate was near minimum recommended dose.

Indications

Procainamide may be useful in suppressing premature ventricular complexes and recurrent ventricular tachycardia which cannot be controlled with lidocaine. It is rarely used to treat ventricular fibrillation because it takes so long to achieve adequate levels even intravenously. Procainamide also may be used to convert supraventricular arrhythmias.[81]

Dosage

The IV dose for premature ventricular complexes and ventricular tachycardia is 100 mg every 5 minutes at a rate of 20 mg/min until one of the following is observed: 1) the arrhythmia is suppressed; 2) hypotension ensues; 3) the QRS complex is widened by 50% of its original width; or 4) a total of 1 g of drug has been injected.[78] The maintenance infusion rate is 1–4 mg/min. Therapeutic blood levels are in the range of 4–10 μg/mL.[82] Dosage should be reduced in patients with left ventricular dysfunction and/or renal failure. The plasma procainamide concentration should be monitored in patients who have renal failure, in patients who are on a constant infusion of 3 mg/min or more for 24 hours or longer, and in patients who are on chronic oral therapy.

An alternative approach to the administration of procainamide uses a loading dose of 17.0 mg/kg given as an infusion over 1 hour, followed by a maintenance infusion of 2.8 mg/kg/hr. In patients with cardiac or renal dysfunction, the loading dose is reduced to 12.0 mg/kg and the maintainance dose is decreased to 1.4 mg/kg/hr.[82] Therapeutic concentrations in plasma are achieved in about 15 minutes and are sustained by the maintenance infusion.[82]

Precautions

Procainamide is a ganglionic blocker with potent vasodilating and modest negative inotropic effects, especially in patients with left ventricular dysfunction.[78,82,83] Procainamide-induced hypotension is most pronounced after rapid intravenous injection, or when high plasma procainamide concentrations are present.[83] Thus, monitoring of the arterial blood pressure and the ECG are essential during intravenous administration. Adverse effects observed on the ECG include widening of the QRS complex and lengthening of the PR or the QT interval. Atrioventricular conduction disturbances, including heart block, or cardiac arrest may follow. Intravenous procainamide must be administered cautiously to patients with acute myocardial infarction.

Bretylium

No antiarrythmic agent has been proven to be superior to defibrillation alone for the treatment of ventricular fibrillation. However, there is substantial inferential evidence that bretylium may be useful. Results of studies differ on whether bretylium improves either fibrillation or defibrillation threshold.[56,84,85] Although the effects of bretylium on the fibrillation threshold are similar to those of lidocaine,[56,62] lidocaine may increase defibrillation threshold whereas bretylium does not.[56,57] No difference in clinical outcome or survival has been found in studies that have compared the use of lidocaine and bretylium for treating patients with out-of-hospital VF.[59,60] Since there is no survival benefit from the use of bretylium over lidocaine and since there may be a greater potential for adverse hemodynamic effects with bretylium than with lidocaine, lidocaine is the drug of first choice for all ventricular ectopy. Bretylium should be considered in patients with refractory malignant ventricular arrhythmias.

Bretylium tosylate is an adrenergic neuronal blocking drug introduced in 1950 as an antihypertensive agent. Tolerance to its antihypertensive action and undesirable side effects limited its oral use in the treatment of hypertension.[86] Interest in bretylium was revived in the mid-sixties when it was found to possess antifibrillatory activity.[87]

Mechanisms of Action

Bretylium is a quaternary ammonium compound with both adrenergic and direct myocardial effects.[88,89] Bretylium's adrenergic effects are biphasic. Initially, bretylium releases norepinephrine from adrenergic nerve endings in direct relation to its concentration at the adrenergic terminal.[90] These sympathomimetic effects last approximately 20 minutes[89,91] and consist of transient hypertension, tachycardia and, in some, increases in cardiac

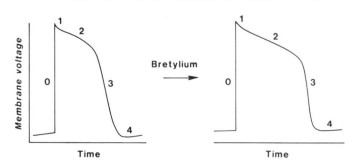

Figure 9. Schematic illustration of normal Purkinje fiber action potential before and after bretylium administration. Drug prolongs duration of action potential and refractory period to greater degree in normal tissue than in ischemic and infarcting tissue. By prolonging refractory period, bretylium may prevent reentry from ischemic zone.

output.[91] Subsequently inhibition of norepinephrine release from peripheral adrenergic terminals results in adrenergic blockade which generally begins 15–20 minutes after injection and peaks 45–60 minutes later.[92] At this time, clinically significant hypotension may develop especially with changes in position.[93] In addition, since bretylium blocks the uptake of norepinephrine into adrenergic nerve terminals, it will potentiate the action of exogenous catecholamines.[88]

The antiarrhythmic action of bretylium is poorly understood. It elevates ventricular fibrillation threshold (the tendency for ventricular fibrillation to occur) as does lidocaine.[62,88] This effect is observed in both normal and in infarcted myocardium, and appears independent of bretylium's adrenergic effects.[93] It also increases the action potential duration and effective refractory period in normal ventricular muscle and Purkinje fibers without lengthening the effective refractory period relative to action potential duration (see Figure 9).[94] Thus, its electrophysiological actions are different from those observed with other antiarrhythmic agents. In general, bretylium does not suppress Phase 4 depolarization or the spontaneous firing of Purkinje fibers.[94] Thus, its effects may be more dependent on bretylium's adrenergic effects than originally thought.[84]

In infarcted canine hearts 1–2 days after coronary artery occlusion, bretylium produces prolongation of action potential duration throughout the normal conduction system, but very little increase in infarcted regions where action potential duration is already prolonged. This results in a reduction of the disparity in action potential duration and refractory period between normal and infarcted regions, reducing the ability for reentry to occur (see Figure 10).[95]

Action Potential Characteristics of Purkinje Cells

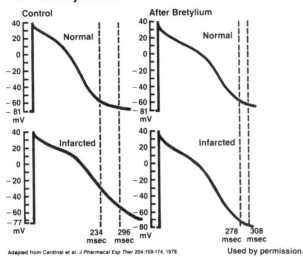

Adapted from Cardinal et al: *J Pharmacal Exp Ther* 204:159-174, 1978.

Used by permission.

Figure 10.   Effects of infarction and bretylium on Purkinje fibers from canine hearts 1–2 days after coronary artery occlusion. Action potentials in infarcted zones (control, lower left) have lower resting potentials and prolonged durations. This disparity may permit reentrant excitation. Bretylium prolongs duration of action potential and refractory period, primarily in surrounding normal tissue and, to a lesser extent, in the infarcted area. This results in a reduction in disparity in action potential duration and refractory period between infarcted and normal tissue. Reentrant excitation is less likely to occur with more equalized recovery times.

Bretylium also produces an early transient improvement in the amplitude and upslope of Phase 0 of the action potential (increased amplitude and increased dV/dt max) in Purkinje fibers in infarcted regions, which improves conduction velocity[95] probably related to the initial release of catecholamines.[88,92] Since ventricular fibrillation may result from competing wave fronts,[96] improved conduction induced transiently by bretylium could conceivably prevent this competition and thus reduce the propensity for ventricular fibrillation to develop.

Indications

Clinically, bretylium has been useful in treating both ventricular fibrillation and ventricular tachycardia refractory to other therapy, including lidocaine, procainamide, and repeated shocks.[59,97] In the absence of data that bretylium is superior to lidocaine in the treatment of either ventricular tachycardia or ventricular fibrillation (Figure 11), to simplify initial pharmacological therapy and to avoid potentially adverse hemodynamic responses to bretylium,[98] it is not recommended as first-line treatment. Bretylium should be considered for use when lidocaine and electrical countershock fails to convert VF, VF recurs despite therapy with lidocaine, or lidocaine and procainamide have not controlled ventricular tachycardia accompanied by a palpable pulse.

Dosage

In ventricular fibrillation, 5 mg/kg undiluted bretylium is given rapidly IV. After 1–2 minutes to permit access to the central circulation, defibrillation is attempted again. If ventricular fibrillation persists, the dose can be increased to 10 mg/kg and repeated at 15- to 30-minute intervals to a maximum dose of 30 mg/kg.[88]

In refractory or recurrent ventricular tachycardia, 500 mg of bretylium (l0 mL) can be diluted to 50 mL, and 5–10 mg/kg can be injected IV over a period of 8–10 minutes. In the conscious patient, hypotension, nausea, and vomiting may follow more rapid injection. If ventricular tachycardia persists, a second dose of 5–10 mg/kg can be given in 1–2 hours and, if necessary, every 6–8 hours thereafter.[99] Alternatively, bretylium can be administered as a continuous infusion at a rate of 2 mg/min.[87] While the onset of action of bretylium in ventricular fibrillation seems to be within a few minutes, in ventricular tachycardia it may be delayed for 20 minutes or more.

Precautions

Postural hypotension is the most common adverse reaction. It is observed in as many as 60% of patients, although the mean arterial pressure infrequently falls more than 20 mmHg.[87] Treatment includes assumption of a supine, or if necessary, Trendelenberg position, and IV fluids. In some cases a vasopressor such as norepinephrine may be required. Hypotension may be

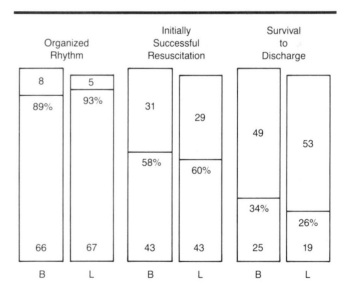

Figure 11.   Outcome in a randomized clinical trial comparing bretylium (B, 74 patients) and lidocaine (L, 72 patients) in out-of-hospital ventricular fibrillation. Percentages indicate restoration of organized rhythm, initially successful resuscitation, and survival to discharge. There were no significant differences between the two groups. Adapted from Haynes RE, Chinn TL, Copass MK, Cobb LA: Comparison of bretylium tosylate and lidocaine in management of out of hospital ventricular fibrillation: A randomized clinical trial. *Am J Cardiol* 48:353-356, 1981.

refractory to epinephrine.[100] Hypertension and tachycardia may also occur, but these effects are transient due to the initial stimulation of norepinephrine release from adrenergic nerve terminals.[88] Nausea and vomiting also may occur after rapid injection in the awake patient.

Bretylium is relatively contraindicated in the treatment of arrhythmias accompanying digitalis toxicity, because catecholamines are thought to exacerbate digitalis toxicity.[90] However, because this effect is transient, bretylium may be of benefit in such patients.[90]

Verapamil

The inhibition of slow channel activity in cardiac and vascular smooth muscle results in several clinically useful effects which differ substantially from one agent to the other.[100,101] Verapamil is highly effective for treating patients who have a supraventricular tachycardia.[102-106]

Mechanisms of Action

Verapamil is a derivative of papaverine.[107,108] The therapeutic usefulness of verapamil is due to its slow-channel-blocking properties, especially on cardiac and vascular smooth muscle.[106] It blocks the slow inward current due to changes in both calcium and sodium flux.[109] Verapamil is a negative inotrope that causes a reduction in myocardial oxygen consumption.[106,110] Its negative inotropic effects are counterbalanced in part by a reduction in systemic vascular resistance and impedence (afterload) caused by its vasodilator effect on vascular smooth muscle. Verapamil also causes coronary vasodilation.[111,112]

Verapamil slows conduction and prolongs refractoriness in the AV node, making it useful in the termination of supraventricular tachycardias that utilize the AV node as part of their reentrant pathway. It will also slow the ventricular response to atrial flutter and fibrillation.[104,113,114] It depresses the amplitude of action potentials in the upper and middle regions of the AV node.[115] The AH interval and the effective functional refractory periods of the AV node lengthen after verapamil is administered.[116] In patients with the typical form of AV nodal tachycardia, verapamil terminates the arrhythmia by blocking conduction in the slow antegrade limb of the reentrant circuit.[116] Because it blocks slow response action potentials, it has the potential to be of benefit in treating arrhythmias associated with ischemia.[117]

Indications

In emergency cardiac care, verapamil is used primarily in the treatment of paroxysmal supraventricular tachycardia (PSVT)[102-106] that does not require cardioversion. The electrophysiological actions of verapamil on the AV node account for its effectiveness in promptly terminating PSVT. The most common form of PSVT is due to sustained reentry within the AV node. The next most common type uses the AV node for at least one limb of its reentrant circuit.[118] When used for properly defined indications, verapamil terminates 90% or more of episodes of PSVT in adults[102-106] and in infants.[119] The drug is also useful in slowing the ventricular response to atrial flutter and fibrillation.[103-107,114]

Verapamil has minimal effects on the bypass tracts of patients with the Wolff-Parkinson-White syndrome.[120] However, due to the reduced AV conduction, the refractory period of the bypass tract during antegrade conduction may be shortened.[120-122] In some patients, verapamil may shorten the refractory period of the accessory pathway due to a reflex increase in adrenergic tone in response to peripheral vasodilation.[122] Thus, the ventricular response to atrial fibrillation may be accelerated in response to verapamil (Figure 12)[121,122] and ventricular fibrillation can occur.[123-126] Verapamil should be avoided in patients with Wolff-Parkinson-White and atrial fibrillation or flutter. Because a reciprocating tachycardia could degenerate into atrial fibrillation, patients with WPW syndrome who are being treated with verapamil for PSVT should be closely monitored continuously and a defibrillator should be immediately available.[123,127]

Verapamil is not effective for the treatment of ventricular tachycardia; it may induce severe hypotension and predispose to the development of ventricular fibrillation.[128] If one cannot be certain of the origin of a wide-QRS tachycardia by ECG criteria it is prudent to assume that the rhythm is ventricular tachycardia until proven otherwise and verapamil should be avoided.[128,129]

Dosage

Single Dose

0.075–0.15 mg/kg body weight (max: 10 mg) given as IV bolus over 1-minute period. Peak therapeutic effects occur within 3–5 minutes of bolus injection.

Repeat Dose

0.15 mg/kg body weight (max: 10 mg) 30 minutes after first dose if initial response is not adequate.

Older Patients

In older patients the IV dose should be administered over at least a 3-minute period.

Age 8–15 Years

0.1–0.3 mg/kg body weight (total single dose range: 2–5 mg) administered as an IV bolus over 1-minute period. Repeat dose: 0.1–0.2 mg/kg body weight (total single dose range: 2–5 mg) 15–30 minutes after first dose if initial response is not adequate.

A

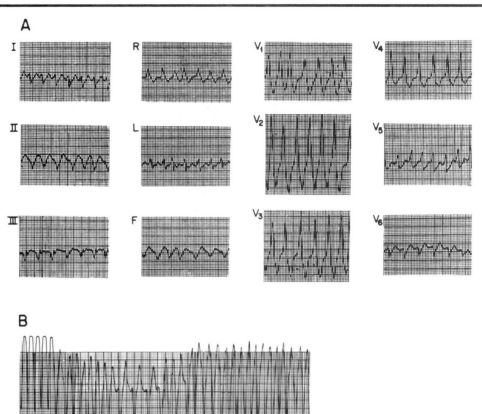

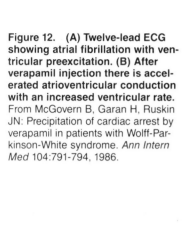

Figure 12. (A) Twelve-lead ECG showing atrial fibrillation with ventricular preexcitation. (B) After verapamil injection there is accelerated atrioventricular conduction with an increased ventricular rate.
From McGovern B, Garan H, Ruskin JN: Precipitation of cardiac arrest by verapamil in patients with Wolff-Parkinson-White syndrome. *Ann Intern Med* 104:791-794, 1986.

B

Precautions

A transient decrease in arterial pressure due to peripheral vasodilatation should be expected in response to verapamil.[102] Cardiac output usually remains unchanged, reflecting the balance between the intrinsic negative inotropic effects of the drug, its reflex sympathetic response, and vasodilatation.[102,130] This is also true in patients with mild-to-moderate left ventricular dysfunction as well.[131] However, in patients with severely reduced left ventricular function, IV verapamil may induce hemodynamic compromise.[131]

Verapamil can be used safely and effectively in patients receiving digitalis. Unless there is evidence of impaired AV conduction, prior treatment with digitalis is not a contraindication to the use of IV verapamil.[132] However, the concomitant use of IV beta-adrenergic blocking agents is a contraindication since the hemodynamic and electrophysiological effects of these agents will be synergistic.[107] Caution is also recommended when the IV verapamil is given to a patient receiving beta blockers orally. Verapamil should be avoided or used with caution in patients with sick sinus syndrome or AV block in the absence of a pacemaker.[106] In patients with

acute pump failure precipitated by supraventricular tachycardia, therapy with verapamil is not contraindicated since alleviation of the tachycardia removes the cause of the hemodynamic compromise. When this is not the case, severe heart failure is a contraindication to the use of verapamil.

Bradycardia can occur if cardioversion is done proximate to the administration of verapamil.

Sodium Bicarbonate (NaHCO₃)

Mechanisms of Action

During cardiopulmonary arrest, hypoxia-induced anaerobic metabolism results in the generation of lactic acid and the development of metabolic acidosis. At the same time, ventilatory failure leads to carbon dioxide retention (hypercarbia) and respiratory acidosis. The acidotic state accompanying arrest of ventilation and circulation usually is of mixed metabolic and respiratory origin. Prompt and efficient ventilation via an endotracheal tube is essential for the elimination of carbon dioxide as well as for oxygenation. Effective ventilation and circulation of blood during CPR are the means available for preventing and managing the acidemia associated with cardiac arrest.[133]

Sodium bicarbonate reacts with hydrogen ions to form water and carbon dioxide to buffer metabolic acidosis. The major problem with its use is that it has a high carbon dioxide content (260–280 mmHg for each 50 mEq).[134] The carbon dioxide crosses rapidly into cells causing a paradoxical worsening of intracellular hypercarbia and acidosis.[135] Bicarbonate crosses into cells much more slowly.[136]

Although metabolic acidosis lowers the threshold for induction of ventricular fibrillation, it has no effect on defibrillation threshold;[137,138] and the inhibitory effect of metabolic acidosis (as opposed to respiratory acidosis[139]) on the action of catecholamines has not been documented to occur at pH values encountered during cardiac arrest and in the presence of the very large doses of epinephrine used in resuscitation. Administration of sodium bicarbonate does not facilitate ventricular defibrillation or survival in cardiac arrest.[140,141]

Indications

The absence of proven efficacy and the numerous adverse effects associated with sodium bicarbonate have led to a reconsideration of its role in cardiac resuscitation. Sodium bicarbonate should be used, if at all, only after application of more definitive and better substantiated interventions, such as prompt defibrillation, effective chest compression, endotracheal intubation and hyperventilation with 100% oxygen, and the use of drugs such as epinephrine and lidocaine. These interventions will usually take approximately 10 minutes; thereafter, sodium bicarbonate therapy, although not recommended, can be considered in specific clinical circumstances such as documented preexisting metabolic acidosis with or without hyperkalemia.

Dosage

When sodium bicarbonate is used, 1 mEq/kg should be given initially. A maximum of one-half this dose may be given for subsequent doses, which should not be given more frequently than every 10 minutes. After resuscitation, bicarbonate adminstration should be determined by measurements of arterial pH and PCO_2.

Precautions

In the past, too much emphasis has been placed on the administration of sodium bicarbonate during cardiac arrest. The crucial role of carbon dioxide tension has been underemphasized. *In vitro,* even partial respiratory

compensation of metabolic acidosis can prevent intracellular acidosis.[142] Sodium bicarbonate administration results in the rapid generation of carbon dioxide:

$$HCO_3^- + H^+ \rightleftharpoons H_2CO_3 \rightleftharpoons CO_2 + H_2O$$

and carbon dioxide is a rapidly acting and potent negative inotrope.[143,144] The performance of the ischemic heart is closely related to tissue PCO_2 and is minimally related to the level of extracellular pH.[144] Cardiac muscle performance is depressed by increases in arterial PCO_2 presumably due to the paradoxically intracellular acidosis that is induced.[145,146] While hydrogen ions induced during metabolic acidosis also exert a negative inotropic action, this effect is much slower in onset and may not be fully manifest until 30 minutes have elapsed from onset of an acidosis to a magnitude equivalent to that induced more rapidly by carbon dioxide.[144] The rapid onset of a carbon dioxide-induced intracellular acidosis is directly related to the rapidity with which carbon dioxide diffuses intracellularly.[144] Intracellular carbon dioxide tension during experimental acute myocardial ischemia has been shown to rise in excess of 300 mmHg, and corresponding intracellular pH falls to as low as 6.1.[147,148] Liberation of carbon dioxide and its rapid intracellular diffusion after sodium bicarbonate administration worsen intracellular acidosis during cardiopulmonary resuscitation. Cerebrospinal fluid acidosis and central venous acidosis result from sodium bicarbonate administration during CPR (Figure 13).[135,149]

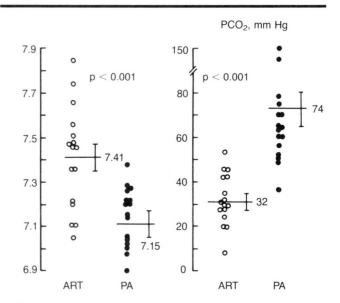

Figure 13. Differences in systemic arterial (ART) and pulmonary artery (PA) pH and PCO_2 in 16 patients during cardiopulmonary resuscitation. Measurements were made at a median of 23 minutes after onset of arrest. Average dose of $NaHCO_3$ ($\pm$ SEM) was 130 $\pm$ 30 mEq over a median interval of 23 minutes. Numerical mean values for each measurement are indicated on the graph. Mixed venous acidemia from CO_2 retention is evident. $NaHCO_3$ would be expected to worsen this acidosis from CO_2 formation. From Weil MH, Rackow EC, Trevino R, Grundler W, Falk JL, Griffel MI: Difference in acid–base state between venous and arterial blood during cardiopulmonary resuscitation. *N Engl J Med* 315:153-156, 1986.

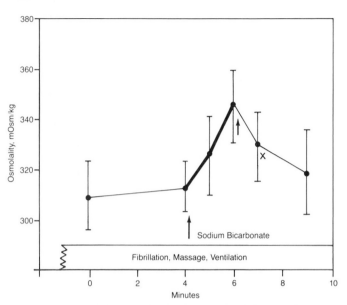

Figure 14. Arterial osmolality in six patients during cardiac resuscitation. Note significant and persistent rise in osmolality after sodium bicarbonate administration. (x's indicate $P < .05$; + $P < .01$). From Bishop RL, Weisfeldt ML: Sodium bicarbonate administration during cardiac arrest. Effect on arterial pH, PCO_2, and osmolality. *JAMA* 235:506-509, 1976.

Other adverse effects from sodium bicarbonate include hypernatremia and hyperosmolality (Figure 14).[150,151] Severe hyperosmolal states during resuscitation may compromise survival.[150] Shift in the oxyhemoglobin saturation curve caused by sodium bicarbonate can inhibit oxygen release to the tissues.

Morphine

Mechanisms of Action

Morphine is effective treatment for ischemic chest pain and for acute pulmonary edema.[152] It manifests both analgesic and hemodynamic effects.[153] It increases venous capacitance and reduces systemic vascular resistance, relieving pulmonary congestion. In doing so, it reduces intramyocardial wall tension, which decreases myocardial oxygen requirements.[154,155] Morphine's hemodynamic effects may be mediated by sympatholytic effects on the central nervous system since they are most pronounced in patients with heightened sympathetic activity.[153,156]

Indications

Morphine is the drug of choice for the treatment of pain and anxiety associated with acute myocardial infarction. It is also useful for treating patients with acute cardiogenic pulmonary edema.

Dosage

Morphine should be administered intravenously in small incremental doses of 2–5 mg every 5–30 minutes, until the desired effect is achieved.

Precautions

Morphine, like many other narcotic analgesics, is a respiratory depressant. Small incremental doses at frequent intervals make serious depression less likely than a single large bolus. Excessive narcosis can be reversed with intravenous naloxone (0.4–0.8 mg). Hypotension is most common and most severe in volume depleted patients and in patients who are dependent on elevated systemic resistance for maintenance of blood pressure.[155] Hypotension and an inappropriate heart rate response which appears to be vagally mediated also has been described.[157]

Calcium Chloride

Mechanisms of Action

Calcium ions increase the force of myocardial contraction.[158] In response to electrical stimulation of muscle, calcium ions enter the sarcoplasm from the extracellular space.[159,160] Calcium ions contained in the sarcoplasmic reticulum are rapidly transferred to the sites of interaction between the actin and myosin filaments of the sarcomere to initiate myofibril shortening.[161] Thus, calcium increases myocardial contractile function. Calcium's positive inotropic effects are modulated by its action on systemic vascular resistance. Calcium may either increase or decrease systemic vascular resistance.[162-164] In normal hearts, calcium's positive inotropic and vasoconstricting effects produce a predictable rise in systemic arterial pressure.[162,165]

Indications

There are no data demonstrating a beneficial effect from the administration of calcium salts during cardiopulmonary resuscitation.[166-168] In theory, the high levels of calcium in the blood induced by the administration of calcium salts may induce reperfusion injury and may adversely effect the neurologic outcome of the patient.[167] Calcium salts should not be used during resuscitation except for the treatment of acute hyperkalemia, hypocalcemia, or calcium channel blocker toxicity and hypermagnesemia.[170]

Dosage

A 10-mL prefilled syringe or ampule of 10% solution of calcium chloride contains 13.6 mEq of calcium (100 mg = 1 mL). Calcium chloride can be given intravenously in a dose of 2–4 mg/kg of 10% solution and repeated if considered necessary at 10-minute intervals. Two other calcium salts are available, calcium gluceptate and calcium gluconate. Calcium gluceptate can be given in a dose of 5–7 mL; the dose of calcium gluconate is 5–8 mL. Calcium chloride is preferable because it produces consistently higher and more predictable levels of ionized calcium in plasma.[171]

Precautions

If the heart is beating, rapid administration of calcium can produce slowing of the cardiac rate. Calcium must be used cautiously in the digitalized patient because it increases ventricular irritability and may precipitate digitalis toxicity. In the presence of sodium bicarbonate, calcium salts will precipitate as carbonates. Thus, these drugs cannot be administered together. Calcium may produce vasospasm in coronary and cerebral arteries.

References

1. Ornato JP, Bryson, Donovan PJ. et al: Measurement of ventilation during cardiopulmonary resuscitation. *Crit Care Med* 11:79-82, 1983.
2. Wynne JW, Modell JH: Respiratory aspiration of stomach content. *Ann Intern Med* 87:466-474, 1977.
3. Ayres SM: Mechanisms and consequences of pulmonary edema. Cardiac lung, shock lung, and principles of ventilatory therapy in adult respiratory distress syndrome. *Am Heart J* 103:97-112, 1982.
4. Madias JE, Madia NE, Hood WB, Jr: Precordial ST-segment mapping. 2. Effects of oxygen inhalation on ischemic injury on patients with acute myocardial infarction. *Circulation* 53:411-417, 1976.
5. Otto CW, Yakaitis RW: The role of epinephrine in CPR: A reappraisal. *Ann Intern Med* 13(part 2):840-843, 1984.
6. Michael JR, Guerci AD, Koehler RC, Shi AY, Tsitlik J, Chandra N, Niedermeyer E, Rogers MC, Traystman RJ, Weisfeldt ML: Mechanisms by which epinephrine augments cerebral and myocardial perfusion during cardiopulmonary resuscitation in dogs. *Circulation* 69:822-835, 1984.
7. Koehler RC, Michael JR, Guerci AD, Chandra N, Schleien CL, Dean JM, Rogers MC, Weisfeldt ML, Traystman RJ: Beneficial effect of epinephrine infusion on cerebral and myocardial blood flows during CPR. *Ann Emerg Med* 14:744-749, 1985.
8. Otto CW, Yakaitis RW, Ewy GA: Spontaneous ischemic ventricular fibrillation in dogs: A new model for the study of cardiopulmonary resuscitation. *Crit Care Med* 11:883-887, 1983.
9. Otto CW, Yakaitis RW: The role of epinephrine in CPR: A reappraisal. *Ann Emerg Med* 13:840-843, 1984.
10. Livesay JJ, Follette DM, Fey KH, et al: Optimizing myocardial supply/demand balance with alpha-adrenergic drugs during cardiopulmonary resuscitation. *J Thorac Cardiovasc Surg* 76:244-251, 1978.
11. Ralston SH: Alpha agonist drug usage during CPR. *Ann Emerg Med* 13:786-788, 1984.
12. Yakaitis RW, Otto CW, Blitt CD: Relative importance of alpha- and beta-adrenergic receptors during resuscitation. *Crit Care Med* 7:293-296, 1979.
13. Holmes HR, Babbs CF, Voorhees WD, Tacker WA, DeGaravilla B: Influence of adrenergic drugs upon vital organ perfusion during CPR. *Crit Care Med* 8:137-140, 1980.
14. Brillman JA, Sanders AB, Otto CW, et al: Outcome of resuscitation from fibrillatory arrest using epinephrine and phenylephrine in dogs. *Crit Care Med* 13:912-913, 1985.
15. Brown CG, Werman HA, Davis EA, et al: Comparative effects of epinephrine and phenylephrine on regional cerebral blood flow during cardiopulmonary resuscitation. *Ann Emerg Med* 15:635, 1986. Abstract.
16. Brown CG, Werman HA, Davis EA, et al: Effect of high- dose phenylephrine versus epinephrine on regional cerebral blood flow during cardiopulmonary resuscitation. *Ann Emerg Med* 15:14, 1986. Abstract.
17. Brown CG, Werman HA, Hamlin R, et al: The comparative effects of methoxamine and epinephrine on regional cerebral blood flow in a swine model. *Crit Care Med* 14:333, 1986. Abstract.
18. Steen PA, Tinker JH, Pluth JR, et al: Efficacy of dopamine, dobutamine, and epinephrine during emergence from cardiopulmonary bypass in man. *Circulation* 57:378-381, 1978.
19. Sato Y, Matsuzawa H, Eguchi S: Comparative Study of Effects of adrenaline, dobutamine, and dopamine on systemic hemodynamics and renal blood flow in patients following open heart surgery. *Jpn Circ J* 46:1059-1063, 1982.
20. Gonzalez ER, Ornato JP, Garnett AR, et al: Enhanced vasopressor response after 3- and 5-mg doses of epinephrine during CPR in humans (abstract). *Am J Emerg Med* 4:418, 1986.
21. Kosnik JW, Jackson RE, Keats S, Tworek RM, Freeman SB: Dose-related response of aortic diastolic pressure during closed-chest massage in dogs. *Ann Emerg Med* 14:204-208;1985.
22. Dal Santa G: Absorption capacity of the airway and lungs, in Dal Santa G (ed): *Nonrespiratory Function of the Lung and Anesthesia.* Boston, Little Brown and Co., 1977, vol 15.
23. Roberts JR, Greenburg MI, Knaub MA, et al: Blood levels following intravenous and endotracheal epinephrine administration. *JACEP* 8:53-56, 1979.
24. Chernow B, Holbrook P, D'Angona DS Jr, Zaritsky A, Casey LC, Fletcher JR, Lake CR: Epinephrine absorption after intratracheal administration. *Anesth Analg* 63:829-832, 1984.
25. Roberts JR, Greenburg MI, Knaub M, Baskin SI: Comparison of the pharmacological effects of epinephrine adminstered by intravenous and endotracheal routes. *JACEP* 7:260, 1978.
26. Hasegawa EA: The endotracheal administration of drugs. *Heart Lung* 15:60-63, 1986.
27. Mace SE: Effect of technique of administration on plasma lidocaine levels. *Ann Emerg Med* 15:522, 1986.
28. Lindemann R: Endoctracheal administration of epinephrine during cardiopulmonary resuscitation (letter). *Am J Dis Child* 136:753, 1982.
29. Steen PA, Tinker JH, Pluth JR, et al: Efficacy of dopamine, dobutamine, and epinephrine during emergence from cardiopulmonary bypass in man. *Circulation* 57:378-384, 1978.
30. Newton DW, Fung EY, Williams DA: Stability of five catecholamines and terbutaline sulfate in 5% dextrose injection in the absence and presence of aminophylline. *Am J Hosp Pharm* 38:1314-1319, 1981.
31. Zaritsky AL, Chernow B: Catecholamines, sympathomimetics, in Chernow B, Lake CR (eds): *The Pharmacological Approach to the Critically Ill Patient.* Baltimore, Williams & Wilkins, 1983, pp 481-509.
32. Packer M, Gottlieb SJ, Kessler PD: Hormone-electrolyte interactions in the pathogenesis of lethal cardiac arrhythmias in patients with control of arrhythmias. *Am J Med* 80(suppl 4A)23-29, 1986.
33. Brown DC, Lewis AJ, Criley JM: Asystole and its treatment: The possible role of the parasympathetic nervous system in cardiac arrest. *J Am Coll Emerg Phys* 8:11,448, 1979.
34. Dauchot P, Gravenstein JS: Bradycardia after myocardial ischemia and its treatment with atropine. *Anesthesiology* 44:501-518, 1976.
35. Epstein SE, Goldstein RD, Redwood DR, et al: The early phase of acute myocardial infarction: Pharmacologic aspects of therapy (NIH Conference). *Ann Intern Med* 78:1918-1925,1973.
36. Myerburg RJ, Estes D, Zaman L, et al: Outcome of resuscitation from bradyarrhythmic or asystolic prehospital cardiac arrest. *J Am Coll Cardiol* 4:1118, 1984.
37. Stueven HA, Tonsfeldt DJ, Thompson BM, et al: Atropine in asystole: Human studies. *Ann Emerg Med* 13:815, 1984.
38. Ornato JP, Gonzalez ER, Morkunas AR, Coyne MR, Beck CL: Treatment of presumed asystole during pre-hospital cardiac arrest. *Am J Emerg Med* 3:395-399, 1985.
39. Iseri LT, Humphrey SB, Siner EJ: Pre-hospital bradyasystolic cardiac arrest. *Ann Intern Med* 88:741-745, 1978.
40. Coon GA, Clinton JE, Ruiz E. Use of atropine for bradyasystolic prehospital cardiac arrest. *Ann Emerg Med* 10:462-467, 1981.
41. O'Rourke GW, Greene NM: Autonomic blockade and the resting heart rate in man. *Am Heart J* 80:469-474, 1970.
42. Kottmeier CA, Gravenstein JS: The parasympathomimetic activity of atropine and atropine methylbromide. *Anesthesiology* 29:1125-1133, 1968.

43. Prete MR, Hannan CJ, Burkle FM: Plasma atropine concentrations via the intravenous, endotracheal, and intraosseous routes of administration (abstract). *Ann Emerg Med* 15:644, 1986.

44. Greenburg MI, Mayeda DV, Chrzanowski R, et al: Endotracheal administration of atropine sulfate. *Ann Emerg Med* 11:546-548, 1982.

45. Knoebel SB, McHenry PL, Phillips JR, et al: Atropine-induced cardioacceleration and myocardial blood flow in subjects with and without coronary artery disease. *Am J Cardiol* 33:327-332, 1974.

46. Richman S: Adverse effect of atropine during myocardial infarction. Enhancement of ischemia following intravenously administered atropine. *JAMA* 228:1414-1416, 1974.

47. Massumi RA, Mason DT, Amsterdam EA, et al: Ventricular fibrillation and tachycardia after intravenous atropine for treatment of bradycardias. *N Engl J Med.* 287:336-338, 1972.

48. Lunde P: Ventricular fibrillation after intravenous atropine for treatment of sinus bradycardia. *Acta Med Scand* 199:369-371, 1976.

49. Cooper MJ, Abinader EG: Atropine-induced ventricular fibrillation: Case report and review of the literature. *Am Heart J* 97:225-228, 1979.

50. Weiner N: Atropine, scopolamine, and related antimuscarinic drugs, in Gillman AG, Goodman LS, Gilman A (eds): *The Pharmcologic Basis of Therapeutics.* New York, Macmillan, Inc., 1980, pp 120-137.

51. Collinsworth KA, Kalman SM, Harrison DC: The clinical pharmacology of lidocaine as an anti-arrhythmic drug. *Circulation* 50:1217-1230, 1974.

52. Kupersmith J, Antman EM, Hoffman BF: *In vivo* electrophysiologic effects of lidocaine in canine acute myocardial infarction. *Circ Res* 36:84-91, 1975.

53. El-Sherif N, Scherlag BJ, Lazzara R, et al: Re-entrant ventricular arrhythmias in the late myocardial infarction period. IV. Mechanism of action of lidocaine. *Circulation* 56:395-402, 1977.

54. Kupersmith J: Electrophysiological and antiarrhythmic effects of lidocaine in canine acute myocardial ischemia. *Am Heart J* 97:360-366, 1979.

55. Spear JF, Moore EN, Gerstenblith G: Effect of lidocaine on the ventricular fibrillation threshold in the dog during acute ischemia and premature ventricular contraction. *Circulation* 46:65-73, 1972.

56. Kerber RE, Pandian NG, Jensen SR, Constantin L, Kieso RA, Melton J, Hunt M: Effect of lidocaine and bretylium on energy requirement for transthoracic defibrillation. Experimental studies. *J Am Coll Cardiol* 7:397-405, 1986.

57. Dorian P, Fain ES, Davy JM, Winkle RA: Lidocaine causes a reversible, concentration-dependent increase in defibrillation energy requirements. *J Am Coll Cardiol* 8:327-332, 1986.

58. Harrison EE: Lidocaine in prehospital countershock refractory ventricular fibrillation. *Ann Emerg Med* 10:420-430, 1981.

59. Haynes RE, Chinn TL, Copass MK, et al: Comparison of bretylium tosylate and lidocaine in management of out-of-hospital ventricular fibrillation. A randomized clinical trial. *Am J Cardiol* 48:353-356, 1981.

60. Olson DW, Thompson BM, Darin JL, Milbrath MH: A randomized comparison study of bretylium tosylate and lidocaine in resuscitation of patients from out-of-hospital ventricular fibrillation in a paramedic system. *Ann Emerg Med* 13:807-810, 1984.

61. Anderson JL: Antifibrillatory versus antiectopic therapy. *Am J Cardiol* 54:7A-13A, 1984.

62. Chow MSS, Kluger J, DiPersio DM, et al: Antifibrillatory effects of lidocaine and bretylium immediately post cardiopulmonary resuscitation. *Am Heart J* 110:938-943, 1985.

63. Lie KI, Wellens HJ, van Capelle FJ: Lidocaine in the prevention of primary ventricular fibrillation. A double-blind, randomized study of 212 consecutive patients. *N Engl J Med* 291:1324-1326, 1974.

64. DeSilva RA, Hennekens CH, Lown B, Casscells W: Lignocaine prophylaxis in acute mycoardial infarction. An evaluation of randomized trials. *Lancet* 2:855-858, 1981.

65. Koster RW, Dunning AJ: Intramuscular lidocaine for prevention of lethal arrhythmias in the prehospitalization phase of acute myocardial infarction. *N Engl J Med* 313:1105-1110, 1985.

66. Carruth JE, Silverman ME: Ventricular fibrillation complicating acute myocardial infarction: Reasons against the routine use of lidocaine. *Am Heart J* 104:545-550, 1982.

67. Dunn HM, McComb JM, Kinney CD, Campbell NPS, Shanks RG, MacKenzie G, Adgey AAJ: Prophylactic lidocaine in the early phase of suspected myocardial infarction. *Am Heart J* 110:353-362, 1985.

68. Benowitz N, Forsyth RP, Melmon KL, Rowland M: Lidocaine disposition kinetics in monkey and man. I. Prediction of a perfusion model. *Clin Pharmacol Ther* 16:87-98,1974.

69. Benowitz NL: Clinical applications of the pharmacokinetics of lidocaine. In Melmon KL (ed): *Cardiovascular Drug Therapy.* Philadelphia, FA Davis Co, 1976, pp 77-101.

70. Stargel WW, Shand DG, Routledge PA, Barchowsky A, Wagner GS: Clinical comparison of rapid infusion and multiple injection methods for lidocaine loading. *Am Heart J* 102:872-876, 1981.

71. Thomson PD, Melmon KL, Richardson JA, et al: Lidocaine pharmacokinetics in advanced heart failure, liver disease, and renal failure in humans. *Ann Intern Med* 78:499-508, 1973.

72. Thomson PD, Rowland M, Melmon KL: The influence of heart failure, liver disease, and renal failure on the disposition of lidocaine in man. *Am Heart J* 82:417-421, 1971.

73. Davison R, Parker M, Atkinson AJ: Excessive serum lidocaine levels during maintenance infusions: Mechanisms and prevention. *Am Heart J* 104:203-208, 1982.

74. Pfeifer HJ, Greenblatt DJ, Koch-Weser J: Clinical use and toxicity of intravenous lidocaine. A report from the Boston collaborative drug surveillance program. *Am Heart J* 92:168, 1976.

75. Chow MS, Ronfeld RA, Hamilton RA, Helmink R, Fieldman A: Effect of external cardiopulmonary resuscitation on lidocaine pharmacokinetics in dogs. *J Pharmacol Exp Ther* 224:531-537, 1983.

76. Lown B: Lidocaine to prevent ventricular fibrillation (editorial). *N Engl J Med* 313:1154-1155, 1985.

77. Kunkel FW, Rowland M, Scheinman MM: Effects of intravenous lidocaine infusion (LI) on atrioventricular (AV) and intraventricular (IV) conduction in patients with bilateral bundle branch block (BBB). *Circulation* 48(suppl 4):188, 1973.

78. Giardina EG, Heissenbuttel RH, Bigger JT Jr: Intermittent intravenous procainamide to treat ventricular arrhythmias. *Ann Intern Med* 78:183-193, 1973.

79. Kastor JA, Josephson ME, Guss SB, et al: Human ventricular refractoriness. II. Effects of procainamide. *Circulation* 56:462-467, 1977.

80. Arnsdorf MF: Electrophysiologic properties of antidysrhythmic drugs as a rational basis for therapy. *Med Clin North Am* 60:213-232, 1976.

81. Fenster PE, Comess KA, Marsh R, et al: Conversion of atrial fibrillation to sinus rhythm by acute intravenous procainamide infusion. *Am Heart J* 106:501-506, 1983.

82. Lima JJ, Conti DR, Goldfarb AL, et al: Safety and Efficacy of Procainamide Infusions. *Am J Cardiol* 43:98-105, 1979.

83. Harrison DC, Sprouse JH, Morrow AG: The antiarrhythmic properties of lidocaine and procainamide. Clinical and physiologic studies of their cardiovascular effects in man. *Circulation* 28:486-491, 1963.

84. Euler DE, Scanlon PJ: Mechanism of the effect of bretylium on the ventricular fibrillation threshold in dogs. *Am J Cardiol* 55:1396-1401, 1985.

85. Koo CC, Allen JD, Pantridge JF: Lack of effect of bretylium tosylate on electrical ventricular defibrillation in a controlled study. *Cardiovasc Res* 18:762-767, 1984.

86. Dollery CT, Emslie-Smith D, McMichael J: Bretylium tosylate in the treatment of hypertension. *Lancet* 1:296-299, 1960.

87. Leveque PE: Antiarrhythmic action of bretylium. *Nature* 207:203-204, 1965.

88. Koch-Weser J: Drug Therapy: Bretylium. *N Engl J Med* 300:473-477, 1979.

89. Patterson E, Lucchesi BR: Bretylium: A prototype for future development of antidysrhythmic agents. *Am Heart J* 106:426-431, 1983.

90. Markis JE, Koch-Weser J: Characteristics and mechanism of inotropic and chronotropic actions of bretylium tosylate. *J Pharmacol Exp Therapy* 178:94-102, 1971.

91. Heissenbuttel RH, Bigger JT Jr: Bretylium tosylate: A newly available antiarrhythmic drug for ventricular arrhythmias. *Ann Intern Med* 91:229-238, 1979.

92. Sasyniuk BI: Symposium on the management of ventricular dysrhythmias. Concept of reentry versus automaticity. *Am J Cardiol* 54:1A-6A, 1984.

93. Anderson JL: Symposium on the management of ventricular dysrhythmias. Antifibrillatory versus antiectopic therapy. *Am J Cardiol* 54:7A-12A, 1984.

94. Bigger JT Jr, Jaffe CC: The effect of bretylium tosylate on the electrophysiologic properties of ventricular muscle and Purkinje fibers. *Am J Cardiol* 27:82-92, 1971.

95. Cardinal R, Sasyniuk BI: Electrophysiological effects of bretylium tosylate on subendocardial Purkinje fibers from infarcted canine hearts. *J Pharmacol Exp Ther* 204:159-174, 1978.

96. Ideker RE, Klein GJ, Harrison L, et al: Epicardial mapping of the initiation of ventricular fibrillation induced by reperfusion following acute ischemia. *Circulation* 57-58 (Suppl 2):64, 1978.

97. Holder DA, Sniderman AD, Fraser G, et al: Experience with bretylium tosylate by a hospital cardiac arrest team. *Circulation* 55:541-544, 1977.

98. Euler DE, Zeman TW, Wallock ME, Scanlon PJ: Deleterious effects of bretylium on hemodynamic recovery from ventricular fibrillation. *Am Heart J* 112:25-31, 1986.

99. Anderson JL: Bretylium tosylate: Profile of the only available class III antiarrhythmic agent. *Clin Ther* 7:205-224, 1985.

100. Ellrodt G, Chew CY, Singh BN: Therapeutic implications of slow-channel blockade in cardiocirculatory disorders. *Circulation* 62:669-679, 1980.

101. Antman EM, Stone PH, Muller JE, et al: Calcium channel blocking agents in the treatment of cardiocirculatory disorders. Part I: Basic and clinical electrophysiologic effects. *Ann Intern Med* 93:875-885, 1980.

102. Singh BN, Collett JT, Chew CY: New perspectives in the pharmacologic therapy of cardiac arrhythmias. *Prog Cardiovasc Dis* 22:243-301, 1980.

103. Weiss AT, Lewis BS, Halon DA, Hasin Y, Gotsman MS: The use of calcium with verapamil in the management of supraventricular tachyarrhythmias. *Int J Cardiol* 4:275-284, 1983.

104. Waxman HL, Myerburg RJ, Appel R, Sung RJ: Verapamil for control of ventricular rate in paroxysmal supraventricular tachycardia and atrial fibrillation or flutter: A double-blind randomized cross-over study. *Ann Intern Med* 94:1-6, 1981.

105. Sung RJ, Elser B, McAllister RG Jr: Intravenous verapamil for termination of re-entrant supraventricular tachycardias. *Ann Intern Med* 93:682-689, 1980.

106. McGoon MD, Vlietstra RE, Holmes DR, Osborn JE: The clincial use of verapamil. *Mayo Clin Proc* 57:495-510, 1982.

107. Singh BN, Ellrodt G, Peter CT: Verapamil: A review of its pharmacological properties and therapeutic use. *Drugs* 15:169-197, 1978.

108. Rosen MR, Wit AL, Hoffman BF: Electrophysiology and pharmacology of cardiac arrhythmias. VI. Cardiac effects of verapamil. *Am Heart J* 89:665-673, 1975.

109. Shigenobu K, Schneider JA, Sperelakis N: Verapamil blockade of slow Na + and Ca + + responses in myocardial cells. *J Pharmacol Exp Ther* 190:280-288, 1974.

110. Nayler WG, Szeto J: Effect of verapamil on contractility, oxygen utilization, and calcium exchangeability in mammalian heart muscle. *Cardiovasc Res* 6:120-128, 1972.

111. Haeusler G: Differential effect of verapamil on excitation-contraction coupling in smooth muscle and on excitation-secretion coupling in adrenergic nerve terminals. *J Pharmacol Exp Ther* 180:672-682, 1972.

112. Winbury MM, Howe BB, Hefner MA: Effect of nitrates and other coronary dilators on large and small coronary vessels: A hypothesis for the mechanism of action of nitrates. *J Pharmacol Exp Ther* 168:70-95, 1969.

113. Hwang MH, Danoviz J, Pacold I, Rad N, Loeb HS, Gunnar RM: Double-blind crossover randomized trial of intravenously adminstered verapamil. Its use for atrial fibrillation and flutter following open heart surgery. *Arch Intern Med* 144:491-494, 1984.

114. Plumb VJ, Karp RB, Kouchoukos NT, Zorn GI, James TN, Waldo AL: Verapamil therapy of atrial fibrillation and atrial flutter following cardiac operation. *J Thorac Cardiovasc Surg* 83:590-596, 1982.

115. Wit AL, Cranefield PF: Effect of verapamil on the sinoatrial and atrioventricular nodes of the rabbit and the mechanism by which it arrests reentrant atrioventricular nodal tachycardia. *Circ Res* 35:413-425, 1974.

116. Wellens HJ, Tan SL, Bar FW, et al: Effect of verapamil studied by programmed electrical stimulation of the heart in patients with paroxysmal reentrant supraventricular tachycardia. *Br Heart J* 39:1058-1066, 1977.

117. Spear JF, Horowitz LN, Moore EN, et al: Verapamil-sensitive "slow-response activity in infarcted human ventricular myocardium, abstracted. *Circulation* 54(suppl 2):71-75, 1976.

118. Josephson ME, Kastor JA: Supraventricular tachycardia: Mechanisms and management. *Ann Intern Med* 87:346-358, 1977.

119. Soler-Soler J, Sagrista-Sauleda J, Cabrera A, et al: Effect of verapamil in infants with paroxysmal supraventricular tachycardia. *Circulation* 59:876-879, 1979.

120. Spurrell RA, Krikler DM, Sowton E: Effects of verapamil on electrophysiological properties of anomalous atrioventricular connexion in Wolff-Parkinson-White syndrome. *Br Heart J* 36:256-264, 1974.

121. Gulamhusein S, Ko P, Carruthers SG, Klein GJ: Acceleration of the ventricular response during atrial fibrillation in the Wolff-Parkinson-White syndrome after verapamil. *Circulation* 65:348-354, 1982.

122. Harper RW, Whitford E, Middlebrook K, Federman J, Anderson S, Pitt A: Effects of verapamil on the electrophysiologic properties of the accessory pathway in patients with the Wolff-Parkinson-White syndrome. *Am J Cardiol* 50:1323-1330, 1982.

123. McGovern B, Garan H, Ruskin JN: Precipitation of cardiac arrest by verapamil in patients with Wolff-Parkinson-White syndrome. *Ann Intern Med* 104:791-794, 1986.

124. Gulamhusein S, Ko P, Klein GJ: Ventricular fibrillation following verapamil in the Wolff-Parkinson-White syndrome. *Am Heart J* 106:145-147, 1983.

125. Jacob AS, Nielsen DH, Gianelly RE: Fatal ventricular fibrillation following verapamil in Wolff-Parkinson-White syndrome with atrial fibrillation. *Ann Emerg Med* 14:159-160, 1985.

126. Klein GJ, Bashore TM, Sellers TD, Pritchett ELC, Smith WM, Gallagher JJ: Ventricular fibrillation in the Wolff-Parkinson-White syndrome. *N Engl J Med* 301:1080-1085, 1979.

127. Sung RJ, Castellanos A, Mallon SM, Bloom MG, Gelbrand H, Myerburg RJ: Mechanisms of spontaneous alternation between reciprocating tachycardia and atrial flutter-fibrillation in the Wolff-Parkinson-White syndrome. *Circulation* 56:409-416, 197.

128. Stewart RB, Bardy GH, Greene HL: Wide complex tachycardia: Misdiagnosis and outcome after emergent therapy. *Ann Intern Med* 104:766-771, 1986.

129. Morady F, Baerman JM, DiCarlo LA, DeBuitleir M, Krol RB, Wahr DW: A prevalent misconception regarding wide-complex tachycardias. *JAMA* 254:2790-2792, 1985.

130. Ferlinz J, Easthope JL, Aronow WS: Effects of verapamil on myocardial performance in coronary disease. *Circulation* 59:313, 1979.

131. Chew CY, Hecht HS, Collett JT, et al: Influence of severity of ventricular dysfunction on hemodynamic responses to intravenously administered verapamil in ischemic heart disease. *Am J Cardiol* 47:917-922, 1981.

132. Schamroth L, Krikler DM, Garrett C: Immediate effects of intravenous verapamil in cardiac arrhythmias. *Br Med J* 1:660-662, 1972.

133. Fillmore SJ, Shapiro M, Killip T: Serial blood gas studies during cardiopulmonary resuscitation. *Ann Intern Med* 2:465-469, 1970.

134. Nieman JT, Rosborough JP: Effects of acidemia and sodium bicarbonate therapy in advanced cardiac life support. *Ann Emerg Med* 13(part 2):781-784, 1984.

135. Berenyi KG, Wolk M, Killip T: Cerebrospinal fluid acidosis complicating therapy of experimental cardiopulmonary arrest. *Circulation* 52:319-324, 1975.

136. Hyneck ML: Simple acid-base disorders. *Am J Hosp Pharmacol* 42:1992-2004, 1985.

137. Gerst PH, Fleming WH, Malm JR: Increased susceptibility of the heart to ventricular fibrillation during metabolic acidosis. *Circ Res* 19:63, 1966.

138. Kerber RE, Pandian NE, Hoyt R, et al: Effect of ischemia, hypertrophy, hypoxia, acidosis and alkalosis on canine defibrillation. *Am J Physiol* 244:H825, 1983.

139. Houle DB, Weil MH, Brown EB, Campbell GS: Influence of respiratory acidosis on ECG and pressor response to epinephrine, norepinephrine, and metaraminol. *Proc Soc Exp Biol Med* 94:561, 1957.

140. Minuck M, Sharma GP: Comparison of THAM and sodium bicarbonate in resuscitation of the heart after ventricular fibrillation in dogs. *Anesth Analg* 56:38, 1977.

141. Guerci AD, Chandra N, Johnson E, Hayburn B, Wurmb E, Taitlik J, Halperin HR, Siu C, Weisfeldt ML: Failure of sodium bicarbonate to improve resuscitation from ventricular fibrillation in dogs. *Circulation* 74(suppl IV):IV75-IV79, 1986.

142. Adler S, Roy A, Relman AS: Intracellular acid-base regulation. II. The interaction between CO_2^- tension and extracellular bicarbonate in the determination of muscle cell pH. *J Clin Invest* 44:21-30, 1965.

143. Poole-Wilson PA, Langer GA: Effects of acidosis on mechanical function and Ca^{2+} exchange in rabbit myocardium. *Am J Physiol* 236:H525, 1979.

144. Weisfeldt ML, Bishop RL, Greene HL: Effects of pH and PCO_2 on performance of ischemic myocardium, in Roy PE, Rona G (eds): *Recent Advances in Studies on Cardiac Structure and Metabolism,* vol 10. Baltimore, Unviersity Park Press, 1975, p 355.

145. Cingolani HE, Faulkner SL, Mattiazzi AR, Bender HW, Graham TP: Depression of human myocardial contractility with "respiratory" and "metabolic" acidosis. *Surgery* 77:427, 1975.

146. Cingolani HE, Mattiazzi AR, Blesa ES, Gonzalez NC: Contractility in isolated mammalian heart muscle after acid base changes. *Circ Res* 26:269, 1970.

147. Flaherty JT, Schaff HV, Goldman R, Gott VL: Metabolic and functional effects of progressive degrees of hypothermia during global ishcemia. *Am J Physiol* 236:H839, 1979.

148. Flaherty JT, Weisfeldt ML, Bulkley BH, Gardner TJ, Gott VL, Jacobus WE: Mechanisms of ischemic myocardial cell damage assessed by phosphorus-31 nuclear magnetic resonance. *Circulation* 65:561, 1982.

149. Weil MH, Rackow EC, Trevino R, Grundler W, Falk JL, Griffel MI: Difference in acid-base state between venous and arterial blood during cardiopulmonary resuscitation. *N Engl J Med* 315:153-156, 1986.

150. Mattar JA, Weil MH, Shubin H, et al: Cardiac arrest in the critically ill. II. Hyperosmolal states following cardiac arrest. *Am J Med* 56:162-168, 1974.

151. Bishop RL, Weisfeldt ML: Sodium bicarbonate administration during cardiac arrest. Effect on arterial pH, pCO_2, and osmolality. *JAMA* 235:506, 1976.

152. Todres D: The role of morphine in acute myocardial infarction. *Am Heart J* 81:566-670, 1971.

153. Zelis R, Mansour EJ, Capone RJ, et al: The cardiovascular effects of morphine. The peripheral capacitance and resistance vessels in human subjects. *J Clin Invest* 54:1247-1258, 1974.

154. Ward JM, McGrath RL, Weil JV: Effects of morphine on the peripheral vascular response to sympathetic stimulation. *Am J Cardiol* 29:659-666, 1972.

155. Alderman EL: Analgesics in the acute phase of myocardial infarction. *JAMA* 229:1646-1648, 1974.

156. Lee G, DeMaria AN, Amsterdam EA, et al: Comparative effects of morphine, meperidine and pentazocine on the cardiocirculatory dynamics in patients with acute myocardial infarction. *Am J Med* 60:949-955, 1976.

157. Semenkovich CF and Jaffe AS: Adverse effects due to morphine sulfate — challenge to previous clinical doctrine. *Am J Med* 79:325-330, 1985.

158. Niedergerke R: The rate of action of calcium ions on the contraction of the heart. *J Physiol* 138:506-515, 1957.

159. Weber A, Herz R, Reiss I: Role of calcium in contraction and relaxation of muscle. *Fed Proc* 23:896-900, 1964.

160. Borle AB: Calcium metabolism at the cellular level. *Fed Proc* 32:1944-1950, 1973.

161. Legato MJ: The myocardial cell: New concepts for the clinical cardiologist, editorial. *Circulation* 45:731-735, 1972.

162. Shapira N, Schaff HV, White RD, Pluth JR: Hemodynamic effects of calcium chloride injection following cardiopulmonary bypass: Response to bolus injection and continuous infusion. *Ann Thorac Surg* 37:133-140, 1984.

163. Nerothin DD, Kaane PB: Calcium — vasodilator or vasoconstrictor? *Anesth Analg* 63:175-284, 1984.

164. Stanley TH, Isen-Amaral JI, Liu WS, et al: Peripheral vascular versus direct cardiac effects of calcium. *Anesthiology* 45:46-58, 1976.

165. Eriksen C, Sorensen B, Bille-Brahe NE, Skovsted P, Lunding M: Haemodynamic effects of calcium chloride administered intravenously to patients with and without cardiac disease during neurolept anaesthesia. *Acta Anaesthesiol Scand* 27:13-17, 1983.

166. Stueven H, Thompson BM, Aprahamian C, et al: Use of calcium in prehospital cardiac arrest. *Ann Emerg Med* 12:136, 1983.

167. Stueven HA, Thompson BM, Aprahamian C, et al: Calcium chloride: Reassessment of use in asystole. *Ann Emerg Med* 13:820, 1984.

168. Harrison EE, Amey BD: Use of calcium in electromechanical dissociation. *Ann Emerg Med* 13:844, 1984.

169. Dembo DH: Calcium in advanced life support. *Crit Care Med* 9:358, 1981.

170. Hariman RJ, Mangiardi LM, McAllister RG, Surawicz B, Shabetal R, Kishida H: Reversal of the cardiovascular effects of verapamil by calicum and sodium: Differences between electrophysiologic and hemodynamic responses. *Circulation* 59:797-804, 1979.

171. White RD, Goldsmith RS, Rodriquez R, et al: Plasma tonic calcium levels following injection of chlorine, gluconate and gluceptate salts of calcium. *J Thorac Cardiovasc Surg* 71:609-613, 1976.

Cardiovascular Pharmacology II

Chapter 8

The drugs considered in this chapter are used primarily to treat congestive heart failure, hypotension, hypertension, and cardiogenic shock associated with acute ischemic heart disease, including acute myocardial infarction. In addition to morbidity associated with these complications themselves, they exacerbate the imbalance between myocardial oxygen supply and demand and increase the likelihood of myocardial ischemia and further hemodynamic decompensation. An aggressive approach to treatment frequently requiring the use of potent, rapid acting, parenteral agents that can be titrated to desired hemodynamic endpoints is essential. A detailed understanding of the pharmacology and proper use of these agents is required to permit rapid hemodynamic improvement and to avoid morbidity. The drugs may be classified as follows:

Inotropic Vasoactive Agents

Norepinephrine (levarterenol, L-norepinephrine)
Dopamine
Dobutamine
Isoproterenol
Amrinone
Digitalis

Vasodilators/Antihypertensives

Sodium nitroprusside
Nitroglycerin
Propranolol
Metoprolol

Diuretics

Furosemide

Cardiovascular Adrenergic Receptors

Adrenergic receptors regulate cardiac, vascular, bronchiolar, and gastrointestinal smooth muscle tone. These receptors were first described by Ahlquist, who studied the effects of various catecholamines on tissue.[1] There are three types of adrenergic receptors: alpha-adrenergic (alpha-1 and alpha-2), beta-adrenergic (beta-1 and beta-2), and dopaminergic.[2-4] Catecholamines differ from one another in their binding affinity for adrenergic receptors (Table 1).

Alpha-1 receptors are present in the postsynaptic region of neurons and vascular smooth muscle. The stimulation of the vascular receptor leads to vasoconstriction. Alpha-1 receptors in myocardium mediate

Table 1. Sympathomimetic Amines

Drug and arrhythmic potential	Usual IV dosage		Adrenergic effects	
			Alpha	Beta
Epinephrine (Adrenaline) + + +	0.5–1.0 mg cardiac arrest	Small doses	+	+ + .
	1–4 μg/min inotropic/pressor support	Large doses	+ +	+ + +
Norepinephrine (Levophed) + +	2–12 μg/min	Small doses	+ +	+
		Large doses	+ + +	+ +
Dopamine (Intropin) + +	2–20 μg/kg/min	Small doses	+	+ *
		Large doses	+ + +	+ +
Dobutamine (Dobutrex) +	2.5–20.0 μg/kg/min		0/+	+ + +
Isoproterenol (Isuprel) + + +	2–10 μg/min		0	+ + +
Amrinone	2–20 μg/kg/min		0	0

*Increases renal and splanchnic blood flow.

positive inotropic and negative chronotropic effects.[5] The influence of clinically available agonists on alpha-1 receptors in order of relative potency are phenylephrine, norepinephrine, and epinephrine.[6]

Presynaptic alpha-2 receptors modulate alpha-receptor tone in large blood vessels[7] and provide a counter-regulatory mechanism for alpha-1 receptor activity. When these receptors are stimulated, release of norepinephrine is inhibited, decreasing alpha-adrenergic activity by limiting norepinephrine accumulation. In the central nervous system, stimulation of the alpha-2 receptors inhibits reflex arcs in the locus ceruleus, leading to peripheral vasodilation.[8,9] Alpha-2 postsynaptic receptors also can mediate arteriolar and venous vasoconstriction.[7]

Stimulation of beta-1 receptors increases heart rate and myocardial contractility. Beta-2 stimulation causes vasodilation and leads to relaxation of bronchial, uterine, and gastrointestinal smooth muscle. Beta-2-receptor activity also modulates fat metabolism and glycogenolysis and drives potassium intracellularly, inducing hypokalemia.[10] This effect may play an important role in the induction of arrythmias during ischemia and help to explain the beneficial effects of beta-adrenergic blockade both acutely and for secondary prevention of cardiac events after myocardial infarction. Beta-adrenergic-receptor stimulation results in renin release, which is inhibited by high doses of beta-blocking agents.

Stimulation of dopaminergic receptors by low concentrations of dopamine results in renal and mesenteric vasodilation. At higher concentrations, the alpha-adrenergic effects of dopamine induce renal and mesenteric vasoconstriction.

Coronary arteries possess both alpha- and beta-adrenergic receptors.[11,12] Histochemical studies suggest that alpha receptors predominate in the larger epicardial coronaries and that beta-receptors predominate in the smaller arteries.[13] Stimulation of alpha receptors (e.g., by agents like norepinephrine or dopamine or by stimulation of sympathetic nerves) produces coronary vasoconstriction.[12-15] Coronary vasoconstriction usually is promptly antagonized by local metabolic factors such as adenosine, which are elaborated in response to cardiac work.[16] In patients with coronary artery disease, the extent of coronary vasoconstriction to a given stimulus may be enhanced.[17] Thus, catecholamines with alpha-agonist properties must be used with caution, if at all, in patients with acute ischemic disease. Alpha-2 postsynaptic receptors may be particularly important in mediating coronary vasospasm. Calcium channel blockers blunt alpha-2-receptor-mediated vasoconstriction, one reason for their efficacy in antagonizing coronary vasoconstriction.[7] Stimulation of beta receptors generally results in coronary vasodilation.

Adrenergic tone is in balance and to some extent modulated by the parasympathetic nervous system, which has effects on electrophysiologic function[18] and coronary vasomotion.[19] Other mechanisms such as an imbalance between vasoactive platelet mediated products such as thromboxane A2 and prostacylin also have been postulated for abnormalities in coronary vasomotion other than automomic influences.[20]

Norepinephrine

Mechanisms of Action

Norepinephrine is a naturally occurring catecholamine that differs chemically from epinephrine only by the absence of a methyl group on the terminal amine. Epinephrine and norepinephrine are approximately equipotent in their ability to stimulate beta-1 (cardiac) receptors, but their relative stimulatory effects on alpha-1 and beta-2 receptors are quite different. Norepinephrine is a potent alpha-receptor agonist with minimal effect on beta-2 receptors. Norepinephrine increases myocardial contractility due to its beta-1-adrenergic effects while its potent alpha-adrenergic effects lead to arterial and venous vasoconstriction.[21]

Norepinephrine's positive inotropic and vasopressor effects have been used in the treatment of refractory shock. However, the increased vascular resistance induced by norepinephrine may counteract its inotropic effects. Norepinephrine increases blood pressure predominantly by elevating systemic vascular resistance and, therefore, may not improve and may actually diminish cardiac output. Because norepinephrine increases myocardial oxygen demand, it can exacerbate myocardial ischemia, especially if coronary vasoconstriction is induced by stimulation of coronary alpha receptors. Norepinephrine should be used as an agent of last resort in the medical management of patients with ischemic heart disease.[22]

Indications

Norepinephrine is used for the treatment of hemodynamically significant hypotension that is refractory to other sympathomimetic amines. Norepinephrine is more likely to be useful when total peripheral resistance is low. Hypotension and low systemic vascular resistance occur rarely[23] in patients with acute myocardial infarction but are more common in patients with sepsis. The use of norepinephrine should be considered a temporizing measure; successful management requires not only support of the blood pressure but also correction of the underlying abnormalities.

Dosage

Norepinephrine bitartrate USP is available in 4-ml ampules containing 1 mg norepinephrine base per milliliter (2 mg norepinephrine bitartrate/mL). It should be mixed in either 5% dextrose and water or saline to provide a concentration of 8 μg/ml of the norepinephrine base or 16 μg/ml of norepinephrine bitartrate. Norepinephrine should be infused through a central venous catheter to minimize the risk of extravasation (see "Precautions"). Infusions of 2 μg/min are generally used as a starting dose. The infusion rate is then titrated to achieve the desired effect, which usually is the maintenance of an adequate blood pressure (one reasonable criterion is a systolic pressure of at least 90 mmHg) at the lowest possible dose. The average adult dose is 2–12 μg/min; higher doses may be needed to maintain an adequate blood pressure. The use of this drug should be viewed as a temporizing measure, and the dose should be reduced and/or the infusion discontinued as soon as possible. Only rarely will treatment need to continue for hours or days. Norepinephrine should be tapered slowly to avoid abrupt and severe hypotension. Norepinephrine should be administered via a volumetric infusion system that ensures a precise flow rate.

Precautions

Because peripheral blood pressure measurements are often inaccurate when severe vasoconstriction is present, central intraarterial pressure monitoring may be necessary for accurate determination of arterial pressure.[24] If the central and peripheral pressures are the same, the use of arterial monitoring should be discontinued. When continuous invasive arterial blood pressure monitoring is not used, cuff or doppler blood pressure should be monitored every 5 minutes during titration and then at 5-minute intervals. Hemodynamic monitoring should be carried out to assess changes in cardiac output, pulmonary occlusive pressure, and peripheral arterial resistance.

Norepinephrine is contraindicated when hypotension is due to hypovolemia except as a temporizing measure to maintain coronary and cerebral perfusion pressure until volume replacement can be achieved.

Norepinephrine increases myocardial oxygen requirements without producing a compensatory increase in coronary blood flow. This can be deleterious in patients with myocardial ischemia or infarction. Norepinephrine may precipitate arrhythmias.

Ischemic necrosis and sloughing of superficial tissues will result if extravasation of norepinephrine occurs. If extravasation occurs, phentolamine, 5–10 mg diluted in 10–15 ml of saline solution, should be infiltrated into the area to antagonize vasoconstriction and to minimize necrosis and sloughing.

Dopamine

Mechanisms of Action

Dopamine hydrochloride is a chemical precursor of norepinephrine that stimulates dopaminergic, beta-2-adrenergic, and alpha-adrenergic receptors in a dose-dependent fashion.[21] Dopamine also stimulates the release of norepinephrine. In low doses (1–2 μg/kg/min) dopamine produces vasodilation of renal, mesenteric, and cerebral arteries by stimulation of dopaminergic receptors. Urine output may increase while heart rate and blood pressure are usually unchanged. In the dosage range of 2–10 μg/kg/min, dopamine stimulates both beta-1- and alpha-adrenergic receptors as well. Increases in cardiac output due to the enhanced myocardial contractility induced by beta-adrenergic stimulation reflexly antagonize, in part, alpha-adrenergic-mediated vasoconstriction. This results in enhanced cardiac output and only modest increases in systemic vascular resistance and preload. At doses above 10 μg/kg/min, the alpha-adrenergic effects of dopamine predominate. This results in renal, mesenteric, and peripheral arterial and venous vasoconstriction with marked increases in systemic vascular resistance and preload. Doses above 20 μg/kg/min produce hemodynamic effects that are similar to those of norepinephrine.

As with all vasoactive agents, there is substantial variability in the response to dopamine. Accordingly, the drug must be titrated to hemodynamic effect. Dopamine increases myocardial work without significantly increasing coronary blood flow in a compensatory manner.[25] The imbalance between oxygen supply and demand may result in myocardial ischemia.

Indications

The primary indication for dopamine is hemodynamically significant hypotension in the absence of hypovolemia. One reasonable definition for the presence of significant hypotension is a systolic arterial pressure of less than 90 mmHg accompanied by evidence of poor tissue perfusion, oliguria, or mental status changes. Dopamine should be used at the lowest dose necessary to ensure adequate perfusion of vital organs. In the immediate postresuscitation period, higher doses may be required to induce the transient hypertension recommended to improve cerebral perfusion.

Dopamine's vasopressor effects at higher infusion rates elevate the pulmonary artery occlusive pressure and may induce or exacerbate pulmonary congestion despite a rise in cardiac output. Vasodilators can be used to reduce preload and improve cardiac output by antagonizing the increased vascular resistance induced by dopamine. The combination of dopamine and nitroprusside produces hemodynamic effects similar to those of dobutamine.[26]

Dosage

Dopamine is available for intravenous use only. The contents of 1 or 2 ampules (400 mg/ampule) should be mixed in 250 ml of 5% dextrose. This yields a concentration of 1,600 or 3,200 μg/ml, respectively. The initial rate of infusion is from 2 to 5 μg/kg/min. This rate may be increased until blood pressure, urine output, and other parameters of organ perfusion improve. The lowest infusion rate that results in satisfactory hemodynamic performance should be used to minimize side effects. Monitoring central hemodynamics is essential for proper use of dopamine in patients who have ischemic heart disease or congestive heart failure and should be instituted prior to or as soon as possible after the initiation of treatment. Dopamine should be administered via a volumetric infusion pump to ensure precise flow rates.

Precautions

Dopamine will increase heart rate and may induce or exacerbate supraventricular and ventricular arrhythmias. On occasion, these effects may require reduction in the dose of therapy or even discontinuation of the infusion. Despite improvement in hemodynamics, myocardial oxygen consumption and myocardial lactate production may increase in response to higher doses of dopamine, indicating that coronary blood supply is not sufficiently augmented to compensate for the increased cardiac work. This imbalance between supply and demand would be expected to induce or exacerbate myocardial ischemia.[25] Nausea and vomiting are frequent. Dopamine may produce cutaneous tissue necrosis and sloughing similar to that produced by norepinephrine if interstitial extravasation occurs. Treatment for extravasation is similar to that described for norepinephrine.

Monoamine oxidase inhibitors such as isocarboxazid (Marplan), pargyline hydrochloride (Eutonyl), tranylcypromine sulfate (Parnate), and phenelzine sulfate (Nardil) are no longer used as extensively as in the past but may potentiate the effects of dopamine. Therefore, individuals receiving these agents should be treated with no more than one tenth of the usual dopamine dose. Agents with similar hemodynamic effects, e.g., the initial effects of bretylium tosylate, may be synergistic with dopamine.[27] Although the mechanism is unknown, patients receiving phenytoin may experience hypotension during concomitant administration of dopamine.[28] Dopamine, like other catecholamines, may result in serious acute hypertension in patients with pheochromocytoma and is contraindicated. Dopamine should not be added to solutions containing sodium bicarbonate or other alkaline IV solutions since dopamine is slowly inactivated at alkaline pH. The kinetics of this reaction are slow enough that dopamine and alkaline solutions (aminophylline, phenytoin, sodium bicarbonate) that are administered over a short period of time can be infused through the same venous catheter.[29] Dopamine should be tapered gradually to avoid an acute hypotensive response.

Dobutamine

Mechanisms of Action

Dobutamine is a synthetic sympathomimetic amine that exerts its potent inotropic effects by stimulating beta-1- and alpha-adrenergic receptors in the myocardium.[30] Its minor stimulation of peripheral alpha receptors is antagonized by more potent beta-2 stimulation, and mild vasodilation usually is induced. Peripheral resistance also falls reflexly in response to increases in cardiac output. In conventional clinical doses, dobutamine is less apt to induce tachycardia than either isoproterenol or dopamine. However, dobutamine will increase heart rate at higher doses. Renal and mesenteric blood flow usually increase as cardiac output increases, but unlike dopamine, dobutamine does not produce renal and mesenteric vasodilation via dopaminergic receptors. Pulmonary occlusive pressure usually decreases.[31] The net hemodynamic effects of dobutamine are similar to those of dopamine combined with a vasodilator such as nitroprusside.[26] Cardiac output increases and peripheral resistance and the pulmonary occlusive pressure decreases.

Dobutamine's beneficial hemodynamic effects and its lack of induction of endogenous norepinephrine release minimize its effects on myocardial oxygen demand, resulting in a more favorable balance between oxygen supply and demand than with either norepinephrine or dopamine.[30] Dobutamine's positive inotropic effect is balanced also by increased coronary blood flow.[25] For these reasons, when titrated to avoid significant increases in heart rate, dobutamine does not increase infarct size or elicit arrhythmias.[32] Heart rate may decrease as hemodynamics improve. Since vasodilatation occurs in response to increased cardiac output, blood pressure may change very little. Accordingly, direct measurement of central hemodynamics, including cardiac output, are required to accurately assess the response to dobutamine.

Dopamine and dobutamine have been used together.[33-35] The combination of moderate doses of both drugs maintain arterial pressure better with less of an increase in pulmonary occlusive pressure and, thus, less pulmonary congestion than dopamine alone.[35] Thus, the combination may result in better hemodynamics in patients with cardiogenic shock.[34] Unfortunately, the prognosis in cardiogenic shock is not improved by the use of inotropic and vasoactive drugs, but these agents can be used to maintain vital organ perfusion while other interventions (PTCA or open heart surgery) that can salvage the myocardium are undertaken.

Indications

Dobutamine is useful in the treatment of patients with pulmonary congestion and low cardiac output or in hypotensive patients in whom vasodilators cannot be used for fear of further lowering of the blood pressure. Dobutamine and moderate volume loading are the treatment of choice in patients with hemodynamically significant right ventricular infarction.[36]

Dosage

Dobutamine may be effective at low doses (e.g., 0.5 μg/kg/min). The usual dose range is from 2.5 to 20.0 μg/kg/min. Doses should be guided by measurement of hemodynamic parameters; the smallest effective dose should be used. One should attempt to avoid increases in heart rates of more than 10% from initial values. Two ampules of dobutamine (500 mg/ampule) should be mixed in 250 ml of 5% dextrose in water or normal saline. Dobutamine should be administered via a volumetric infusion pump to ensure precise flow rates.

Precautions

Dobutamine may cause tachycardia, arrhythmias, and fluctuation in the blood pressure, which can provoke myocardial ischemia, especially at higher doses. Other side effects include headache, nausea, and tremor.

Isoproterenol

Mechanisms of Action

Isoproterenol hydrochloride is a synthetic sympathomimetic amine with nearly pure beta-adrenergic-receptor activity.[21] Its potent inotropic and chronotropic properties frequently result in increased cardiac output despite a reduction in mean blood pressure due to peripheral vasodilation and venous pooling. However, isoproterenol markedly increases myocardial oxygen requirements and may induce or exacerbate myocardial ischemia. Newer inotropic agents that are less prone to induce ischemia or arrhythmias have replaced isoproterenol in most clinical settings.

Indications

Isoproterenol is indicated for the immediate and temporary control of hemodynamically significant and atropine refractory bradycardia in the patient who still has a pulse. Electronic pacing provides better control than isoproterenol without increasing myocardial oxygen consumption. If pacing is available, it should be used instead of isoproterenol, or as soon as possible after isoproterenol has been given as a temporizing measure. When used for chronotropic support, isoproterenol may exacerbate ischemia and/or hypotension. Isoproterenol's vasodilatory effects lower coronary perfusion pressure during cardiac arrest and increase the mortality rate in experimental animal models.[37] Thus, its use is contraindicated in the treatment of cardiac arrest.

Dosage

The dose needed for chronotropic support is usually small (more than 10 μg/min is rarely necessary). The initial starting dose is 2 μg/min, with gradual titration of the dose upward until a heart rate of approximately 60 beats/min is reached. One milligram of isoproterenol is diluted in 500 ml of 5% dextrose and water to yield a concentration of 2 μg/ml. Isoproterenol should be administered via a volumetric infusion pump to ensure a precise flow rate.

Precautions

Because isoproterenol increases myocardial oxygen requirements, it should be avoided in patients with ischemic heart disease. Isoproterenol's potent chronotropic properties can induce serious arrhythmias, including ventricular tachycardia and fibrillation. Isoproterenol may also exacerbate tachyarrhythmias due to digitalis toxicity or hypokalemia.

Amrinone

Mechanisms of Action

Amrinone is a rapid-acting inotropic agent available for parenteral use. Amrinone is a phosphodiesterase inhibitor. Its inotropic and vasodilator effects are not reversed by adrenergic blocking drugs or by NE depletion.[38] Amrinone has been studied extensively in patients with congestive cardiomyopathy, but its efficacy in patients with ischemic heart disease is not established.[39] Amrinone's net hemodynamic effects are similar to those of dobutamine. Cardiac output increases and peripheral resistance and preload are diminished at doses between 2 and 20 μg/kg/min. Higher doses produce a tachycardia similar to that observed with dobutamine.[39,40] Amrinone can exacerbate ischemia induced by coronary occlusion.[41] Thus, it should be used with caution, if at all, in patients with ischemic heart disease. Because hemodynamic benefit is usually not associated with changes in heart rate and/or blood pressure, the monitoring of central hemodynamics is essential for proper titration or dose.

Indications

Amrinone should be considered for use in patients with severe congestive heart failure refractory to diuretics, vasodilators, and conventional inotropic agents.

Dosage

A loading dose of amrinone of 0.75 mg/kg is given over 2–3 minutes, followed by a 2–20 μg/kg/min infusion titrated to hemodynamic effect. The monitoring of central hemodynamic pressures is essential for proper titration. Amrinone should be administered by an infusion system that ensures a precise flow rate.

Precautions

Amrinone can induce or worsen myocardial ischemia. Hemodynamic monitoring is essential since changes in central hemodynamics may be substantial in the absence of changes in heart rate or blood pressure. Dosage should be adjusted frequently to achieve improvement at the lowest possible dose. Amrinone can cause thrombocytopenia in 2–3% of patients. The fall in platelet count is usually modest, rarely associated with significant bleeding, and usually resolves when the drug is discontinued. Platelet reduction appears to be dose dependent and is due to a decrease in platelet survival time. Other side effects include gastrointestinal upset, myalgia, fever, hepatic dysfunction, and ventricular irritability. Because amrinone contains metabisulfite, its use is contraindicated in patients allergic to bisulfites.

The Tapering of Vasoactive Drugs

Inotropic and vasoactive agents should be tapered gradually under close supervision. They should not be discontinued abruptly since some of these agents may deplete myocardial catecholamines and several contract intravascular volume. The infusion rate should be reduced gradually, and intravascular fluid should be repleted if necessary to avoid hypotension.

Digitalis

Mechanisms of Action

Digitalis is used to increase myocardial contraction and control the ventricular response to atrial flutter and fibrillation. Digitalis' mild positive inotropic effect is due to the inhibition of membrane-bound sodium potassium ATPase. This effect alters calcium flux and increases the concentration of calcium in the sarcoplasmic reticulum, which, in turn, increases contractility.[42] Digitalis' inotropic effects do not depend on catecholamine liberation and are unaffected by beta-adrenergic receptor blockade.[43] Digitalis evokes vasoconstriction in coronary and mesenteric vascular beds.[44]

Digitalis exerts direct and indirect effects on the sinoatrial and atrioventricular nodes. It directly and indirectly (via increasing vagal tone) depresses impulse conduction through the AV node. It increases the rate of atrial conduction.

The proper dose of digitalis depends on the route of administration and the desired effect. Higher doses are often required to control the ventricular response to atrial fibrillation than for other indications. Digitalis toxicity is more common when the serum level is high, but toxicity may be present with low serum levels and it may be absent despite elevated levels because it is the myocardial tissue level of the glycoside that determines toxicity and not the circulating blood level.[45]

Indications

Digitalis helps control the ventricular response to atrial fibrillation or atrial flutter and may convert paroxysmal supraventricular tachycardia to normal sinus rhythm. It may also convert atrial flutter to atrial fibrillation. Digoxin may be used for supraventricular rhythm disturbances if the patient is hemodynamically stable and does not require emergent electrical cardioversion. Digoxin's inotropic effects are less potent than those of parenteral inotropes, and it may cause significant toxicity and adverse drug interactions in critically ill patients.[46] Thus, digitalis preparations have little role in the management of acute congestive heart failure.

Dosage

Digoxin can be administered either orally or intravenously. Intravenous digoxin administration avoids the problem of gastrointestinal absorption and produces a more rapid onset of action and peak effect than oral administration. With intravenous digoxin, effects are seen within 5–30 minutes, and peak effects in 1.5–3 hours. In nonemergency situations, treatment can be initiated orally. Regardless of route of administration, digoxin's relatively long elimination half-time (36 hours) necessitates the administration of an initial loading dose. Loading doses of digoxin in the range of 10–15 µg/kg lean body weight generally provide therapeutic effect with minimum risk of toxicity.[47]

The maintenance dose is affected by body size and renal function. Clinical guides to the adequacy of digitalization include control of supraventricular arrhythmias and improvement in congestive heart failure. The uses of the other digitalis preparations have been reviewed elsewhere.[42]

Precautions

Digitalis toxicity is a common and important problem occurring with an incidence varying from 7 to 20%.[48,49] Virtually every rhythm disturbance has been described with digitalis toxicity, but the most frequent include atrial and ventricular premature complexes, ventricular bigeminy, and ventricular tachycardia. Accelerated junctional rhythm or nonparoxysmal junctional tachycardia, paroxysmal atrial tachycardia with 2:1 AV block, and high levels of atrioventricular block are less common but characteristic of digitalis excess. Noncardiac manifestations of digitalis toxicity include anorexia, nausea, vomiting, diarrhea, visual disturbances, and mental status changes including psychosis, lassitude, and agitation. Toxicity is more frequent in patients with hypokalemia, hypomagnesmia, and/or hypercalcemia.[49]

When digitalis toxicity is suspected, the drug must be stopped and the serum level should be measured. Normal levels do not exclude toxicity. Correction of coexistant hypokalemia is an important consideration. The serum potassium level should be increased until it is normal unless heart block is present. Caution is necessary in patients with heart block since it can be worsened by the administration of potassium. Additional treatment may include the use of lidocaine, phenytoin and/or propranolol for control of ventricular or supraventricular arrhythmias.[50,51] A temporary pacemaker may be required to treat high-grade AV block. Catecholamines are relatively contraindicated since they may aggravate the potential for serious ventricular arrhythmias. Electrical cardioversion can be dangerous in the setting of clinical digitalis toxicity with arrhythmias and can precipitate a fatal ventricular arrhythmia. Cardioversion should be reserved for the treatment of life-threatening, hemodynamically significant arrhythmias. If cardioversion is necessary in a digitalis intoxicated patient, the lowest possible energy levels (10–20 J) should initially be tried.[52] Anti-digoxin antibodies are now available and are the treatment of choice for massive digoxin overdose or refractory digitalis toxicity.[53] In the future, it is likely they will become widely used for the treatment of all types of digitalis toxicity.

Massive overdoses of digitalis may induce hyperkalemia.[54] Because it induces mesenteric and coronary vasoconstriction, digitalis may induce ischemia and/or mesenteric infarction.[44] Multiple drug interactions with digitalis, the most common being quinidine's property of raising the digitalis blood level two- to fourfold, have been described.[47]

Sodium Nitroprusside

Mechanisms of Action

Sodium nitroprusside is a potent peripheral vasodilator with effects on both arterial and venous smooth muscle. Its effects are seen almost immediately and cease within minutes after the infusion is stopped. Nitroprusside is metabolized by red blood cells to hydrocyanic acid, which is converted to thiocyanate by the liver and excreted by the kidneys. Hepatic and/or renal dysfunction can affect the clearance of the drug and its potentially injurious metabolites, cyanide and thiocyanate.[55]

Nitroprusside is used in the emergency treatment of hypertension and heart failure. Nitroprusside reduces blood pressure by reducing peripheral arterial resistance and by increasing venous capacitance and, thus, preload. Arterial effects are not lost even when preload is markedly diminished, although tachycardia ensues.[56] In the absence of heart failure, cardiac output either falls or remains unchanged. When heart failure is present, nitroprusside generally increases cardiac output by diminishing vascular impedence and thus increasing stroke volume.[57] The increase in stroke volume usually is sufficient to maintain the systemic blood pressure at or only slightly below the pretreatment level. In patients with left ventricular failure, nitroprusside-induced tachycardia suggests an inadequate (relative or absolute) left ventricular filling pressure.[58] The hemodynamic improvement induced in the presence of left ventricular failure and/or hypertension may be of particular significance to patients with ischemic heart disease. Nitroprusside reduces myocardial work and may therefore mitigate ischemia. However, there are some data that suggest that nitroprusside also may reduce coronary perfusion to ischemic myocardium,[59] which may counterbalance some or all of the beneficial effects on myocardial work.

Numerous studies have reported improvement in left ventricular function, tissue perfusion, cardiac output, and clinical status in patients with low cardiac outputs and high systemic vascular resistances.[60,61] Nitroprusside tends to reduce pulmonary occlusive pressure to a greater extent than dobutamine because of its more potent venodilating effects and its ability to enhance diastolic relaxation of the left ventricle.[62,63]

Indications

Sodium nitroprusside is the parenteral treatment of choice for hypertensive emergencies when immediate reduction of peripheral resistance is necessary. It reduces blood pressure rapidly, is easily titratable, is generally well tolerated, and can be rapidly reversed if necessary simply by discontinuing the infusion. It is also very useful in the treatment of patients with acute left ventricular failure. Nitroprusside may be used when heart failure and pulmonary congestion is acute or poorly controlled by diuretic therapy. Combined therapy with dopamine and nitroprusside frequently is more effective than the use of either agent alone. The net hemodynamic effects of this combination are similar to the effects of dobutamine.[26]

Dosage

The contents of a 50-mg vial of nitroprusside can be dissolved in 2–3 ml of dextrose in water and then mixed with 250–1,000 ml of dextrose in water depending on the concentration desired. No diluent other than dextrose in water should be used. The solution must be wrapped promptly in aluminum foil or another opaque material to protect the solution from deteriorating with exposure to light. The freshly prepared solution may have a very faint brownish tint. Nitroprusside in aqueous solution will react with a variety of substances to form highly colored reaction products. Should this occur, the infusion should be replaced. Once prepared, the solution, should be used immediately.[55] Treatment should begin with an infusion rate of 0.5 μg/kg/min titrated to the desired endpoint. Hemodynamic monitoring is essential for proper titration when treating congestive heart failure. The average therapeutic dose of nitroprusside ranges from 0.5 to 8.0 μg/kg/min. Nitroprusside should be administered by an infusion system that ensures a precise flow rate.

Precautions

The monitoring of central hemodynamic pressures is essential when treating congestive heart failure both for safety and to assure proper titration of effect. Systemic arterial pressure must be monitored frequently. At times this may require the use of an intraarterial pressure line. Hypotension is the most common adverse reaction seen with nitroprusside. Nitroprusside-induced hypotension may precipitate myocardial ischemia, infarction, or stroke. Deterioration of the ventilation–perfusion relationship and hypoxemia can occur.[64,65] Elderly patients may be more sensitive to the drug; such patients should be treated with lower doses. The possibility that the effects of nitroprusside on coronary blood flow may exacerbate ischemia despite reduced myocardial work is controversial. Since in the presence of congestive heart failure intravenous nitroglycerin has a similar hemodynamic profile but improves ischemia, many recommend its use in preference to nitroprusside.[66,67]

Nitroprusside is metabolized to thiocyanate by the liver. Thiocyanate intoxication due to nitroprusside is uncommon unless large doses of nitroprusside are given (greater than 8 μg/kg/min), prolonged infusions (greater than 2–3 days) are given, or the patient has renal failure. Blood levels should be monitored when high or prolonged dosage regimens are used or renal failure is present. If blood thiocyanate levels remain below 10 mg/100 ml, continued use of the agent is usually safe. Signs of thiocyanate toxicity include tinnitus, visual blurring, mental status changes, nausea, abdominal pain, hyperreflexia, and seizures. Cyanide toxicity is a rare complication of nitroprusside therapy in patients with hepatic dysfunction.[55]

Nitroglycerin

Mechanisms of Action

Nitroglycerin relaxes vascular smooth muscle by binding to specific vascular receptors and causing the formation of disulfide bonds.[68] Nitrate preparations differ principally in their rate of onset, duration of action, potency, and route of administration. Although nitrates have multiple uses, only the use of sublingual and intravenous nitroglycerin for the treatment of angina pectoris, acute myocardial infarction, and left ventricular failure will be discussed here.

Nitroglycerin is effective in relieving angina pectoris. Relief usually occurs in 1–2 minutes but may take as long as 10 minutes.[69] In the past, this response has been considered so predictable that it was suggested as a clinical diagnostic test for angina,[70] although it is now known that other conditions (such as esophageal spasm) can respond to nitrate therapy as well. Nitrates relieve angina pectoris in part by dilating the smooth muscle of the venous system, which inhibits venous return leading to a decrease in ventricular volume, ventricular pressure, and wall stress. The decrease in left ventricular work and wall tension usually results in improved subendocardial perfusion.

Nitroglycerin dilates large coronary (conduit) arteries, antagonizes vasospasm, and increases coronary collateral blood flow to ischemic myocardium.[71,72] These effects are particularly important when myocardial ischemia is due to abnormal coronary vasomotion.[73] Sublingual nitroglycerin decreases left ventricular filling pressure without significantly lowering systemic vascular resistance. Cardiac output usually falls in response to the decreased preload or remains the same when left ventricular filling pressure is normal at the time of administration.[74,75]

In patients with congestive heart failure, intravenous nitroglycerin reduces left ventricular filling pressure and systemic vascular resistance.[76-78] The decline in ven-

tricular volume and systolic wall tension decreases myocardial oxygen requirements and usually reduces myocardial ischemia.[79] The net effect is an increase in cardiac output. When compared to nitroprusside, intravenous nitroglycerin produces a slightly greater reduction of preload and a slightly lesser reduction of impedance.[80] Nitroglycerin loses its arterial effects when preload is reduced.[81] In comparison, nitroprusside retains its arterial effects even if preload is reduced.[56] Nitroglycerin does not usually increase heart rate if preload is adequate.

Indications

Sublingual nitroglycerin is the drug of choice for the treatment of an anginal episode. It is effective for exertional as well as rest angina. For suspected angina pectoris, one tablet (0.3–0.4 mg) should be given sublingually. The dose may be repeated twice at 5-minute intervals as needed. If the pain is not gone after three sublingual tablets, the patient should seek medical attention immediately. With unstable angina pectoris or myocardial infarction, intravenous administration of nitroglycerin is preferred. Although oral nitrates have been shown to result in a similar reduction in the frequency of anginal pain in patients with unstable angina, oral administration produces variable bioavailability and has a delayed onset of action.[82] Patients with coronary vasospasm ("Prinzmetal's variant angina") usually respond promptly to sublingual nitroglycerin.

Nitroglycerin is the parenteral agent of choice for the emergency treatment of congestive heart failure, particularly in patients with ischemic heart disease. In patients with congestive heart failure intravenous nitroglycerin and sodium nitroprusside exert similar beneficial hemodynamic effects.[80] Both lower systemic arterial resistance and increase venous capacitance. Intravenous nitroglycerin has slightly more potent venous effects and nitroprusside slightly more potent arterial effects. Arterial dilation with nitroglycerin is more critically dependent on preload.[56,81] Thus, either agent can be used to improve hemodynamics. Intravenous nitroglycerin is preferred in the setting of acute ischemic heart disease because of its potent anti-ischemic effects. Intravenous nitroglycerin may reduce infarct size when it is used to treat congestive heart failure[83] associated with infarction and in patients with inferior wall infarction.[84,85] However, there are insufficient data to warrant the routine use of nitroglycerin to limit infarct size.[86]

Nitroglycerin must be used with caution in patients with acute myocardial infarction because it may induce hypotension, which can compromise coronary artery perfusion and aggravate myocardial ischemia. In most studies of patients with infarction no more than a 10% reduction in blood pressure has been deemed appropriate.[84,85] The only studies evaluating the response of the chest pain of patients with acute infarction have not shown a benefit from intravenous nitroglycerin.[84,87] However, it is likely that nitroglycerin would be effective for recurrent angina after infarction.

Dosage

When used sublingually, the recommended starting dose of nitroglycerin is 0.3–0.4 mg. The drug is less effective orally because of deactivation in the liver. A dose of 0.3 or 0.4 mg can be repeated at 5–minute intervals to a total dose of three tablets if discomfort is unrelieved.

Intravenous nitroglycerin may be administered by bolus or by continuous infusion.[88] A 50-μg bolus of nitroglycerin may be administered prior to the initiation of a continuous nitroglycerin infusion at a rate of 10–20 μg/min. The infusion should be increased by 5 or 10 μg/min every 5–10 minutes until the desired hemodynamic or clinical response is achieved (e.g., fall in systemic vascular resistance or left ventricular filling pressure or relief of chest pain). In general, most patients respond to 50–200 μg/min. An occasional patient may require up to 500 μg/min. A convenient dilution for intravenous use is obtained when two 20-mg vials are diluted in 250 ml, resulting in a concentration of 160 μg/ml. Nitroglycerin should be administered by an infusion system that ensures a precise flow rate.

Recent data strongly suggest that the maintenance of sustained high plasma levels of nitroglycerin will rapidly induce tolerance. Thus, intermittent dosing, with nitrate-free periods, and the use of the lowest possible effective dose is strongly recommended.[89]

Precautions

Headache is a common consequence of therapy with nitroglycerin. Blood pressure may fall, resulting in nausea, giddiness, faintness, or syncope. Such symptoms are often aggravated by the erect position. Patients should be instructed to sit or lie down when taking nitroglycerin and to use the smallest dose that will relieve angina. Hypotension in a recumbent patient often responds to elevation of the legs. Patients usually accommodate to both the hypotensive effects and the headaches with chronic therapy. Hypotension and bradycardia following nitroglycerin usually are responsive to atropine.[90] Nitroglycerin may cause methemoglobinemia and ventilation–perfusion mismatch, which can result in hypoxemia.[91] The most serious risk is hypotension sufficient to produce ischemia of heart, brain, kidney, or other organs, particularly in those patients where perfusion is impaired because of arterial obstruction. Hypotension is best treated with fluid administration. The rapid titration of intravenous nitroglycerin in patients with congestive heart failure requires hemodynamic monitoring to assure efficacy and safety.

Beta Blockers: Propranolol and Metoprolol

Mechanisms of Action

Beta blocking agents attenuate the effects of circulating catecholamines by blocking their ability to bind to beta receptors. Both propranolol and metoprolol are available for intravenous use. Propranolol hydrochloride is a nonselective agent (effects both beta-1 and beta-2 receptors) with no intrinsic sympathomimetic activity.[92,93] Because it is nonselective, it has effects on both cardiac and pulmonary systems. Metoprolol is a beta-1-selective agent, which means that at low doses it inhibits mostly beta-1 receptors.[93] At higher doses, however, so-called selective agents lose most, if not all, of their selectivity.[93,94] Both agents will reduce heart rate, blood pressure, myocardial contractility, and therefore, myocardial oxygen consumption. These effects on myocardial work explain the effectiveness of these agents in the treatment of angina pectoris and hypertension.

Beta blockers also can help to control arrhythmias that are dependent on catecholamine stimulation for their initiation and/or propagation, perhaps in part by antagonizing beta-2-mediated hypokalemia.[10,95] Propranolol may control recurrent episodes of ventricular tachycardia or ventricular fibrillation refractory to other antiarrhythmics, especially when the arrhythmias are caused by myocardial ischemia. Beta blockers are useful also in the treatment of atrial fibrillation, atrial flutter, and paroxysmal supraventricular tachycardia involving the AV nodal conduction by reducing AV nodal conduction and, thus, slowing ventricular response of these rhythm disturbances. Beta blockers may terminate and/or prevent the reoccurrence of these arrhythmias. In addition to beta-blocking activity, some beta blockers have a quinidine-like effect on myocardial membranes and the cardiac action potential.[96,97]

The effects of competitive inhibition of beta-receptor sites by beta blockers is dependent, in part, on receptor number and the level of circulating catecholamines. In addition, differences in the metabolism of these agents between individual patients explain the lack of correlation between dose or plasma level and response. Oral administration results in substantially different pharmacokinetics than intravenous administration.[98]

Indications

The primary emergency indication for beta blockers in the emergency cardiac care circumstance is for control of recurrent ventricular tachycardia, recurrent ventricular fibrillation, and/or rapid supraventricular arrhythmias refractory to other therapy. Beta blockers are most effective when these arrhythmias are attributable to excess beta-adrenergic stimulation or are precipitated by myocardial ischemia.

Beta blockers are useful in patients with hypertension and tachycardia if left ventricular function is not severely depressed. Their use early in the setting of acute myocardial infarction is controversial. Although some studies have suggested a reduction in myocardial infarct size and/or mortality if beta blockers are administered early after the onset of acute myocardial infarction,[99-103] the routine use of beta blockers for the treatment of acute myocardial infarction is not recommended.[86] Several studies have now conclusively shown that the chronic use of beta-blocking agents reduces the mortality of patients after myocardial infarction, and their use is recommended as prophylaxis for patients at risk after myocardial infarction if there are no strong contraindications to their use.[104]

Dosage

Intravenous beta blockers should be administered slowly with frequent and careful monitoring of the blood pressure, electrocardiogram, and clinical response. A small test dose is recommended. Propranolol may be given intravenously in small doses (1–3 mg) every 5 minutes. The total dose of propranolol should not exceed 0.1 mg/kg. The plasma half-life of propranolol is 3.5–6 hours, but it does not correlate with pharmacologic effect during chronic therapy. The drug is ineffective when administered by intramuscular injection. Metoprolol is given in 5-mg aliquots every 5 minutes to a maximum dose of 15 mg. Its plasma half-life is 3–4 hours; however, its biological half-life is longer.[98]

Precautions

The principal adverse effects of beta-blocking agents are precipitation of hypotension, congestive heart failure, and bronchospasm. Caution must be exercised when therapy is considered for critically ill patients who may be dependent on beta-adrenergic receptor support. Therapy may be hazardous when cardiac function is depressed, as is usually the case after cardiac arrest. Congestive heart failure precipitated by beta blockade can usually be managed with diuretics, vasodilators, and/or inotropic agents. In patients with reactive airway disease, beta-adrenergic blockers may produce serious and even fatal bronchoconstriction. Should bronchospasm occur, it can be managed often by the administration of sympathomimetics and aminophylline. Treatment with beta blockers is contraindicated in patients who exhibit significant atrioventricular block and/or bradycardia. Atropine may restore an adequate heart rate when bradycardia is induced by beta blockers. Isoproterenol or a temporary transvenous pacemaker is the treatment of choice for atropine-resistant bradycardia.

These adverse effects may be synergistic with those of other agents and chronotropic with similar actions. For example, the negative inotropic effects of calcium blockers are synergistic with those of beta blockers. In addition, drug interactions are common. For example, the reduction in blood flow induced by beta blockers will inhibit the clearance of agents that are metabolized in the liver.[92,93]

Furosemide

Mechanisms of Action

Furosemide is a potent, rapidly acting diuretic that inhibits reabsorption of sodium and chloride in the ascending loop of Henle.[105] In patients with pulmonary edema during myocardial infarction, intravenous furosemide exerts direct venodilating effects that reduce venous return and, thus, central venous pressures.[106] This effect is seen prior to the onset of a diuresis that begins roughly 10 minutes after treatment and reaches peak effect in about 30 minutes. The diuretic effects last for about 6 hours. These reductions in central volumes induced by diuresis are generally associated with a decline in cardiac output.[107]

In patients with chronic heart failure and excess extravascular fluid, diuresis may be induced in part by changes in osmolarity. When this occurs, the egress of extravascular fluid into the intravascular space results in no net change in intravascular volume.[108] In addition, a generalized pressor response has been described when large doses of furosemide are administered intravenously to patients with chronic heart failure.[109]

In patients with acute myocardial infarction and other disease states associated with abnormal left ventricular compliance, diuretics must be used cautiously since small changes in volume may induce large changes in left ventricular pressure.[107] This may reduce cardiac output and/or induce hypotension, which can reduce coronary perfusion. Because the effects of diuretics on preload are synergistic with those of morphine and nitrates, combination therapy should be used with caution.

Indications

In emergency cardiac care setting, furosemide is indicated for the emergency treatment of pulmonary congestion associated with left ventricular dysfunction.

Dosage

A 20- to 40-mg intravenous dose of furosemide (or 0.5 mg/kg as an initial dose and up to 2.0 mg/kg in toto) is recommended. It should be injected slowly over a period of at least 1–2 minutes. Patients who fail to respond to bolus administration of furosemide may respond to continuous infusions of this drug.[110-113] Furosemide infusions at rates of 0.25–0.75 mg/kg/hr may produce adequate diuresis even in patients with renal dysfunction.[112]

Precautions

Dehydration and hypotension can result. Sodium, potassium, calcium, and magnesium depletion are common and may pose a serious threat to patients with coronary heart disease as well as those receiving digitalis. Hyperosmolality and metabolic alkalosis can occur. Furosemide is a sulfonamide derivative and may induce allergic reactions in patients with sensitivity to sulfonamides.

References

1. Ahlquist RP: A study of adrenotropic receptors. *Am J Physiol* 153:586-600, 1948.
2. Lands AM, Arnold A, McAuliff JP, et al: Differentiation of receptor systems activated by sympathomimetic amines. *Nature* 214:597-598, 1967.
3. Langer SZ: Presynaptic receptors and their role in the regulation of transmitter release. Sixth Gaddum memorial lecture, National Institute for Medical Research, Mill Hill, Jan 1977. *Br J Pharmacol* 60:481-497, 1977.
4. Lefkowitz RJ: Beta-adrenergic receptors: Recognition and regulation. *N Eng J Med* 295:323-328,1976.
5. Schumann HJ, Wagner J, Knorr A, et al: Demonstration in human atrial preparations of alpha adrenoceptors mediating positive inotropic effects. *Naunyn Schmidebergs Arch Pharmacol* 302:333-336, 1978.
6. Langer SZ, Hicks PE: Alpha-adrenoreceptor subtypes in blood vessels: Physiology and pharmacology. *J Cardiovasc Pharmacol* 6(suppl 4):S547-S558, 1984.
7. Mehta J, Lopez LM: Calcium-blocker withdrawal phenomenon: increase in affinity of alpha2 adrenoceptors for agonist as a potential mechanism. *Am J Cardiol* 58:242-246, 1986.
8. Haeusler G: Cardiovascular regulation by central adrenergic mechanisms and its alteration by hypotensive drugs. *Circ Res* 36 (supp l):I223-I232,1975.
9. Shaw J, Hunyor SN, Korner PI: The peripheral circulatory effects of clonidine and their role in the production of arterial hypotension. *Eur J Pharmacol* 14:101-111, 1971.
10. Brown MJ, Brown DC, Murphy MB: Hypokalemia from beta-2 receptor stimulation by circulating epinephrine. *N Engl J Med* 309:1414-1419, 1983.
11. Haddy FJ: Physiology and pharmacology of the coronary circulation and myocardium, particularly in relation to coronary artery disease. *Am J Med* 47:274-286, 1969.
12. Dempsey PJ, Cooper T: Pharmacology of the coronary circulation. *Ann Rev Pharmacol Toxicol* 12:99-110, 1972.
13. King MP, Angelakos ET, Uzgiris I: Innervation of the coronaries, abstracted. *Fed Proc* 30:613, 1971.
14. Berne RM: Regulation of coronary blood flow. *Physiol Rev* 44:1-29, 1964.
15. Feigl EO: Sympathetic control of coronary circulation. *Circ Res* 20:262-271, 1967.
16. Katori M, Berne RM: Release of adenosine from anoxic hearts: Relationship to coronary flow. *Circ Res* 19:420-425,1966.
17. Mudge GH, Goldberg S, Gunther S, et al: Comparison of metabolic and vasoconstrictor stimuli on coronary vascular resistance in man. *Circulation* 59:544-550, 1979.
18. Levy MN, Martin PJ, Stuesse SL: Neural regulation of the heart beat. *Ann Rev Physiol* 43:443-453, 1981.
19. Vedernikov YP: Mechanisms of coronary spasm of isolated human epicardial coronary segments excised 3 to 5 hours after sudden death. *J Am Coll Cardiol* 8(suppl 1):42a-49a, 1986.
20. Shepherd JT, Vanhoutte PM: Mechanisms responsible for coronary vasospasm. *J Am Coll Cardiol* 8:50a-54a, 1986.
21. Weiner N: Norepinephrine, epinephrine, and the sympathomimetic amines, in Gilman AG, Goodman LS, Rall TW, Murad F (eds): *Goodman and Gilman's The Pharmacological Basis of Therapeutics.* New York, Macmillan Publishing Co, 1985, pp 145-180.
22. Sobel BE, Braunwald E: The management of acute myocardial infarction, in Braunwald E (ed): *Heart Disease: A Textbook of Cardiovascular Medicine.* Philadelphia, W.B. Saunders Co, 1984, pp 1301-1333.
23. Ross J Jr, Frahm CJ, Braunwald E: The influences of intracardiac baroreceptors on venous return, systemic vascular volume and peripheral resistance. *J Clin Invest* 40:563-572, 1961.
24. Cohn JN: Blood pressure measurement in shock. Mechanism of inaccuracy in auscultatory and palpatory methods. *JAMA* 199:118-122, 1967.
25. Mueller HS, Evans R, Ayers S: Effect of dopamine on hemodynamics and myocardial metabolism in shock following acute myocardial infarction in man. *Circulation* 57:361-365, 1978.
26. Keung ECH, Siskind SJ, Sonneblick EH, et al: Dobutamine therapy in acute myocardial infarction. *JAMA* 245:144-146, 1981.
27. Anderson JL: Bretylium tosylate: Profile of the only available class III antiarrhythmic agent. *Clin Ther* 7:205-224, 1985.
28. Bivins JA, Rapp RP, Griffin WO Jr, et al: Dopamine-phenytoin interaction: a cause of hypotension in the critically ill. *Arch Surg* 113:245-249, 1978.
29. Newton DW, Fung EY, Williams DA: Stability of five catecholamines and terbutaline sulfate in 5% dextrose injection in the absence and presence of aminophylline. *Am J Hosp Pharm* 38:1314-1319, 1981.
30. Leier CV: Acute inotropic support, in Leier CV (ed): *Cardiotonic Drugs: A Clinical Survey.* New York, Marcel Dekker, 1986, pp 49-84.
31. Stoner JD, Bolen JL, Harrison DC: Comparison of dobutamine and dopamine in treatment of severe heart failure. *Br Heart J* 39:536-539, 1977.
32. Gillespie TA, Ambos HD, Sobel BE, et al: Effects of dobutamine in patients with acute myocardial infarction. *Am J Cardiol* 39:588-594, 1977.
33. Francis GS, Sharma B, Hodges M: Comparative hemodynamic effects of dopamine and dobutamine in patients with acute cardiogenic collapse. *Am Heart J* 103:995-999, 1982.
34. Richards C, Ricome JL, Rimailho A, et al: Combined hemodynamic effects of dopamine and dobutamine in cardiogenic shock. *Circulation* 67:620-626, 1983.
35. Maekawa K, Liang C, Hood WB: Comparison of dobutamine and dopamine in acute myocardial infarction. Effects of systemic hemodynamics, plasma catecholamines, blood flows and infarct size. *Circulation* 67:750-759, 1983.
36. Dell'Italia LJ, Starling MR, Blumhardt R, et al: Comparative effects of volume loading, dobutamine, and nitroprusside in patients with predominant right ventricular infarction. *Circulation* 72:1327-1335, 1985.
37. Niemann JT, Haynes KS, Garner D, et al: Post-countershock pulseless rhythms: response to CPR, artificial cardiac pacing, and adrenergic agonists. *Ann Emerg Med* 15:112-120, 1985.
38. Mancini D, Lejemtel T, Sonnenblick E: Intravenous amrinone for the treatment of the failing heart. *Am J Cardiol* 56:9b-15b, 1985.
39. Taylor SH, Verma SP, Hussain M, et al: Intravenous amrinone in left ventricular failure complicated by acute myocardial infarction. *Am J Cardiol* 56:29B-32B, 1985.
40. Klein NA, Siskind SJ, Frishman WH, et al: Hemodynamic comparison of intravenous amrinone and dobutamine in patients with chronic congestive heart failure. *Am J Cardiol* 48:170-175, 1981.
41. Rude RE, Kloner RA, Maroko PR, et al: Effects of amrinone on experimental acute myocardial ischemic injury. *Cardiovasc Res* 14:419-427, 1980.
42. Hoffman BF, Bigger JT Jr: Digitalis and allied cardiac glycosides, in Gilman AG, Goodman LS, Gilman A, et al (eds): *Goodman and Gilman's The Pharmacological Basis of Therapeutics,* ed 6. New York, Macmillan Publishing Co, 1980, pp 729-760.
43. Fawaz G: Effect of reserpine and pronethalol on the therapeutic and toxic actions of digitalis on the dog heart-lung preparation. *Br J Pharmacol* 29:302-308, 1967.
44. Smith TW, Antman EM, Freidman PL, et al: Digitalis glycosides: Mechanisms and manifestations of toxicity, Part II. *Prog Cardiovasc Dis* xxvi:495-540, 1984.
45. Ordog GJ, Benaron S, Bhasin V, et al: Serum digoxin levels and mortality in 5,100 patients. *Ann Emerg Med* 16:32-39, 1987.
46. Goldstein RA, Passamani ER, Roberts R: A comparison of digoxin and dobutamine in patients with acute infarction and cardiac failure. *N Engl J Med* 303:846-850, 1980.
47. Smith TW, Antman EM, Freidman PL, et al: Digitalis glycosides: mechanisms and manifestations of toxicity, Part I. *Prog Cardiovasc Dis* xxvi:413-458, 1984.
48. Sodeman WA: Diagnosis and treatment of digitalis toxicity. *N Engl J Med* 273:35-37;93-95, 1965.
49. Chung EK: *Digitalis Intoxication.* Baltimore, Williams and Wilkins Co, 1969.

50. Lang TW, Bernstein H, Barbieri F, et al: Digitalis toxicity: treatment with diphenylhydantoin. *Arch Intern Med* 116:573-580, 1965.

51. Hilmi KI, Regan TJ: Relative effectiveness of antiarrhythmic drugs in treatment of digitalis induced ventricular tachycardia. *Am Heart J* 76:365-369, 1968.

52. Kleiger R, Lown B: Cardioversion and digitalis. Clinical studies. *Circulation* 33:878-887, 1966.

53. Smith TW, Butler VP Jr, Haber E, et al: Treatment of life-threatening digitalis intoxication with digoxin-specific FAB antibody Fragments. *N Engl J Med* 307:1357-1362, 1982.

54. Bismuth C, Gaultier M, Conso F, Efthymiou ML: Hyperkalemia in acute digitalis poisoning: Prognostic significance and therapeutic implications. *Clin Toxicol* 6:153-162, 1973.

55. Cohn JN, Burke LP: Nitroprusside. *Ann Intern Med* 91:752-757, 1979.

56. Franciosca JA, Duerkman BW, Wiler M, Silverstein SR: Optimal left ventricular filling pressure during nitroprusside infusion for congestive heart failure. *Am J Med* 74:457-464, 1983.

57. Guiha NH, Cohn JN, Mikulic E, et al: Treatment of refractory heart failure with infusion of nitroprusside. *N Engl J Med* 291:587-592, 1974.

58. Miller RR, Vismara LA, Williams DO, et al: Pharmacological mechanisms for left ventricular unloading in clinical congestive heart failure. Differential effects of nitroprusside, phentolamine, and nitroglycerin on cardiac function and peripheral circulation. *Circ Res* 39:127-133, 1976.

59. Flaherty JT: Comparison of intravenous nitroglycerin and sodium nitroprusside in acute myocardial infarction. *Am J Med* 74(6B): 53-60, 1983.

60. Franciosa JA, Guiha NH, Limas CH, et al: Improved left ventricular function during nitroprusside infusion in acute myocardial infarction. *Lancet* 1:650-653, 1972.

61. Chatterjee K, Parmley WW, Ganz W, et al: Hemodynamic and metabolic responses to vasodilator therapy in acute myocardial infarction. *Circulation* 48:1183-1193, 1973.

62. Fuch RM, Rutler DL, Powell WJ: Effects of dobutamine on venous capacity, abstracted. *Clin Res* 24:218a, 1976.

63. Grossman W, Brodie B, Mann T, et al: Effects of sodium nitroprusside on left ventricular diastolic pressure-volume relations. *Circulation* 52 (suppl 2):35, 1975.

64. Mookherjee S, Warner R, Keighley J, et al: Worsening of ventilation perfusion relationship in the lungs in the face of hemodynamic improvement during nitroprusside infusion, abstracted. *Am J Cardiol* 39:282,1977.

65. Brodie TS, Gray R, Swan HJC, et al: Effect of nitroprusside on on arterial oxygenation, intrapulmonic shunts, and oxygen delivery, abstracted. *Am J Cardiol* 37:123, 1976.

66. Yacobi A, Amann AH, Baoske DM: Pharmaceutical considerations of nitroglycerin. *Drug Intell Clin Pharm* 17:255-261, 1983.

67. Jaffe AS, Roberts R: The use of intravenous nitroglycerin in cardiac disease. *Pharmacotherapy* 2:273-280, 1982.

68. Needleman P, Corr PB, Johnson EM: Drugs used for the treatment of angina: organic nitrates, calcium channel blockers and β-adrenergic antagonists, in Gilman AG, Goodman LS, Rall TW, Murad F (ed): *Goodman and Gilman's The Pharmacological Basis of Therapuetics*. Macmillan Publishing Co, 1985, pp 806-826.

69. Hill NS, Antman EM, Green LH, et al: Intravenous nitroglycerin: review of pharmacology, indications, therapeutic effects, and complications. *Chest* 79:69-73, 1981.

70. Horowitz LD, Herman MV, Gorlin R: Clinical response to nitroglycerin as a diagnostic test for coronary artery disease. *Am J Cardiol* 29:149-153, 1972.

71. Cohen MV, Downey JM, Sonnenblick EH, et al: The effects of nitroglycerin on coronary collaterals and myocardial contractility. *J Clin Invest* 52:2836-2847, 1973.

72. Malindzak GS, Green HD, Stagg PL: Effects of nitroglycerin on flow after partial constriction of the coronary artery. *J Appl Physiol* 29:17-22, 1970.

73. Hillis LD, Braunwald E: Coronary-artery spasm. *N Engl J Med* 299:695-702, 1978.

74. Kotter V, Von Leiter ER, Wunderlich J, et al: Comparison haemodynamic effects of phentolamine, sodium nitroprusside, glyceryl trinitrate in acute myocardial infarction. *Br Heart J* 39:1196-1204, 1977.

75. Miller RR, Vismara LA, Williams DO, et al: Pharmacological mechanisms for left ventricular unloading in congestive heart failure. Differential effects of nitroprusside, phentolamine, and nitroglycerine on cardiac function and peripheral circulation. *Circ Res* 39:127-133, 1976.

76. Gold HK, Leinback RC, Sanders CA: Use sublingual nitroglycerin in congestive failure following acute myocardial infarction. *Circulation* 46:839-845, 1972.

77. Kovick RB, Tillisch JH, Berens SC, et al: Vasodilator therapy for chronic left ventricular failure. *Circulation* 53:322-328, 1976.

78. Gray R, Chatterjee K, Vyden J, et al: Hemodynamic and metabolic effects of isosorbide dinitrate in chronic congestive heart failure. *Am Heart J* 90:346-352, 1975.

79. Greenberg H, Dwyer EM, JR, Jameson AG, et al: Effects of nitroglycerine on the major determinants of myocardial oxygen consumption. An angiographic and hemodynamic assessment. *Am J Cardiol* 36:425-432, 1975.

80. Leir CV, Ambach D, Thompson MJ, et al: Central and regional hemodynamic effects of intravenous isosorbide dinitrate, nitroglycerin and nitroprusside in patients with congestive heart failure. *Am J Cardiol* 48:1115-1123, 1981.

81. Bussmann WD, Schofer H, Kaltenbach M: Effects of intravenous nitroglycerin on hemodynamics and ischemic injury in patients with acute myocardial infarction. *Eur J Cardiol* 8:61-74, 1978.

82. Curfman GD, Heinsimer JA, Lozner EC, et al: Intravenous nitroglycerin in the treatment of spontaneous angina pectoris: A prospective, randomized trial. *Circulation* 67:276-282, 1983.

83. Bussmann WD, Passek D, Seidel W, Kaltenbach M: Reduction of ck and mb indexes of infarct size by intravenous nitroglycerine. *Circulation* 63:615-622, 1981.

84. Jaffe AS, Geltman EM, Tiefenbrunn AJ, et al: Reduction of infarct size in patients with inferior infarction with intravenous glyceryl trinitrate. *Br Heart J* 49:452-460, 1983.

85. Flaherty JT, Becker LC, Bulkley BH, et al: A randomized prospective trial of intravenous nitroglycerin in patients with acute myocardial infarction. *Circulation* 68:576-588, 1983.

86. Standards and guidelines for cardiopulmonary resuscitation (CPR) and emergency cardiac care (ECC). *JAMA* 255:2841-3044,1986.

87. Mikolich JR, Nicoloff NB, Robinson PH, et al: Relief of refractory angina with continuous intravenous infusion of nitroglycerin. *Chest* 77:375-379, 1980.

88. Leinbach RC, Gold HK: Intermittent and continuous nitroglycerine infusions for control of myocardial ischemia. *Circulation* 56 (suppl 3):194, 1977.

89. Abrams J: Tolerance to organic nitrates. *Circulation* 74:1181-1185, 1986.

90. Come PC, Pitt B: Nitroglycerin-induced severe hypotension and bradycardia in patients with acute myocardial infarction. *Circulation* 54:624-628, 1976.

91. Weygandt GR, Kopman EA, Bauer S, et al: The cause of hypoxemia induced by nitroglycerin, abstracted. *Am J Cardiol* 43:427, 1979.

92. Shand DG: Drug therapy: propranolol. *N Engl J Med* 293:280-285, 1975.

93. Koch-weser J: Drug therapy: metoprolol. *N Engl J Med* 301:698-703, 1979.

94. Prichard BNC: Beta-adrenergic receptor blockade in hypertension, past, present and future. *Br J Clin Pharmacol* 5:379-399, 1978.

95. Nordrehaug JE: Malignant arrhythmia in relation to serum potassium in acute myocardial infarction. *Am J Cardiol* 56:20d-23d, 1985.

96. Davis LD, Temte, JV: Effects of propranolol on the transmembrane potentials of ventricular muscle in purkinje fibers of the dog. *Circ Res* 22:661-667, 1968.

97. Woosley RL, Kornahauser D, Smith R, et al: Suppression of chronic ventricular arrhythmias with propranolol. *Circulation* 60:819-827, 1979.

98. Frishman WH: Drug therapy: Beta-adrenergic antagonists — new drug new indications. *N Engl J Med* 305:500-506, 1981.

99. Peter T, Norris RN, Clarke ED, et al: Reduction of enzyme levels by propranolol after acute infarction. *Circulation* 57:1091-1095, 1978.

100. Hjalmarson A, Herlitz J, For the goteborg metropolol trial group. The goteberg metropolol trial in acute myocardial infarction. *Am J Cardiol* 53:(suppl i): 1d-50d, 1984.

101. The Miami Trial Research Group: Metropolol in acute myocardial infarction (Miami). A randomized placebo-controlled intervention trial. *Eur Heart J* 6:199-226, 1985.

102. The International Collaborative Study Group. Acute myocardial infarct size reduction by timolol administration. *Am J Cardiol* 57:28f-33f, 1986.

103. ISIS-I (first international study of infarct survival) collaborative group. Randomized trial of intravenous atenolol among 16,027 cases of suspected acute myocardial infarction: ISIS-I. *Lancet* 2:57-66, 1986.

104. Frishman WT, Furberg CD, Friedewald WT: Beta-adrenergic blockage for survivors of acute myocardial infarction. *N Engl J Med* 310:830-837, 1984.

105. Mudge GH: Diuretics and other agents employed in the mobilization of edema fluid, in Gilman AG, Goodman LS, Gilman A, et al (eds): *Goodman and Gilman's The Pharmacological Basis Of Therapeutics.* New York, Macmillan Publishing Co Inc, 1980, pp 892-915.

106. Dikshit K, Vyden JK, Forrester JJ, et al: Renal and extra-renal hemodynamic effects of furosemide in congestive heart failure after acute myocardial infarction. *N Engl J Med* 288:1087-1090, 1973.

107. Biddle TL, Yu PN, Effects of furosemide on hemodynamics and lung water in acute pulmonary edema secondary to myocardial infarction. *Am J Cardiol* 43:86-90, 1979.

108. Schuster CJ, Weil MH, Besso J, et al: Blood volume following diuresis induced by furosemide. *Am J Med* 76:585-592, 1984.

109. Francis GS, Siegal RM, Goldsmith SR, et al: Acute vasoconstrictive responses to intravenous furosemide in patients with chronic congestive heart failure. *Ann Intern Med* 103:1-6, 1985.

110. Lawson DH, Gray JM, Henry DA, et al: Continous infusion of furosemide in refractory edema. *Br J Med* 2:476, 1978.

111. Copeland JG, Campbell DW, Platchetka JR, et al: Diuresis with continous infusion of furosemide after cardiac surgery. *Am J Surg* 146:796-799, 1983.

112. Amiel SA, Blackburn AM, Rubens RD: Intravenous infusion of furosemide as treatment for ascites in malignant disease. *Br Med J* 288:1041, 1984.

113. Krasna MJ, Scott GE, Scholz PM, et al: Postoperative enhancement of urinary output in patients with acute renal failure using continuous furosemide therapy. *Chest* 89:294-295, 1986.

Acid–Base Balance

Chapter 9

In a chemical reaction an acid donates a hydrogen ion (H^+) while a base accepts a hydrogen ion. The balance between hydrogen donors (acids) and hydrogen acceptors (bases) must be maintained within a narrow range for proper bodily function. The most frequently used measure of acid–base status is the pH, a value that is inversely related to the logarithm of the concentration of hydrogen ions (Figure 1).

The "normal" H^+ concentration is 40 ± 5 nEq/L, which corresponds to a pH of 7.40 ± 0.05 units. The term "acidosis" refers to a state in which the H^+ concentration is increased to more than 45 nEq/L, corresponding to a pH of less than 7.35; while "alkalosis" refers to a decrease in H^+ concentration to below 35 nEq/L (pH > 7.45).

A marked increase or decrease in body pH is potentially harmful. Acidosis diminishes myocardial contractility, reduces the vascular response to catecholamines, and may interfere with the actions of other pharmcological agents. Alkalosis inhibits the release of oxygen from red blood cells.

Because pH is related to the logarithm of H^+ concentration, small changes in pH represent marked changes in H^+ concentration. For example, a pH fall from 7.40 to 7.10 (a change of 0.30 pH units) corresponds to a doubling of the H^+ concentration (from 40 to 80 nEq/L). If the pH falls another 0.30 pH unit (to 6.80), the H^+ concentration doubles again (to 160 nEq/L). Conversely, an increase in pH of 0.30 units corresponds to a 50% reduction in the H^+ concentration.

In the emergency cardiac care circumstance, acute acidosis is generally the dominant concern. The emphasis of this chapter will be on the problems of acidosis to a greater extent than alkalosis and to acute rather than chronic alterations in acid–base status.

Acid is a normal waste product of cellular metabolism. During aerobic metabolism (metabolism dependent on oxygen), the body produces two forms of acid:

1. Carbon dioxide (CO_2), which is a "volatile" acid (can be excreted by the lungs); and
2. Metabolic acids that must be neutralized ("buffered") by circulating endogenous base compounds and/or secreted by the kidney to maintain normal acid–base homeostasis.

Carbon dioxide is easily eliminated from the body when circulation, renal function, and ventilation are normal. When these fuctions are abnormal or when the load of CO_2 is excessive, acidosis can result.

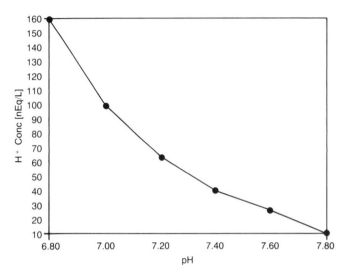

Figure 1. Graphic representation of the relation of pH values to H^+ concentration.

Metabolic acids such as lactic acid are of a larger molecular size than CO_2. Such acids result from the metabolism of amino acids, fats, and carbohydrates, and they are buffered by circulating buffer systems in plasma. Some of the other metabolic acids (e.g., inorganic phosphoric and sulfuric acids) are eliminated primarily by renal excretion. Acidosis occurs only when excessive quantities of these acids are produced or the body's buffering systems or renal function are abnormal.

There are two ways in which bases can accumulate: excessive ingestion of a base (e.g., bicarbonate) or the loss of excess acid. The latter may occur when hypokalemia is present and H^+ is renally excreted in preference to potassium or when H^+ depletion occurs secondary to vomiting. These changes are compensated for by changes in ventilation, renal excretion, and by the circulating buffer systems of the body.

Buffer Systems in the Body

The pH is determined by the interplay of two factors: 1) processes that raise or lower the H^+ concentration and 2) defense mechanisms (buffer systems) that respond to changes in the H^+ concentration to maintain the pH of body fluids at a normal value.

Buffers that stabilize the pH of human blood acutely include plasma proteins, hemoglobin, phosphate, ammonium, and bicarbonate. The carbonic acid

(H_2CO_3)–bicarbonate (HCO_3^-) buffer system is particularly important for rapid fine-tuning adjustments in the body pH, but as with all buffering systems, it requires adequate hemodynamic, renal, and pulmonary function.

Physiologic human buffer systems usually consist of a weak acid or base in equilibrium with the salt of that acid or base. This principle is expressed diagrammatically in the following equation:

weak base + strong acid $\leftrightarrows$ neutral salt + weak acid

For example, if strong metabolic acids are released into the blood stream, sodium bicarbonate (a weak base) will combine with the H^+ of the strong acid to form carbonic acid (a weaker acid) and a neutral salt. If the strong metabolic acid is lactic acid the equation will now appear as

H^+ lactate + $NaHCO_3^-$ $\leftrightarrows$ H_2CO_3 + Na lactate
(strong acid) (weak base)   (weak acid) (neutral salt)

In general, the H^+ contributed by any strong acid can combine with HCO_3^- to form carbonic acid (H_2CO_3). Carbonic acid then dissociates to release water (H_2O) and carbon dioxide (CO_2) via the following reaction in the presence of the enzyme carbonic anhydrase.

$$H^+ + HCO_3^- \leftrightarrows H_2CO_3 \leftrightarrows H_2O + CO_2$$

The normal ratio of bicarbonate to carbonic acid is 20:1. As long as this ratio is maintained, the pH will be normal.

In order for the carbonic acid system to function normally, CO_2 must be delivered to the lungs, where it crosses the alveolar capillary membrane into the alveolar spaces and can be removed by ventilation. Thus, for this system, two major factors might decrease its ability to acutely eliminate an acid load and lead to a change in the 20:1 ratio of bicarbonate to carbonic acid:

1. Poor tissue or pulmonary circulation, and
2. Inadequate ventilation.

The bicarbonate–carbonic acid buffer system equation can move in either direction, depending on the concentrations on either side of the equation. For practical purposes, inadequate carbonic anhydrase activity in plasma is not of concern. The bicarbonate buffer system can correct modest increases in H^+ concentration by eliminating more CO_2, as long as circulation and ventilation are adequate.

The other buffer systems operate on principles similar to that of the bicarbonate–carbonic acid system. For the phosphate system, a neutral salt (NaCl) and a weak acid ($NaHPO_4$) are formed in response to a H^+ load. The weak acid is subsequently excreted by the kidneys. Proteins can act as either acids or bases, releasing or binding H^+ as needed. The hemoglobin buffer system operates in large part through the carbonic acid reaction within the red blood cell itself.

The principle of buffering excess bases is the same as that for acids. If a strong base such as sodium hydroxide enters the system, it is neutralized by combining with carbonic acid to form a weaker base and water:

$$NaOH + H_2CO_3 \rightarrow NaHCO_3 + H_2O$$

The bicarbonate formed in this reaction is excreted by the kidneys.

Buffer systems reduce, but do not eliminate, the hazards of acidosis or alkalosis in response to an acute increase or decrease in the H^+ concentration. The rate of reaction of buffer systems in plasma is rapid, and they participate in almost instantaneous chemical processes. However, these systems, most commonly those that neutralize excess acid, can become depleted. When this occurs, the term "base deficit" is applied. This temporary compromise in the buffering capacity of plasma causes an exacerbation in the pH fall following an acid load. Fortunately, there are additional pulmonary and renal compensatory mechanisms that can (over time) restore acid–base balance by conserving buffers and helping to eliminate excess acids or bases in the system.

Proper interpretation of the etiology of an acid–base disturbance requires analysis of the partial pressure of carbon dioxide in arterial ($PaCO_2$) and/or venous ($PvCO_2$) blood. Normal $PaCO_2$ is 35–45 mmHg (mean 40 mmHg). The $PaCO_2$ provides an important measure of the adequacy of pulmonary ventilation and gas exchange because it varies inversely with the minute ventilation (the product of the respiratory rate and the tidal volume). If minute ventilation increases, $PaCO_2$ decreases; if ventilation decreases, $PaCO_2$ increases.

An increase in ventilation is known as hyperventilation. Tachypnea (rapid breathing) is not synonymous with "hyperventilation". Each breath or tidal volume (VT) is made up of dead space ventilation (VD) (air entering portions of the tracheobronchial tree where no gas exchange occurs) and effective alveolar ventilation (VA). When breathing is rapid but shallow, tidal volume is reduced. Since dead space cannot decrease, alveolar ventilation must decrease. The net effect of rapid breathing may be a reduction in effective ventilation with a progressive rise in $PaCO_2$. True hyperventilation is present only when minute ventilation increases.

An acute increase in the $PaCO_2$ will cause an increase in the concentration of carbonic acid; an acute decrease in the $PaCO_2$ has the opposite effect. Neither perturbation will change the overall HCO_3^- content of the buffer system because an acid cannot react with its own salt (carbonic acid cannot react with its own salt, sodium bicarbonate). Only the ratio between bicarbonate and carbonic acid changes (the ratio is normally 20:1) as the relative amounts of chemicals change on one side of the equation or the other. The bicarbonate concentration can change over time due to increased or decreased renal bicarbonate resorption as long as renal function is normal and there is a normal concentration of circulating plasma cations (Na$^+$, K$^+$). By manipulating respiratory excretion (ventilation) or renal excretion, the normal 20:1 ratio and a normal pH can be maintained. If either of these systems fail, the ability of the buffer systems to compensate for acidosis or alkalosis is severely compromised.

The role of the kidneys in the maintenance of acid–base homeostasis is to secrete acid and to reabsorb bicarbonate. In addition, the kidneys excrete phosphate, chloride, and ammonia associated with a H$^+$ ion. Although it takes up to 24 hours for renal regulation to occur, it is an important part of the acid–base system.

Clinical Blood Gas Analysis

Blood gas analysis measures the following parameters in blood:

1) Oxygen tension (PO$_2$);
2) pH;
3) Carbon dioxide (PCO$_2$) tension.

It can be performed on arterial (then designated PaCO$_2$ and PaO$_2$) or venous (PvCO$_2$ and PvO$_2$) blood. The serum HCO$_3$ concentration can be estimated if the pH and the PCO$_2$ are known, using Figure 1 to determine the H$^+$ concentration:

$$HCO_3^- \text{ concentration} = \frac{24 \times PCO_2}{[H^+]}$$

Normally, the arterial PCO$_2$ tension (PaCO$_2$) is 40 $\pm$ 5 mmHg. A PaCO$_2$ above 45 mmHg (hypercarbia) is usually caused by inadequate ventilation (hypoventilation). A PaCO$_2$ below 35 mmHg (hypocarbia) usually signifies hyperventilation. The combination of acidosis and a high PaCO$_2$ is termed "respiratory acidosis". It is presumed that the acidosis is due to inadequate ventilatory function because the PaCO$_2$ is high. Acidosis due to the buildup of metabolic acid (H$^+$) and accompanied by a normal or low PaCO$_2$ is termed "metabolic acidosis" because it is presumed that it is occurring despite normal or increased ventilation. The combination of an alkalotic pH and a low PaCO$_2$ is usually due to respiratory alkalosis or increased ventilation with the loss of excessive amounts of CO$_2$ and H$^+$. Alkalosis due to a buildup of HCO$_3^-$ accompanied by a normal or high PaCO$_2$ is usually due to metabolic alkalosis (frequently volume depletion and/or hypokalemia) and the increased PaCO$_2$ is an attempt at respiratory compensation.

Arterial blood gas analysis may reflect only acute changes due to buffering or also more chronic compensatory changes in renal and/or respiratory function. When there is chronic elevation of the PaCO$_2$, the excretion of HCO$_3^-$ by the kidneys is decreased, resulting in a buildup of HCO$_3^-$ to buffer the extra acid load and to restore a normal pH. Metabolic acidosis

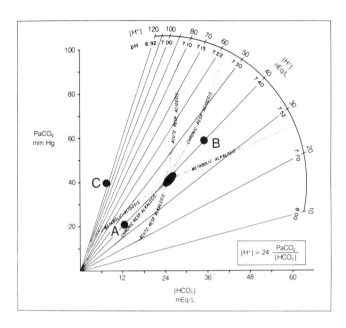

Figure 2. **Acid–base map describing the relationships among arterial pH, H$^+$ concentration, PCO$_2$, and HCO$_3^-$ concentration.** The dark area in the center represents the range of normal values for these parameters; the stippled areas represent the different simple acid–base disturbances. Points A, B, and C indicate three mixed acid–base disorders. (From Harrington JT, Cohen JJ, Kassirer JP: Mixed acid–base disturbances, in Cohen JJ, Kassirer JP (eds): *Acid/ Base*. Boston, Little, Brown and Co, 1982.)

is frequently compensated by respiratory alkalosis (hyperventilation). Metabolic alkalosis is frequently compensated by respiratory acidosis (hypoventilation, increased PaCO$_2$ — which preserves the 20:1 ratio of bicarbonate to carbonic acid). Respiratory acidosis (hypoventilation) is compensated by metabolic alkalosis (renal preservation of bicarbonate), and respiratory alkalosis (hyperventilation) is compensated by excretion of bicarbonate.

When two primary acid–base disturbances occur simultaneously, the term "mixed acid–base disturbance" is used. In this circumstance, the pH changes cannot be explained by only one abnormality. An easy way to determine if there is more than one abnormality is to plot the values on a chart which delineates what values would be expected if a pure respiratory or metabolic acidosis or alkalosis were present (Figure 2).

Acid–Base Balance and Cardiopulmonary Resuscitation

Acid–Base Changes During CPR

Cardiac output during CPR is low, averaging only one quarter to one third of normal,[1] and results in a severe fall in tissue oxygen delivery. Faced with a critical shortage of oxygen, cells shift to a less efficient form of energy production known as anaerobic metabolism. This form of metabolism increases the production of lactic acid, a source of H^+.[2] Fortunately, the buildup of lactic acid during CPR is slow.[3-5]

During anaerobic metabolism, the carbon dioxide concentration increases far more rapidly inside cells than in the blood. Anoxic arrest of the heart causes a progressive increase in the PCO_2 concentration inside heart muscle cells that may reach very high levels (90–475 mmHg).[6] Above an intramyocardial PCO_2 of 475 mmHg, the high PCO_2 contributes to electromechanical dissociation. This problem can be corrected only by restoring or improving coronary blood flow during cardiopulmonary resuscitation.

Intracellular carbon dioxide diffuses from the cells into the capillary blood and returns to the heart and lungs in venous blood. Central (mixed) venous blood during CPR is acidotic (pH approximately 7.15) and hypercarbic ($PvCO_2$ approximately 74 mmHg).[7] With hyperventilation during resuscitation, carbon dioxide is removed from the relatively small amount of blood flowing through the lungs. Thus, the blood passing through the lungs and into the arterial circulation is relatively cleansed of carbon dioxide and is less acidotic than venous blood. Arterial blood pH during well-performed CPR in humans is usually normal, slightly acidotic, or even mildly alkalotic.[5,7-9] However, venous blood remains acidotic because pulmonary blood flow is only a quarter to a third of normal (this phenomenon of venous acidosis in the face of arterial alkalosis has been termed the "venous paradox").[7]

When a patient receiving CPR is severely acidotic on the arterial side, it is usually due to inadequate ventilation/oxygenation.[9] The best solution is to improve the mechanical technique of CPR and to hyperventilate the patient. If severe acidosis is present despite hyperventilation, correct intubation, and properly performed external chest massage, an alternate method for providing assisted circulation (open-chest compressions or venoarterial bypass), may need to be considered.

Pharmacologic Buffers During CPR

In the past, administration of sodium bicarbonate ($NaHCO_3$) was recommended during CPR in the belief that it would increase the amount of HCO_3^- available to buffer the H^+ produced during anaerobic metabolism.

However, sodium bicarbonate itself contains and releases a large amount of CO_2 into the blood (the PCO_2 of $NaHCO_3$ is 260–280 mmHg).[7] The CO_2 released when bicarbonate is given diffuses into cells more quickly than does HCO_3^-, causing a paradoxical rise in intracellular PCO_2, a further fall in intracellular pH, and further impairment in cellular function.

The adverse effects caused by elevated intracellular PCO_2 have been most clearly demonstrated in the central nervous system. Paradoxical acidosis of cerebrospinal fluid occurs following sodium bicarbonate therapy.[10] Intracerebral acidosis caused by the administration of $NaHCO_3$ may be responsible for some of the prolonged periods of confusion following successful cardiac resuscitation. When the PCO_2 of heart muscle cells is increased (as occurs following the administration of $NaHCO_3$), cardiac contractility, cardiac output, and blood pressure all decrease in experimental models.[7,11-13]

Sodium bicarbonate can cause other potentially harmful effects as well,[4,14,15] including hyperosmolality, alkalemia, and sodium overload. With rare exception,[16] sodium bicarbonate has not been shown to improve survival from cardiac arrest in experimental animals.[17-19] It is not recommended for the routine initial cardiac arrest management even for unwitnessed arrests. Bicarbonate should not be used until other more proven interventions (such as defibrillation, cardiac compression, support of ventilation including intubation) and pharmacologic therapies (such as epinephrine and antiarrhythmic agents) have been employed. It is estimated that these interventions usually require at least 10 minutes during the routine resuscitation sequence.

In certain unusual circumstances, such as in patients with known preexisting metabolic acidosis with or without hyperkalemia or in the treatment of severe hypercalcemia, bicarbonate may be of benefit and should be used earlier in the resuscitation sequence. During prolonged CPR, sodium bicarbonate, though not recommended, may be used at the discretion of the team leader. If it is to be used, an initial dose of 1 mEq/kg is recommended. No more than half of the original dose should be given for any subsequent dose. Repeat doses should not be given any more frequently than every 10 minutes.

In the postresuscitation phase of management, bicarbonate administration should be guided by arterial blood gas measurement. During low blood flow states as exist during CPR, however, arterial blood gas measurement is a poor index of the severity of cellular acidosis.[7]

Alternate buffer agents have not yet been shown to improve survival during cardiac resuscitation, although some of these agents have the advantage of not exacerbating intracellular acidosis. THAM (tromethamine, tris-buffer) is a potent amine buffer which actively binds H ions. It combines with carbonic acid (H_2CO_3), increasing the amount of bicarbonate anion (HCO_3^-) available in the blood. THAM penetrates into cells and may neutralize acidic ions in the intracellular fluid. In dogs, THAM can effectively correct the metabolic acidosis during cardiac arrest.[20] Anecdotal reports suggest that it may be of value during prolonged cardiac resuscitation in humans.[21]

Dichloroacetate (DCA) reduces the serum lactate concentration by stimulating pyruvate dehydrogenase, the enzyme that catalyzes the rate-limiting step in the oxidation of lactate to pyruvate.[22] It is a safe and effective adjunct in the treatment of patients with lactic acidosis,[22] but its value during CPR is unexplored.

Conclusion

Acidosis, particularly at the intracellular level, plays an important role in determining the survival of patients receiving CPR. The only preventive and corrective treatment that is of proven benefit is properly performed CPR and effective airway management.

Pharmacological buffers have not yet been shown to be of value. The potential risks of sodium bicarbonate therapy outweigh its advantages for the average patient receiving CPR during initial resuscitation efforts. Alternate buffer agents show promise, but further investigation is needed before they can be recommended during cardiac resuscitation.

References

1. Del Guercio LRM, Feins NR, Cohn JD, et al: Comparison of blood flow during external and internal cardiac massage in man. *Circulation* 32:(suppl):I171-I180, 1965.
2. Weil MH, Afifi AA: Experimental and clinical studies on lactate and pyruvate as indicators of the severity of acute circulatory failure (shock). *Circulation* 41:989-1001, 1970.
3. Weil MH, Trevino RP, Rackow EC: Sodium bicarbonate during CPR. Does it help or hinder? editorial. *Chest* 88:487, 1985.
4. Bishop RL, Weisfeldt ML. Sodium bicarbonate administration during cardiac arrest. *JAMA* 235:506-509, 1976.
5. Grundler W, Weil MH, Yamaguchi M, et al: The paradox of venous acidosis and arterial alkalosis during CPR, abstracted. *Chest* 86:282, 1984.
6. MacGregor DC, Wilson GJ, Holness DE, et al: Intramyocardial carbon dioxide tension: a guide to the safe period of anoxic arrest of the heart. *J Thorac Cardiovasc Surg* 68:101-107, 1974.
7. Weil MH, Rackow EC, Trevino R, et al: Difference in acid-base state between venous and arterial blood during cardiopulmonary resuscitation. *N Engl J Med* 315:153-156, 1986.
8. McGill JW, Ruiz E: Central venous pH as a predictor of arterial pH in prolonged cardiac arrest. *Ann Emerg Med* 13:684-687, 1984.
9. Ornato JP, Gonzalez ER, Coyne MR, et al: Arterial pH in out-of-hospital cardiac arrest. *Am J Emerg Med* 3:498-502, 1985.
10. Niemann JT, Rosborough JP: Effects of acidemia and sodium bicarbonate therapy in advanced cardiac life support. *Ann Emerg Med* 13:781-784, 1984.
11. Berenyi KJ, Wolk M, Killip T: Cerebrospinal fluid acidosis complicating therapy of experimental cardiopulmonary arrest. *Circulation* 52:319-324, 1975.
12. Clancy RL, Cingolani HE, Taylor RR, et al: Influence of sodium bicarbonate on myocardial performance. *Am J Physiol* 212:917-923, 1967.
13. Huseby JS, Bumprecht DG: Hemodynamic effects of rapid bolus sodium bicarbonate on myocardial performance. *Am J Physiol* 212:917-923, 1967.
14. Graf H, Leach W, Arieff AI: Evidence for a detrimental effect of bicarbonate therapy in hypoxic lactic acidosis. *Science* 227:754-756, 1985.
15. Mattar JA, Weil MH, Shubin H, et al: Cardiac arrest in the critically ill (II: Hyperosmolar states following cardiac arrest). *Am J Med* 56:162-168, 1974.
16. Redding JS, Pearson JW: Resuscitation from ventricular fibrillation. *JAMA* 203:255-260, 1968.
17. Yakaitis RW, Thomas JD, Mahaffey JE: Influence of pH and hypoxia on the success of defibrillation. *Crit Care Med* 3:139-142, 1975.
18. Redding JS, Pearson JW: Metabolic acidosis: a factor in cardiac resuscitation. *Southern Med J* 60:926-932, 1967.
19. Guerci AD, Chandra N, Johnson E, et al: Failure of sodium bicarbonate to improve resuscitation from ventricular fibrillation in dogs. *Circulation* 74:IV75-IV79, 1986.
20. Minuck M, Sharma GP: Comparison of THAM and sodium bicarbonate in resuscitation of the heart after ventricular fibrillation in dogs. *Anesth Analg* 56:38-45, 1977.
21. Lee WH Jr, Darby TD, Aldinger EE, et al: Use of THAM in the management of refractory cardiac arrest. *Am Surg* 28:87-89, 1962.
22. Stacpoole PW, Harman EM, Curry SH, et al: Treatment of lactic acidosis with dichloroacetate. *N Engl J Med* 309:390-396, 1983.

Catheter- and Infusion-Related Sepsis: The Nature of the Problem and Its Prevention

Chapter 10

An estimated 2,000,000 nosocomial infections occur annually in hospitals in the United States. Ten percent are bacteremias or disseminated infections which prolong the hospital stay four days per patient.[1] Forty-five percent of all nosocomial infections are device-related infections, and about one quarter of these are due to infusion fluids, intravascular catheters, and monitoring devices. Since approximately 12% of all hospital patients have an indwelling needle and another 12% have a plastic catheter in place, these frequent infections can be expected to continue as exposures to invasive medical devices increase. Measures to prevent such device-related infections should maximize the risk:benefit ratio associated with these devices; all device-related infections should be preventable.

Classification of Intravascular-Device-Related Infections

Categories of infections related to intravascular devices use include the following:

1. Significant vs. insignificant catheter colonization without obvious infection.
2. Local cutaneous infection.
3. Local vascular infection.
4. Bacteremia.
5. Complicated bacteremia (i.e., endocarditis).

The pathogenesis of device-related infections is as follows: 1) During manufacture, devices may be contaminated, directly introducing microorganisms into the patient when used. 2) The device may interrupt epithelial barriers and provide microorganisms direct access to the bloodstream or deep tissues. 3) During use, devices may support growth of bacteria and act as reservoirs.

Bacteremia, the most important infection complication related to infusion therapy, occurs in 35,000 patients annually, with a case-fatality rate of approximately 30%. Sepsis from catheter contamination occurs ten times more commonly than infusion-related infections. Intrinsic fluid contamination (which may occur during manufacture) probably occurs in approximately 0.1% of units produced, whereas contamination of infusion fluid during use occurs in approximately 2.0–10.0% of all infusions. The majority of infections related to intravascular catheters are caused by *Staphylococcus aureus* and *Staphylococcus epidermidis*, with infections caused by enterococci, aerobic gram-negative bacilli, and Candida occurring less frequently.[2,3]

Risk Factors for Device-Related Infections

Type of Catheter

Bacteremia occurs in approximately 0.1–0.2% of patients with scalp vein needles, whereas it occurs in up to 8.0% of patients with plastic catheters in place. Although early reports documented an incidence as high as 27% of infusion-related bacteremia in patients on total parenteral nutrition with plastic catheters, other studies suggest that the incidence may be reduced to 7%.[4-8]

Percutaneous vs. Cutdown Insertion

Recent studies have demonstrated that the incidence of infection with percutaneous femoral venous and arterial catheters inserted and cared for using proper aseptic technique is not different from catheters inserted at other sites.[2,8-12] Venous and arterial catheters inserted by surgical cutdown may be associated with up to a ninefold increase in the incidence of bacteremia compared to catheters inserted by direct puncture.[2,13,14]

Length of Time in Place

The colonization rate of intravascular catheters increases in direct proportion to indwelling time.[3,4,11,15-17] With venous cannulation, the rate of positive catheter cultures and associated bacteremia increases markedly after 2–3 days.[3,4,11,18]

Arterial catheters also have an increased incidence of positive catheter cultures after 2–4 days; and in one series, 16 local infections occurred in 23 patients in whom the catheter had been left in place for more than 4 days. In addition, bacteremia occurred only in those patients who had catheters left in for more than 4 days.[4,11,12,14,16]

Pulmonary artery catheters can be left in place for approximately 3 days before evidence of positive catheter-tip culture commonly occurs.[16] One study documented an increased incidence of positive cultures of blood drawn through the distal port of the pulmonary artery catheter in patients after 3 days.[19] Two other studies showed no correlation between the length of time that the catheter was in place and the incidence of positive catheter-tip cultures.[10,20] However, in one of the studies, no pulmonary artery catheter in place for 2 days or less had a positive culture of the catheter tip.[10] In the other study, all catheters had been inserted for fewer than 3 days, and the incidence of positive catheter cultures decreased with shorter insertion times.[20]

Failure to Conform to Aseptic Technique During Insertion

There is a strong correlation between the cutaneous flora of patients and the microorganisms recovered from tips of their intravascular catheters.[4,10] It has been hypothesized that microorganisms gain access to the tip of the cannula both at the moment of insertion and, subsequently, by migrating along the interface between catheter and tissue. In addition, intravenous (IV) cannulas can be contaminated during the time of insertion by microorganisms on the hands of hospital personnel. Almost half of personnel randomly sampled may carry gram-negative bacilli on their hands, and approximately 10% may carry *S. aureus*. However, when serial cultures are performed, all persons at various times may carry gram-negative bacilli, and two thirds may carry *S. aureus* on their hands.[21-23] Washing the hands with soap and water and employing mechanical friction for at least 15 seconds is sufficient to remove most transiently acquired bacteria.[23]

Failure to Clean and Redress the Insertion Site

If the skin at the insertion site is not cleansed and redressed periodically while the catheter is in place, the potential for catheter colonization and infection is increased.[4,10] In addition, during cleansing, the site can be inspected for evidence of phlebitis or infection.

Antibiotic Therapy

Systemic antibiotics do not decrease the rate of colonization of the catheter tip or of bacteria but may increase the incidence of resistant gram-negative bacteria or fungi. Antibiotic ointment or povidone–iodine ointment at the skin site may reduce infection when used for insertions requiring a cutdown and may be efficacious for percutaneous insertion.[4,13,24]

Condition of Patient

Patients with severe acute or chronic illness and trauma have a loss of many host defense mechanisms, which predisposes them to infections with microorganisms of low virulence. It is important to remember that the most likely sources of pathogens in these patients are the personnel caring for them.[4,21-23] Patients with preexisting bacteremia have an increased incidence of positive cultures from catheter tips. The loosely organized clot that quickly forms around the intravascular segment of the plastic catheter may serve as a trap for circulating microorganisms. However, microorganisms from anatomically distant sites of infection such as tracheostomy, the urinary tract, or surgical wounds may become established on the cannula tip in the absence of recognized bacteremia.[4]

Motion of Catheter

To-and-fro motion of the catheter after insertion may facilitate entry of cutaneous microorganisms into the catheter wound and encourage the development of phlebitis by traumatizing the vein.[4]

Phlebitis

The presence of phlebitis at the insertion site greatly increases the incidence of infection.[25] Phlebitis occurs more commonly when veins of the lower extremity are used. In addition, the type and size of the cannulating device influence the incidence of phlebitis. There is a tenfold greater incidence of phlebitis with the use of plastic catheters as opposed to steel needles.[2,7] Shorter catheters in peripheral veins seem to produce more phlebitis than longer central venous catheters.[26] A catheter of large diameter may inflict greater irritation to the vessel wall than does a narrow-diameter catheter. The incidence of phlebitis is increased by the duration of cannulation and by the infusion of hypertonic fluids or various drugs. Although there is a 12-fold increase in the incidence of infection in the presence of phlebitis, bacteremia can occur in the absence of phlebitis.[3,14]

Type of Fluid Infused

Klebsiella, Enterobacter, Serratia, and *Pseudomonas cepacia* show rapid growth within 24 hours in 5% dextrose in water.[27] Minute quantities of blood added to glucose-containing solutions buffer the fluid significantly and provide organic nutrients for more fastidious microorganisms incapable of growth in unaltered fluid. Blood products may also be a source of introduced microorganisms incapable of growth in unaltered fluid, which are often Klebsiella. Hypertonic glucose solutions support the growth of Candida; sepsis due to this microorganism is a common complication of hyperalimentation.[3] Lipid emulsions support rapid growth of a variety of microorganisms.[28] Most contamination of infusion fluid is probably extrinsic, excluding isolated outbreaks caused by intrinsic contamination at time of manufacture. Since the infusion fluid can be contaminated at the time that agents are added before administration, a significant potential hazard exists and a rigid aseptic protocol is required during preparation of these infusions.[4,27]

Reported rates of in-use contamination of infusion fluids have ranged from 3 to 38%. Microorganisms are probably introduced most frequently during manipulation of infusion apparatus by personnel or patients. The presence of Klebsiella has been demonstrated frequently on the hands of both hospital personnel and patients. The rate of fluid contamination is directly proportional to the duration of infusion therapy, and microorganisms capable of growth in IV fluid can persist for days in delivery tubing despite serial replacements of the bottle.[23,27-29]

Manipulation of the Delivery System

Manipulation of any component within the IV delivery system may result in contamination. This includes addition of medications to the bottle, injection of medications into the tubing, administration of blood products, irrigation of an occluded cannula or catheter, manipulation to reposition a pulmonary artery catheter, and the use of the IV system to obtain blood samples.[3,4,20,30]

Presence of Monitoring Devices Within the Infusion System

Transducers for monitoring pressure are a potential source of bacteremia, especially when reusable domes are employed. Contamination of reusable domes can occur with blood from an infected patient, from contaminated detergent or flushing solution, or from inadequate sterilization procedures.[31-35] The interiors of disposable domes can become contaminated, presumably from bacteria on the diaphragm of the transducer, which gain access to the fluid within the domes. Donowitz, et al.,[35] have shown that as the disposable dome is screwed onto the transducer head, the fluid used as the coupling medium between the dome and the transducer runs out and into the hands of the individual assembling the unit. If the coupling fluid is contaminated with bacteria from the transducer head, the microorganisms may be transferred to the stopcocks and open ports as these are manipulated, introducing the bacteria into the fluid-filled system. Failure to sterilize the heads of the transducers, leaving them moist between use, and using dextrose and water as the contact medium between the heads and the disposable domes favors growth of microorganisms. Dextrose and water, sometimes also used as the flushing solution, supports growth of any microorganisms that might gain access to the fluid within the domes.[33]

Three-way stopcocks within the infusion system frequently have been shown to be contaminated with microorganisms. These microorganisms may come from the hands of personnel during frequent manipulations of the stopcocks, from the syringe that is used either to flush or to draw blood specimens, from residual blood that may remain in the extra port where it may serve as a breeding ground for bacteria, and from failure either to treat the stopcock with strict aseptic techniques or to keep a sterile cap on the stopcock when not in use.[35-38] Calibrated plastic chambers that permit the administration of fluid in precise volume and require frequent manipulation, both to fill and to add medications, are another potential source of contamination.[39]

Reuse of Catheters

Endotoxic reactions without bacteremia can occur if intravascular catheters are sterilized and reused. The detergicide used to flush the catheters may fail to eliminate all contaminants. Following final sterilization, which kills the organisms, high levels of residual endotoxin may persist. Even though endotoxin may not be present on the interior of the catheters, it may be evidenced on the outer surfaces, thus predisposing the patient to fever, chills, and hypotension when these catheters are inserted into the vascular space.[40]

Measures to Deal with Catheter- and Infusion-Related Infections[41,42]

Is the Invasive Device Necessary?

Since catheter-infusion-related sepsis can be eliminated altogether by not using these invasive devices, one must always ascertain the need for them. Then the need must be reevaluated daily and the device removed as soon as it is no longer required.

Choice of a Cannula

Scalp vein needles produce lower rates of infection; however, plastic catheters provide a more secure avenue in the critically ill patient. Intravenous cannulation of the lower extremities should be avoided because of the higher incidence of associated complications.

Cannula Insertion

Hands should be thoroughly washed and care taken not to touch the needle or the skin when inserting the intravascular cannula. For optimal asepsis, the procedure should be conducted as a minor surgical procedure: The operator should wear sterile gloves, hair cover, and mask; and the area of catheter insertion should be surrounded with sterile drapes.

Cannulas that are inserted in an emergency without proper asepsis must be replaced at the earliest opportunity.

The site chosen for cannula placement must be prepared with an effective antiseptic and properly shaved as indicated. For placement of a peripheral line, tincture of iodine (2% iodine and 70% alcohol) should be liberally applied, allowed to dry for at least 30 seconds, then washed off with 70% alcohol. Both of these agents should be applied with friction, working from the center of the field to the periphery. An iodophor (povidone–iodine) may be substituted but must not be washed off with alcohol. Prior to the insertion of lines into central veins or into areas that have a greater potential for contamination, such as the groin, the skin should be scrubbed for 2–4 minutes with an iodophor. In the rare case that iodine preparations cannot be tolerated for placement of the peripheral line, vigorous prolonged washing (at least 1 minute) with 70% alcohol is acceptable. However, this may not be adequate for placement of central lines.

Cannula Care

After venous or arterial catheterization is established, the cannula should be securely anchored to prevent irritating to-and-fro motion and to avoid transport of cutaneous bacteria into the puncture wound. A topical antiseptic, such as povidone–iodine, that does not favor the selective growth of resistant bacteria and Candida should be applied to the puncture site.

All venous, arterial, and pulmonary arterial catheters and their insertion sheaths should be removed after 72 hours. (Central venous lines used only for hyperalimentation may be left in place for a longer time, as long as there are no signs of local or systemic infection.) The insertion site should be inspected at least every 48 hours with aseptic technique, the dressing should be changed, and a topical antiseptic ointment should be reapplied. If signs of inflammation, phlebitis, or purulent infection are detected, the catheter must be removed immediately. Central venous catheters and insertion sheaths (such as for pulmonary artery catheters) can be exchanged over a guidewire[43-45] if no other site for vascular access is available and there is no evidence of local or systemic catheter-related sepsis. Introducers should not be left in place for this purpose. However, it is imperative that the tip of the removed catheter or sheath be cultured quantitatively (see below); and if the culture is positive, the new catheter or sheath must be removed and a different site cannulated.

Prevention of Contamination and Care of the Delivery System

Intravenous fluid containers should be examined before use and discarded if turbidity or precipitate is detected. Glass bottles should be inspected, since fungal and bacterial contamination can occur through a crack so small that fluid does not leak. Bottles lacking a vacuum when opened should not be used, and plastic bags should be gently squeezed to detect punctures. Every container should be clearly labelled with the patient's name, added medications, and time of opening.

Intravenous fluids should be used as soon as possible after opening, and no bottle or bag should be left in place for more than 24 hours. Infusions of lipid emulsions should be completed within 12 hours. Administration sets should be changed every 24 hours, or at the very minimum, every 48 hours.[46,47] The bottles and tubing should also be changed when cannulas are replaced and after administration of blood products or lipid emulsions. Although a 0.45-μ filter will block the passage of all fungi and bacteria except for some types of pseudomonas and aberrant bacteria, a 0.22-μ filter will block all bacteria; a pump is often necessary, however, to ensure adequate flow. Care should be taken to avoid contaminating the system when inserting and manipulating filters, but there are no controlled clinical trials to verify the effectiveness of filters in reducing infection.[48]

Measures to Prevent Transducer-Related Infection

All hospital personnel must recognize that transducers may be a potential source of nosocomial infection. Since reusable transducers and domes must be cleaned with soap and water, rinsed, and then sterilized with ethylene oxide gas or glutaraldehyde between use, there always exists a potential for improper cleaning and contamination. It is recommended that disposable rather than reusable domes be used and that the disposable ones not be resterilized and reused.

To ensure that transducers remain sterile while being calibrated and set up for use, only experienced personnel who are trained in aseptic technique should be given these responsibilities. A simple arrangement of tubing and stopcocks should be used in the monitoring system, and as many components of the system as possible should be disposable and presterilized. Use only sterile manometers to calibrate sterile transducers.

Because transducers may become contaminated during in-use manipulation, the need for aseptic technique when handling monitoring systems should be stressed to hospital personnel. The system should not be opened for blood drawing, administration of medications, or other procedures, and blood should not be allowed to back up or reflux into transducers. When unavoidable, blood samples can be drawn through a stopcock placed near the intravascular catheter, but tubing should never be disconnected for blood drawing. Stopcocks should be treated as a sterile field to be covered with a sterile cap or syringe when not in use, and they should be manipulated only after a thorough washing of hands. Blood should not be allowed to remain in the stopcock port.[31,38]

Use of a sterile heparinized solution administered by a continuous flush valve may help maintain catheter patency and reduce the need for the potentially contaminating manipulations engendered by a clotted catheter tip. Because of potential contamination, monitoring systems should not be filled from multidose vials of heparin. Solutions containing glucose, which is an excellent culture medium for any contaminant, should not be used for flushing.

Routine replacement of transducers, manifolds, connecting tubing, and fluids for flushing the system may reduce the risk of transducer-associated infections. No controlled studies have documented the effectiveness or need for this recommendation, but it is based on similar recommendations made for IV fluid therapy.[46,47] Since transducers are expensive and often in short supply, it may not always be possible to replace all components of the monitoring system every 24–48 hours.

The use of disposable chamber domes with transducers may not entirely eliminate the infection hazard.[31,32] If the permanent transducer heads are not cleaned with disinfecting solution such as glutaraldehyde, organisms can grow on the transducer head and may be transferred from the site to fluid within the disposable domes from the operator's hands, with subsequent contamination of intravascular pressure monitoring lines. The permanent transducer head diaphragms should be disinfected before use, and glucose-containing solutions should not be used as the coupling medium between the disposable dome and the transducer diaphragm.

Management of Suspected Infusion-Associated Sepsis

Many infections occur without any local inflammation. If fever of obscure origin develops in any patient with a venous or arterial catheter in place, blood cultures must be obtained from at least two independent venipunctures. Furthermore, the infusion fluid system, including the transducer and tubing administration sets, the container, and the catheter (or catheters) must be immediately discontinued. After the skin of the catheter site is cleansed with an effective antiseptic, the catheter should be aseptically removed. For short catheters, the entire length, beginning several millimeters inside the former skin surface–catheter interface should be amputated using sterile scissors. With long catheters, two 5-cm segments should be cut — the proximal one inside the former skin–catheter interface, the other being the catheter tip. Each segment should be placed in a separate, appropriately labelled sterile container. A semiquantitative assessment of catheter contamination can be obtained by rolling the amputated segment across a blood agar plate.[48] Any pus from the insertion site should be Gram's stained and cultured. When bacteremia related to contaminated fluid is suspected, fluid should be aseptically withdrawn from the IV line and cultured.

The single most important therapeutic step for the patient with infusion-associated sepsis is discontinuation of the catheter and the infusion system. Catheter removal alone may result in dramatic clinical improvement. Empiric antimicrobial therapy should be administered to presumably septic, critically ill patients pending culture and antimicrobial susceptibility results. Therapy should include administration of agents with activity against both penicillinase-producing staphylococci and multiple drug-resistant gram-negative bacilli. If suppurative thrombophlebitis is suspected, the site of the venipuncture must be explored and the involved vein excised.[24]

The possibility of transducer-related infection should be considered in any monitored patient with bacteremia or fungemia of unknown or undetermined origin. Suspicion should be heightened when infection is poorly responsive to appropriate antimicrobial therapy as long as the transducer is in place but resolves after the monitoring equipment is removed. When monitor-related infections are suspected, potential common sources of contamination such as IV fluids or medications should be tested, suspected monitoring devices should be cultured, monitoring practices and sterilization procedures should be reviewed, and environmental or patient culture specimens should be obtained as indicated by clinical epidemiologic findings.[30-32,36,38,50]

References

1. Dixon RE: Effect of infections on hospital care. Ann Intern Med 89:749-753, 1978.
2. Stamm WE: Infections related to medical devices. Ann Intern Med 89:764-769, 1978.
3. Maki DG: Nosocomial Bacteremia. An Epidemiologic Overview. Amer J Med 70:719-732, 1981.
4. Maki DG, Goldman DA, Rhame FS: Infection control in intravenous therapy. Ann Intern Med 79:867-887, 1973.
5. Ryan JA, Abel RM, Abbott WM, et al: Catheter complications in total parenteral nutrition: A prospective study of 200 consecutive patients. N Engl J Med 290:757-761, 1974.
6. Band JD, Alvarado CJ, Maki DG: A semiquantitative culture technique for identifying infection due to steel needles used for intravenous therapy. Am J Clin Pathol 72:980-984, 1979.
7. Tully JL, Friedland GH, Baldini LM, Goldman DA: Complications of intravenous therapy with steel needles and teflon catheters. Am J Med 70:702-706, 1981.
8. Bozzetti F, Terno G, Camerini E, Baticci F, Scarpa D, Pupa A: Pathogenesis and predictability of central venous catheter sepsis. Surgery 91:383-389, 1982.
9. Thomas F, Burke JP, Parker J, Orme JF, Gardner RM, Clemmer TP, Hill GA, MacFarlane P: The risk of infection related to radial vs. femoral sites for arterial catheterization. Crit Care Med 11:807-812, 1983.
10. Singh S, Nelson N, Acosta I, Check F, Puri VK: Catheter colonization and bacteremia with pulmonary and arterial catheters. Crit Care Med 10:736-739, 1982.
11. Pinilla JC, Ross DF, Martin T, Crump H: Study of the incidence of intravascular catheter infection and associated septicemia in critically ill patients. Crit Care Med 11:21-25, 1983.
12. Ersoz CJ, Hedden M, Lain L: Prolonged femoral arterial catheterization for intensive care. Anesth Analg 49:160, 1970.
13. Moran JM, Atwood RP, Rowe MI: A clinical and bacteriologic study of infections associated with venous cutdowns. N Engl J Med 272:554-559, 1965
14. Band JD, Maki DG: Infections caused by arterial catheters used for hemodynamic monitoring. Am J Med 67:735-741, 1979.
15. Samsoondar W, Freeman JB, Coultish I, Oxley C: Colonization of Intravascular Catheters in the Intensive Care Unit. Am J Surg 149:730-732, 1985.
16. Kaye W, Wheaton M, Potter-Bynoe G: Radial and pulmonary artery catheter-related sepsis, abstracted. Crit Care Med 11:249, 1983.
17. Damen J, Bosten D: A prospective analysis of 1400 pulmonary artery catheterizations in patients undergoing cardiac surgery. Acta Anaesthesiol Scand 30:386-392, 1986.
18. Freeman R, King B: Analysis of results of catheter tip cultures in open-heart surgery patients. Thorax 30:26-30, 1975.
19. Applefeld JJ, Caruthers TE, Reno DJ, et al: Assessment of the sterility of long-term cardiac catheterization using the thermodilution Swan-Ganz catheter. Chest 74:377-380, 1978.
20. Prachar H, Dittel M, Jobst CH, et al: Bacterial contamination of pulmonary artery catheters. Intensive Care Med 4:79-82, 1978.
21. Maki DG: Control of colonization and transmission of pathogenic bacteria in the hospital. Ann Intern Med 89:777-780,1978.
22. Schimpff SC, Miller RM, Polakavetz S, et al: Infection in the severely traumatized patient. Ann Surg 179:352-357, 1974.
23. Steere AC, Mallison GF: Handwashing practices for the prevention of nosocomial infections. Ann Intern Med 83:683-690, 1975.
24. Maki DG, Band JD: A comparative study of polyantibiotic and iodophor ointments in prevention of vascular catheter-related infection. Am J Med 70:739-744, 1981.
25. Stein JM, Pruitt BA Jr: Suppurative thrombophlebitis. A lethal iatrogenic disease. N Engl J Med 282:1452-1455, 1970.

26. Giuffrida DJ, Bryan-Brown CW, Lumb PD, et al: Central vs. Peripheral Venous Catheters in Critically Ill Patients. *Chest* 90(6):806-809, 1986.
27. Maki DG, Martin WT: Nationwide epidemic of septicemia caused by contaminated infusion products. IV: Growth of microbial pathogens in fluids for intravenous infusions. *J Infect Dis* 131:267-272, 1975.
28. Melly MA, Meng HC, Schaffner W: Microbial growth in lipid emulsions used in parenteral nutrition. *Arch Surg* 110:1479-81, 1975.
29. Maki DG, Hassemer CA: Endemic rate of fluid contamination and related septicemia in arterial pressure monitoring. *Amer J Med* 70:733-738, 1981.
30. Gibilisco PA, Lopez GA, Appleman MD, et al: In Vitro Contamination of "Piggyback/Heparin Lock" Assemblies: Prevention of Contamination with a Closed, Positive Locking Device (Click-Lock). *JPEN* 10(4):431-434, 1986.
31. Weinstein RA, Stamm WE, Kramer L, et al: Pressure monitoring devices. Overlooked source of nosocomial infection. *JAMA* 236:936-938, 1976.
32. Weinstein RA, Emori TG, Anderson RL, et al: Pressure transducers as a source of bacteremia after open heart surgery. *Chest* 69:338-344, 1976.
33. Buxton AE, Anderson RL, Klimek J, et al: Failure of disposable domes to prevent septicemia acquired from contaminated pressure transducers. *Chest* 74:508-513, 1978.
34. Maki DG, Band JD: Septicemia from disposable pressure-monitoring chamber domes. "Beware of Greeks Bearing Gifts," editorial *Chest* 74:486-487, 1978.
35. Donowitz LG, Marsik FJ, Howyt JW, et al: Serratia Marcescens bacteremia from contaminated pressure transducers. *JAMA* 242:1749-1751, 1979.
36. Walrath JM, Abbott NK, Caplan E, et al: Stopcock: Bacterial contamination in invasive monitoring systems. *Heart Lung* 8:100-104, 1979.
37. Dryden GE, Briekler J: Stopcock contamination. *Anesth Analg* 58:141-142, 1979.
38. Stamm WE, Colella JJ, Anderson RL, et al: Indwelling arterial catheters as a source of nosocomial bacteremia. An outbreak caused by Flavobacterium species. *N Engl J Med* 292:1099-1102, 1975.
39. Duma RJ, Warner JF, Dalton HP: Septicemia from intravenous infusions. *N Engl J Med* 284:257-160, 1971.
40. Endotoxic reactions associated with the reuse of cardiac catheters. *Morbidity Mortality Weekly Rep* 28:25-27, 1979.
41. Goldman DA, Maki DG, Rhame FS, et al: Guidelines for infection control in intravenous therapy. *Ann Intern Med* 79:848-850, 1973.
42. Simmons BP: Guidelines for prevention of intravascular infections: Guideline for prevention of intravenous therapy-related infections; Guideline for prevention of infections related to intravascular pressure monitoring systems. *Hospital Inf Control* 9:28J-28T, 1982.
43. Ruggiero RP, Aisenstein TJ: Central Catheter Exchange — Indications and Technique. *Nutr Support Services* 1(5):16-18, 1981.
44. Bozzetti F, Terno G, Bonfati G, et al: Prevention and Treatment of Central Venous Catheter Sepsis by Exchange via a Guidewire. *Ann Surg* 198:48-52, 1983.
45. Gregory JA, Schiller WR: Subclavian Catheter Changes Every Third Day in High Risk Patients. *Am Surgeon* 51:534:536, 1985.
46. Buxton AE, Highsmith AK, Garner JA, et al: Contamination of intravenous infusion fluid: Effects of changing administration sets. *Ann Intern Med* 90:764-768, 1979.
47. Band JD, Maki DG: Safety of changing intravenous delivery systems at longer than 24 hour intervals. *Ann Intern Med* 91:173-178, 1979.
48. Control of infections from intravenous infusions. *Med Lett Drugs Ther* 15:105-107, 1973.
49. Maki DG, Weise CE, Sarafin HW: A semiquantitative culture method for identifying intravenous-catheter-related infarction. *N Engl J Med* 296:1305-1309, 1977.
50. Center for Disease Control: National nosocomial infections study. Annual Summary, 1974. Atlanta, US Center for Disease Control, issued March 1977.

Intravenous Techniques

Chapter 11

Intravenous (IV) cannulation is a means to gain direct access to the venous circulation, either peripheral or central. There are several indications for IV cannulation:

1. To administer drugs and fluids.
2. To obtain specimens of venous blood for laboratory determinations.
3. To insert catheters into the central circulation, including the right heart and pulmonary artery, for physiological monitoring and electrical pacing.

An essential part of advanced life support is proficiency in gaining direct access to the venous circulation, as early as possible, to establish an IV lifeline to administer essential drugs and fluids and assure their immediate uptake and distribution.[1]

Many drugs can be administered by the intramuscular or subcutaneous route, however, absorption of the drug from the tissues into the capillary blood perfusing the tissue is dependent upon blood flow. In low cardiac output states, blood is shunted away from skin and muscle, which markedly impairs uptake and distribution of the drug. If the drug is administered IV, access to the circulation is assured.

Intramuscular injections cause a release of creatine phosphokinase (CPK) from the local area of muscle into the circulation and may thereby alter the diagnostic capability of using the serum activity of that enzyme to detect myocardial necrosis.[2,3]

The following discussion is concerned with percutaneous IV techniques that do not require a cutdown:

1. Peripheral venipuncture
   a. Arm vein
   b. Leg vein
   c. External jugular vein
2. Central venipuncture
   a. Femoral vein
   b. Internal jugular vein
   c. Subclavian vein

After a brief description of various available needles, cannulas, and catheters, and a discussion of general principles of IV therapy, the specific anatomy, indications, performance criteria, and complications for each of the techniques will be detailed.

Intravenous Cannulas

There are essentially three types of cannulas: 1) hollow needles (including those attached to a syringe and the butterfly type), 2) indwelling plastic catheters inserted over a hollow needle, and 3) indwelling plastic catheters inserted either through a hollow needle or over a guidewire which is previously introduced through a needle.

Plastic catheters, rather than hollow needles, should be used for emergency IV therapy since they can be better anchored and permit freer movement of the patient. In patients who need volume expansion, the catheter should be the largest gauge possible. The flow rate through a 14-gauge catheter of 5 cm length averages approximately 125 mL/min; this may be twice the flow through a 16-gauge catheter 20 cm long, and three times the flow through a 20-gauge catheter 3 cm long[4].

The length of the needle and catheter depends on the site of insertion. For cannulation of a peripheral vein, a needle and catheter length of 5 cm is adequate. If a central vein such as the internal jugular or the subclavian is to be cannulated, a needle length of at least 6 or 7 cm is required since the vein may lie up to 5 cm from the point of entry of the needle. The necessary catheter length can be determined by measuring from the point of insertion to the appropriate location on the anterior chest which coincides with the desired position of the tip in the central circulation. For an internal jugular or subclavian insertion, a catheter should be at least 15–20 cm long (see Figure 16).

If a catheter-over-needle-device is used (Figure 1), the venipuncture is made and the catheter is introduced into the vein as the needle is removed. The end of the IV tubing is then connected directly to the end of the plastic catheter. The length of the catheter is limited by the length of the needle required, but the puncture in the vein is exactly the size of the external plastic catheter, which reduces the possibility of blood leaking around the venipuncture site.

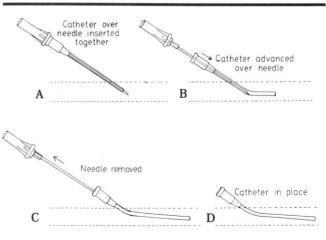

Figure 1. Insertion of catheter over needle.

If a catheter-inside-needle unit is used (Figure 2), the catheter is pushed into the vein through the needle after venipuncture; the needle is retracted to the external end of the catheter (where it remains), and the IV tubing is attached to it. Great caution must be exercised that the catheter is not retracted through the needle, since the sharp tip of the needle may shear off the end of the catheter and produce a catheter-fragment embolus.

A third alternative is to use a guidewire (Seldinger technique)[5] (Figure 3). This is a valuable technique when used properly but can lead to perforation of a major vessel even when done by an experienced individual. Individuals who are not extensively trained in the proper use of a guidewire should not use one. The guidewire must be several centimeters longer than the catheter to be placed, and the diameter of the wire must be small enough to allow it to pass through both the needle and the catheter. At all times during insertion of a catheter over a guidewire, the end of the guidewire must extend beyond the end of the catheter that remains outside the patient; this prevents the wire from sliding all the way into

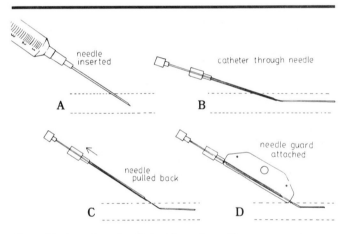

Figure 2.   Insertion of catheter through needle.

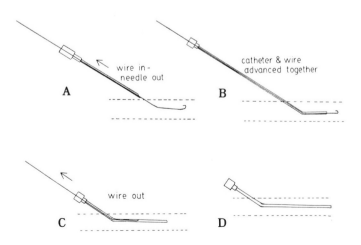

Figure 3. Insertion of catheter over guidewire (Seldinger technique).

the catheter and being lost within the circulation. The tip of the guidewire must be flexible; a J-tip facilitates passage of the wire through the tortuous vessels. After the venipuncture is made with the needle, the flexible-tipped or J-tipped guidewire is inserted through the needle. If the guidewire does not pass easily into the vein, it should be removed, a syringe reattached to the needle, and the needle advanced or withdrawn until it is within the lumen of the vein. Once the guidewire is successfully placed through the needle into the vein, the needle is removed and the catheter is inserted over the guidewire. When the catheter is in place, the guidewire is removed and the infusion tubing is connected to the catheter. The use of a guidewire eliminates the hazard of a catheter-fragment embolus, it allows the wire to be withdrawn if it does not pass into the vein easily, and it permits repositioning of the needle within the vein without having to remove the needle altogether.

A guidewire may also be employed with a catheter-over-needle device. Once the needle is in the vein, the guidewire is inserted through the needle. The outer catheter is then passed over the wire into the vein, and the needle and wire are removed.

A guidewire may be used to introduce a dilator and sheath for insertion of an intracardiac catheter. Once the guidewire is in the vein, the needle is removed. After making a small incision in the skin at the insertion site, the dilator and sheath are passed over the wire into the vein. The dilator and guidewire are then removed, leaving the sheath in place. The size of the sheath is determined by the size of the catheter to be introduced.

General Principles of IV Therapy

Principles Common to All IV Techniques[1]

Cannulation of either a peripheral or a central vein is preferable to intracardiac injection during CPR. If an internal jugular or subclavian central venous line is in place at the time of the arrest, then it should be used for drug administration. If no vein has been cannulated prior to the arrest, cannulation of an antecubital vein should be the site of first choice since CPR may have to be interrupted if either jugular or subclavian veins are chosen.

If circulation is not rapidly restored after initial drug administration via a peripheral line, a central line should be placed, with minimum interruption of CPR, by an experienced operator. In the intubated patient the internal jugular site should require less interruption of external chest compression during placement than the subclavian route. The central circulation can be entered from the external jugular with the use of a J-wire. However, external jugular venous cannulation requires interruption of ventilation during cannulation unless an endotracheal tube is in place. The increased risk of complications reported to be associated with the placement of central lines should be noted, especially for patients receiving thrombolytic therapy. In addition, it constitutes a relatively strong contraindication to the initiation of thrombolytic therapy.

Distal wrist and hand veins and distal saphenous veins in the legs are the least favorable sites for drug administration during cardiac arrest since blood flow from the distal extremities is markedly diminished. Femoral veins are best avoided unless a long catheter can be passed above the diaphragm.

In an emergency situation where speed is essential, especially outside the hospital, strict aseptic technique may be impossible. After the patient becomes stabilized, the cannula must be removed and replaced under sterile conditions.

If the patient is awake, it is preferable that the overlying skin be anesthetized, using 1% lidocaine without epinephrine, prior to inserting a large-bore cannula. In addition, a scalpel or the sharp tip of a smaller needle (such as 18-gauge) can be used to make a small skin incision through which the larger cannula will pass more easily.

After the catheter is inserted, sterile infusion tubing with injection sites near the tip of the tubing is attached. The other end of the tubing is connected to a container of sterile 5% dextrose in water. Ideally, this container should be a plastic bottle or bag, either of which is nonbreakable and easily carried on the litter with the patient. In fact, if a plastic bag is used, it can be placed under the patient's shoulders during transportation, and the weight of the patient will keep the infusion going at the preset rate. The plastic bag should be squeezed before use to detect any punctures that may lead to contamination of the contents; no drug should be added to the solution that may be absorbed by the plastic.[6] To keep the IV line open, the rate of infusion should be set at 10 mL/hr.

Complications Common to All IV Techniques

All techniques share the following complication risks. Where specific complications occur with any one technique, those conditions will be listed with the description of that technique. Local complications include hematoma formation, cellulitis, thrombosis, and phlebitis. Systemic complications include sepsis, pulmonary thromboembolism, air embolism, and catheter-fragment embolism.

Peripheral Veins

The most common areas used for IV therapy are in the hands and arms. Favored sites are the dorsum of the hands, the wrists, and the antecubital fossae. Preferred locations for IV therapy in the legs are the long saphenous veins. However, as described above, of these

peripheral veins, only the antecubital veins should be used for drug administration during CPR.[1]

Anatomy: Upper Extremities[7,8]
(Figure 4)

On the dorsum of the hand, a series of veins arise from the digital veins which run parallel to the long axis of the hand, interconnected by a series of arches which form the dorsal plexus. At the radial side of the dorsal plexus, a thick vein, the superficial radial vein, runs laterally up to the antecubital fossa and joins the median cephalic vein to form the cephalic vein. Other superficial veins on the ulnar aspect of the forearm run to the elbow and join the median basilic vein to form the basilic vein. The median vein of the forearm bifurcates into a Y in the antecubital fossa, laterally becoming the median cephalic, and medially becoming the median basilic.

The basilic vein passes up the inner side of the arm, becoming deep at the lower third of the arm. As it continues cephalad, it joins the brachial vein to become the axillary vein. The cephalic vein continues laterally up the arm, crosses anteriorly, and becomes deep in the interval between the pectoralis major and the deltoid muscles; after a sharp angulation, it joins the axillary vein at a 90° angle, an anatomic detail which makes the cephalic vein unsuitable for insertion of central venous or pulmonary artery catheters.

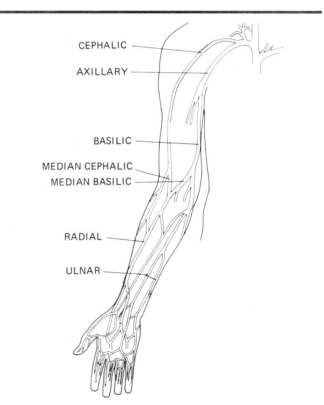

Figure 4. Anatomy of veins of upper extremity.

Anatomy: Lower Extremities[7,8]
(Figure 5)

The long saphenous vein begins on the inner side of the foot, receiving branches from the dorsal venous arch of the foot. It travels upward in front of the medial malleolus of the tibia to the groove between the upper medial end of the tibia and the calf muscle, and passes backward behind the internal condyle of the femur. It then runs somewhat outward and upward on the inner side of the front of the thigh to 1½ in. (3.8 cm) below the inguinal ligament, where it pierces the saphenous opening to end in the femoral vein.

Anatomy: External Jugular Vein[7,8]
(Figure 6)

The external jugular vein is formed below the ear and behind the angle of the mandible where a branch of the posterior facial vein joins the posterior auricular vein. The external jugular vein then passes downward and obliquely backward across the surface of the sterno-mastoid muscle, pierces the deep fascia of the neck just above the middle of the clavicle, to end in the subclavian vein lateral to the anterior scalene muscle. There are valves and other veins entering the external jugular vein at the entrance to the subclavian vein. There are also valves in the external jugular vein about 4 cm above the clavicle.

Technique: Arm or Leg Vein

Since the largest of the superficial veins of the arm are in the antecubital fossa, these should be selected initially if the patient is in circulatory collapse or cardiac arrest (Figure 7). In the stable patient, however, if accessible, the more distal veins of the arm may be selected first (Figure 8). Similarly, the long saphenous vein at the medial malleolus may be utilized first, but can be entered at any point along its course. Generally, a point between the junction of two veins is chosen for entry, since here the vein is more stabilized and venipuncture is more easily accomplished. The steps for initiating IV therapy of the arm or leg vein follow:

1. Apply tourniquet proximally.
2. Locate vein and cleanse the overlying skin with alcohol or povidone–iodine.
3. Anesthetize the skin if a large-bore cannula is to be inserted in an awake patient.
4. Hold vein in place by applying pressure on vein distal to the point of entry.
5. Puncture the skin with bevel of needle upward about 0.5–1.0 cm from the vein; enter the vein either from the side or from above.
6. Note blood return and advance the catheter either over or through the needle, depending on the type of catheter–needle device being employed. Remove tourniquet.

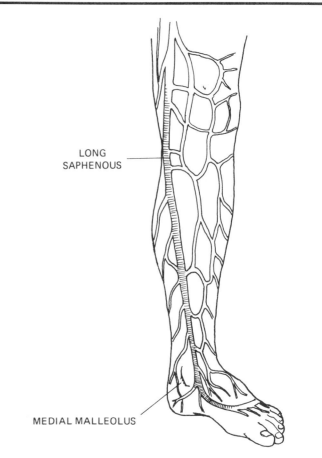

Figure 5. Anatomy of long saphenous vein of leg.

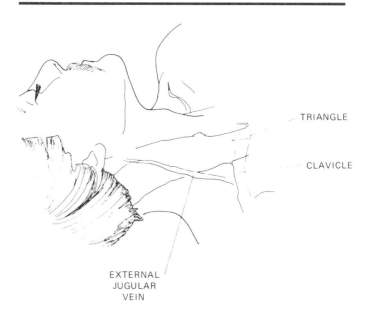

Figure 6. Anatomy of external jugular vein.

7. Withdraw and remove the needle and attach the infusion tubing.
8. Cover the puncture site with povidone–iodine ointment and a sterile dressing. Tape dressing in place.

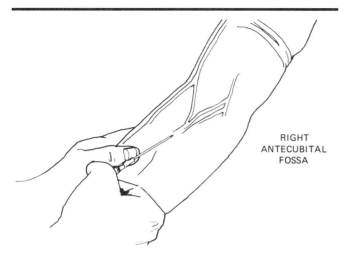

Figure 7.   Antecubital venipuncture.

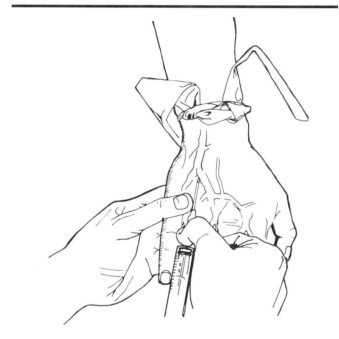

Figure 8.   Venipuncture of dorsal hand vein.

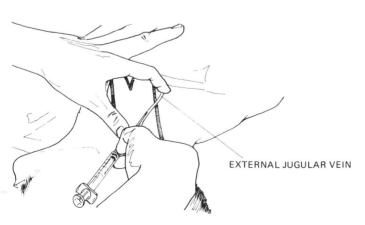

Figure 9.   External jugular venipuncture.

Technique: External Jugular Vein[9]
(Figure 9)

The steps for initiating IV therapy of the external jugular vein follow:

1. Place the patient in a supine, head-down position to fill the external jugular vein; turn the patient's head toward the opposite side.
2. Cleanse and anesthetize the skin as described previously.
3. Align the cannula in the direction of the vein with the point aimed toward the ipsilateral shoulder.
4. Make venipuncture midway between the angle of the jaw and the mid-clavicular line, "tourniqueting" the vein lightly with one finger above the clavicle.
5. Proceed as described in the section on technique for arm and leg veins.

Using Peripheral Veins for IV Therapy

Advantages

The technique is easy to master. Antecubital vein cannulation usually provides an effective route for the administration of drugs during cardiac arrest so that central cannulation or intracardiac injection may be unnecessary. If basic life support measures are underway, antecubital vein catheterization does not interfere with continuing ventilation and chest compression.

After administration of a drug during CPR, the arm should be raised and a 50-mL bolus of fluid administered to facilitate access to the central circulation. One to two minutes should be allowed for agents to reach the central circulation.

Disadvantages

In circulatory collapse, it may be difficult or impossible to establish an access from a peripheral vein. Recent studies have demonstrated a significant delay in the arrival of a drug at the heart when peripheral IV sites are used for injection during CPR, even when effective chest compression is being performed.[10,11] In addition, peak drug levels are lower when peripheral sites are used than when a drug is administered via a central vein,[10,12] and there is some delay for drugs to reach the central circulation. Hypertonic or irritating solutions should not be administered through a peripheral vein, since pain and phlebitis will result. Even if isotonic solutions are used, however, the incidence of phlebitis is still high if the long saphenous vein is used.

Femoral Vein

Anatomy[7,8]

The femoral vein lies in the femoral sheath, medial to the femoral artery immediately below the inguinal ligament. If a line is drawn between the anterior superior iliac spine and the symphysis pubis, the femoral artery runs directly across the midpoint; medial to that point is the femoral vein. If the femoral artery pulse is palpable, the artery can be located with a finger and the femoral vein will lie immediately medial to the pulsation (Figure 10). (If a pulse cannot be felt with cardiac compression, the CPR team should be informed.)

The femoral vein is formed from both the deep and superficial (saphenous) veins of the legs; it extends above the inguinal ligament as the external iliac and becomes the common iliac after being joined by the internal iliac. Both common iliacs join to become the inferior vena cava (Figure 11).

Technique

The steps for initiating IV therapy of the femoral vein follow:

1. Cleanse the overlying skin with povidone–iodine; it is especially important in this site because the danger of contamination is great. If the puncture is being performed electively, first shave the hair around the area. Drape the area.
2. Locate the femoral artery either by its pulsation or by finding the midpoint of a line drawn between the anterior superior iliac spine and the symphysis pubis.
3. Infiltrate the skin with lidocaine if the patient is awake.
4. Make the puncture with the needle attached to a 5- or 10-mL syringe two fingers' breadths below the inguinal ligament, medial to the artery, directing the needle cephalad at a 45° angle with the skin or frontal plane (some prefer to enter at a 90° angle) until the needle will go no farther (Figure 12).
5. Maintain suction on the syringe, and pull the needle back slowly until blood appears in the syringe, indicating that the lumen of the vein has been entered.
6. Lower the needle more parallel to the frontal plane, remove the syringe, and insert the catheter.

Using the Femoral Vein for IV Therapy

Advantages

As with an arm vein, if basic life support is being carried out, there is no need for interruption. The femoral vein can be entered when more peripheral veins are collapsed. Once the femoral vein is cannulated, there is easy access to the central circulation so that a long catheter can be passed above the diaphragm.[1]

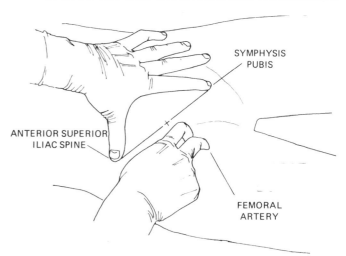

Figure 10. Femoral artery runs directly across the midpoint of line drawn between anterior superior iliac spine and symphysis pubis.

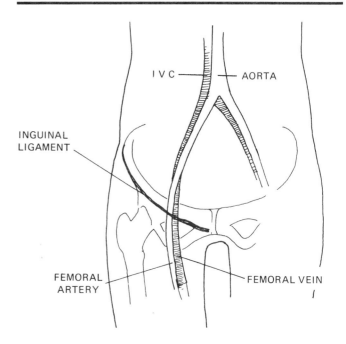

Figure 11. Anatomy of femoral vein. Femoral vein lies medial to femoral artery below inguinal ligament.

Disadvantages

Easy location of the vein depends on the presence of the femoral artery pulse; in the absence of an arterial pulse, practice is required to cannulate the femoral vein. However during CPR, the femoral vein pulsates and is easier to palpate than the femoral artery since arterial flow is low.[13] The complication rate, especially involving thrombosis and infection, may be higher than for more peripheral veins. Given the reduced blood flow to the lower extremities, when the femoral vein is cannulated, a long catheter must be advanced into the thoracic cavity.[13]

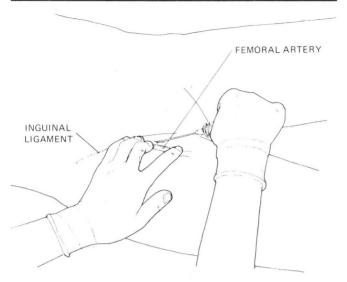

Figure 12. Femoral venipuncture.

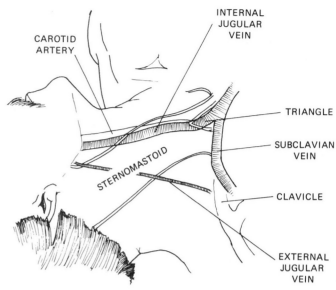

Figure 13. Anatomy of internal jugular vein.

Specific Complications

Hematoma may occur, either from the vein itself or from the adjacent femoral artery. Thrombosis and phlebitis may extend not only to involve the deep veins, but may extend proximally to the iliac veins or the inferior vena cava. When this occurs, use of the femoral vein may preclude the subsequent use of the saphenous vein.

Inadvertent cannulation of the femoral artery during cardiac arrest may not be recognized since femoral arterial pressure and oxygen tension may be so low that the aspirated blood resembles blood from the femoral vein. Infusion of a potent vasopressor such as epinephrine into the femoral artery will cause ischemic injury to the involved limb.

Internal Jugular and Subclavian Veins

Anatomy

Internal Jugular Vein[7,8,14] (Figure 13)

The internal jugular vein emerges from the base of the skull, enters the carotid sheath posterior to the internal carotid artery, and runs posteriorly and laterally to the internal and common carotid artery. Finally, near its termination, the internal jugular vein is lateral and slightly anterior to the common carotid artery.

The internal jugular vein runs medial to the sternomastoid muscle in its upper part, posterior to it in the triangle between the two inferior heads of the sternomastoid in its middle part, and behind the anterior portion of the clavicular head of the muscle in its lower part, where it ends just above the medial end of the clavicle by being joined by the subclavian vein.

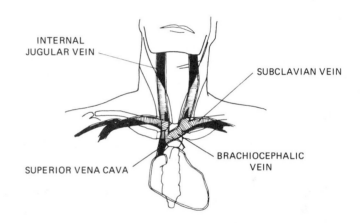

Figure 14. Anatomy of the subclavian vein.

Subclavian Vein[7,8,15] (Figure 14)

The subclavian vein, which in the adult is approximately 3–4 cm long and 1–2 cm in diameter, begins as a continuation of the axillary vein at the lateral border of the first rib, crosses over the first rib, and passes in front of the anterior scalene muscle. The anterior scalene muscle is approximately 10–15 mm thick and separates the subclavian vein from the subclavian artery which runs behind the anterior scalene muscle. The vein continues behind the medial third of the clavicle where it is immobilized by small attachments to the rib and clavicle. At the medial border of the anterior scalene muscle and behind the sterno-costoclavicular joint, the subclavian unites with the internal jugular to form the innominate, or brachiocephalic, vein. The large thoracic

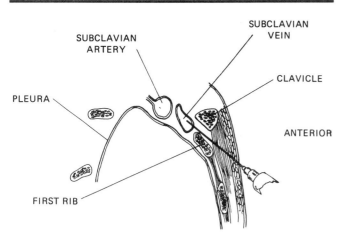

Figure 15. In sagittal section through medial third of clavicle, both apical pleura and subclavian artery can be seen immediately posterior to subclavian vein. (Adapted from Davidson, et al: *Lancet* 2:1140, 1963. Used by permission.)

duct on the left and the smaller lymphatic duct on the right enter the superior margin of the subclavian vein near the internal jugular junction. On the right, the brachiocephalic vein descends behind the right lateral edge of the manubrium, where it is joined by the left brachiocephalic vein which crosses over behind the manubrium. On the right side, near the sternal–manubrial joint, the two veins join together to form the superior vena cava. Medial to the anterior scalene muscle, the phrenic nerve, the internal mammary artery, and the apical pleura are in contact with the postero-inferior side of the subclavian vein and the jugulo-subclavian junction. In a sagittal section through the medial third of the clavicle, both the apical pleura and the subclavian artery can be seen immediately posterior to the subclavian vein[16] (Figure 15).

Indications for Internal Jugular and Subclavian Venipuncture

Since the internal jugular and subclavian veins remain patent when peripheral veins are collapsed, their cannulation allows emergency access to the venous circulation when IV therapy is urgently required. Cannulation of these veins is also used to gain access to the central circulation for measurement of central venous pressure, for administration of hypertonic or irritating solutions, and for passing catheters into the heart and pulmonary circulation.

Technique: General Principles[10-12,14-26]

The steps for initiating therapy of the internal jugular and subclavian veins follow:

1. A needle at least 6 cm long with a 16-gauge catheter at least 15–20 cm long is usually selected. If the catheter is to be inserted through the needle, the needle must be 14-gauge. If the Seldinger technique is employed, a thin wall 18-gauge needle will accept a standard guidewire.

2. Determine the depth of catheter placement by measuring from the point of insertion to the following surface markers on the chest wall (Figure 16):
   a. Sternoclavicular joint — subclavian vein.
   b. Midmanubrial area — brachiocephalic vein.
   c. Manubrial–sternal junction — superior vena cava.
   d. Five centimeters below the manubrial–sternal junction — right atrium of the heart.

3. Place the tip of the catheter above the right atrium for administration of fluids.

4. Place the patient in a supine, head-down position (Trendelenberg) of at least 15° to distend the veins and reduce the chance of air embolism. Extend the patient's head and turn it away from the side of venipuncture.

5. Cleanse the area around the site of puncture with povidone–iodine and drape as for any surgical procedure. Wear sterile gloves. Ideally, a face mask and a hair cover should be worn also.

6. If the patient is awake, infiltrate the skin with lidocaine.

7. Mount the needle on a 5- or 10-mL syringe containing 0.5–1.0 mL saline solution or lidocaine. After the skin has been punctured with the bevel of the needle upward, flush the needle to remove an occasional skin plug.

8. As the needle is slowly advanced, maintain negative pressure on the syringe. As soon as the lumen of the vein is entered, blood will appear in the syringe; advance the needle a few millimeters farther to

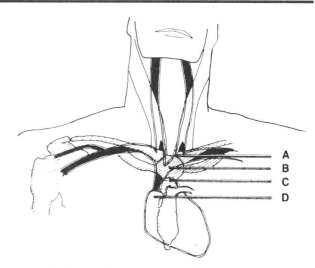

Figure 16. Surface markers on chest wall to determine depth of catheter placement: sternoclavicular joint — subclavian vein (A), midmanubrial area — brachiocephalic vein (B), manubrial-sternal junction — superior vena cava (C), and 5 cm below manubrial-sternal junction — right atrium (D).

obtain a free flow of blood. Rapid backward movement of the plunger and the appearance of bright red blood indicates that an artery has been entered. Completely remove the needle and apply pressure, if possible, to the puncture site for at least 10 minutes.

9. Occasionally, the vein will not be entered despite the fact that the needle has been inserted to the appropriate depth. Maintain negative pressure on the syringe and slowly withdraw the needle; blood may suddenly appear in the syringe, indicating that the needle is now in the lumen of the vein. If no blood appears, completely remove the needle and reinsert it, directing it at a slightly different angle depending on the site of venipuncture.

10. Remove the syringe from the needle, with the finger occluding the needle to prevent air embolism. (A 5-cm water pressure difference across a 14-gauge needle will allow the introduction of approximately 100 mL of air per second.[27]) If the patient is breathing spontaneously, remove the syringe during exhalation. If the patient is being artificially ventilated either with a bag–valve unit or with a mechanical ventilator, remove the syringe during the inspiratory (positive-pressure) cycle. Quickly insert the catheter or guidewire through the needle to a predetermined point and remove the needle.

11. If the catheter is inserted through the needle, never pull the catheter backward through the needle, as the sharp end may shear off the tip of the catheter, producing a catheter-fragment embolus.

12. It is occasionally impossible to advance the plastic catheter despite the fact that the needle tip is within the vein. Since the catheter must not be withdrawn through the needle, the needle and the catheter must be removed together and the venipuncture attempted again. The use of the flexible straight or J-tipped guidewire should eliminate this problem. Insert the guidewire through the needle into the vein, remove the guidewire, attach the syringe and, while maintaining negative pressure on the syringe, reposition the needle until it is in the vein; remove the syringe and insert the guidewire once again. If the guidewire passes freely into the vein, remove the needle and then pass the catheter over the guidewire into the vein.

13. Where feasible, affix the catheter to the skin with a suture, making certain that the catheter is not compressed by the suture.

14. Attach the IV tubing to the catheter.

15. Apply povidone–iodine ointment to the puncture site and tape the catheter in place.

Technique: Internal Jugular[14]

The right side of the neck is preferred for venipuncture for three reasons:[17]

1. The dome of the right lung and pleura is lower than the left.
2. There is more or less a straight line to the atrium.
3. The large thoracic duct is not endangered.

Three alternate approaches will be described: posterior, central, and anterior. In trained hands, each is an effective means to cannulate the internal jugular vein. The route chosen depends on the experience and the preference of the operator. In general, the central approach is the easiest to learn and to do. The following three approaches assume that the patient is in the supine, head-down (Trendelenberg) position as described above.

Posterior Approach[18,19]

The steps for initiating the posterior approach to internal jugular cannulation follow (Figure 17):

1. Introduce the needle under the sternomastoid muscle near the junction of the middle and lower thirds of the lateral (posterior) border (5 cm above the clavicle or just above the point where the external jugular vein crosses the sternomastoid muscle).
2. Aim the needle caudally and ventrally (anteriorly) toward the suprasternal notch at an angle of 45° to the sagittal and horizontal planes and with 15° forward angulation in the frontal plane.
3. The vein should be entered within 5 to 7 cm.

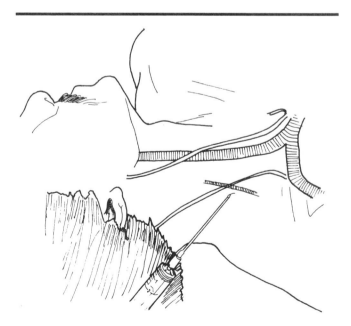

Figure 17. Posterior approach for internal jugular venipuncture.

Central Approach[21,28]

The steps for initiating the central approach to internal jugular cannulation follow (Figure 18):

1. Locate by observation and palpation the triangle formed by the two heads (sternal and clavicular) of the sternomastoid muscle and the clavicle. It may be helpful to have the awake patient lift his or her head slightly off the bed to make the triangle more visible. In some patients with large or obese necks, it may be difficult to identify the triangle. Palpate the suprasternal notch and slowly move laterally, locating first the sternal head of the sternomastoid muscle, the clavicle, the triangle itself, and finally, the clavicular head of the sternomastoid muscle.
2. Occasionally the carotid arterial pulse will be palpable within the triangle. Place two fingers along the artery and retract it medially. This maneuver identifies both the location of the artery (so that inadvertent puncture is avoided) and the position of the internal jugular vein, which is lateral to the artery.
3. Insert the needle at the apex of the triangle formed by the two heads of the sternomastoid muscle and the clavicle.
4. Direct the needle caudally and laterally, parallel to the medial border of the clavicular head of the sternomastoid muscle toward the ipsilateral nipple at a 45° to 60° angle with the frontal plane.
5. If the vein is not entered after the needle has been inserted a few centimeters, slowly withdraw the needle, maintaining a negative pressure on the syringe. If the vein is still not entered, withdraw the needle completely; reinsert it, directing it 5° to 10° more in the lateral direction. If still unable to enter the vein, direct the needle more in line with the sagittal plane. However, do not direct the needle medially (across the sagittal plane), since the carotid artery will be punctured.

Anterior Approach[22]

The steps for initiating the anterior approach to internal jugular cannulation follow (Figure 19):

1. Place the left index and middle fingers (if from the right side) on the carotid artery and retract it medially away from the anterior border of the sternomastoid muscle.
2. Introduce the needle between the index and middle fingers at the midpoint of this anterior border (5 cm above the clavicle and 5 cm below the angle of the mandible).
3. Forming a posterior angle of 30° to 45° with the frontal plane, direct the needle caudally toward the ipsilateral nipple and toward the junction of the middle and medial thirds of the clavicle.

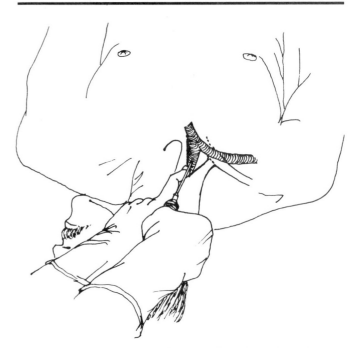

Figure 18. Central approach for internal jugular venipuncture.

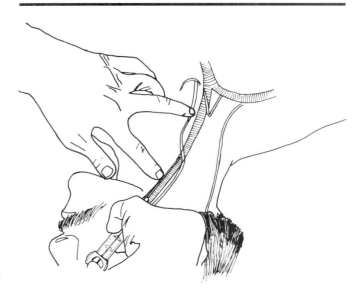

Figure 19. Anterior approach for internal jugular venipuncture.

Technique: Subclavian Vein

Two approaches for cannulation of the subclavian vein will be described: the direct infraclavicular subclavian puncture, and indirect cannulation of the subclavian vein via the external jugular vein with a guidewire.

Infraclavicular Subclavian Approach[15]

The steps for initiating the direct infraclavicular subclavian puncture follow (Figure 20):

1. The patient must be in a supine, head-down position of at least 15°.
2. Introduce the needle 1 cm below the junction of the middle and medial thirds of the clavicle.
3. Hold the syringe and needle parallel to the front plane (the plane of the back of the patient).
4. Direct the needle medially and slightly cephalad, behind the clavicle toward the posterior–superior aspect of the sternal end of the clavicle.
5. Establish a good point of reference by firmly pressing the fingertip into the suprasternal notch to locate the deep side of the superior aspect of the clavicle, and direct the course of the needle slightly behind the fingertip.
6. Once the lumen of the vein has been entered, rotate the bevel of the needle caudally and clockwise 90°, thus facilitating the downward turn that the catheter must negotiate into the brachiocephalic vein.

Cannulation of Subclavian Vein via the External Jugular Vein With a J-Wire[29]

The steps for initiating indirect cannulation of the subclavian vein by way of the external jugular vein with a guidewire follow:

1. Prepare the patient and make the venipuncture into the external jugular vein as described previously. Use a needle through which the J-wire will pass.
2. Insert a flexible J-tipped wire that fits through both the needle and the catheter (this should be tested before the venipuncture is done) and advance the J-wire into the external jugular and subclavian veins. Gentle manipulation may be necessary to pass the device through venous valves and tortuous vessels. At no time should the wire be forced.
3. With several centimeters of wire still protruding from the distal end of the needle, remove the needle from the vein. Hold the wire near the skin insertion site as soon as it appears, to prevent the wire from being inadvertently pulled out of the vein.
4. Make a small skin incision with a scalpel to facilitate insertion of the catheter through the skin.
5. Slide the catheter over the wire up to the point of insertion. Make certain that several centimeters of wire are protruding from the other end of the catheter. Slowly advance the catheter and the wire into the vein. As soon as the catheter is in place, remove the wire.
6. Affix the catheter, and dress the insertion site as previously described.

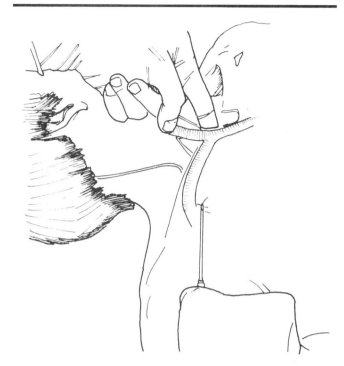

Figure 20. Infraclavicular subclavian venipuncture.

Using Direct Internal Jugular and Subclavian Venipuncture

Advantages[14-26]

Since puncture does not depend on visually locating these veins, rapid access to the circulation is possible even if peripheral veins are collapsed. These approaches also allow direct access to the central circulation.

The internal jugular approach may be preferred to the subclavian puncture since with the former there is less risk of pleural puncture, and hematomas which may form in the neck are visible and compressible. Internal jugular venipuncture may be easier to perform during CPR. It also may be easier to insert a balloon-tipped flow-directed pulmonary artery catheter via the right internal jugular vein since it is a straight shot from the insertion site to the right atrium.

The subclavian route may be preferred, however, since with prolonged subclavian cannulation, more subsequent neck movement may be possible than with the internal jugular approach.

Disadvantages

Because of the proximity of the carotid and subclavian arteries, the apical pleura, lymphatic ducts, and various nerves, these structures can be damaged by inexperienced operators. Techniques for internal jugular and subclavian venipuncture also require more training than for peripheral venipuncture, and the complication rate is much higher. This may be of particular importance in patients receiving treatment with thrombolytic agents.

If basic life support is being performed, the presence of an additional operator at the head or chest of the patient may crowd those performing ventilation and chest compression, and either make CPR more difficult to perform or require that it be interrupted altogether to cannulate the veins.

Using Subclavian Cannulation via the External Jugular Vein

Advantages

The technique is easy to learn and perform. The venipuncture itself is no different from any other peripheral venipuncture, but training and practice is required to use guidewires and insert central catheters safely.

Disadvantages

The complication rate of the external jugular puncture is not different from any other peripheral venipuncture. However, the wire or the catheter may perforate any of the veins along the course of the insertion. During CPR, this technique has the same disadvantages as internal jugular and subclavian venipuncture.

Specific Complications[14-17,30-33]

Local

Bleeding with resultant hematoma may occur from perforating either the vein itself or an adjacent artery. If a hematoma appears on one side of the neck, it is hazardous to attempt puncture on the opposite side, since a bilateral hematoma in the neck can severely compromise the airway. Any adjacent structure may be damaged, including artery, nerve, or lymphatic duct. If the patient has an endotracheal tube with an inflated cuff in place, it is even possible to perforate the trachea with the needle and deflate the cuff. Thrombosis of the vein around the catheter may occur, especially with prolonged catheterization. Thrombosis may extend to the superior vena cava and lead to vena cava obstruction and pulmonary thromboembolism.

Systemic

Pneumothorax is a common complication; a follow-up chest x-ray film must be obtained as soon as possible. The position of the catheter tip must be verified by x-ray film before infusing blood, hyperalimentation fluids, and other preparations. Infiltration of fluid into the mediastinum or pleural cavity may occur from an extruded catheter. Bleeding from an injured vein or adjacent artery may lead to hemothorax. Air embolism may occur during insertion, or it may occur when the IV administration set becomes disconnected from the catheter hub. The use of three-way stopcocks or extension tubes increases the risk of disconnection. If the catheter tip is in the right atrium or the right ventricle, it may induce cardiac arrhythmias; during manipulation of the patient, perforation of the right atrium or the right ventricle may occur, producing cardiac tamponade. To avoid these complications, the catheter tip should be outside the right atrium in the superior vena cava. Catheters that remain in place longer than three days may cause local and systemic infection (bacteremia). See Chapter 10.

References

1. Standards and Guidelines for Cardiopulmonary Resuscitation (CPR) and Emergency Cardiac Care (ECC). *JAMA* 255:2905-2989, 1986.
2. Sobel BE, Shell WE: Serum enzyme determinations in the diagnosis and assessment of myocardial infarction. *Circulation* 45:471-482, 1972.
3. Meltzer HY, Mrozak S, Boyer M: Effect of intramuscular injections on serum creatine phosphokinase activity. *Am J Med Sci* 259:42-48, 1970.
4. Graber D, Dailey RH: Catheter flow rates updated. *JACEP* 6:518, 1977.
5. Seldinger SI: Catheter replacement of the needle in percutaneous arteriography; a new technique. *Acta Radiol* 39:368-376, 1953.
6. Plastic containers for IV solutions. *Med Lett* 17:43-44, 1975.
7. Hamilton CM (ed): *Textbook of Human Anatomy.* London, MacMillan & Co Ltd 1956.
8. Gray H: *Anatomy of the Human Body,* ed 28, Goss CM (ed). Philadelphia, Lea & Febiger, 1966.
9. Venipuncture of the jugular vein. Procedure Sheet, Orange County California, Mobile Intensive Care Training Division, 1974.
10. Kuhn GJ, White BC, Swetnam RE, et al: Peripheral vs central circulation times during CPR: A pilot study. *Ann Emerg Med* 10:417-419, 1981.
11. Hedges JR, Barsan WB, Doan LA, et al: Central versus peripheral intravenous routes in cardiopulmonary resuscitation. *Am J Emerg Med* 2:385-390, 1984.
12. Barsan WG, Levy RC, Weir H: Lidocaine levels during CPR: Differences after peripheral venous, central venous, and intracardiac injections. *Ann Emerg Med* 10:73, 1981.
13. Neiman JT, Rosborough JP, Hauskuecht et al: Pressure-synchionized cineangiography during experimental cardiopulmonary resuscitation *Circulation* 64:985-991, 1981.
14. Defalque RJ: Percutaneous catheterization of the internal jugular vein. *Anesth Analg* 53:116-121, 1974.
15. Moosman DA: The anatomy of infraclavicular subclavian vein catheterization and its complications. *Surg Gynecol Obstet* 136:71-74, 1973.
16. Wilson F, Nelson JH Jr, Moltz A: Methods and indications for central venous pressure monitoring. *Am J Obstet Gynecol* 101:137-151, 1968.
17. McConnell RY, Fox RT: Experience with percutaneous internal jugular-innominate vein catheterization. *California Med* 117:1-6, 1972.
18. Jernigan WR, Gardner WC, Mahr MM, et al: Use of the internal Jugular vein for placement of central venous catheter. *Surg Gynecol Obstet* 130:520-524, 1970.
19. Brinkman AJ, Costley DO: Internal Jugular venipuncture. *JAMA* 223:182-183, 1973.
20. Garcia JM, Mispireta LA, Pinho RV: Percutaneous supraclavicular superior vena cava cannulation. *Surg Gynecol Obstet* 134:839-841, 1972.

21. Daily PO, Griepp RB, Shumway NE: Percutaneous internal jugular vein cannulation. *Am Med Assoc Arch Surg* 101:534-536,1970.

22. Mostert JW, Kenny GM, Murphy GP: Safe placement of central venous catheter into internal jugular veins. *Am Med Assoc Arch Surg* 101:431-432, 1970.

23. Yoffa D: Supraclavicular subclavian venepuncture and catheterization. *Lancet* 2:615-617, 1965.

24. Man B, Kraus L: The clinical value of subclavian vein catheterization. *Angiology* 24:649-655, 1973.

25. Buchsbaum HJ, White AJ: The use of subclavian central venous catheters in gynecology and obstetrics. *Surg Gynecol Obstet* 136:561-563, 1973.

26. Craig RG, Jones RA, Sproul GJ, et al: The alternate methods of central venous system catheterization. *Am Surg* 34:131-134, 1968.

27. Flanagan JP, Grandisaria IA, Gross RJ, et al: Air embolus — a lethal complication of subclavian venipuncture. *N Engl J Med* 281:488-489, 1969.

28. Kaplan JA, Miller ED: Internal jugular vein catheterization. *Anesth Rev* 3:21-23, 1976.

29. Blitt CD, Wright WA, Petty WC, et al: Central venous catheterization via the external jugular vein. A technique employing the J-wire. *JAMA* 229:817-818, 1974.

30. Marshal JP, Chadwick SJ, Meyers DS: Catheter perforation of the right ventricle. A complication of endoscopy. *N Engl J Med* 290:890-891, 1974.

31. Peters JL, Armstrong R: Air embolism occurring as a complication of central venous catheterization. *Ann Surg* 187:375-378, 1978.

32. Peters JL: Central-venous-catheters Luer locks, letter. *Lancet* 2:430-431, 1978.

33. Gibson RN, Hennessy OF, Collier N, Hemingway AP. Major complications of central venous catheterization: A report of five cases and a brief review of the literature. *Clin Radiol* 36:205-208, 1985.

Credit is given to Monte Deignan, Greg Jennings, and Peter Miniscalco for artwork and photography.

Invasive Monitoring Techniques

Chapter 12

Part I: Introduction to Arterial Cannulation

Indications

The primary indication for arterial cannulation is to ensure accurate blood pressure measurements. Placement of an intraarterial catheter allows one to 1) continuously monitor arterial pressure, 2) avoid the discomfort and injury from frequent arterial punctures, 3) sample arterial blood without disturbing the steady state, 4) determine cardiac output utilizing Indocyanine Green dye (becoming less necessary given modern non-invasive technology, e.g., blood pressure and oximetry devices). To use intraarterial monitoring safely and effectively, the operator must be skilled in the technique, and the staff must be familiar with the catheter and transducer system in order to eliminate air bubbles, prevent clots and contamination, correctly calibrate the system, and avoid artifacts.

Rationale for Intraarterial Pressure Monitoring

The patient in shock with an elevated systemic vascular resistance may manifest a significant discrepancy between pressure obtained by auscultatory and palpatory methods compared to intraarterial pressure.[1] Central intraarterial systolic pressure may be as much as 150 mmHg higher than the pressure recorded with a sphygmomanometer. In hypotensive patients with normal or decreased systemic vascular resistance, there should be no discrepancy between pressure obtained with a cuff and intraarterial pressure unless localized atherosclerosis is present.

The Korotkoff sounds that are heard over the brachial artery as the arm cuff is deflated are probably due to vibrations of the arterial wall set in motion by intermittent flow through the compressed segment. Absence of these sounds indicates that either flow is insufficient or the vessel wall itself has been altered so that sounds are not transmitted. With increased arterial constriction in hypotensive states, diastolic runoff is slowed; following release of pressure in the cuff at the onset of flow, there is a decreased pressure gradient. With a decreased gradient there is no intermittent turbulence-producing jet flow through the obstructed segment, and therefore, no sounds are produced. The increased wall tension from vasoconstriction may also make the wall less likely to vibrate and produce sounds.[1] Failure to recognize that

low cuff pressure does not necessarily indicate arterial hypotension may lead to dangerous errors in therapy.

Any patient who requires titrated intravenous (IV) vasopressors or vasodilators for improved hemo-dynamics should have blood pressure continuously recorded. However, only if intense vasoconstriction is present is an intraarterial line of importance.

Direct vs. Indirect Arterial Pressure Measurements[2-6]

Variance of 5–20 mmHg

A disparity of 5–20 mmHg is probably within the expected range for direct and indirect pressure measurements. Directly recorded pressure may be slightly greater than indirectly recorded pressure for several reasons. As the arterial pressure pulse wave passes to the periphery, there are marked changes in its form. The pulse wave arrives later, the ascending limb becomes steeper, and the systolic pressure becomes higher, whereas the diastolic pressure is lower. The mean arterial pressure, however, is unchanged. The major factors responsible for changes in the arterial pulse contour are 1) distortion of the components of the pulse waves as they travel peripherally, 2) different rates of transmission of various components of the pulse wave, 3) amplification or distortion of different components of the pulse by standing or reflected waves, 4) differences in elastic behavior and in the caliber of the arteries, 5) conversions of some kinetic energy to hydrostatic energy, and 6) changes that occur in the arterial catheter and the extension line from the catheter to the transducer. There may also be a disparity in measurements if cuff size and placement are inappropriate. Finally, the transducer may be improperly calibrated or zeroed.

When indirect pressure is recorded to be greater than direct pressure, this phenomenon is most likely due to either equipment malfunction or technical error. If the arterial waveform is damped, it suggests a problem with the tubing: air bubbles or blood in the line or the transducer dome, clotting at the catheter tip, mechanical occlusions of the catheter or the tubing, or loose or open connections. If the arterial waveform is normal, other causes must be excluded: improper cuff size and placement, failure to calibrate the sphygmomanometer and the transducer, or an error in electrically and mechanically zeroing the transducer.

Variance of 20–30 mmHg

When there is a disparity of 20–30 mmHg between cuff pressure and intraarterial pressure, all factors listed above may be responsible. In addition, the auscultatory method may lead to lower readings in the patient with severe vasoconstriction, such as in shock or hypothermia. Another possible source of error is the fact that the cuff reads pressure from beat to beat, while the digital recording on the electronic monitor reads the highest pressure every 3–7 seconds. In the presence of occlusive peripheral disease, the pressure recorded in a peripheral artery, such as the radial or the dorsalis pedis, may be significantly lower than the cuff pressure taken more proximally.

Variance of Greater Than 30 mmHg

When the disparity is greater than 30 mmHg, the most common problem is overshoot of the apparent systolic pressure (Figure 1A,B) caused by the resonance of the catheter system. This more commonly occurs when the heart rate is rapid, when the rate of rise of pressure (dP/dt) is rapid, and when the natural frequency of the catheter system is low. It can be anticipated that the longer and more compliant the extension tubing and the lower the natural frequency, the greater the error in measurement. This can be minimized by using stiff extension tubing as short as possible.

Intraarterial pressure may be significantly higher than cuff pressure when a single end-hole catheter is in a narrow artery with high flow. When the catheter faces the flow, kinetic energy is converted to potential energy, falsely elevating the measured blood pressure.

The disparity between the direct and indirect pressure measurements can be minimized by observing the following procedures:[2,6]

1. Allow the transducer and amplifier to warm up for at least 10 minutes before starting to zero and calibrate the system.
2. Mechanically zero the transducer.
3. Purge all air from the pressure system.
4. Check all fittings for tightness.
5. Electrically zero and calibrate the system with a mercury manometer or a water column.[7]
6. Use stiff, noncompliant extension tubing of shortest possible length, and avoid use of more than one stopcock between catheter and transducer.
7. Avoid draining blood samples the full length of the plumbing system.
8. Maintain the catheter so that clotting does not occur.
9. Place the extension tubing near the patient with care to prevent a pulsating line.
10. Recheck the mechanical and electrical zero position, and recalibrate the system, if necessary, when the level of the patient is changed.

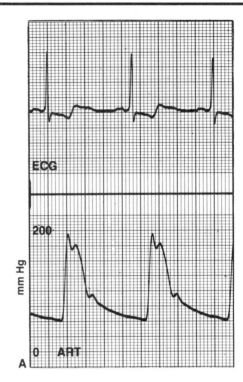

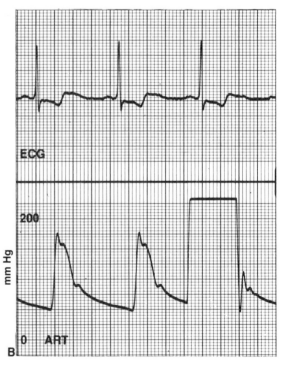

Figure 1. **(A) Overshoot of apparent systolic pressure (ART) due to resonance from 72-inch-long extension tubing.** Recorded pressure is 195 mmHg. (B) Systolic pressure (ART) recorded with 6-inch extension tubing in same patient. The recorded systolic pressure is 175 mmHg which correlated with cuff systolic pressure of 170 mmHg.

11. Avoid making adjustments to the amplifier except at time of calibration.
12. Check the zero setting (both electrically and mechanically) and calibration at least once per shift.

Use of Doppler Device for Blood Pressure Monitoring[8-10]

A Doppler device and an arm cuff may be used noninvasively to measure blood pressure. The Doppler transducer, which should be an instrument with high frequency output (10 MHz), is placed over the radial artery at the wrist, and a blood pressure cuff of appropriate size is placed around the upper arm. The cuff is inflated until the Doppler signal disappears, and then slowly deflated until blood flow is again audible; this is the systolic pressure. A change in the signal can be recognized as the diastolic pressure. The Doppler signal can be heard clearly and recorded, even at low levels of systolic pressure, when the Korotkoff sounds are not audible and the pulse is not palpable. However, it should be noted that in patients with hypotension, diastolic pressure measurements may be difficult to determine by this method. Doppler measurement of blood pressure over the radial artery correlates well with intraarterial pressure in the radial artery even in patients with hypotension. With intense vasoconstriction, neither the Doppler nor the intravascular radial arterial pressure will reflect aortic pressure, and a more centrally placed line, such as one in the femoral or the axillary artery, may be required.

Indirect Blood Pressure Monitoring by Automatic Oscillometry

Automatic indirect blood pressure determinations can be performed via automatic oscillometry. Automatic oscillometry is a technique that uses a double air bladder enclosed in a cuff to determine the arterial blood pressure of the extremity within the cuff. The cuff is positioned over an artery, and the proximal bladder is inflated to occlude blood flow, while residual air volume is maintained in the distal bladder. In a stepwise fashion the proximal bladder is deflated and restoration of blood flow causes arterial wall oscillations that are sensed by the distal bladder. A microprocessor then assesses the transmitted signals and determines systolic blood pressure, diastolic blood pressure, and mean blood pressure.[11] The accuracy of the data generated suffers from the same vagaries as other nonautomatic blood pressure determinations. Cuff size and fit, extremes of blood pressure, and obesity may cause errors of measurement.[12-15]

In a study by Venus, et al., a comparison of indirect automatic blood pressure determination vs. blood pressure determination via direct radial arterial cannulation was done. In 109 determinations they found that there were no significant differences in mean arterial blood pressure between the two techniques. However, the indirect determination underestimated systolic blood pressure by 9.2 ± 16.4 mmHg and overestimated diastolic blood pressure by 8.7 ± 10.6 mmHg. They concluded that automatic indirect blood pressure monitoring was adequate for routine monitoring of mean arterial pressure, but for hemodynamic titration of vasoactive drugs, direct intraarterial measurements should be considered.[16]

In a study by Johnson, et al., evaluating five automatic blood pressure monitors compared to measurements made from direct arterial line monitoring, the correlation coefficient ranged from 0.7 to over 0.9. However, they concluded that in critically ill patients, especially those who were hypotensive, where peripheral recordings may themselves not correlate with central pressure, indirect monitorings were inadequate and direct monitoring necessary.[17]

Site Selection

An artery suitable for placing an indwelling catheter for continuous monitoring of intraarterial pressures should have the following characteristics: 1) The vessel should be large enough to measure pressure accurately without the catheter occluding the artery or producing thrombosis. 2) The artery should have adequate collateral circulation should occlusion occur. 3) There should be easy access to the site for nursing care. 4) It should not be in an area prone to contamination.

The axillary artery is a large artery with excellent collateral flow, so that thrombosis should not lead to any serious sequelae. It can be used to monitor central arterial pressure. However, embolism of air or thrombus which forms about the catheter tip may produce ischemic injury to the brain or the hand. The femoral artery also can be used. The femoral pulse still may be palpable when the radial pulses are lost in patients with marked hypotension. It also reflects intraaortic pressure better than peripheral arteries.[1] Caution is advised in the presence of occlusive arterial disease.

The radial artery can also be used for cannulation and is probably safe and free from significant potential complications if careful attention is directed to demonstrating adequate ulnar collateral flow prior to cannulation. Even though thrombosis of the radial artery at the catheter site is common (as noted later), ischemic injury of the hand is rare if there is adequate ulnar collateral flow. (See "Modified Allen Test".)

The dorsal pedal arteries are without significant cannulation hazards if collateral flow is demonstrated to the remainder of the foot through the posterior tibial artery. Since thrombosis, which might follow brachial artery cannulation, may lead to significant ischemic injury of the lower arm and hand, the brachial artery should not routinely be used.

Complications of Arterial Catheterization

The major complications of arterial cannulation are ischemia and necrosis secondary to either thrombosis or embolism. Ischemia is manifested by pain (either at rest or when using the involved extremity), pallor, and paresthesias. Necrosis is manifested by obvious tissue death. Whether ischemia or necrosis distal to the area of obstruction does or does not occur depends on the presence of collateral flow and the rate of recanalization. Other complications include hemorrhage, infection, vasovagal syncope, aneurysms, and arteriovenous fistula — the complications that may occur with cannulation of any artery. Complications following cannulation of specific arteries will be discussed as a separate topic in the sections pertaining to each artery.

Thrombosis

The longer the cannula is in place, the greater the incidence of thrombosis; radial artery cannulas left in place longer than 48 hours markedly increase the incidence of thrombosis.[18-21] Yet, cannulation of the femoral artery with a long, thin catheter for up to 16 days was not associated with any thrombotic complications in one published series of studies.[22,23] The larger the size of the cannula relative to the diameter of the arterial lumen, the greater the incidence of thrombosis. This may relate both to the fact that the larger cannula relative to vessel size may produce more intimal damage, and that the larger cannula in a small vessel occupies most of the lumen and in itself obstructs the flow. A large 18-gauge catheter in a small vessel would occupy most of the lumen, whereas a smaller 20-gauge catheter in a large vessel might occupy only 15–20% of the lumen.[24] A 20-gauge catheter produces the lowest incidence of thrombosis in the radial artery.[24-26]

One study indicated that the incidence of dysfunction of the catheter as manifested by damping of the arterial waveform was not different with either 18-gauge or 20-gauge catheters. However, the dysfunction was invariably due to thrombosis with the larger catheter; with the smaller catheter it was usually due to kinking.[24] The shape of the cannula and the material from which the cannula is made also influences the incidence of thrombosis. Nontapered catheters induce a lower incidence of thrombus formation compared to tapered catheters,[25,27] and catheters made of Teflon have been shown to invoke the lowest incidence of thrombosis.[24,26] Repeated attempts at puncturing the radial artery not only may lead to thrombosis in the absence of an indwelling catheter but also increase the incidence of thrombosis with an indwelling catheter.[19,27] Hypotension and low cardiac output, the use of vasopressors, peripheral arteriosclerotic occlusive disease, diabetes mellitus, Raynaud's disease, hypothermia, autoimmune diseases with vasculitis, and excessive and prolonged pressure on the artery to control bleeding following catheter removal predispose to thrombosis and the ischemic sequelae of thrombosis.[19,28]

With intermittent flushing, the incidence of thrombosis is increased. A continuous flush system should be used to insure catheter patency, prevent thrombosis, and minimize the incidence of embolism. Several systems are now available which allow a continuous flow of 3.0 mL/hr when the system is pressurized to 300 mmHg. A valve can be opened that provides a flush at 1.5 mL/sec.[29] With the flush valve closed, the resistance in the system is so high that the pressure measured within the system does not differ by more than 2% from the pressure at the tip of the catheter.[29,30] However, since air will pass easily through the flow system, it must be removed from the bag before pressurization. The solution for continuous irrigation should have heparin added; a concentration of 2–4 units/mL appears adequate. By opening the flush valve and then rapidly closing it, a square wave is generated on the arterial waveform which indicates that no clot or bubbles are present in the system (Figure 2A). If clots, bubbles, or loose connections are present, the square wave response will be damped significantly[31] (Figure 2B).

Embolism

Embolism may occur from small clots that form around the tip of the catheter, or by air and particulate matter introduced into the system. Emboli are more common when intermittent flushing of the catheter is done by hand; if hand flushing is required, a few milliliters of blood should be withdrawn through the stopcock to clear the system of air or clot before flushing. A continuous flush system that eliminates the need for intermittent flushing minimizes the problem of embolism.[25,29]

Hemorrhage

If any connection in the arterial line between the patient and the transducer opens or becomes disconnected, rapid exsanguination of the patient may follow unless the situation is promptly recognized. A bleeding diathesis, due either to anticoagulation or a disease process, increases the incidence of hemorrhage from the puncture site. Bleeding may occur around the catheter if a needle larger than the catheter was used to introduce the catheter, or it may occur following catheter removal. Hypertension, especially with a rapid rise of the systolic upstroke (dP/dt) within the artery, may also increase the incidence of bleeding. Hematoma following removal of an arterial catheter is common, may not appear for 1–2 days following removal of the cannula, and may persist for 7–10 days. The incidence and size of the hematoma can be minimized with the application of pressure to the cannulation site for 10 minutes after withdrawal of the catheter.[28,29]

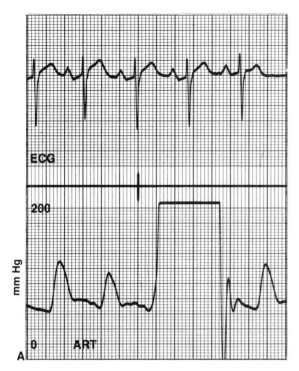

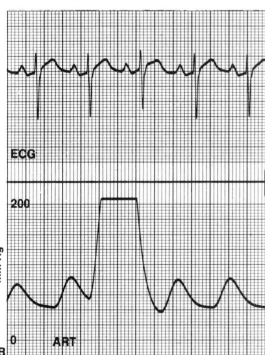

Figure 2. (A) Normal arterial waveform (ART) with normal square wave response during rapid flushing with continuous flush system. (B) Significantly damped square wave response in arterial waveform when clots, bubbles, or loose connections are present.

Infection

The most obvious risk factor for catheter-related infection appears to be the length of time the catheter resides in the vessel; most infections are caused by arterial catheters left in place for more than 72 hours.[32] Arterial catheters inserted by cutdown involve an increased incidence of infection compared to catheters inserted percutaneously.[32] There are many other risk factors for catheter-related infection; these are described in Chapter 10.

Vasovagal Reactions

Hypotension with bradycardia may occur during arterial puncture and can be reversed promptly with atropine.[33]

Part II: Arterial Cannulation Sites, Techniques, and Complications

Cannulation of the Femoral Artery

Anatomy

The femoral artery (Figure 3) continues from the external iliac artery beneath the inguinal ligament in the leg. If a line is drawn from the anterior superior iliac spine to the symphysis pubis, the femoral artery passes through the midpoint of that line at the level of the inguinal ligament. Lateral to the femoral artery is the femoral nerve, and medial to the artery within the femoral sheath is the femoral vein.[34] (See Figures 10 and 11, Chapter 11.)

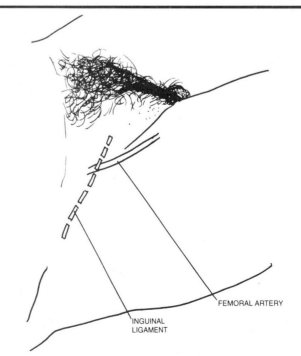

Figure 3.   Anatomy of the femoral artery.

Equipment Needed

1. A 19- or 20-gauge Teflon catheter, 16 cm long. The catheter should be long enough to extend through the skin well into the artery so that it does not become dislodged with patient movement.
2. A flexible guidewire small enough to pass through the catheter and needle.
3. A 20-gauge needle, 5 cm long.
4. Other equipment as for any arterial cannulation.

Technique (See Figure 4)

1. Identify the femoral artery and choose a site approximately 2 cm below the inguinal ligament or near the inguinal fold.
2. Shave the groin and cleanse the skin with povidone–iodine.
3. Wear sterile gloves, mask, and a hair cover.
4. Cover the area around the insertion site with sterile drapes. If the Seldinger technique is used, the sterile field should be large enough to allow manipulation of the guidewire and catheter without risk of contamination.
5. Place the index, middle, and fourth fingers of one hand along the course of the femoral artery beyond the inguinal ligament. The use of three fingers not only indicates the location of the artery but also demonstrates its course. If the index finger is spread away from the middle and ring fingers, which are held together, the insertion site is between the index and the middle fingers.
6. Infiltrate the overlying skin with 1% lidocaine without epinephrine if the patient is awake.
7. If the Seldinger technique is used, enter the skin and artery at about a 45° angle. As soon as a free flow of blood spurts from the end of the needle, insert the wire through the needle well into the artery; then remove the needle. If the artery is not entered with the initial attempt, insert the needle deeply until it can go no further through both the anterior and posterior walls of the artery and then slowly withdraw the needle until free arterial flow is obtained. The wire must pass without any resistance whatsoever to indicate that it is in the lumen of the artery. Inserting the wire against resistance may lead to intramural insertion or dissection.
8. If the artery is not entered, withdraw the needle completely. Again determine the location of the femoral artery and make another attempt.
9. If the artery is entered with the needle but the wire cannot be passed, remove the needle and maintain pressure over the artery for at least 5–10 minutes before the next attempt is made.
10. If the wire passes easily into the artery, remove the needle and insert the catheter over the wire; then remove the wire from the catheter and attach the connecting tubing to the end of the catheter.

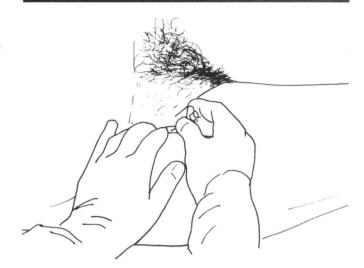

Figure 4. Cannulation of the femoral artery.

11. Suture the catheter in place with 3-0 silk.
12. Cover the insertion site with povidone–iodine ointment and a sterile dressing.
13. If a catheter-over-needle device is used, insert both in the same manner as above; when free arterial flow is obtained through the end of the needle, advance the catheter into the artery while holding the needle in place. Finally, remove the needle. Subsequent care is the same as when the catheter is inserted via the Seldinger method.

Complications

Thrombosis: The larger the catheter used, the greater the incidence of thrombosis; when the femoral artery is used for cardiac catheterization via the Judkins technique, thrombosis following catheterization may be as high as 1–4%.[35-39] Although rare with 19- or 20-gauge catheters,[22,23] thrombosis of the femoral artery may occur in the presence of peripheral vascular disease, following repeated attempts at insertion of catheters into the artery, and following prolonged, excessive pressure to control bleeding after catheter removal.

Embolism: A thrombus that forms about the catheter in the femoral artery may embolize to the lower leg and the foot, producing gangrene.[40] To detect emboli early, the pulses of the femoral, popliteal, posterior tibial, and dorsalis pedis arteries should be checked frequently, ideally with a Doppler flow meter. If there is evidence of loss of pulses or diminution in peripheral pulses, the femoral artery catheter must be removed.

Hematoma and Hemorrhage: Hematoma is common following removal of the femoral arterial catheter but can be minimized by maintaining pressure over the femoral artery for approximately 10 minutes following removal of the catheter. However, the femoral pulse must not be completely obliterated by pressure since this will predispose the patient to thrombosis.[38,41] Above the inguinal ligament, the femoral artery joins the external iliac artery, which slopes abruptly backward as it ascends. If the artery is punctured above the inguinal ligament, it becomes difficult to tamponade the vessel to control bleeding. Since the posterior wall of the artery is commonly punctured during insertion, this occurrence may lead to unrecognized retroperitoneal hemorrhage.[39,42]

Arteriovenous Fistula: A fistula between the femoral artery and the femoral vein may be produced, especially with larger catheters such as are used for cardiac catheterization and angiography.[36,39] A false aneurysm may also follow femoral arterial catheterization.

Cannulation of the Axillary Artery

Anatomy

The axillary artery (Figure 5) is a continuation of the subclavian artery as it leaves the root of the neck at the lateral border of the first rib to enter the axilla. As the axillary artery leaves the axilla at the lower border of the teres major muscle, it enters the arm as the brachial artery. The axillary artery, vein, and the three cords of the bracheal plexus form a neurovascular bundle within the axillary sheath. Because of the extensive collateral circulation that exists between the thyrocervical trunk of the subclavian artery and the subscapular artery, which is a branch of the distal axillary artery, ligation or thrombosis of the axillary artery usually will not lead to compromise of flow to the distal arm.[43,44] Since the axillary is a large artery (almost the size of the femoral artery) and is close to the aorta, pulsation and pressure are maintained even in the presence of peripheral vascular collapse with marked peripheral vasoconstriction.

Equipment Needed

1. Since the axillary artery may be cannulated with either the Seldinger technique or a catheter-over-needle device, the cannula required depends on the method used. For the Seldinger technique, a 19- or 20-gauge Teflon catheter 16 cm long, a flexible guidewire that fits both needle and catheter, and a 20-gauge needle 5 cm long will be necessary. The catheter-over-needle device should have a 20-gauge catheter at least 2½ inches (6.4 cm) long.
2. Other equipment is the same as for other arterial cannulation.

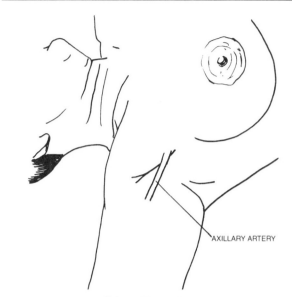

Figure 5. Anatomy of the axillary artery.

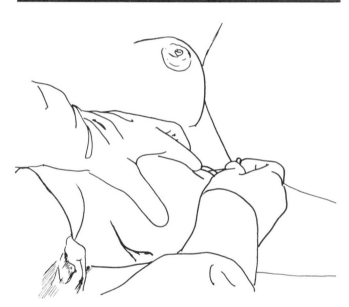

Figure 6. Cannulation of the axillary artery.

Technique[44,45] (See Figure 6)

1. Immobilize the arm; it should be hyperabducted and externally rotated more than 90° from the patient's body.
2. Stand at the patient's side, either above or below the abducted arm.
3. Locate the artery within the axilla.
4. Shave and cleanse the skin with povidone–iodine solution.
5. Wear sterile gloves, mask, and hair cover and drape the area with sterile towels.
6. Infiltrate the skin with 1% lidocaine without epinephrine if the patient is awake.

7. Insert the needle into the artery as high as possible within the axilla.

8. If the Seldinger technique is used, once free arterial flow is obtained, pass the wire through the needle into the artery and remove the needle.

9. If the catheter-over-needle device is used, remove the needle and slowly withdraw the catheter once blood appears (indicating that the tip is in the lumen), then advance the catheter into the artery.

10. If after three attempts the artery is not entered, discontinue the procedure on that side and choose another site for arterial puncture.

11. If successful, secure the catheter in place with a 3-0 or 4-0 silk suture.

12. Apply povidone–iodine ointment to the skin at the site of insertion and cover it with a sterile dressing.

Complications

Thrombosis: Because of extensive collateral circulation, thrombosis of the axillary artery should not lead to any ischemic or necrotic sequelae. Moreover, with 19- or 20-gauge catheters, thrombosis is rare.[23,44-46]

Embolism: Although thrombosis of the axillary artery may not lead directly to injury to the distal arm, it is still possible that a thrombus which forms about the catheter tip may embolize to the radial or ulnar circulation. In the absence of adequate collateral flow through the superficial palmar arch, this could produce ischemic injury to the hand.

Since the right axillary artery arises from the right brachiocephalic trunk in direct communication with the common carotid artery, it is quite possible that air, clot, or particulate matter may embolize to the brain during flushing. It may be safer to use the left axillary artery rather than the right, but in either instance, flushing should be performed gently, with minimum volume and with careful attention to prevent the introduction of air or a clot into the system. Irrigation with a continuous flow system should be used.

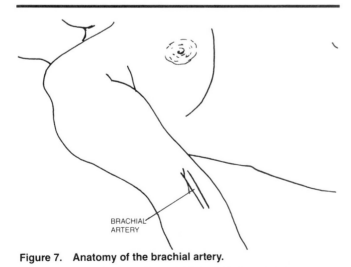

Figure 7. Anatomy of the brachial artery.

Neurological Complications: During attempts at axillary arterial puncture, direct injury to the cords of the brachial plexus may occur, or an axillary sheath hematoma may lead to nerve compression and injury.[45] The axillary artery, therefore, should not be used for intraarterial monitoring in patients with bleeding diatheses.

Cannulation of the Brachial Artery

Anatomy

The brachial artery (Figure 7) extends into the arm as a continuation of the axillary artery. It passes down the upper inner arm just under the medial edge of the biceps muscle. In the antecubital fossa, just above the elbow crease, it is easily palpable medial to the biceps tendon and lateral to the median nerve. In the lower part of the antecubital fossa, the brachial artery divides into the radial artery and the ulnar artery. There are anastomoses around the elbow from the inferior ulnar collateral artery above to branches of the ulnar artery below.[43] However, if collateral circulation is inadequate, obstruction of the brachial artery may be catastrophic, leading to loss of the forearm and hand.

Equipment Needed

1. A 20-gauge Teflon catheter-over-needle, nontapered shaft, 1½–2 inches (3.8–5.1 cm) in length (or a longer 20-gauge catheter may be inserted with the Seldinger technique).

2. Arm board to prevent the arm from flexing at the elbow.

3. Other equipment the same as for radial artery cannulation.

Technique (See Figure 8)

1. Locate brachial artery medial to the biceps tendon above the elbow crease.

2. Cleanse the overlying skin with povidone–iodine solution.

3. Wear sterile gloves (plus mask and hair cover for optimal asepsis) and drape the area with sterile towels.

4. Infiltrate the overlying skin with 1% lidocaine without epinephrine if the patient is awake.

5. Immobilize the artery with two or three fingers.

6. Insert the catheter-over-needle device at about a 30° angle to the surface of the skin and advance the catheter and needle stylet into the artery until blood appears in the hub of the needle.

7. While holding the needle in the fixed position, advance the catheter-over-needle into the artery.

8. Remove the needle and attach the hub of the catheter to connecting tubing.

9. Tie the catheter in place with 3-0 or 4-0 silk sutures.

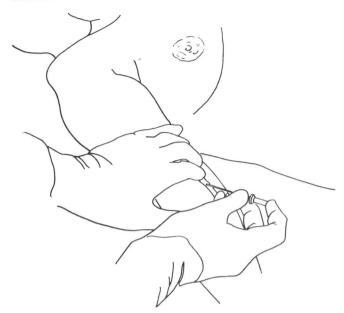

Figure 8.   Cannulation of the brachial artery.

10. Apply povidone–iodine ointment to the skin at the site of insertion and cover it with a sterile dressing.
11. Make certain that the arm is immobilized to prevent flexion at the elbow.

Complications

Thrombosis and Embolism: Barnes, et al., reported brachial artery catheterization in 1,000 patients with no objective ischemia of the distal arm.[47] However, the duration of catheter placement was not described. The same group reported that of 54 patients who had brachial artery catheterization for 1–3 days with an 18-gauge Teflon catheter connected to a continuous flush system, 2 patients had evidence of ulnar artery obstruction and 1 had evidence of radial artery obstruction. Nevertheless, neither of the 2 patients had any symptoms or signs of ischemia of the hand. Another group reported a study of 25 patients in whom an 18-gauge polyethylene catheter was inserted in the brachial artery for an average of 11.5 hours.[48] Angiography, both before catheter removal and 6 months later, revealed a high incidence of early and late vascular abnormalities: 14 of the 25 subjects had absent peripheral pulses and vascular abnormalities after removal of the catheter. Of 11 patients who were studied 6 months later, 4 had evidence of vascular irregularities and narrowing of the brachial artery at the puncture site. They had, nonetheless, regained peripheral pulses.

Neurological Complications: Subfascial bleeding after percutaneous puncture of the artery has been reported[49] in patients on anticoagulant therapy and may lead to median nerve neuropathy and Volkman's contracture. Increasing pain, swelling, or minimal evidence of neuropathy in the area of distribution of the median nerve (such as paresthesias or weakness) are indications for both immediate reversal of anticoagulation treatment and fasciotomy. To prevent this complication, the brachial artery should not be used for cannulation in patients with bleeding diatheses.

Cannulation of the Radial Artery

Anatomy[34]

The radial artery (Figure 9), a branch of the brachial artery, extends down the anterior radial aspect of the forearm where, after sending a branch to the palm, it disappears deep to the abductor pollicis longus tendon just beyond the distal end of the radius. From there, it continues across the floor of the anatomical snuffbox into the dorsum of the hand. At the wrist, the radial artery is palpable in a longitudinal groove formed by the tendon of the flexor carpi radialis medially and the distal radius laterally. The ulnar artery, the other major branch of the brachial artery, extends down the ulnar aspect of the forearm to the wrist, where it is sheltered by the tendon of the flexor carpi ulnaris. At the wrist, the ulnar artery is palpable just lateral to this tendon. The superficial palmar arch is formed from a continuation of the ulnar artery into the hand; both the deep palmar arch and the dorsal arch are a continuation of the radial artery. Mozersky, et al., studied 140 hands using a Doppler flow probe and found that the superficial palmar arch was predominantly supplied by the ulnar artery in only 88% of the cases; 12% of the hands had either poor collateral flow or an incomplete palmar arch with no collateral circulation whatsoever.[50]

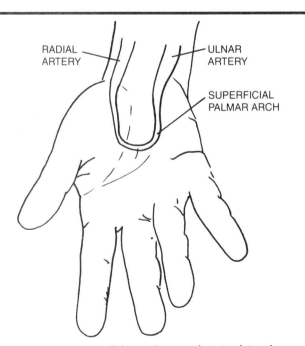

RADIAL ARTERY

ULNAR ARTERY

SUPERFICIAL PALMAR ARCH

Figure 9.   Anatomy of radial and ulnar arteries at wrist and superficial palmar arch.

Assessment of Ulnar Collateral Circulation

Since radial artery cannulation is commonly associated with radial artery thrombosis, continued viability of the hand in such a situation depends on collateral flow via the superficial arch from the ulnar artery. If collateral flow is incomplete or absent, ischemic injury to the hand will follow radial artery thrombosis. It is therefore absolutely essential that, prior to cannulating a radial artery, the presence of collateral flow be demonstrated.[51] Four methods for determining the presence of collateral circulation are described.

The Modified Allen Test:[52] The modified Allen test (Figure 10) differs from Allen's original description[53] in 1929 and is performed as follows:

1. If the patient's hands are not warm, they should be immersed in warm water to make pulsations more easily demonstrable.
2. Have the patient open and close his hand, held overhead or out in front, several times to exsanguinate it and then clench the fist tightly closed. If the patient is unconscious or under anesthesia, clench the fist passively for him.
3. Occlude both the radial and the ulnar artery; then have the patient lower and open his hand. When the hand is open, it should be relaxed; hyperextension of the wrist or hand should be avoided since it increases the tension of the palmar fascia, which compresses arterial microcirculation. Failure to relax the hand, or hyperextending the hand at the wrist, may cause a falsely abnormal Allen test.
4. Release the pressure over the ulnar artery and observe the open hand for return of color: Return within 6 seconds indicates patency of the ulnar artery and an intact arch. Delay of color from 7 to 15 seconds indicates that the ulnar artery filling is slow. Persistant blanching for up to 15 seconds or more indicates an incomplete ulnar arch. Those hands that have delayed or absent return of color with release of ulnar compression should not be used for radial artery cannulation.
5. To test for patency of the radial artery, repeat the test but release pressure over the radial artery instead of the ulnar artery.

Modified Allen Test With Doppler Plethysmography:[50,54] A Doppler instrument can be used to detect patency of the ulnar and radial artery by placing the probe over the artery to be examined. The normal arterial velocity signal is multiphasic, with a prominant systolic component and one or more diastolic sounds. If the artery examined is obstructed, velocity distal to the obstruction is attenuated, with a resultant decrease in the systolic component and loss of the normal diastolic sounds.

The continuity of the palmar arch may be assessed by noting the response of the arterial velocity in either the radial or ulnar artery during a period of compression of the opposite artery. Normally, the arterial velocity signal is increased in response to compression of the opposite artery at the wrist. If there is a lack of continuity between the radial and ulnar circulations in the hand, arterial compression will not result in an increase in velocity in the opposite artery. A similar response would result if the artery being compressed were congenitally absent or occluded by disease.

Doppler Assessment of the Superficial Palmar Arch (See Figure 11):

1. Place the probe between the heads of the third and fourth metacarpals, acutely angulated in the transverse plane.
2. Advance the probe proximally until maximal signal is

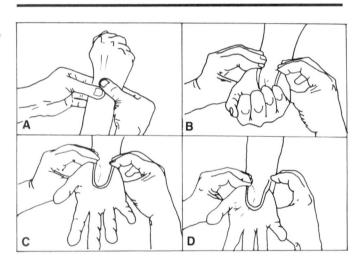

Figure 10. Modified Allen test. While patient's hand is held overhead with fist clenched to exsanguinate it, both radial and ulnar arteries are compressed (A). The hand is lowered (B) and opened (C). Pressure is then released over ulnar artery (D). Color should return to hand within 6 seconds, indicating patent ulnar artery and intact superficial palmar arch.

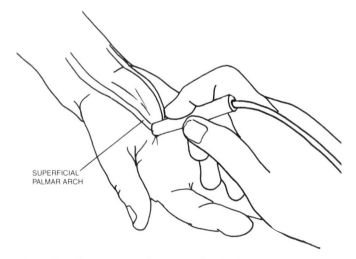

SUPERFICIAL PALMAR ARCH

Figure 11. Assessment of the superficial palmar arch with Doppler instrument.

obtained. The superficial palmar arch is usually found proximal to a line drawn along the medial edge of the outstretched thumb; the superficial palmar arch is the most distal palmar arch.

3. Compress the radial artery once the arch is identified; if there is no change or an actual increase in the signal following compression, it confirms that the palmar arch is complete and that it could be supplied (to a greater or lesser degree) by the ulnar artery. If the signal disappears when the radial artery is compressed, the arch is incomplete with no antegrade collateral circulation.

Method Using Plethymography:[55]

1. Place a finger pulse transducer over the patient's thumb and observe the resulting pulse contour on an oscilloscope.
2. Compress both the radial and ulnar arteries, which should result in immediate loss of the pulse on the monitor.
3. Release the pressure over the ulnar artery. Normally, there is an almost immediate return of the pulse contour on the monitor screen. The presence of pulsations in the thumb while the radial artery is still compressed is evidence of adequate ulnar artery circulation and an indication that the radial artery can be cannulated safely. Failure of the pulse to return after release of compression of the ulnar artery indicates that there is inadequate ulnar collateral circulation and that cannulation of that radial artery should be avoided.

Equipment Needed

1. A 20-gauge Teflon catheter-over-needle with non-tapered shaft, 1¼–2 inches (3.2–5.1 cm) in length.
2. Short arm board and roll of gauze.
3. Povidone-iodine solution.
4. Lidocaine 1% without epinephrine and 3-mL syringe with 25-gauge needle.
5. Sterile gloves and sterile drapes (face mask and hair cover for optimal asepsis).
6. Fluid-filled connecting tubing to transducer.

Technique (See Figure 12)

1. The patient's hand should be supported and dorsiflexed at the wrist approximately 60°, with both the hand and the lower forearm secured to a board. A roll of gauze behind the wrist will maintain dorsiflexion.
2. Locate the radial artery just proximal to the head of the radius.
3. Cleanse the area with povidone-iodine solution.
4. Wear sterile gloves and drape the area with sterile towels.

5. Infiltrate the skin over and to the sides of the radial artery with 1% lidocaine without epinephrine if the patient is awake.
6. A small skin incision at the point of insertion may facilitate entry of the catheter-needle device, but with a 20-gauge needle this is usually not necessary. Insert the catheter-over-needle device at about a 30° angle to the surface of the skin and advance the catheter and needle stylet into the artery until blood appears in the hub of the needle.
7. While holding the needle in the fixed position, advance the catheter-over-needle into the artery.
8. Remove the needle and attach the hub of the catheter to connecting tubing.
9. Tie the catheter securely in place with 3-0 or 4-0 silk sutures.
10. Remove packing from under the back of the wrist if used, and fix the wrist in a neutral position to the board. This is essential since one or two full flexions of the wrist joint can completely destroy an arterial line, and securing the hand in a dorsiflexed position for a prolonged period may lead to neuromuscular injury to the hand.
11. Apply povidone–iodine ointment to the skin at the site of insertion, and cover with a sterile dressing.

Complications

Thrombosis: Thrombosis is common, occurring in more than 50% of radial artery cannulations in some series.[17,20,24-27,33,56-58] Although the incidence of thrombosis is high, ischemic and necrotic complications are much less common, occurring in less than 1% of the patients with radial artery cannulas. However, one study group reported persistent ischemic symptoms in the hands of 50% of patients with radial arterial thrombosis.[21] Patient's with vasospastic (Raynaud's) disease and those with inadequate ulnar arches frequently exhibit ischemic and necrotic signs and symptoms

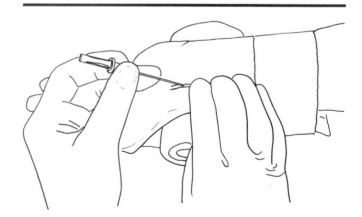

Figure 12. Cannulation of the radial artery.

following cannulation of radial arteries.[19,20,51] If there are frequent small emboli issuing from the site of catheter insertion to the distal vessels of the digits, they may lead to ischemic and necrotic symptoms even in the presence of an intact palmar collateral circulation. Thrombosis may occur several days following catheter removal. Despite the fact that thrombosis of the radial artery is frequent, patients whose progress has been followed for several months generally show evidence of recanalization.[18,20,51]

To prevent complications that might follow thrombosis of the radial artery, it is important not only to demonstrate adequate ulnar collateral circulation prior to insertion of the radial catheter but also to monitor daily the radial artery at the site of insertion with a Doppler instrument. Decreased or absent velocity signals may be due either to the catheter obstructing flow in the radial artery or, more commonly, to the presence of a thrombus at the site of catheterization. If the Doppler signal is lost or ischemic changes appear, the cannula should be removed.

Spasm has been implicated as a cause of obstruction to flow in the hand and may occur both during cannulation and following removal of the cannula.[1,59] However, Crossland and Neviaser reported that all instances of impaired circulation to the hand following radial artery cannulations were found to be due to thrombosis rather than to spasm.[51] If, following catheter removal, flow does not return to the hand after 1 hour, the artery should be explored for probable thrombectomy.[51,60] The radial pulse may still be palpable distal to a complete occlusion; in one series with a complete occlusion, the distal pulse was palpable in 64% of the subjects, while 10% had a radial pulse equal to the opposite radial pulses.[26]

Embolism: Embolism, both distally and cephalad, occurs less commonly than thrombosis. Although distal emboli may be demonstrated with angiography in up to 25% of patients following radial artery cannulation, objective and symptomatic digital ischemia is uncommon.[18,25,51,61] Whereas thrombosis with inadequate collateral flow to the hand is manifested by a pale and/or cold hand, emboli commonly produce cold and purple spots on the digits. These symptoms usually clear within approximately 1 week but may lead to digital gangrene, necessitating the amputation of fingers or, rarely, the entire hand.

Vigorous flushing with large volumes of flushing solution, especially when trying to correct a partially obstructed catheter with a damped arterial tracing, may allow the flushing solution to reach the central circulation and lead to either air or small-clot embolism in the brain. Lowenstein, et al., showed that it took only 7 mL of fluid vigorously flushed as a bolus into a radial catheter to reach the central circulation of the aortic arch; the volume of flushed solution correlated with arm length and patient height.[61] It is recommended that, if intermittent flushing is performed, meticulous care be used to avoid introducing any air bubbles into the system and that no more than 2 mL solution be flushed at any one time, and then at a relatively slow rate. Since a continuous flow system delivers approximately 1.5 mL/sec when the flush valve is open, flushes should be restricted to 2 seconds or less.[29,61,62]

Necrosis of Overlying Skin: Necrosis of the skin proximal to the site of insertion may also occur. The blood supply to the skin of the distal forearm arises directly from small branches of the radial artery without any collateral circulation. If the tip of the catheter interferes with these small branches, ischemia to the overlying skin may follow.[63,64] If temporarily localized blanching of the skin appears with intermittent flushing, the tip of the catheter should be repositioned until blanching no longer occurs. The following steps should be employed to decrease the incidence of skin necrosis: 1) The most distal site possible should be chosen for radial artery cannulation. 2) The smallest catheter size possible should be used to cause the least amount of obstruction of the lumen. 3) Prolonged cannulation should be avoided to prevent propagation of a thrombus from the catheter itself.

Aneurysm: Mathieu, et al., reported an aneurysm of the radial artery in a patient cannulated with an 18-gauge catheter. The catheter, which was inserted after repeated attempts at puncture, remained in place for 10 days; 18 days following removal of the catheter, an aneurysm of the radial artery was noted. It was repaired without sequelae.[65]

Cannulation of the Dorsalis Pedis Artery

Anatomy

The dorsalis pedis artery (Figure 13) extends subcutaneously as a continuation of the anterior tibial artery down the dorsum of the foot parallel and lateral to the extensor hallucis longus tendon. The lateral plantar artery, which is the terminal branch of the posterior tibial artery, is the other major artery supplying the foot. In most individuals, it supplies collateral flow via the main arterial arch of the foot, which is analogous to the palmar arch of the hand. However, in approximately 12% of the population, the dorsalis pedis artery is absent, usually bilaterally.[66-69]

Demonstration of Collateral Flow

Prior to cannulating the dorsalis pedis artery, it must be determined that adequate collateral flow to the distal foot is present. The foot should be warm, and immersion in water may be necessary. The simple procedure, which is analogous to the Allen test, follows:

1. Occlude the dorsalis pedis artery; then blanch the great toe by compressing the toenail for several seconds.

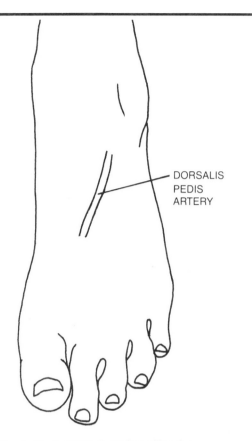

Figure 13. Anatomy of the dorsalis pedis artery.

2. Release pressure on the nail and observe for flushing; a rapid return of color indicates adequate collateral flow.[67]

A Doppler flow meter may also be used to assess flow in both the dorsalis pedis artery and the posterior tibial artery.[70]

Equipment Needed

1. A 20-gauge Teflon catheter-over-needle device with a nontapered shaft, approximately 1½ inches (3.8 cm) long.
2. Other equipment as for radial artery cannulation.

Technique (See Figure 14)

1. Check for presence of a dorsalis pedis artery pulse and for presence of adequate collateral flow as previously defined.
2. Cleanse the overlying skin with povidone–iodine solution.
3. Wear sterile gloves and drape the area with sterile towels.
4. Infiltrate the overlying skin with 1% lidocaine without epinephrine if the patient is awake.
5. Insert the catheter as for radial arterial cannulation.
6. Suture the catheter to the skin with 3-0 or 4-0 silk.
7. Cover the insertion site with povidone–iodine ointment and a sterile dressing.
8. Tape the line to the catheter firmly to the foot.

Complications

Thrombosis:[70] Thrombosis may occur in approximately 7% of those arteries cannulated. It can be recognized during cannulation by noting blanching of the great and second toes lasting longer than 15 seconds with compression of the posterior tibial artery. Occlusion can be confirmed with the Doppler technique by demonstrating retrograde flow distal to the site of cannula insertion in the dorsalis pedis artery, and with loss of the signal upon occlusion of the posterior tibial artery.

Part III: Bedside Pulmonary Artery Catheterization

Catheterization of the pulmonary artery can be performed easily and rapidly at the bedside using a balloon-tipped flow-directed thermodilution catheter. Continuous monitoring of the intravascular waveform allows the operator to follow the course of the catheter through the right heart and into the pulmonary artery to the wedge position. Although in a large number of patients this can be done without fluoroscopy, access to a fluroscope is advised.

Indications[71-76]

There are several general indications for pulmonary artery catheterization in critically ill patients. These include:

1. Measurement of right atrial (RA), pulmonary arterial (PA), and pulmonary artery occlusive pressures (PAOP);
2. Measurement of cardiac output by thermodilution (in addition, cardiac output can be determined by the Indocyanine Green indicator dilution technique, with

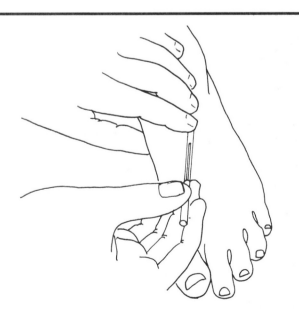

Figure 14. Cannulation of the dorsalis pedis artery.

injection either from the right atrium or the pulmonary artery, and sampling from a peripheral artery); and

3. Sampling of pulmonary arterial (mixed venous) blood.

With the data derived from the above measurements, one can evaluate both right and left ventricular function. This includes defining hemodynamic subsets,[77] separating cardiogenic from noncardiogenic pulmonary edema, diagnosing acute mitral regurgitation[77] and ruptured intraventricular septum,[78] and determining the response to therapeutic interventions with serial measurements.

Rationale

In the past, left heart filling pressure or occlusive pressure was estimated from the level of central venous pressure, clinical examination, and chest x-ray; cardiac output from mixed venous oxygen saturation or content; and intrapulmonary shunt from the difference between calculated alveolar and the measured arterial oxygen tensions — $(A - a)DO_2$, with A = alveolar; a = arterial; DO_2 = oxygen difference. Direct measurement is more accurate. The following section will develop the rationale for pulmonary artery catheterization and is based on the following principle: if one needs to know PAOP, cardiac output, or intrapulmonary shunt, each must be measured. Pulmonary artery catheterization allows this to be done.

Measurement of Occlusive Pressure

The level of the PAOP is a determinant of pulmonary congestion and the transfer of fluid from the pulmonary capillary bed to the interstitial space and alveoli. Measurement of PAOP allows a differential diagnosis between different forms of pulmonary edema and the establishment of physiologic limits beyond which fluid loading must not be allowed to proceed.[79,80] In the absence of either mechanical ventilation with positive end-expiratory pressure (PEEP) or obstruction in the pulmonary veins, PAOP pressure closely approximates left atrial mean pressure within ± 2 mmHg. In the additional absence of obstruction at the mitral valve, such as occurs with mitral stenosis or left atrial myxoma, PAOP also closely approximates mean left ventricular diastolic pressure.[81] However, in the presence of elevated left ventricular end-diastolic pressure (the height of ventricular filling pressure just before ventricular contraction) caused either by an increase in end-diastolic volume or a decrease in left ventricular compliance, PAOP does not as accurately reflect left ventricular end-diastolic pressure, which may significantly exceed mean PAOP. The height of the pulmonary artery a wave or the pulmonary capillary a wave, if recorded, is the most consistent accurate indirect index for sudden changes in

actual left ventricular end-diastolic pressure.[82,83] Nevertheless, the PAOP reflects mean left ventricular diastolic pressure and is therefore a useful index to estimate not only the possible risk of the development of pulmonary edema[79,83] but also left ventricular preload. On the other hand, preload is defined as end-diastolic volume, not pressure. In critically ill patients, ventricular compliance is altered, and there may be no correlation between pressure and volume, making it impossible to estimate left ventricular preload from PAOP.[84,85]

In the absence of marked tachycardia or pulmonary vascular disease, pulmonary artery diastolic pressure is equivalent to PAOP with the PA diastolic pressure exceeding the PAOP by no more than 5 mmHg; in this case, both reflect mean left ventricular filling pressure. By comparing pulmonary artery diastolic pressure with mean PAOP, it can be determined whether pulmonary vascular disease (with elevated pulmonary vascular resistance) is present and whether pulmonary artery diastolic pressure will reliably reflect mean left ventricular filling pressure. If the pulmonary artery diastolic pressure and the PAOP differ by less than 5 mmHg, the pulmonary artery diastolic pressure may be used to monitor mean left ventricular diastolic pressure. This may be especially important when the balloon ceases to function and PAOP can no longer be obtained. Unfortunately, increased pulmonary vascular resistance is common among the critically ill and this approximation frequently cannot be used.

In the presence of acute mitral regurgitation with the transmission of the large V wave into the pulmonary capillary and pulmonary arterial bed (Figure 15), mean PAOP pressure may exceed pulmonary artery diastolic pressure.[86] However, this would be detected by the presence of a large V wave on the downslope of the pulmonary artery pressure tracing or on the PAOP tracing. In this circumstance, the Z point (the pressure immediately after the A wave) will correlate best with left atrial pressure.[87] If PAOP exceeds PA diastolic pressure and a large V wave is absent, care must be taken to determine that one is actually measuring PAOP pressure rather than mean or damped pulmonary artery pressure (Figure 16), or a pseudo-occlusive pressure (see Figure 22).

Central venous or right atrial pressure can be measured easily by inserting a catheter into the superior vena cava or right atrium. Before the advent of pulmonary artery flotation catheters, central venous pressure frequently was used to estimate left ventricular filling pressures. However, Forrester, *et al.*, showed that in patients with acute myocardial infarction, central venous pressure does not reflect left ventricular filling pressure.[88] The level of central venous pressure correlates poorly both with the level of PAOP and with radiologic evidence of left ventricular failure. Furthermore, directional changes in central venous pressure are often of no value

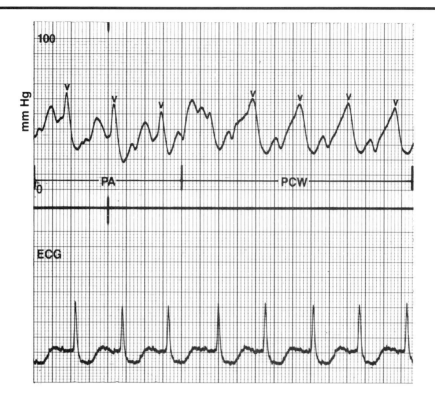

Figure 15. V waves in acute mitral regurgitation. V wave can be seen immediately following systolic pulmonary artery (PA) waveform but is more prominent on PAOP (PCW) waveform. The second wave in PA tracing can be identified as v wave; it peaks at same time, following R wave of ECG (0.4 second), as v wave on wedge tracing. Mean PAOP is higher than PA diastolic pressure.

in following the results of acute blood volume manipulation. There are several factors that increase central venous pressure.[89] The major determinants are pumping effectiveness of the right heart (central venous pressure is elevated with right ventricular failure) and increased venous return caused by either 1) decreased resistance to blood flow from the arteries to the veins, or 2) an increased ratio of blood volume to vascular blood holding capacity. Elevation of external cardiac pressure such as by cardiac tamponade, positive-pressure breathing,

pneumothorax, and obstructive pulmonary disease increases central venous pressure as well.

In the presence of normal right heart function, acute deterioration of left ventricular function will not be reflected in changes in central venous pressure. In critically ill patients, there may be no correlation between central venous pressure and PAOP, but PAOP may change while central venous pressure remains unchanged or moves in the opposite direction. This suggests that there may be discrepancies in function between the right and left sides of the heart in such patients.[90-92]

There are limitations to the use of the chest x-ray films in predicting the hemodynamic status of patients with acute myocardial infarction.[93,94] There is a good correlation between the level of PAOP and the development of interstitial and alveolar pulmonary edema, both occurring as PAOP rises above 20–25 mmHg. However, there may be a significant delay of up to 12 hours between the onset of elevation of the occlusive pressure and clinical and radiologic evidence of pulmonary edema. There may also be a significant lag between the lowering of occlusive pressure and the clearing of the x-ray film manifestations of pulmonary edema. This lag may persist as long as 4 days. These delays in appearance

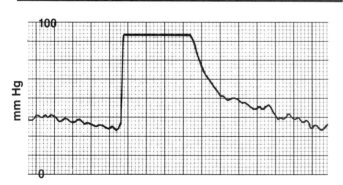

Figure 16. Damped pulmonary artery (PA) pressure tracing and damped square wave response during rapid flushing with continuous flush system.

and clearing of pulmonary edema on chest x-ray films are probably related to the fact that during the acute phase of myocardial infarction the hemodynamics change rapidly. It may take several hours for enough edema fluid to accumulate to be visible on chest x-ray film, and several days for the fluid to be resorbed.[93,94]

Even the clinical examination may fail to separate patients whose PAOP are high from those whose occlusive pressures are low. In one study,[95] 39% of patients who developed hypotension during the course of acute myocardial infarction were found to have low PAOP pressures. Yet a third of these patients with low occlusive pressures had third heart sounds on physical examination, and two thirds had abnormal pulmonary findings on chest x-ray film, including pulmonary vascular redistribution and frank pulmonary edema. Since the therapy in these patients was to expand the blood volume, treatment directed toward pulmonary edema based on the findings of the clinical examination would have been inappropriate. Because of the difficulty in estimating the PAOP even under stable circumstances, in the unstable situation, especially when rapidly activating vasoactive agents are being employed, serial measurement of the PAOP is essential.

The Need for Measuring Cardiac Output

Extreme reductions of cardiac output are manifested by signs of tissue hypoperfusion; hypotension may or may not be present. However, significant reduction of cardiac output may occur without these clinical findings and with the reading of a normal blood pressure. Blood pressure is the product of cardiac output and systemic vascular resistance; as cardiac output falls, blood pressure may be maintained by an elevation of systemic vascular resistance. In some patients, systemic vascular resistance becomes markedly elevated so that blood pressure is high despite a significantly decreased cardiac output. On the other hand, a patient may develop hypotension and still have a markedly elevated cardiac output, with the primary defect being a fall in systemic vascular resistance. Only by knowing left ventricular filling pressure, cardiac output, and calculated systemic vascular resistance can one rationally develop a therapeutic program.

The mixed venous O_2 content is commonly used to follow changes in cardiac output. According to the Fick relationship, cardiac output (CO) is equal to oxygen consumption (VO_2) divided by the arteriovenous oxygen content difference [$C(a-v)O_2$].

$$CO = \frac{VO_2}{C(a-v)O_2}$$

As long as oxygen consumption and the arterial oxygen content remain constant, the level of mixed venous oxygen content may accurately reflect the arteriovenous oxygen content difference and, thereby, cardiac output. There may be conditions, however, that alter the mixed venous oxygen content other than changes in cardiac output.

The oxygen content of blood is primarily a function of the hemoglobin concentration and oxygen saturation. With depression of either the hemoglobin or the oxygen saturation of arterial blood, arterial oxygen content will be reduced. If oxygen consumption and cardiac output are stable according to the Fick relationship, arteriovenous oxygen content difference must also remain constant. Yet, mixed venous oxygen content will be lower in this situation as well, independent of changes in cardiac output. For example, if arterial oxygen content (CaO_2) is reduced from 20 to 15 vol%, and $C(a-v)O_2$, cardiac output, and oxygen consumption remain the same, mixed venous content (CvO_2) will decrease by 5 vol% as well. Thus, in the absence of a change in cardiac output (or oxygen consumption), the fall in CvO_2 would suggest that cardiac output had fallen when, in fact, the only change may have been due to a fall in arterial oxygen content, i.e., a change due to a decrease in either hemoglobin or oxygen saturation.

On the other hand, patients may have changes in oxygen consumption caused by fever, seizures, shivering, or agitation as well as by excessive circulating catecholamines. According to the Fick equation, if cardiac output remains the same and oxygen consumption increases, arteriovenous oxygen content difference must increase and mixed venous oxygen content will fall. In conclusion: while simply following the mixed venous oxygen content may be helpful, it may also give misleading information regarding cardiac output.

Use of central venous oxygen content instead of mixed venous oxygen content in critically ill patients with shock or heart failure also introduces significant error, since there is a poor correlation in these patients between the level of mixed venous oxygen content and central venous oxygen content.[96,97] Obtaining mixed venous blood through a pulmonary artery catheter eliminates most sources of error that might arise.

If the goal of fluid resuscitation is to achieve an adequate cardiac output, PAOP alone cannot be considered a reliable guide to define the end point of resuscitation, and cardiac output must be measured. Nevertheless, the measurement of PAOP is important because it will detect the early onset of congestive heart failure or fluid overload[98-100] and guide the determination of optimal fluid administration. A ventricular function curve can be drawn during volume loading if stroke volume (cardiac output divided by heart rate) is measured at different levels of PAOP (Figure 17). The occlusive pressure that provides the best stroke volume then can be determined ("optimal filling pressure").[101,102]

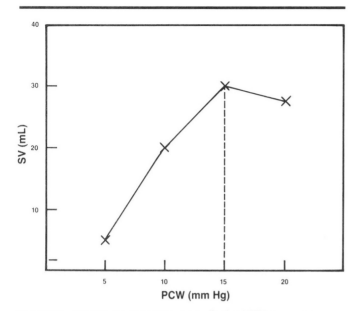

Figure 17. Ventricular function curve. Optimal filling pressure (dotted line) is PAOP (PCW) that produces highest stroke volume (SV).

One other pitfall must be described. The thermodilution technique measures the output of the right side of the heart, which is normally equal to that of the left. However, in the presence of an intracardiac shunt, right ventricular output does not equal left ventricular output; considerable error may be introduced in assuming that thermodilution cardiac output reflects systemic flow. Fortunately, one can determine the fraction of left-to-right or right-to-left shunt according to standard formulas and can correct the value for thermodilution cardiac output with this fraction to obtain systemic cardiac output.[76]

The Need for Measuring Intrapulmonary Shunt (Qs/Qt)

The difference between the calculated alveolar oxygen tension and the measured arterial oxygen tension, i.e., $(A-a)DO_2$, has been commonly employed as an indicator of the magnitude of venous mixture and intrapulmonary shunting. Only if mixed venous oxygen content is normal will the alveolar arterial oxygen tension difference correlate with intrapulmonary shunt. In critically ill patients, mixed venous oxygen content cannot be assumed to be normal, and the alveolar-arterial oxygen difference may reflect changes in mixed venous oxygen content rather than changes in intrapulmonary shunt.

The mixture that is pumped from the left ventricle is blood that is fully oxygenated as it passes through ventilated alveoli, and mixed venous blood which bypasses ventilated alveoli through right-to-left shunts (Figure 18). Any condition that increases intrapulmonary shunting will lower the arterial oxygen content and thereby increase the $(A-a)DO_2$.

Approximately 5% of right ventricular output is normally shunted from right to left through the lungs. Therefore, if mixed venous blood is markedly desaturated with a low oxygen content, even moderate amounts of this very desaturated blood passing through normal anatomic shunts (or slightly increased physiologic shunts) will contaminate fully oxygenated blood and lower the arterial oxygen content. This will also cause a widened alveolar arterial oxygen difference. If one assumes that the widened $(A-a)DO_2$ is due to a large right-to-left intrapulmonary shunt, when indeed it is due to mixed venous blood with a markedly lowered oxygen content bypassing alveoli through normal or slightly increased shunts, therapy directed toward intrapulmonary shunting (such as positive end-expiratory pressure) would be inappropriate and perhaps deleterious. Therefore, if it is necessary to know the magnitude of the intrapulmonary shunt for optimal therapy, it must be calculated. For the calculation, mixed venous oxygen content must be measured. Using an assumed arteriovenous oxygen content difference to determine the mixed venous oxygen content without actual measurement should be avoided since it will introduce a significant error in the shunt calculation.[103]

Technique

The following discussion includes a description of the catheter itself, the technique of insertion, and finally, pitfalls and complications of pulmonary artery catheterization.

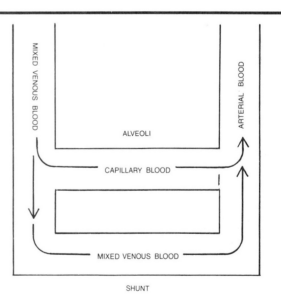

Figure 18. Mixed venous blood perfusing functioning alveolar units equilibrates with alveolar oxygen (capillary blood), but mixed venous blood that passes through intrapulmonary shunts is unchanged (mixed venous blood). Arterial blood is mixture of capillary blood and shunted mixed venous blood. Oxygen tension and content of arterial blood are therefore determined by both volume (quantity) and oxygen content (quality) of capillary blood and shunt blood.

Description of the Pulmonary Artery Catheter

Both 5 F and 7 F radiopaque pulmonary artery catheters are available, but the standard thermodilution catheter for adults is made only in 7 F size. This thermodilution catheter is 100 cm long and is marked with black rings at 10-cm intervals measured from the tip. It contains three lumens and a wire. The distal lumen terminates at the tip of the catheter and is used for measuring pulmonary artery and PAO pressure as well as for blood sampling. A proximal lumen terminates approximately 30 cm from the tip of the catheter and is used for injecting the thermal bolus into the right atrium for thermodilution cardiac output, for measuring right atrial or central venous pressure, for fluid and drug administration, and for blood sampling. There is a third lumen that terminates in a balloon near the catheter tip. The balloon is inflated with 1.25–1.50 mL air. This distention facilitates advancement of the catheter during insertion and allows measurement of PAOP once the catheter is in the pulmonary artery. The wire terminates in a thermistor bead 3.5–4.0 cm proximal to the tip and provides electrical connections between the thermistor and the cardiac output computer. This thermistor allows continuous measurement of pulmonary artery blood temperature (body core temperature) as well as measurement of cardiac output by thermodilution. Many of the catheters require a specific computer for determination of cardiac output by thermodilution, although some are made to function with cardiac output computers of different manufacturers. Catheters made by different manufacturers may vary slightly and the reader is advised to consult the package insert for the catheter being used.

Recently, 7.5 F catheters have become available with either an additional right atrial lumen for fluid administration or a right ventricular lumen for fluid administration, pressure monitoring, or passing a probe for pacing the right ventricle.

Equipment Needed for Insertion

The following checklist summarizes equipment needed for catheterization:

1. Pulmonary artery catheter.
2. Two three-way stopcocks to connect to the proximal right atrial and the distal pulmonary arterial ports.
3. Pressure monitoring lines to be connected to the transducer.
4. Syringe for balloon inflation.
5. Equipment for percutaneous catheter sheath insertion or cutdown.
6. Sterile gowns, drapes, gloves, mask, and hair cover.
7. Transducer/oscilloscope equipment.

Preparation

If the patient is on mechanical ventilation prior to catheter insertion, the ventilatory settings and alarms should be checked, the connecting tubing emptied of water, and the trachea suctioned. Since insertion of the pulmonary artery catheter may cause cardiac dysrhythmias, an IV line must be in place. Lidocaine, atropine, and a defibrillator must be available at the bedside, and the patient should be monitored continuously with an electrocardiogram. The transducer and connecting tubing should be set up, the transducer leveled, and the electrical equipment tested, zeroed, and calibrated before the catheter is inserted.

Careful preparation of the area of insertion with povidone–iodine solution, as for any other surgical procedure, should be performed. Since the catheter may remain in the patient for several days, strict attention to aseptic technique during insertion is vital to minimizing subsequent infection (see Chapter 10). The operator and assistants should be fully gowned and should wear hair covers, face masks, and sterile gloves. In addition, once the area of insertion is adequately prepared with antiseptic solution, the largest possible area should be draped. This generally includes most of the bed on which the patient is lying. Such meticulous preparation allows the operator to have a large sterile area on which to keep all equipment and to test the catheter. It also minimizes the chance of contamination of the long, coiled catheter during insertion.

Site of Insertion

The pulmonary artery catheter can be inserted through a cutdown into a median basilic vein in the antecubital fossa, or it may be inserted percutaneously via an insertion sheath through either the internal jugular vein, the subclavian vein, or the femoral vein. The choice of site of insertion depends on the skill and preference of the operator as well as the urgency of the situation. As a rule, percutaneous catheter insertion can be performed in a shorter period of time than by a venous cutdown. However, the use of the venous cutdown avoids the hazards of pneumothorax and hemorrhage that exist with internal jugular or subclavian insertions. The major difficulty with insertion of the catheter through a cutdown in the antecubital fossa is that the catheter tends to become dislodged more easily with motion of the arm, requiring the patient's arm to be restrained. However, the venous cutdown has become the preferred route in cardiovascular patients because puncture of vessels in noncompressible regions is dangerous if thrombolytic agents have been given and represent a contraindication to their use for several days.[104]

It may be more difficult to insert the catheter through the femoral vein; the catheter has to traverse a long distance before arriving at the right heart and tends to become deflected by the various veins entering the inferior vena cava. In addition, the femoral approach may place the patient at greater risk for catheter-related infection. If the femoral approach is used, careful skin preparation and attention to aseptic technique should minimize the risk of infection, as with other sites of insertion.

Testing of the Catheter Prior to Insertion

Once the insertion site has been prepared and the patient and the bed are draped, the catheter should be removed from its container, using sterile technique. With some cardiac output computers, the thermistor can be tested by connecting the catheter connector cable from the cardiac output computer to the thermistor attachment at the end of the catheter. Either the ambient room temperature will be displayed on the computer or an indicator for thermistor continuity will appear. Since the products of various manufacturers differ, the operator must be familiar with his or her own equipment.

The balloon is tested by inflating it to the recommended inflation volume. For general purposes, testing should be with air, but if there is a possibility of right-to-left shunt within the heart, carbon dioxide should be used. Never use liquid for balloon inflation. In order to be certain there are no leaks in the balloon, it can be inflated under water. If air bubbles appear around the balloon, the catheter should be discarded. A three-way stopcock should be attached to both the right atrial or CVP (proximal) and pulmonary artery (distal) lumen, and pressure monitoring lines attached to the stopcocks and to the transducers. Both lumens should be flushed with sterile saline solution containing 2–4 units of heparin per milliliter so that fluid remains in the catheter and the lumens are free of air bubbles.

Inserting the Catheter

There are several principles to be followed in catheter insertion. To avoid damage to the catheter or the balloon when inserting it through a cutdown, employ a vessel dilator or disposable vein guide. Never use forceps on the catheter. To avoid damaging the balloon during percutaneous insertions through a catheter introducer, use an 8 F catheter sheath for the 7 F pulmonary artery catheter. Some manufacturers, however, provide catheters with a tapered tip that can be passed through an introducer that is the same French size as the catheter. The specific instructions for each catheter should be consulted. During insertion, the balloon should be fully inflated when the catheter is in the right ventricle; this will minimize ventricular irritability. Do not exceed the recommended volume for balloon inflation as balloon rupture can result. Always deflate the balloon prior to withdrawing the catheter to avoid damage to intracardiac structures.

In order to determine the distance of insertion before reaching the level of the superior vena cava and the right atrium, use surface markers as illustrated in Figure 16, Chapter 11. The distance from the tip of the catheter to the point of skin insertion can be noted using the markers on the catheter for every 10-cm length. Generally, if the catheter is inserted from the internal jugular or the subclavian vein, it should be in the right atrium after about 15–20 cm. If the catheter is inserted from the arm, the right atrium should be reached after advancing the catheter approximately 40 cm if from the right, and 50 cm if from the left, antecubital fossa.

Introduce the catheter by cutdown or percutaneously through a suitable sheath. As the catheter approaches the central circulation either from above or from below, it may be helpful to partially inflate the balloon with approximately half the recommended volume to facilitate its passage.

While monitoring the pressure waveform from the distal lumen, gently advance the catheter into the vena cava and the right atrium. Once the catheter is in the right atrium, inflate the balloon to its full volume. With continuous waveform monitoring, advance the catheter carefully through the right atrium into the right ventricle, the pulmonary artery, and to the pulmonary artery wedge position (Figure 19).

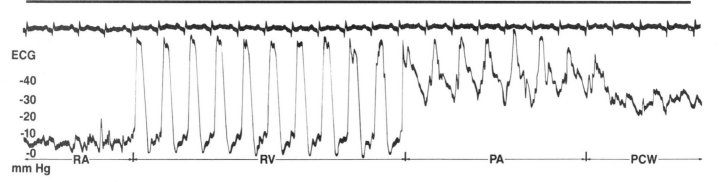

Figure 19. Pressure waveforms recorded as pulmonary artery catheter is advanced through right atrium (RA) and right ventricle (RV) into pulmonary artery (PA) and to PAOP (PCW) position.

When the catheter is in the vena cava, the waveform is usually relatively damped. If the patient is asked to cough, there should be an abrupt increase in pressure, indicating that the catheter tip is within the veins of the thorax. When the catheter enters the right atrium, the amplitude of the waveform should be unchanged, but venous waves should still be recognized. As the catheter passes the tricuspid valve and enters the right ventricle, there is an abrupt increase in systolic pressure which falls rapidly toward zero and then plateaus prior to the next abrupt rise with systole. The diastolic waveform in the right ventricle has the appearance of a square root sign. When the catheter enters the pulmonary artery, the systolic pressure remains the same (in the absence of obstruction at the pulmonic valve), but the waveform is that of an arterial pressure with a dicrotic notch and a gradual fall during diastole before the next abrupt upstroke. The diastolic pressure is higher in the pulmonary artery than in the right ventricle. When the catheter reaches the occlusive position, the waveform should again become damped with the appearance of a and v waves; the mean PAOP should be equal to or less than pulmonary artery diastolic pressure. Once the proper position is reached, the balloon should be deflated, at which time the waveform should be equal to or less than pulmonary artery diastolic pressure. Once the occlusive position is reached, the balloon should be deflated, at which time the waveform should abruptly change from that of occlusive pressure to that of the pulmonary artery.

The following are criteria to confirm proper position:

1. The ability to flush the catheter before inflating the balloon, which excludes the possibility of catheter obstruction.
2. The disappearance of the typical pulmonary artery pressure tracing when the balloon is inflated and its reappearance promptly after deflation.
3. The presence of a PAOP lower than or equal to pulmonary artery diastolic pressure.[105]
4. Oxygen tension or saturation of blood drawn from the occlusive position greater than or equal to that of systemic arterial blood.

In the average-sized adult, if the catheter is inserted from the internal jugular or the subclavian vein, the pulmonary artery should be entered after about 50 cm of the catheter has been inserted; if from the arm or the femoral vein, the pulmonary artery should be entered after about 70 cm of catheter has been inserted. Insertion of the catheter beyond this length without reaching the pulmonary artery suggests that the catheter is coiling up either in the right atrium or the right ventricle. If the pulmonary artery is not entered, deflate the balloon and withdraw the catheter back to the right atrium. Since the 7 F catheter has a preformed curve to the tip, it is important to insert the catheter with the curve pointing in such a way to easily pass through the right atrium, the right ventricle, and into the pulmonary artery.

Once the occlusive position has been reached, alternately inflate and deflate the balloon and position the catheter so that PAOP waveform can be obtained with full inflation of the balloon. Always inflate the balloon slowly while monitoring the waveform, and stop inflation once wedge waveform appears. Inflation beyond this point may lead to pulmonary artery rupture.

In conditions of low-output state, tricuspid regurgitation, or pulmonary hypertension, it may be difficult or impossible to pass the catheter into the pulmonary artery. On occasion, having the patient take deep breaths will facilitate the passage of the catheter; if unsuccessful, fluoroscopy will have to be used.

As the catheter remains in the vascular compartment, it softens. At times it may be necessary to flush the catheter with cold solution in order to stiffen it and make passage easier. In addition, if several attempts at passage are unsuccessful, it may be necessary to remove and replace the catheter.

Cardiac arrhythmias that appear during insertion of the catheter usually disappear once the catheter is withdrawn from that chamber or passed through that chamber into the next. Arrhythmias most commonly occur when the catheter is in the right ventricle; therefore, when the catheter is in this position, the balloon must be inflated so that the catheter tip is completely covered, reducing the likelihood of stimulating the right ventricular endocardium and producing cardiac arrhythmias. If the arrhythmia does not cease following withdrawal of the catheter, drug therapy or countershock may have to be used. In addition, transient right bundle branch block may occur as the catheter tip passes through the right ventricle. This condition can be especially hazardous in a patient who has preexisting left bundle branch block since it may cause complete heart block.[106] In such patients it is prudent to insert a temporary transvenous pacing catheter before attempting insertion of a pulmonary artery catheter.

Once the catheter is in place in the pulmonary artery, secure the catheter with suture. If a catheter sheath introducer was used, it may have to be pulled back, although now sheaths are made with side ports and can be left in place if fluid is continuously infused via the port. Each time the catheter or sheath is manipulated, and while the catheter is being secured, reconfirm that PAOP can be obtained to assure that the catheter has not been moved. A soon as the catheter is secured, obtain a chest x-ray film to document the location of the catheter tip. This procedure will exclude the presence of pneumothorax or other complications if the insertion was by way of the internal jugular or subclavian technique. If the catheter was inserted from the arm, immobilize the arm.

The pulmonary artery waveform must be continuously monitored so that inadvertant wedging can be recognized immediately and the catheter withdrawn. Failure to withdraw the catheter from an occlusive position may lead to pulmonary infarction.

After the catheter has been in place for some time, if the tip has slipped back toward the pulmonic valve so that occlusive pressures can no longer be obtained, do not advance the catheter. Bacteria may be introduced from either that part of the catheter outside the patient or from the skin insertion site itself. Recently, special catheter sleeves have been developed that are said to allow the catheter to be repositioned aseptically. There is little data to provide reassurance that repositioning of a catheter, especially after 24–48 hours, can be accomplished aseptically with the sleeves.

Pitfalls[107]

Despite the fact that a specific numerical value, relating either to intravascular pressure or cardiac output, can be obtained with hemodynamic monitoring, one must continually be wary of the error within the system. Such error can be introduced at many points — from the transducer, the connecting tubing, the catheter itself, the balloon, the location of the catheter tip within the chest, and from the effects of changes in intrathoracic pressure. Several of these pitfalls will be discussed in the following section.

The Transducer

The transducer must be calibrated frequently using a mercury manometer with a sterile connector. It should be calibrated at least prior to each use and perhaps daily while in use. The dome must be screwed on tightly to ensure contact between the dome and the transducer diaphragm. The fluid-filled system must be completely free of air.

Zero Reference Point

The level of the right atrium is the standard zero reference point for the transducer. The level of the right atrium, or the phlebostatic axis (Figure 20), is defined as

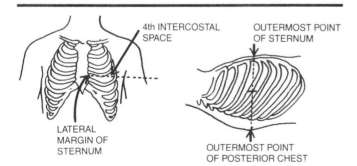

Figure 20. Level of right atrium, or phlebostatic axis, is the junction between transverse plane of body passing through fourth intercostal space at lateral margin of sternum and a frontal plane of body passing through midpoint of line from outermost point of sternum to outermost point of posterior chest. (Adapted from Woods, et al,[108] Used by permission.)

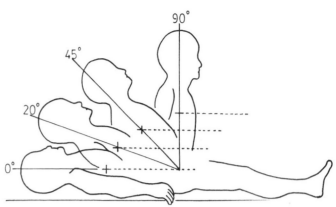

Figure 21. Phlebostatic level (. . . . .) passes through phlebostatic axis (+) and is parallel with horizon as patient moves from supine to erect sitting position. (Adapted from Woods, et al.[108] Used by permission.)

the junction between the transverse plane of the body passing through the fourth intercostal space at the lateral margin of the sternum, and a frontal plane of the body passing through the midpoint of a line from the outermost point of the sternum to the outermost point of the posterior chest.[109,110] With the patient supine, this is the midaxillary line. However, in a position other than supine, the transducer can be zeroed at the phlebostatic level (a plane which rotates about the phlebostatic axis as the patient moves from a flat to an erect position). The phlebostatic level passes through the axis and is parallel with the horizon. If the transducer is zeroed at this phlebostatic level, there should be no significant change in pressures measured with the patient being either supine or erect (Figure 21). However, a recent study defining the effect of body position on pulmonary artery and PAOP demonstrated that there is little change in pressures when the patient is either supine or elevated to 45°; but when the patient is erect with legs dangling over the edge of the bed, there may be a slight decrease in intravascular pressures as measured at the phlebostatic axis. Nevertheless, the difference in pressure between the supine position and the erect sitting position may be only 1 or 2 mmHg.[108]

Although it may not be possible to accurately compare absolute values from patient to patient using the phlebostatic axis, at least the patient can serve as his own control; and changes in pressures will have an accurate reference point. The phlebostatic axis should be marked with indelible ink on each patient.

Location of the Catheter Tip Relative to the Left Atrial Level

Close approximation of left atrial pressure by PAOP requires a blood-filled segment of pulmonary vasculature to serve as an extension of the catheter system. When any part of the system distal to the catheter tip is emptied of blood, PAOP no longer reflects left atrial pressure. Whether pulmonary capillaries contain blood is a function of pulmonary artery pressure, alveolar pressure, left atrial pressure, and the hydrostatic relation of these vessels to the left atrium. Several studies have shown that pulmonary artery catheters placed below the left atrium correctly record PAOP that are equal to left atrial pressures at all levels of positive end-expiratory pressure (PEEP). However, pulmonary artery catheters placed above the left atrium may record PAOP higher than left atrial pressure in the presence of PEEP.

In the zones of the lung where alveolar pressure exceeds both pulmonary artery and pulmonary venous pressure, the collapsible pulmonary capillaries are closed with no flow (Zone 1).[111,112] In the center of the lung, where alveolar pressure is greater than pulmonary venous pressure but less than pulmonary arterial pressure, flow is determined by the difference between pulmonary arterial and alveolar pressure (Zone 2). In the lower zones of the lung, all capillaries are held open because pulmonary venous pressure is higher than alveolar pressure, and flow is determined by the difference between pulmonary artery pressure and pulmonary venous pressure (Zone 3).

A pulmonary artery catheter located in Zones 1 or 2 will not reflect left atrial pressure. Zone 1 is without perfusion before the balloon is inflated, and the vascular segment downstream from the catheter in Zone 2 will change to Zone 1 as soon as the balloon is inflated. In both instances, alveolar pressure exceeds PCW pressure. A catheter located in the upper or midzones of the lung will also detect a change in alveolar pressure transmitted to its tip with each increment of PEEP, since its initial downstream pressure is alveolar pressure.

When a catheter is referenced to atmosphere at the vertical height of the left atrium and is not in the lower zones (Zone 3), the pressure recorded at the transducer level is a function of the vertical height of the column of fluid in the catheter above the left atrium and any alveolar pressure transmitted to the catheter. Therefore, lateral x-ray films must be taken to establish the position of the catheter with respect to the left atrium. If it is found to be above the left atrium, the catheter should be removed to a position below the left atrium.[113-116]

Recently, Berryhill and Benumof have demonstrated in research with dogs that the discrepancy between PAOP and left atrial pressure appears to be minimized during spontaneous breathing with PEEP (so-called CPAP, or continuous positive airway pressure), even if the catheter tip is above the left atrium.[117] This suggests that PAOP should be measured either during the spontaneous breathing phase of intermittent mandatory ventilation (IMV) or during CPAP.

Balloon Problems

In one study, 15 of 16 catheters located peripherally showed eccentric inflation of the balloon; in 9 of those instances, the waveform did not change on inflation of the balloon.[118] In the remaining 6, the waveform became flat either without a change of pressure or with a gradual increase of pressure. One patient with an eccentric balloon inflation developed hemoptysis following repeated measurements of PAOP. Nine of the 16 balloons inflated normally following withdrawal of the catheter tip to a large branch of the pulmonary artery. In the cadaveric lung, 5 of 10 balloons showed eccentric inflation when the catheter was advanced to a smaller artery, while a normal inflation was observed when the catheter was withdrawn to the large arteries.

The ideal position of the Swan-Ganz catheter is in a large pulmonary artery from which it can advance into the occlusive position on inflation of the balloon but slip back to the previous location on deflation. When located in smaller vessels, particularly at a bifurcation, the catheter may be fixed prematurely (with only partial inflation of the balloon) before the vessel is occluded. Further inflation can cause an eccentricity in the partially inflated balloon if it expands to the less resistant area. A balloon of this type at a bifurcation may not occlude the lumen; it may, instead, force the catheter tip to impinge on a vessel wall, resulting in a loss of pulmonary artery waveform. If a continuous flush system is used, a gradual increase of pressure higher than the mean pulmonary artery pressure may be seen (so-called pseudo-occlusive pressure) in the presence of impingement of the catheter tip (Figure 22). The pressure recorded is the pressure in the flush system, not the pulmonary artery. Repeated overinflation, or forced inflation of the balloon to wedge in a smaller pulmonary artery or a vasoconstricted vessel, may rupture the pulmonary artery, particularly when there is an eccentric inflation of the balloon. Most reports of pulmonary artery rupture are related to catheters that were in peripheral locations.

Catheters that initially are in correct position may subsequently advance peripherally. Poor wedging of the balloon may occur following the introduction of high PEEP, high tidal volume ventilation, positional changes of the patient, coughing, or even movement of the catheter tip with contraction of the heart.[119] Distortion of surrounding lung tissue due to existing disease might also be a causative factor in catheter mislocation.

In addition, forced water injection for cardiac output measurements may relocate the catheter peripherally. Catheter position should be checked daily by x-ray film to insure an accurate wedge and to avoid perforation of the vessel. The balloon should be deflated and the catheter pulled back gradually if 1) the catheter is located peripherally, 2) a pseudo-occlusive pressure tracing is obtained when the balloon is inflated, or 3) the inflation

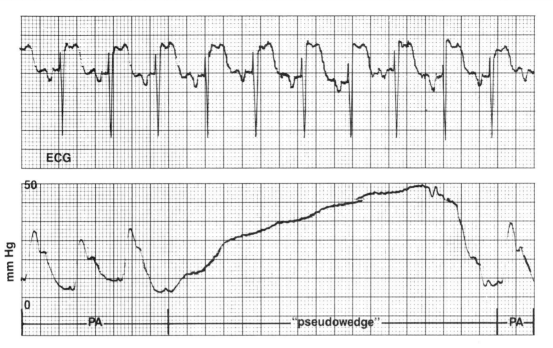

Figure 22. Pseudo-occlusive ("pseudowedge") pressure tracing recorded with inflation of balloon in presence of impingement of catheter tip.

volume necessary to wedge the balloon is significantly less than the maximum recommended. If it is pulled back rapidly, the loop of the catheter in the ventricle will tighten, which may eventually pull the catheter back farther than desired into the main pulmonary artery or even into the right ventricle.

Changes in Intraluminal Pressure With Respiration

During spontaneous breathing, and especially exaggerated during deep breathing, the pressure within the pulmonary artery (the intraluminal pressure) follows intrathoracic pressure. During deep inspiration, the measured intraluminal pressure is significantly lower than during exhalation. If the patient is being treated with mechanical ventilation, intrathoracic pressure will become positive during the inspiratory cycle of the ventilator and falsely elevate intraluminal pressure. If the patient is receiving intermittent mandatory ventilation (IMV), the intrathoracic pressure will become subatmospheric during spontaneous inspiration, thus lowering the measured intraluminal pressure. During the inspiratory cycle of the ventilator, intrathoracic and, therefore, intraluminal pressures are elevated. If an electronic digital pressure readout is used, significant error may be introduced into the reading. The electronic equipment records the highest pressure as the systolic pressure and the lowest pressure as diastolic; both may be incorrect.

Intraluminal pressure should be recorded at end-expiration in all patients, both those breathing spontaneously and those on mechanical ventilation, to eliminate the artifact of the positive-negative intrathoracic pressure swings.[120,121] This may be accomplished either by reading the pressure from the oscilloscope or from a paper writeout. Simultaneous recording of intraluminal pressure and airway pressure may facilitate identifying the point of end-expiration (Figure 23).[121]

Intraluminal vascular pressure minus intrapleural pressure represents transmural, or effective, vascular filling pressure. Change in intraluminal vascular pressures will reflect change in transmural vascular pressures only if intrapleural pressure remains constant. The extent of airway pressure transmission to the intrapleural space will depend on airway resistance and lung and thoracic wall compliance; it may vary greatly from patient to patient. The more intrapleural pressure varies from normal, the greater the error in interpreting intraluminal pressure as a reflection of transmural or effective vascular filling pressure.[122,123]

In a patient with chronic obstructive pulmonary disease with both airway obstruction and loss of lung recoil, markedly positive intrathoracic pressures can be produced during the active process of expiration, and intraluminal vascular pressures recorded as mean or average can be elevated because of the addition of this positive intrathoracic pressure.[124] Similarly, patients treated with positive end-expiratory pressure (PEEP) will have raised intraluminal vascular pressures, yet trans-

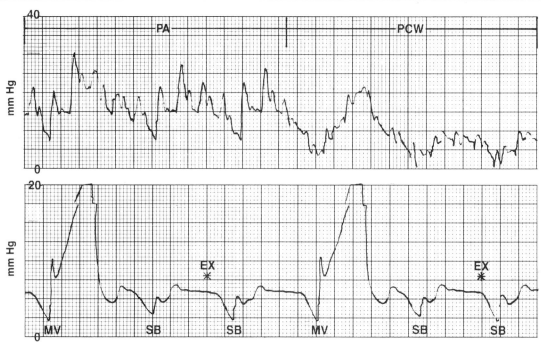

Figure 23. **Changes in pulmonary artery (PA) and PAOP (PCW) pressure induced by changes in intrathoracic pressure during both spontaneous breathing (SB) and intermittent mandatory ventilation (MV).** To eliminate artifact, intraluminal pressures should be recorded at end-expiration (EX). Upper tracing is intraluminal pressure; lower tracing is airway pressure recorded simultaneously (with 7.5 mmHg or 10 cmH$_2$O positive end-expiratory pressure).

mural filling pressure may remain unchanged or actually decreased.

Intrapleural pressure can be measured either by an intrapleural catheter[122,123] or by an esophageal balloon.[125] The intrapleural catheter probably gives a more accurate measurement of intrapleural pressure, but during insertion there is always the hazard of pneumothorax. Supine esophageal pressure reflects intrathoracic pressure with reasonable accuracy if there is proper balloon design and use, although pressures in the supine position may be higher than in the upright position, presumably due to the weight of the contents of the mediastinum.[126,127]

Transmural or effective vascular filling pressure is equal to intraluminal vascular pressure minus intrapleural or intraesophageal pressure. A significant number of patients with acute respiratory failure being treated with mechanical ventilation and PEEP have elevated intraluminal filling pressure, often exceeding 20 mmHg. However, by measuring intrapleural pressure and by calculating the transmural pressure, one may find an actual decrease in cardiac filling pressure, necessitating transfusion in those patients. On the other hand, patients who have decreased lung compliance may not have intrapleural pressure elevated significantly by PEEP; in these patients, elevated intraluminal pressure reflects increased filling pressure, indicating intravascular hypervolemia, congestive heart failure, or both. Despite similar

intraluminal vascular pressure in these two groups of patients, appropriate therapy in each of these extremes is quite different.[122,123] In the patient with chronic obstructive pulmonary disease who exhibits large swings in intrathoracic pressure with spontaneous breathing, transmural pressure is more useful as an estimation of left ventricular function or pulmonary venous hypertension.[124,128]

In a study designed to determine whether there were significant changes in intravascular pressure measured both on and off PEEP, a group of patients with a variety of illnesses (including postoperative complications, pulmonary disease, neurologic disease, and cardiovascular disease) had PAOP recorded. The patients were then disconnected from the ventilator for 10–15 seconds.[129] No significant change was noted in PAOP on and off the ventilator, even with PEEP. However, in 21% of the patients there was a delayed progressive elevation of PAOP throughout the recording. This was observed in the setting of underlying heart disease, presumably reflecting the higher filling pressures required by the failing left ventricle in order to accommodate the increased venous return that resulted from the restoration of intrathoracic pressures to atmospheric levels.[130] Results of the study suggested that it is not necessary to discontinue PEEP or mechanical ventilation to record PAOP.[129] However, in another study, a group of patients was investigated who had acute respiratory failure requiring PEEP ranging from 5 to 25 cmH_2O. It was demonstrated that for every 5 cm of water increase in PEEP, PAOP increased by 1 mmHg. Beyond 25 cm of PEEP, the correlation decreased significantly.[131]

Whether or not PEEP raises intraluminal vascular pressure depends on pulmonary compliance. In the patient with severe respiratory failure with markedly decreased pulmonary compliance, PAOP may not differ much on and off PEEP. On the contrary, the patient with highly compliant lungs will have a marked increase in intraluminal PAOP as PEEP is increased. It may be appropriate to define the alteration in pressure caused by PEEP by measuring PAOP with PEEP, then momentarily disconnecting PEEP to determine the change in PAOP. The patients who show a marked disparity between pressures recorded on and off PEEP might best be managed with an esophageal balloon or an intrapleural catheter to accurately measure effective vascular filling pressure.[122,125]

In the patient treated with PEEP for respiratory failure, even if transmural or effective vascular PAOP is determined by measuring intrapleural pressure, one cannot be certain that this reflects left ventricular preload. Although left ventricular diastolic pressure and PAOP are commonly used to reflect left ventricular preload, preload is defined as left ventricular end-diastolic volume or fiber length. In the presence of acute respiratory failure and high PEEP, pulmonary vascular resistance may be elevated. This leads to right ventricular dilatation, which compresses the left ventricle within the rigid pericardium and alters the pressure–volume relationships (compliance) of the left ventricle. Serial PAOP measurements that become elevated over the course of time may give the misleading impressions of left ventricular failure when, in fact, left ventricular diastolic volume or preload is actually decreased because of the decrease in left ventricular compliance.[132-135]

Errors in the Sampling of Blood From the Pulmonary Artery

Ability to obtain true mixed venous blood from the pulmonary artery depends on the position of the catheter, the flow past the catheter from the more proximal pulmonary artery, the relative resistance to the flow from the pulmonary capillary bed, and the proximity of the tip of the catheter to the gas exchange area. Rapid withdrawal rates of blood from the distal tip of the pulmonary artery catheter may draw in oxygenated blood from the capillary bed and cause falsely elevated mixed venous PO_2 values. However, at withdrawal rates of 3 mL/min, results of one study showed no contamination of pulmonary arterial blood with pulmonary capillary blood.[98] In order to define whether pulmonary arterial blood is contaminated with pulmonary capillary blood, the pulmonary venous CO_2 is measured after ventilation has been stable for more than 10 minutes. If the mixed venous PCO_2 is equal to or lower than a simultaneous arterial PCO_2, it suggests contamination of pulmonary arterial blood by the pulmonary capillary blood. Nevertheless, blood drawn from atelectatic areas of the lung would not be subject to this artifact since equilibrium with alveolar gas is prevented.[136]

Complications of Pulmonary Artery Catheterization

Complications of pulmonary artery catheterization include pulmonary vascular damage (thrombosis, hemorrhage, and pulmonary infarction), entanglement or damage to intracardiac structures, cardiac arrhythmias, endocarditis and sepsis, catheter fracture, balloon malfunction, misplacement of catheters outside the right heart, and electrical hazards. Some of these complications will be discussed in the following section.

Thrombotic Complications

Thrombosis may develop around the catheter and occlude any of the veins through which the catheter has been inserted.[137,138] Heparin bonding of the catheter may reduce the incidence of thrombosis.[139] In a patient who has a pulmonary artery catheter inserted via an antecubital cutdown, or percutaneously via the subclavian or internal jugular veins, the development of unilateral upper extremity edema and/or unilateral neck pain and venous distention should suggest deep venous thrombosis of the upper extremity and possibly the superior vena cava.[137]

Pulmonary infarction may occur from thrombus developing around the catheter (either from its tip or more proximally), with emboli passing to the pulmonary circulation, by embolization of thrombus that has formed within the catheter, or by catheter occlusion of a branch of the pulmonary artery.[140] The incidence of thrombus forming about the pulmonary artery catheter with subsequent pulmonary embolization is increased in patients with disseminated intravascular coagulation,[141] decreased cardiac output, hypotension, and congestive heart failure.[141-143]

There are several observations that might suggest obstruction of the pulmonary vasculature by thrombosis or embolism. Damping of the pressure tracings with only intermittent patency of the catheter present after flushing with saline solution may be observed even with thrombus or embolus restricted to the vascular segment containing the catheter. Manifestations of more extensive vascular obstruction may include falling systemic blood pressure, urine output, and the development of hypercapnia while minute ventilation remains constant (indicating an increase in dead space ventilation); widening of the alveolar-arterial oxygen tension difference, an increase in intrapulmonary shunt, and a shift in the electrical axis of the ECG toward the right.[141]

Persistent wedging of the pulmonary artery catheter may in itself produce pulmonary infarction or may predispose to *in situ* thrombosis. Wedging may occur because of the tendency of the catheter to advance into the lung due to the rhythmic contractions of the heart and the pulsatile propelling force of the blood flow. The loop in the right heart tends to become smaller, causing the end of the catheter to be propelled into narrower pulmonary artery branches; especially during the first 12 hours of catheterization. Persistant inflation of the balloon can occur even though the stopcock is open if the air lumen of the catheter is on the inside of a moderate bend which traps air beyond that point, presumably caused by a pinching off of the air lumen, leaving the balloon filled. In order to prevent pulmonary infarction from persistent wedging of the catheter, the following measures should be taken:

1. Since the catheter loop tends to tighten and the tip migrates into the distal pulmonary artery with time (especially during the first 24 hours), the pulmonary artery waveform should be monitored continuously.
2. Frequent chest x-ray films should be obtained with attention to the position of the catheter tip and to the possibility of air within the balloon.

If a PAOP is obtained with less than the recommended inflation volume on subsequent balloon inflations, it is probable that the catheter has advanced too far and should be partially withdrawn. A constant infusion of heparinized saline solution should be maintained at all times.[140]

A recent study has demonstrated that thrombus may form in the central circulation around pulmonary artery catheters in most, if not all, patients. Pulmonary artery catheters that had been inserted percutaneously via the internal jugular vein preoperatively into patients undergoing cardiac surgery were examined through a right atriotomy approximately 2 hours after insertion. All were found to have thrombus extending from the tip of the catheter along the shaft of the catheter. Each patient had a normal coagulation profile. In all patients, the introducer and the catheter were filled with heparinized saline solution before introduction, and the catheters were rapidly placed into the pulmonary artery. There was no statistical correlation between thrombus size and the hemodynamic status of the patient or the duration of catheter insertion.[144]

Pulmonary Hemorrhage

Pulmonary hemorrhage may occur either as a result of pulmonary infarction or from direct damage to the pulmonary artery, especially in the presence of pulmonary hypertension. The elevated pulmonary artery pressure may force the tip of the catheter (with the balloon inflated) peripherally into a small branch of the pulmonary artery. The pressure gradient across the

segment of the pulmonary artery may then force the tip through the vessel wall. Therefore, in patients with pulmonary hypertension, PAOP measurement should be approached with caution, and length of time in the wedge position should be kept at a minimum.[145,146]

Knotting and Entanglement or Damage to Intracardiac Structures

If the pulmonary artery catheter is withdrawn with the balloon inflated, injury to either the pulmonic or the tricuspid valvular apparatus may follow.[147] Not only has rupture of the cordae tendineae of the tricuspid valve been reported,[147] but the catheter may become looped around the papillary muscle of the tricuspid valve so that removal is impossible.[148] Finally, a knot may form in the distal catheter.[149] To avoid damage to valvular structures during withdrawal, the balloon should be deflated. The incidence of knotting and coiling of the catheter is probably increased with the smaller 5 F catheter. Partially inflating the balloon when the catheter tip reaches the subclavian vein or the superior vena cava during insertion may prevent coiling of the catheter in the right atrium or the right ventricle. If, when attempting to remove the catheter, there is resistance to withdrawal, the attempt should be interrupted and a chest x-ray film obtained to exclude the possibility of knotting or entanglement of the catheter within the heart.

Cardiac Arrhythmias

Atrial and ventricular arrhythmias are common during transit of the catheter through the right heart.[150-152] Tachyarrhythmias may persist even after the catheter is removed. Arrhythmias are usually caused by the bare tip of the catheter impinging upon the endocardium; this possibility can be minimized by making certain that the balloon is fully inflated so that the tip of the catheter is covered. Right bundle branch block can occur during passage of the catheter through the right heart; in a patient with preexisting left bundle branch block, this condition can lead to complete heart block. In a patient with left bundle branch block, a transvenous pacing catheter should be placed prior to inserting a pulmonary artery catheter;[106] or a pulmonary artery catheter with pacing capabilities should be used.

Endocarditis

Septic endocarditis, which involves the right side of the heart due to prolonged pulmonary artery catheterization, occurs rarely. However, aseptic endocarditis and thrombotic endocardial vegetations involving the right side of the heart occur in approximately 30% of autopsied patients who have had a pulmonary artery catheter in place. These aseptic vegetations may be of significance in providing a nidus for subsequent sepsis, as well as a source of pulmonary emboli. Both septic and aseptic endocarditis may be more common in burn patients.[153-157]

Pulmonary-Artery-Catheter-Related Sepsis

Frequent manipulations of the pulmonary artery catheter, as well as leaving the pulmonary catheter in place for more than 3 days, increase the incidence of positive blood cultures drawn through the pulmonary artery catheter and positive cultures from catheter tips.[152,158,159] (See Chapter 10.)

Fracture of Catheter

There is one report of fracture of a pulmonary artery catheter 0.5 cm proximal to the right atrial opening. This catheter was inserted via a cutdown from the right antecubital fossa; difficulty was experienced in passing the catheter. An acceptable waveform was never obtained. When the catheter was withdrawn, the distal point of the catheter beyond the fracture was attached to the proximal part only by the wires leading to the thermistor.[160]

Balloon Rupture

The balloon may be defective prior to insertion, may be damaged during insertion, or balloon rupture may occur while the catheter is in use. Several recommendations for balloon care have been published in *Health Devices*.[161] Since excessive storage temperatures may cause the latex balloons to rupture, the catheters should be stored in well-ventilated areas (away from direct sunlight, nearby heat sources, or chemical fumes) at temperatures no higher than 25° C. An air-filled balloon-tipped catheter should not be used in a patient with an intracardiac right-to-left shunt because systemic air embolism will occur if the balloon ruptures. Use carbon dioxide for balloon inflation in this situation. Test the balloon before catheterization by submerging it in sterile water and inflating it with air. Leave the catheters in original packages until needed and remove them carefully to avoid damage to the balloons. Use care during insertion. Do not exceed maximum inflation volumes. Monitor the pulmonary artery waveform and stop inflation when proper wedging is achieved. The balloon should resist inflation, and the syringe plunger should spring back when released. Failure to wedge the device and the absence of inflation resistance indicate balloon rupture, distention of the pulmonary artery, or displacement of the catheter tip back into the main pulmonary artery or right ventricle.

If balloon rupture is suspected, aspirate into the syringe the same gas volume used for inflation; disconnect the syringe and leave the stopcock open to vent the balloon. If the balloon is broken, a few drops of blood may appear at the inflation port. Remove the catheter immediately since fragments from deteriorating latex form emboli.

Complications Relating to Insertion

Any complications described in Chapter 11 may occur during placement of a pulmonary artery catheter percutaneously into a central vein. Pneumothorax may occur during subclavian venipuncture, and the carotid artery may be entered during internal jugular venipuncture. Even inadvertent placement of the pulmonary artery catheter into the right pleural space has been reported.[162] Injury to nerve or artery may occur during cutdown.

Part IV: Arterial Puncture

Arterial puncture is indicated to obtain a specimen of arterial blood for various laboratory determinations such as arterial gases or lactate.[163,164] If frequent specimens are required or continuous pressure monitoring is indicated, an indwelling arterial line should be used as described in "Arterial Cannulation."

The sites that are commonly used for arterial puncture are the radial artery, the brachial artery, and the femoral artery.

Equipment Needed

The list of equipment and supplies needed for arterial puncture includes:

1. 3- to 5-mL sterile syringe (glass or plastic).
2. 25-gauge 5/8 inch (1.6 cm) needle for radial, brachial, and femoral puncture, or
3. 22-gauge 1½ inch (3.8 cm) needle for femoral puncture in obese patients.
4. Plug for syringe or rubber stopper for end of needle.
5. Heparin — 1,000 units/mL.
6. Povidone–iodine or 70% isopropyl alcohol for skin cleansing.
7. 1% lidocaine without epinephrine.
8. 3-mL syringe — 25-gauge 5/8 inch (1.6 cm) needle for lidocaine.
9. Container of crushed ice (plastic bag, cup, emesis basin, etc.).

Technique

The steps in the process of arterial puncture are as follows:

1. Fill the syringe for drawing arterial specimen with a small amount of heparin. If the syringe is glass, rinse the barrel with heparin and eject the residue from the syringe with the needle pointing upward. Push the plunger home to expel the air and leave only the dead space of the needle and the syringe filled with heparin. If a plastic syringe is used, the syringe does

not need to be rinsed, since heparin does not adhere to the wall of the plastic syringe; however, it is still essential to discard the excess heparin and air, leaving only the dead space filled.

2. For radial artery puncture: Extend the wrist as for insertion of an arterial line; the site of puncture should be ½–1 inch (1.3–2.5 cm) proximal to the wrist crease.

3. For brachial artery puncture: The arm should be extended at the elbow and supinated (palm up); the site of puncture should be slightly above the elbow crease.

4. For femoral artery puncture: The patient should be supine with the legs straight; the puncture should be made distal to the inguinal ligament at the level of the inguinal crease.

5. Wear sterile gloves for optimal asepsis.

6. Cleanse the skin with povidone–iodine or alcohol.

7. Palpate the artery selected. It is usually best to place two or three fingers along the course of the artery, both to locate its position and direction and to immobilize it.

8. Inject lidocaine to raise a skin wheal at the puncture site (optional).

9. Insert the needle for radial (Figure 24) or brachial (Figure 25) artery puncture through the skin wheal at about a 45–60° angle and direct it slowly toward the pulsation. For femoral artery puncture (Figure 26), insert the needle at a 90° angle. Occasionally penetration into the artery can be sensed, but usually puncture is detected by blood slowly entering the syringe as a result of arterial pressure. (This occurs most easily with a glass syringe. If a plastic syringe is used, gentle aspiration may be required.) If blood is not obtained during insertion, slowly withdraw the needle and stop once blood appears. If no blood appears, withdraw the needle altogether and start again.

10. Obtain 2-3 mL of blood and remove the needle from the artery while applying pressure to the site.

11. Pressure should be maintained at the puncture site for at least 5-10 minutes, longer if the patient has a coagulopathy or is hypertensive.

12. Hold the syringe vertically (needle tip upright) and expel any air bubbles.

13. Either remove the needle from the syringe and apply a rubber cap to the end of the syringe, or leave the needle attached and apply the needle cover, or plug the tip into a rubber stopper.

14. Roll the syringe four to five times between the palms of the hands to mix blood with heparin.

15. Place the syringe in ice, and transport it immediately to the laboratory.

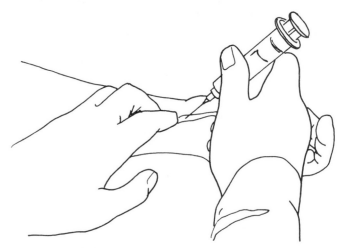

Figure 24.   Radial artery puncture.

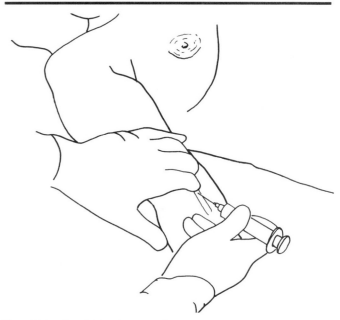

Figure 25.   Brachial artery puncture.

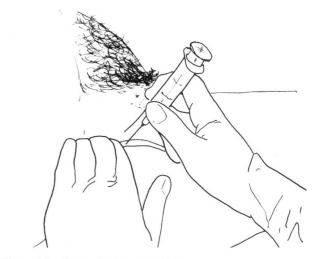

Figure 26.   Femoral artery puncture.

Complications

The major complication of arterial puncture is a hematoma. This generally can be prevented or minimized by using a 25-gauge needle and applying pressure for at least 5–10 minutes after the puncture has been completed. Thrombosis of the artery may occur after repeated punctures, as mentioned in "Arterial Cannulation." Infection is a possible, but uncommon, complication. Injury to an adjacent nerve may occur with attempts at puncturing the femoral or brachial arteries.

Pitfalls

Since heparin has a low PCO_2 and an acidic pH, a quantity of heparin in the syringe in excess of that needed to fill the dead space will lower the PCO_2 and pH of the arterial blood.[165]

Blood gas samples should be analyzed as soon as possible and should be placed in ice for even short delays. The blood sample must be adequately submerged in the ice or ice water. Since blood metabolism occurs in the syringe, the PO_2 and the pH decrease and the PCO_2 increases. The magnitude of the change is determined by both time and temperature. In addition, when the hemoglobin is saturated at a PO_2 above 150 mmHg, a small change in oxygen content represents a large drop in PO_2 because of the shape of the oxygen–hemoglobin dissociation curve. Therefore, unless arterial blood samples are analyzed immediately after they are drawn, they should be immersed in ice.[165,166]

A small amount of air in the syringe may markedly lower PCO_2 since air contains negligible carbon dioxide. The direction of change in PO_2 depends on whether arterial PO_2 initially was lower or greater than ambient oxygen tension.

Vacutainers, even though nitrogen-filled, should not be used for drawing arterial blood gas specimens since they contain measurable amounts of oxygen and will therefore alter arterial PO_2 significantly.[167]

References

1. Cohn JN: Blood pressure measurement in shock. Mechanism of inaccuracy in ausculatory and palpatory methods. *JAMA* 199:118-122, 1967.
2. Harrington DP: Disparities between direct and indirect arterial systolic blood pressure measurements. *Cardiovasc Pulmonary Tech* 6:40, 1978.
3. Hamilton WF, Dow P: An experimental study of standing waves in pulse propagated through the aorta. *Am J Physiol* 125:48-59,1939.
4. Remington JW: Contour changes of the aortic pulse during propagation. *Am J Physiol* 199:331-334, 1960.
5. Nutter DO: Measuring and recording systemic blood pressure, in Hurst JW, Logue RB, Schlant RC, et al (eds): *The Heart, Arteries and Veins,* ed 2. New York, McGraw-Hill Book Co Inc, 1978, pp 217-226.
6. Evaluation: Physiological pressure transducers. *Health Devices* 8:199-204, 1979.
7. Civetta JM: Invasive catheterization, in Shoemaker WC, Thompson WL (eds): *Critical Care, State of the Art,* Fullerton, Calif, The Society of Critical Care Medicine, 1980, vol 1, chap B, pp 18-21.
8. Waltemath CL, Preuss DD: Determination of blood pressure in low-flow states by the Doppler technique. *Anesthesiology* 34:77-79, 1971.
9. Kazamias TM, Gander MP, Franklin DL, et al: Blood pressure measurement with Doppler ultrasonic flowmeter. *J Appl Physiol* 30:585-588, 1971.
10. Harken AH, Smith RM: Aortic pressure versus Doppler-measured peripheral arterial pressure. *Anesthesiology* 38:184-186, 1973.
11. Paulus DA: Noninvasive blood pressure measurement. *Med Instrum* 15:91-94, 1981.
12. Van Bergen FH, Weatherhead DS, Treloar EF, et al: Comparison of indirect and direct methods of measuring arterial blood pressure. *Circulation* 10:481-490, 1954.
13. Berliner K, Fujiy H, Ho Lu D, et al: The accuracy of blood pressure determinations. A comparison of direct and indirect measurements. *Cardiologia* 37:118-128, 1960.
14. Lowry RL, Lichti EL, Eggers GWN Jr: The Doppler: An aid in monitoring blood pressure during anesthesia. *Anesth Analg* 52:531-535, 1973.
15. Geddes LA, Whistler SJ: The error in indirect blood pressure measurement with the incorrect size of cuff. *Am Heart J* 96:4-8, 1978.
16. Venus B, Mathru M, Smith RA, et al: Direct versus indirect blood pressure measurements in critically ill patients. *Heart Lung* 14:228-231, 1985.
17. Johnson CJH, Kerr JH: Automatic blood pressure monitors. *Anaesthesia* 40:471-478, 1985.
18. Bedford RF, Wollman H: Complications of percutaneous radial-artery cannulation: An objective prospective study in man. *Anesthesiology* 38:228-236, 1973.
19. Mandel MA, Dauchot PJ: Radial artery cannulation in 1,000 patients: Precautions and complications. *J Hand Surg* 2:482-485,1977.
20. Palm T: Evaluation of peripheral arterial pressure on the thumb following radial artery cannulation. *Br J Anaesth* 49:819-824, 1977.
21. Little JM, Clarke B, Shanks C: Effects of radial artery cannulation. *Med J Aust* 2:791-793, 1975.
22. Ersoz CJ, Hedden M, Lain L: Prolonged femoral arterial catheterization for intensive care. *Anesth Analg* 49;160-165, 1970.
23. Gurman GM, Kriemerman SI: Cannulation of big arteries in critically ill patients. *Crit Care Med* 13:217-220, 1985.
24. Bedford RF: Radial arterial function following percutaneous cannulation with 18- and 20-gauge catheters. *Anesthesiology* 47:37-39, 1977.
25. Downs JB, Rackstein AD, Klein EF Jr, et al: Hazards of radial-artery catheterization. *Anesthesiology* 38:283-286, 1973.
26. Davis FM: Radial artery cannulation: Influence of catheter size and material on arterial occlusion. *Anaesth Intensive Care* 6:49-53, 1978.
27. Downs JB, Chapman RL Jr, Hawkins IF Jr: Prolonged radial-artery catheterization. An evaluation of heparinized catheters and continuous irrigation. *Arch Surg* 108:671-673, 1974.
28. Arthurs GJ: Case report: Digital ischemia following radial artery cannulation. *Anaesth Intensive Care* 6:54-55, 1978.
29. Shinebourne E, Pfitzner J: Continuous flushing device for indwelling arterial and venous cannulae. *Br J Hosp Med* 9(suppl):64, 1973.
30. Gardner RM, Bond EL, Clark JS: Safety and efficacy of continuous flush systems for arterial and pulmonary artery catheters. *Ann Thorac Surg* 23:534-538, 1977.
31. Gardner RM, Warner HR, Toronto AF, et al: Catheter-flush system for continuous monitoring of central arterial pulse waveform. *J Appl Physiol* 29:911-913, 1970.
32. Band JD, Maki DG: Infections caused by indwelling arterial catheters for hemodynamic monitoring. *Am J Med* 67:735-741, 1979.
33. Gardner RM, Schwartz R, Wong HC: Percutaneous indwelling radial-artery catheters for monitoring cardiovascular function. Prospective study of the risk of thrombosis and infection. *N Engl Med* 290:1227-1231, 1974.
34. Grant JC: *An Atlas of Anatomy,* ed 6. Baltimore, Williams & Wilkins Co, 1972, pp 224-258.
35. Mortensen JD: Clinical sequelae from arterial needle puncture, cannulation, and incision. *Circulation* 35:1118-1123, 1967.

36. Bolasny BL, Killen DA: Surgical management of arterial injuries secondary to angiography. *Ann Surg* 174:962-964, 1971.

37. Shah A, Gnoj J, Fisher VJ: Complications of selective coronary arteriography by the Judkins technique and their prevention. *Am Heart J* 90:353-359, 1975.

38. Colvin MP, Curran JP, Jarvis D, et al: Femoral artery pressure monitoring. Use of the Seldinger technique. *Anaesthesia* 32:451-455, 1977.

39. Christian CM II, Naraghi M: A complication of femoral arterial cannulation in a patient undergoing cardiopulmonary bypass. *Anesthesiology* 49:436-437, 1978.

40. Katz AM, Birnbaum M, Moylan J, et al: Gangrene of the hand and forearm: A complication of radial artery cannulation. *Crit Care Med* 2:270-272, 1974.

41. Williams CD, Cunningham JN: Percutaneous cannulation of the femoral artery for monitoring. *Surg Gynecol Obstet* 141:773-774, 1975.

42. Morris TR, Bouhoutsos J: The dangers of femoral artery puncture and catheterization. *Am Heart J* 89:260-261, 1975.

43. Grant JC: *An Atlas of Anatomy,* ed 6. Baltimore, Williams & Wilkins Co, 1972, pp 1-79.

44. De Angelis J: Axillary arterial monitoring. *Crit Care Med* 4:205-206, 1976.

45. Adler DC, Bryan-Brown CW: Use of the axillary artery for intra-vascular monitoring. *Crit Care Med* 1:148-150, 1973.

46. Bryan-Brown CW, Kwun KB, Lumb PD, et al: The axillary artery catheter. *Heart Lung* 12:492, 1983.

47. Barnes RW, Foster EJ, Janssen GA, et al: Safety of brachial arterial catheters as monitors in the intensive care unit prospective evaluation with the Doppler ultrasonic velocity detector. *Anesthesiology* 44:260-265, 1976.

48. Bjork L, Enghoff E, Grenvik A, et al: Local circulatory changes following brachial artery catheterization. *Vasc Dis* 2:283-292, 1965.

49. Macon WL IV, Futrell JW: Median nerve neuropathy after per-cutaneous puncture of the brachial artery in patients receiving anticoagulants. *N Engl J Med* 288:1396, 1973.

50. Mozersky DJ, Buckley CJ, Haggood CO Jr, et al: Ultrasonic evaluation of the palmar circulation. A useful adjunct to radial artery cannulation. *Am J Surg* 126:810-812, 1973.

51. Crossland SG, Neviaser RJ: Complications of radial artery catheterization. *The Hand* 9:287-290, 1977.

52. Ryan JF, Raines J, Dalton BC, et al: Arterial dynamics of radial artery cannulation. *Anesth Analg* 52:1017-1025, 1973.

53. Allen EV: Thromboangiitis obliterans: Methods of diagnosis of chronic occlusive arterial lesions distal to the wrist with illustrative cases. *Am J Med Sci* 178:237-244, 1929.

54. Kamienski RW, Barnes RW: Critique of the Allen test for continuity of the palmar arch assessed by Doppler ultrasound. *Surg Gynecol Obstet* 142:861-864, 1976.

55. Brodsky JB: A simple method to determine patency of the ulnar artery intraoperatively prior to radialartery cannulation. *Anesthesiology* 42:626-627, 1975.

56. Brown AE, Sweeney DB, Lumley J: Percutaneous radial artery cannulation. *Anesthesiology* 24:532-536, 1969.

57. Slogoff S, Keats AS, Arlund C: On the safety of radial artery cannulation. *Anesthesiology* 59:42-47, 1983.

58. Weiss BM, Gattiker RI: Complications during or following radial artery cannulation: a prospective study. *Intensive Care Med* 12:424-428, 1986.

59. Dalton B, Laver MB: Vasospasm with an indwelling radial artery cannula. *Anesthesiology* 34:194-197, 1971.

60. Cohn JN: Central venous pressure as a guide to volume expansion. *Ann Intern Med* 66:1283-1287, 1967.

61. Lowenstein E, Little JW, Lo HH: Prevention of cerebral embolization from flushing radial-artery cannulas. *N Engl J Med* 285:1414-1415, 1971.

62. Mequid M, Vebilacqua R: Management of arterial cannulas, editorial. *N Engl J Med* 286:376, 1972.

63. Wyatt R, Glaves I, Cooper DJ: Proximal skin necrosis after radial-artery cannulation. *Lancet* 1:1135-1138, 1974.

64. John RW: A complication of radial artery cannulation. *Anesthesiology* 40:598-600, 1975.

65. Mathieu A, Dalton B, Fisher JE, et al: Expanding aneurysm of the radial artery after frequent puncture. *Anesthesiology* 38:401-403, 1973.

66. Barnhorst DA, Barner HB: Prevalence of congenitally absent pedal pulses. *N Engl J Med* 278:264-265, 1968.

67. Johnstone RE, Greenhow DE: Catheterization of the dorsalis pedis artery. *Anesthesiology* 39:654-655, 1973.

68. Huber JF: The arterial network supplying the dorsum of the foot. *Anat Rec* 80:373-391, 1941.

69. Grant JC: *An Atlas of Anatomy,* ed 6. Baltimore, Williams & Wilkins Co, 1972, pp 306-326.

70. Youngberg JA, Miller ED: Evaluation of percutaneous cannulations of the dorsalis pedis artery. *Anesthesiology* 44:80-83, 1976.

71. Swan HJ, Ganz W, Forrester J, et al: Catheterization of the heart in man with use of a flow-directed balloon-tipped catheter. *N Engl J Med* 283:447-451, 1970.

72. Ganz W, Swan HJC: Measurement of blood flow by thermodilution. *Am J Cardiol* 29:241-246, 1972.

73. Ganz W, Donoso R, Marcus HS, et al: A new technique for measurement of cardiac output by thermodilution in man. *Am J Cardiol* 27:392-396, 1971.

74. Forrester JS, Ganz W, Diamond G, et al: Thermodilution cardiac output determination with a single flow-directed catheter. *Am Heart J* 83:306-311, 1972.

75. Alpert JS, Dexter L: Blood flow measurement: The cardiac output, in Grossman W (ed): *Cardiac Catheterization and Angiography.* Philadelphia, Lea & Febiger, 1979, pp 61-71.

76. Franch RH: Cardiac Catheterization, in Hurst JW, Logue RB, Schlant RC, et al (eds): *The Heart, Arteries and Veins,* ed 4. New York, McGraw-Hill Book Co Inc, 1978, pp 479-501.

77. Forrester JS, Diamond G, Chatterjee K, et al: Medical therapy of acute myocardial infarction by application of hemodynamic subsets. *N Engl J Med* 295:1356-1362, 1404-1413, 1976.

78. Meister SG, Helfant RH: Rapid bedside differentiation of ruptured interventricular septum from acute mitral insufficiency. *N Engl J Med* 287:1024-1025, 1972.

79. Swan HJ: Second annual SCCM lecture. The role of hemodynamic-monitoring in the management of the critically ill. *Crit Care Med* 3:83-89, 1975.

80. Swan HJC: What is the role of invasive monitoring procedures in the management of the critically ill?, in Corday E (ed): *Controversies in Cardiology.* Philadelphia, FA Davis Co, 1977, Cardiovascular Clinics, vol 8, No. 1.

81. Walston A II, Kendall ME: Comparison of pulmonary wedge and left atrial pressure in man. *Am Heart J* 86:159-164, 1973.

82. Falicov RE, Resnekov L: Relationship of the pulmonary artery end-diastolic pressure to the left ventricular end-diastolic and mean filling pressures in patients with and without left ventricular dysfunction. *Circulation* 42:65-73, 1970.

83. Fisher ML, DeFelice CE, Parisi AF: Assessing left ventricular filling pressure with flow-directed (Swan-Ganz) catheters. *Chest* 68:542-547, 1975.

84. Sibbald WJ, Driedger AA, Myers ML, et al: Biventricular function in the adult respiratory distress syndrome: Hemodynamic and radio-nuclide assessment, with special emphasis on right ventricular fiunction. *Chest* 84:126-134, 1983.

85. Raper R, Sibbald WJ: Misled by the wedge? The Swan-Ganz catheter and left ventricular preload. *Chest* 89:427-434,1986.

86. Carley JE, Wong BYS, Pugh DM, et al: Clinical significance of the v wave in the main pulmonary artery. *Am J Cardiol* 39:982-985, 1977.

87. Braunwald E, Fishman AP, Cournand A: Time relationship of dynamic events in the cardiac chambers, pulmonary artery and aorta in man. *Circ Res* 4:100-107, 1956.

88. Forrester JS, Diamond G, McHugh TJ, et al: Filling pressures in the right and left sides of the heart in acute myocardial infarction. A reappraisal of central-venous-pressure monitoring. *N Engl J Med* 285:190-193, 1971.

89. Guyton AC, Jones CE: Central venous pressure: Physiological significance and clinical implications. *Am Heart J* 86:431-437, 1973.

90. Civetta JM, Gabel JC: Flow directed, pulmonary-artery catheterization in surgical patients: Indication and modifications of technique. *Ann Surg* 176:753-756, 1972.

91. Rice CL, Hobelman CF, John DA, et al: Central venous pressure or pul-monary capillary wedge pressure as the determinant of fluid replacement in aortic surgery. *Surgery* 84:437-440, 1978.

92. Risk C, Rudo N, Falltrick R, et al: Comparison of right atrial and pulmonary capillary wedge pressures. *Crit Care Med* 6:172-175, 1978.

93. Kostuk W, Barr JW, Simon AL, et al: Correlations between the chest film and hemodynamics in acute myocardial infarction. *Circulation* 48:624-632, 1973.

94. McHugh TJ, Forrester JS, Adler L, et al: Pulmonary vascular congestion in acute myocardial infarction: Hemodynamic and radiologic correlations. *Ann Intern Med* 76:29-33, 1972.

95. Carabello B, Cohn PF, Alpert JS: Hemodynamic monitoring in patients with hypotension after myocardial infarction. The role of the medical center in relation to the community hospital. *Chest* 74:5-9, 1978.

96. Lee J, Wright F, Barber R, et al: Central venous oxygen saturation in shock: A study in man. *Anesthesiology* 36:472-478, 1972.

97. Scheinman MM, Brown MA, Rapaport E: Critical assessment of use of central venous oxygen saturation as a mirror of mixed venous oxygen in severely ill cardiac patients. *Circulation* 40:165-172, 1969.

98. Crexells C, Chatterjee K, Forrester JS, et al: Optimum level of filling pressure in the left side of the heart in acute myocardial infarction. *N Engl J Med* 289:1263-1266, 1973.

99. Russell RO Jr, Rackley CE, Pombo J, et al: Effects of increasing left ventricular filling pressure in patients with acute myocardial infarction. *J Clin Invest* 49:1539-1550, 1970.

100. Shah DM, Browner BD, Dutton RE, et al: Cardiac output and pulmonary wedge pressure. Use for evaluation of fluid replacement in trauma patients. *Arch Surg* 112:1161-1168, 1977.

101. Weisel RD, Vito L, Dennis RC, et al: Clinical applications of thermodilution cardiac output determinations. *Am J Surg* 129:449-454, 1975.

102. Malin CG, Schwartz S: Starling curves as a guide to fluid management in the critically ill. *Heart Lung* 4:588-592, 1975.

103. Horovitz JH, Carrico CJ, Shires GT: Venous sampling sites for pulmonary shunt determinations in the injured patient. *J Trauma* 11:911-914, 1971.

104. American Heart Association: Standards and guidelines for cardio-pulmonary resuscitation (CPR) and emergency cardiac care (ECC). *JAMA* 255:2905-2984, 1986.

105. Sutler PM, Lindauer JM, Fairley HB, et al: Errors in data derived from pulmonary artery blood gas values. *Crit Care Med* 3:175-181, 1975.

106. Abernathy WS: Complete heart block caused by the Swan-Ganz catheter. *Chest* 65:349,1974.

107. Pace NL: A critique of flow directed pulmonary arterial catheterization. *Anesthesiology* 47:455-465, 1977.

108. Woods SL, Mansfield LW: Effect of body position upon pulmonary artery and pulmonary capillary wedge pressure in non-critically ill patients. *Heart Lung* 5:83-90, 1976.

109. Winsor T, Burch GE: Phlebostatic axis and phlebostatic level: Reference levels for venous pressure measurements in man. *Proc Soc Exp Biol* 58:165-169, 1945.

110. Winsor T, Burch GE: Use of the phlebomanometer: Normal venous pressure values and a study of certain clinical aspects of venous hypertension in man. *Am Heart J* 31:387-406, 1946.

111. West JB, Dollery CT, Naimark A: Distribution of blood flow in isolated lung; relation to vascular and alveolar pressures. *J Appl Physiol* 19:713-724, 1964.

112. West JB, Dollery CT: Distribution of blood flow and the pressure-flow relations of the whole lung. *J Appl Physiol* 20:175-183, 1965.

113. Tooker J, Huseby J, Butler J: The effect of Swan-Ganz catheter height on the wedge pressure-left atrial pressure relationships in edema during positive pressure ventilation. *Am Rev Respir Dis* 117:721-725, 1978.

114. Roy R, Powers SR, Feustel P, et al: Pulmonary wedge catheterization during positive end-expiratory pressure ventilation in the dog. *Anesthesiology* 46:385-390, 1977.

115. Benumof JL, Saidman LJ, Arkin DB, et al: Where pulmonary arterial catheters go: Intrathoracic distribution. *Anesthesiology* 46:336-338, 1977.

116. Kane PB, Askanazi J, Neville JF Jr, et al: Artifacts in the measurement of pulmonary artery wedge pressure. *Crit Care Med* 6:36-38, 1978.

117. Berryhill RE, Benumof JL: PEEP-induced discrepancy between pulmonary arterial wedge pressure and left atrial pressure: The effects of controlled vs spontaneous ventilation and compliant vs non-compliant lungs in the dog. *Anesthesiology* 51:303-308, 1979.

118. Shin B, Ayella RJ, McAslan TC: Pitfalls of Swan-Ganz catheterization. *Crit Care Med* 5:125-127, 1977.

119. Shin B, McAslan TC, Ayelia RJ: Problems with measurement using the Swan-Ganz catheter. *Anesthesiology* 43:474-476, 1975.

120. Gooding JM, Laws HL: Interpretation of pulmonary capillary wedge pressure during different modes of ventilation. *Resp Care* 22:161, 1977.

121. Berryhill RE, Benumof JL, Rauscher LA: Pulmonary vascular pressure reading at the end of exhalation. *Anesthesiology* 49:365-368, 1978.

122. Qvist J, Pontoppidan H, Wilson RS, et al: Hemodynamic responses to mechanical ventilation with PEEP: The effect of hypervolemia. *Anesthesiology* 42:45-55, 1975.

123. Downs JB: A technique for direct measurement of intrapleural pressure. *Crit Care Med* 4:207-209, 1976.

124. Rice DL, Awe RJ, Gaasch WH, et al: Wedge pressure measurement in obstructive pulmonary disease. *Chest* 66:628-632, 1974.

125. Milic-Emili J, Mead J, Turner JM, et al: Improved technique for estimating pleural pressure from esophageal balloons. *J Appl Physiol* 19:207-211, 1964.

126. Ferris BG Jr, Mead J, Frank NR: Effect of body position on esophageal pressure and measurement of pulmonary compliance. *J Appl Physiol* 14:321-324, 1959.

127. Knowles JH, Hong SK, Rahn H: Possible errors using esophageal balloon in determination of pressure-volume characteristics of the lung and thoracic cage. *J Appl Physiol* 14:525-530, 1959.

128. Bahler RC, Chester EH, Belman MJ, et al: Multi-disciplinary treatment of chronic pulmonary insufficiency. The influence of intrathoracic pressure variations on increases in pulmonary vascular pressure during exercise in patients with chronic obstructive pulmonary disease. *Chest* 72:703-708, 1977.

129. Davidson R, Parker M, Harison RA: Validity of determinations of pulmonary wedge pressure during mechanical ventilation. *Chest* 73:352-355, 1978.

130. Beach T, Millen E, Grenvik A: Hemodynamic response to discontinuance of mechanical ventilation. *Crit Care Med* 1:85-90, 1973.

131. Kirby RR, Civetta JM, Gallagher TJ, et al: The effect of PEEP upon pulmonary capillary pressures (PCWP). American Society of Anesthesiologists Annual Refresher Course Lecture, 1976, pp 229-230.

132. Pontoppidan H, Wilson RS, Rie MA, et al: Respiratory intensive care. *Anesthesiology* 47:96-116, 1977.

133. Scharf SM, Brown R, Saunders N, et al: Changes in canine left ventricular size and configuration with positive end-expiratory pressure. *Circ Res* 44:672-678, 1979.

134. Laver MB, Straus HW, Pohost GM: Right and left ventricular geometry: Adjustments during acute respiratory failure. *Crit Care Med* 7:509-519, 1979.

135. Jardin F, Farcot J, Boisante L, et al: Influence of positive end-expiratory pressure on left ventricular performance. *N Engl J Med* 304:387-392, 1981.

136. Shapiro HM, Smith G, Pribble AH, et al: Errors in sampling pulmonary arterial blood with a Swan-Ganz catheter. *Anesthesiology* 40:291-295, 1974.

137. Dye LE, Segall PH, Russell RO, et al: Deep venous thrombosis of the upper extremity associated with use of the Swan-Ganz catheter. *Chest* 73:673-675, 1978.

138. Chastre J, Cornud F, Bouchama A, et al: Thrombosis as a complication of pulmonary artery catheterization via the internal jugular vein. Prospective evaluation by phlebography. *N Engl J Med* 306:278-281, 1982.

139. Hoar PF, Wilson RM, Mangano DT, et al: Heparin bonding reduces thrombogenicity of pulmonary artery catheters. *N Engl J Med* 305:993-995, 1981.

140. Foote GA, Schabel SI, Hodges M: Pulmonary complications of the flow-directed balloon-tipped catheter. *N Engl J Med* 290:927-931, 1974.

141. Yorra FH, Oblath R, Jaffe H, et al: Massive thrombosis associated with use of the Swan-Ganz catheter. *Chest* 65:682-684, 1974.

142. Goodman DJ, Rider AK, Billingham ME, et al: Thromboembolic complications with the indwelling balloon-tipped pulmonary arterial catheter. *N Engl J Med* 291:777, 1974.

143. Colvin MP, Savege TM, Lewis CT: Pulmonary damage from a Swan-Ganz catheter. *Brit J Anesth* 47:1107-1110, 1975.

144. Hoar PF, Stone JG, Wicks AE, et al: Thrombogenesis associated with Swan-Ganz catheters. *Anesthesiology* 48:445-447, 1978.

145. Page DW, Teres D, Hartshorn JW: Letter: Fatal hemorrhage from Swan-Ganz catheter. *N Engl J Med* 291:260, 1974.

146. Lapin ES, Murray JA: Hemoptysis with flow-directed cardiac catheterization. *JAMA* 220:1246, 1972.

147. Smith WR, Glauser FL, Jemison P: Ruptured chordae of the tricuspid valve. The consequence of flow-directed Swan-Ganz catheterization. *Chest* 70:790-792, 1976.

148. Schwartz KV, Garcia FG: Entanglement of Swan-Ganz catheter around an intracardiac structure, letter. *JAMA* 237:1198-1199, 1977.

149. Daum S, Schapira M: Intracardiac knot formation in a Swan-Ganz catheter. *Anesth Analg* 52:862-863, 1973.

150. Geha DG, Davis NJ, Lappas DG: Persistent atrial arrhythmias associated with placement of a Swan-Ganz catheter. *Anesthesiology* 39:651-653, 1973.

151. Sprung CL, Jacobs LJ, Caralis PV, et al: Ventricular arrhythmias during Swan-Ganz catheterization of the critically ill. *Chest* 79:413, 1981.

152. Damen J, Bolten D: A prospective analysis of 1400 pulmonary artery catheterizations in patients undergoing cardiac surgery. *Acta Anaesthesiol Scand* 30:380-392, 1986.

153. Pace NL, Horton W: Indwelling pulmonary artery catheters. Their relationship to aseptic thrombotic endocardial vegetations. *JAMA* 233:893-894, 1975.

154. Greene JF Jr, Fitzwater JE, Clemmer TP: Septic endocarditis and indwelling pulmonary artery catheters. *JAMA* 233:891-892, 1975.

155. Ehrie M, Morgan AP, Moore FD, et al: Endocarditis with the indwelling balloon-tipped pulmonary artery catheter in burn patients. *J Trauma* 18:664-666, 1978.

156. Sasaki TM, Panke TW, Dorethy JF, et al: The relationship of central venous and pulmonary artery catheter position to acute right-sided endocarditis in severe thermal injury. *J Trauma* 19:740-743, 1979.

157. Ducatman BS, McMichan JC, Edwards WD: Catheter-induced lesions of the right side of the heart. *JAMA* 253:791-795, 1985.

158. Applefeld JJ, Caruthers TE, Reno DJ, et al: Assessment of the sterility of long-term cardiac catheter position using the thermodilution Swan-Ganz catheter. *Chest* 74:377-380, 1978.

159. Prachar H, Dittel M, Jobst C, et al: Bacterial contamination of pulmonary artery catheters. *Intensive Care Med* 4:79-82, 1978.

160. Parulkar DS, Grundy EM, Bennett EJ: Fracture of a float catheter. A case report. *Brit J Anaesth* 50:201-203, 1978.

161. Latex balloons on wedge-pressure catheters. *Health Devices* 6:123-124, 1977.

162. Carlon GC, Howland WS, Kahn RC, et al: Unusual complications during pulmonary artery catheterization. *Crit Care Med* 6:364-365, 1978.

163. Petty TL, Bigelow DB, Levine BE: The simplicity and safety of arterial puncture. *JAMA* 195:693-695, 1966.

164. Sackner MA, Avery WG, Sokolowski J: Arterial punctures by nurses. *Chest* 59:97-98, 1971.

165. Bageant RA: Variations in arterial blood gas measurements due to sampling techniques. *Resp Care* 20:565-570, 1975.

166. Kemp GL: Questions and answers: Arterial blood samples should be stored in ice for gas analysis. *JAMA* 223:696, 1973.

167. Lang GE, Mueller RG, Hunt PK: Possible error resulting from use of "nitrogen-filled" vacutainers for blood-gas determinations, editorial. *Clin Chem* 19:559-563, 1973.

Credit is given to Peter Miniscalco for artwork and photography.

Invasive Therapeutic Techniques   Chapter 13

Part I: Emergency Cardiac Pacing

A cardiac pacemaker is a device that delivers an artificial stimulus to the heart, causing electrical depolarization and cardiac contraction. Although cardiac contraction may follow mechanical stimulation to the heart such as that from a precordial thump or a needle puncture, for all practical purposes cardiac pacing is accomplished by direct electrical stimulation.

An electrical cardiac pacemaker may be either external or internal. Although emergency cardiac pacing was first successfully accomplished using external electrical stimulation by electrodes applied to the chest wall, the large currents required caused significant muscle contraction, burns of the skin, and pain.[1] Now, modified external noninvasive temporary pacemaker monitor systems have been developed and are available and well tolerated. Large electrodes with high impedance transmit the stimuli across the thorax. Using this technique, the stinging pain of cutaneous sensory nerve stimulus is usually absent, and discomfort from skeletal muscle contraction is greatly reduced.[2]

Internal cardiac pacing may be performed by stimulating either the epicardium or the endocardium. Epicardial pacing requires a thoracotomy in order to apply the pacing electrode to the surface of the heart. This technique is reserved for temporary pacing following cardiac surgery or for long-term permanent pacing. The heart may also be paced by endocardial stimulation; a pacing electrode wire is passed intravenously into the right atrium, coronary sinus, or right ventricle. This technique is most commonly used for emergency cardiac pacing, but it is also used for long-term permanent cardiac pacing. For emergency cardiac pacing, especially when there is no pulse (making insertion of a floating pacemaker catheter impossible), and if external pacing is unsuccessful or unavailable, a transthoracic wire may be passed through a needle that has been inserted through the chest wall into the right ventricular chamber.[3-5] Using this method, ventricular endocardial pacing can be rapidly initiated. In this section, blind insertion (without fluoroscopy) of both transvenous and transthoracic pacemakers will be described.

The Pacemaker System

An electrical cardiac pacemaker has essentially two components: a pulse generator, which may be external or implanted inside the patient for permanent pacing, and a pacing electrode.

Characteristics of an External Pulse Generator[6]

Identifying qualities of the external pulse generator include the following:

1. Output with Variable Amplitude (in milliamperes, or mA): This allows one both to define the threshold for ventricular capture and to alter pacemaker output if the threshold changes.
2. Fixed Mode of Pacing: The pulse generator emits stimuli at regular intervals regardless of cardiac activity. This may lead to competition between pacer stimuli and the intrinsic cardiac signal, causing ventricular arrhythmias, including ventricular fibrillation and/or a decrease in cardiac output.
3. Demand Mode With Variable Sensitivity to Intracardiac QRS Complexes: In the demand mode, a pacemaker rate is selected; if the intrinsic heart rate exceeds the rate of the pacemaker, the pacemaker generator will be inhibited. If a spontaneous QRS complex does not appear after a preset escape interval depending on the rate setting of the pacemaker, the pacemaker will generate a pulse (ventricular-inhibited pacemaker). The ability to vary the sensitivity of the sensing mechanism allows one to determine the QRS complex amplitude at the pacing catheter electrodes at the time of insertion and to follow changes of the amplitude with time. This helps to determine proper catheter placement. In addition, the sensitivity can be adjusted to eliminate outside interference from electrode artifacts and electrical devices.
4. Variable Rate Setting Independent of Amplitude: The rate setting determines the rate that the pacemaker will generate stimuli in both the fixed and the demand mode.
5. Additional Indicators: The external generator should have a pacing indicator needle that functions each time the pacer generates a stimuli; there should also be another indicator that functions each time the pacer is inhibited when the heart is beating at its own intrinsic rate.

Characteristics of an Electrode Catheter

The pacemaker electrode may be either bipolar or unipolar.[6-9] A unipolar system utilizes one electrode in contact with the heart (cathode); an electrical circuit is completed by placing a subcutaneous ground lead (anode) some distance from the heart. A bipolar catheter has the two electrodes in contact with the heart: the distal electrode is the cathode and the proximal electrode is the anode. There is little physiologic difference between the two forms. The pacing threshold may be lower with a unipolar than with a bipolar electrode. The unipolar system is more sensitive to impulses arising in the heart as well as to external electrical interference. The unipolar system will provide more reliable demand function in the presence of small intracardial signals but is ten times more likely to respond to false signals from extraneous electrical interference. The bipolar catheter usually requires fewer repositionings to maintain its capturing function.[10]

The pacing spike is more prominent with the unipolar catheter and may facilitate recognition on the surface ECG. A bipolar system can be converted easily to a unipolar system by disconnecting the proximal (anode) electrode from the pacemaker generator, inserting a metal suture and wire subcutaneously in the chest wall, and attaching this wire to the anode of the pulse generator.

The transvenous pacing catheter may be a thin flexible wire, with or without a balloon tip, or a larger and stiffer catheter. The balloon at the tip of the pacing catheter (as with a balloon-tipped pulmonary artery catheter) directs the catheter tip into the right ventricle and makes blind insertion relatively easy.

Atrial vs. Ventricular Pacing

Cardiac pacing may be accomplished by stimulating either the atrium or the ventricle. Atrioventricular sequential pacing is also employed when a wire is placed in both the right atrium and the right ventricle; the atrium and the ventricle are sequentially paced, mimicking the normal sequence of cardiac contraction. Both atrial pacing in the presence of intact atrioventricular conduction or atrioventricular sequential pacing provide the atrial "kick" that augments ventricular stroke volume.[11] The stroke volume with ventricular pacing may be significantly less in the absence of the atrial kick. However, atrial pacing is difficult since the pacing electrode tends to become easily dislodged and capture is lost. Ventricular pacing is generally easier and more reliable; it, of course, must be employed in the presence of atrioventricular conduction disturbances. On the other hand, atrial pacing is used for overdriving (suppressing) supraventricular tachyarrhythmias.

Indications for Emergency Cardiac Pacing

Emergency cardiac pacing is indicated for treatment of symptomatic bradycardia, for prophylaxis of conduction disturbances that occur during acute myocardial infarction, and for control of tachycardias with overdrive suppression.

Symptomatic Bradycardia

Cardiac output is the product of heart rate and stroke volume. If the rate slows, stroke volume must increase to maintain cardiac output. If cardiac output falls, systemic vascular resistance will rise in order to maintain blood pressure. Although slow heart rates may be well tolerated in individuals with normal hearts, an abrupt slowing of the rate may be followed by failure of these compensatory mechanisms. This situation will lead to symptoms of hypoperfusion and hypotension (including lightheadedness, syncope, and seizures), pulmonary congestion, and increased myocardial ischemia. Such patients are best managed with a cardiac pacemaker to prevent episodes of bradycardia and to allow the use of antiarrhythmic drugs to suppress tachyarrhythmias that may occur in this syndrome.

Prophylactic Pacing in Acute Myocardial Infarction[12-15]

In acute inferior myocardial infarction, the new development of Mobitz Type I second-degree atrioventricular (AV) block is generally not an indication for pacemaker insertion. The development of Mobitz Type II second-degree heart block in inferior wall infarction is an indication for a temporary pacemaker.

The situation with anterior myocardial infarctions is quite different. New onset of second-degree AV block (Mobitz Type I or II) is an indication for insertion of a standby demand pacemaker, since third-degree AV block with an unstable ventricular pacemaker may follow abruptly without any premonitory signs. Another indication for prophylactic pacing in the setting of acute anterior myocardial infarction is a new right bundle branch block. Conduction abnormalities that occur with acute anterior myocardial infarction are often followed by complete atrioventricular block. Following the new onset of isolated left bundle branch block, some physicians prefer to insert a temporary pacemaker, while others prefer only to monitor the patient closely.[13-15]

Overdrive Pacing for Atrial or Ventricular Tachyarrhythmias

Atrial flutter, supraventricular tachycardia, and the tachycardias associated with the Wolff-Parkinson-White (WPW) syndrome may be converted to normal sinus rhythm by atrial pacing.[16-24] Rapid atrial pacing in the treatment of supraventricular tachycardias may 1) immediately revert the supraventricular tachycardia to normal sinus rhythm, 2) transiently convert the rhythm to atrial fibrillation, which may subsequently convert spontaneously to normal sinus rhythm, 3) convert the rhythm to atrial fibrillation with immediate slowing of the ventricular rate, or 4) slow the ventricular rate by increasing the atrial rate in those cases in which tachycardia cannot be terminated or atrial fibrillation cannot be initiated.

Rapid pacing of the atrium is not without significant hazard; it is possible for the pacing catheter to be displaced into the right ventricle with capture of the ventricle and resultant ventricular fibrillation. Overdrive ventricular pacing may be effective in the treatment of refractory ventricular arrhythmias.[7,12,16,17] Ventricular arrhythmias may be prevented by acceleration of the heart rate; however, the rate of overdrive does not have to exceed the rate of the ectopic mechanism and need be only somewhat faster than the normal sinus pacemaker to be effective.

Choice of Catheter for Blind Insertion[3-5,8,10,25-28]

Balloon-Tipped Catheters

A balloon-tipped catheter in the presence of spontaneous circulation may be passed easily and rapidly to the right atrium and the right ventricle. During cardiac arrest, however, passage may be difficult or impossible. The catheter (either 3 F or 5 F) is 100 cm long with two electrodes at the distal tip separated by a latex balloon. At the proximal end of the catheter are two female connector terminals and a Luer adapter with a two-way stopcock for inflation of the balloon. Beginning from the distal tip are ring markers at 10-cm intervals. Both the 3 F and 5 F balloon-tipped catheters are used for insertion from the brachial, internal jugular, or subclavian veins, and the larger (5 F) catheter is also used for insertion from the femoral vein. A balloon-tipped pacing catheter is generally preferred for blind insertion but does require significant blood flow to propel it into the right ventricle.

Semifloating Catheters

The 3 F or 4 F semifloating catheter is similar to the balloon-tipped catheter; it has two bipolar electrodes at the distal tip, but does not have a balloon. This catheter is flexible, yet retains enough stiffness to permit significant control and guidance. Since it does not require blood flow for positioning, it can be passed into the heart during cardiac arrest.

Regular Pacing Catheters

The 6 F and 7 F pacing catheters are generally inserted with fluoroscopy, but they may be easily passed blindly via the femoral vein into the apex of the right ventricle, especially if the distal tip is preformed to a "J" shape. Blood flow is not required for passage of these stiffer catheters.

Transmyocardial Pacing Stylets

The transmyocardial pacing stylet is a unipolar catheter that is inserted transthoracically through a needle into the left or right ventricle. It is a flexible wire with a large J-shaped tip which forms the cathode in contact with the ventricular endocardium. In some types, the anode is located several centimeters proximal to the tip; the anode contacts the chest wall and completes the unipolar loop. An adaptor connected to the proximal end allows the attachment of the stylet to a pulse generator. In other models, the anode consists of a separate electrode that is inserted into the chest wall. Since the transthoracic pacemaker does not require blood flow for insertion, it is easily inserted during cardiac arrest.

Choice of Site for Blind Insertion[3-5,10,25,28]

Antecubital Vein

A median antecubital vein may be entered either percutaneously or by cutdown. Although commonly employed as a site for temporary pacemaker insertion, there are several disadvantages. With arm movement, the intracardiac electrode is commonly displaced, resulting in loss of pacing, extrusion from the ventricle, or myocardial perforation. Since frequent repositioning may be required, sepsis and phlebitis can be more common in this site. Electrode instability is only partially corrected by uncomfortable restraint of the patient's arm.

Internal Jugular or Subclavian Vein

Percutaneous cannulation of either the internal jugular or subclavian vein is easily accomplished. Insertion of the pacemaker via these routes generally provides stable pacing, and the patient may be fully active with no limitation of ambulation or arm motion. The complications of internal jugular and subclavian venipuncture include pneumothorax, carotid or subclavian artery puncture, and brachial plexus injury.

Femoral Vein

Insertion of a catheter percutaneously into the femoral vein is rapid and easy. Since soft catheters may form angles or loops during passage up the inferior cava or may float away from endocardial contact, stiffer catheters are required for insertion via the femoral approach. After insertion, the patient must not flex the cannulated leg rapidly and sharply at the hip; the catheter, which is fixed at the groin, may move forward into the right ventricle, resulting in perforation, or the tip may be deflected from the endocardium with loss of capture. Some physicians restrict ambulation or allow only activity from bed to chair, whereas others allow patients full ambulation and report no complications. Phlebitis and thromboembolism occur rarely despite catheters remaining in place for prolonged periods. However, it is probably best to limit femoral pacemaker longevity to 7–10 days, recognizing that the incidence of catheter-related sepsis increases after 3 days (see Chapter 10).

Transthoracic

Insertion of a pacing catheter directly through the chest wall into the heart is usually reserved for emergency situations in which a floating catheter cannot be inserted, e.g., during cardiac arrest. The technique presents the same hazards as intracardiac injection and pericardiocentesis, which include internal mammary artery, coronary artery, or myocardial laceration, cardiac tamponade, and pneumothorax.

General Principles for Blind Pacemaker Insertion

Aseptic Technique

Since the catheter may remain in the patient for several days, attention to strict aseptic technique during insertion is vital to minimizing subsequent infection. The area of insertion should be carefully prepared with povidone–iodine solution; the operator and assistant should be fully gowned and should wear hair covers, face masks, and sterile gloves. The area around the insertion site must be covered with sterile drapes large enough to prevent contamination of the long catheter. After the catheter is in place, the site should be covered with povidone–iodine ointment and a sterile dressing. Using sterile techniques, the insertion site should be inspected at least every 48 hours for signs of phlebitis or local infection, cleansed, and redressed.

Electrocardiographic Monitoring

During emergency pacemaker insertion, the cardiac rhythm should be continuously monitored with an ECG. An IV catheter must be in place, and resuscitation equipment, including a defibrillator and essential cardiac drugs, should be immediately available at the bedside. If there is excessive atrial or ventricular irritability as the catheter is inserted, it should be withdrawn into the vena cava; once the arrhythmia has subsided, a new attempt at insertion can be made.

Monitoring Catheter-Tip Location (Figure 1)

The limb leads of an ECG machine, which must be properly grounded with less than 10 μA leakage current,[6] are attached to the patient. The V lead is attached to the wire from the distal electrode of the pacing catheter. An electrically safe short cable with an insulated alligator clip on each end, or the special adaptor that is supplied in some pacemaker kits, is used as the connector. The intracardiac ECG is continuously recorded from the catheter tip by setting the lead selector switch of the ECG machine on V.[29] As the catheter approaches the right atrium, large negative P waves and small QRS complexes are recorded. In the low right atrium, the P waves become positive and the QRS complex is more prominent than the P waves. As the catheter enters the right ventricle, a large intracavitary QRS complex is recorded; when the catheter electrode tip touches the endocardial surface of the right ventricle, ST segment elevation is seen, indicating that the catheter should be in proper position for ventricular pacing.

An alternative is to use the pacemaker spike and evidence of ventricular capture to determine the location of the intracardiac catheter. The pacemaker electrodes are attached to a pulse generator. The rate of the generator should be set at a level above the intrinsic cardiac rate, and the amplitude or output should be set at maximum. While recording a surface ECG, the pacemaker is passed into the heart. Contact with the endocardium of the desired chamber (right atrium or right ventricle) is recognized by capture of the pacemaker on the surface ECG.

Determination of Pacing Threshold

Once the pacemaking catheter is in place, as evidenced by ventricular capture, the threshold of stimulation must be determined. The amplitude of the output signal should be gradually decreased until capture is lost; this is the pacing threshold. Ideally, this should be less than 1.0 mA. This low threshold indicates that the electrode is in optimal contact with the endocardium. If the pacing threshold is high and if the need for pacing is not urgent, the catheter should be repositioned until a lower pacing threshold is obtained. However, if the need for pacing is urgent, the output should be turned as high as necessary to achieve capture. Under more controlled conditions (such as with fluoroscopy), the catheter can be repositioned to achieve a lower pacing threshold. The maintenance current for pacing should be set at two to three times the threshold current. The patient, if awake, should be instructed to take deep breaths, cough, and shift his or her position in bed to assess the stability of the pacing site and maintenance of capture.

Demand Mode

The pulse generator should generally be set in the demand mode to avoid competition between the pacemaker and spontaneous rhythm, which may lead to ventricular fibrillation.

Chest X-ray

As soon as the pacemaker is inserted, a chest x-ray must be taken. If the catheter was inserted via the internal jugular or subclavian vein, a pneumothorax must be excluded. A lateral film also should be taken to verify the position of the pacing catheter. The tip of the pacing catheter on the lateral film must point anteriorly, which

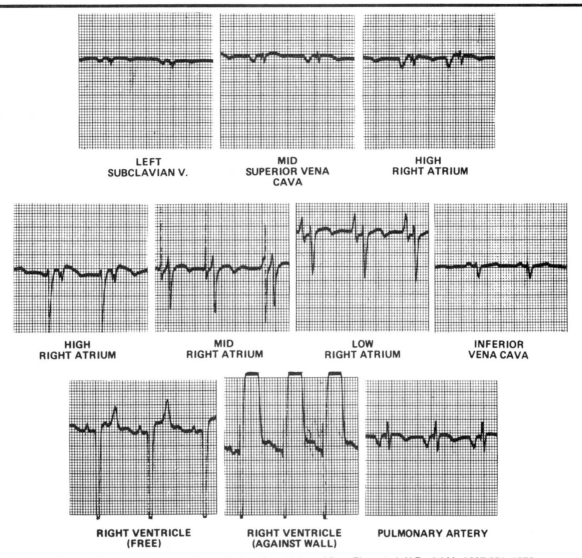

Figure 1. Electrocardiographic monitoring of catheter tip location. (Adapted from Bing, et al: *N Engl J Med* 287:651, 1972. Reprinted by permission of the *New England Journal of Medicine*.)

indicates that the catheter tip is in the right ventricle. If the catheter tip points posteriorly, it may indicate that the catheter tip is in the coronary sinus or has perforated the ventricle.[30]

Blind Catheter Insertion From Subclavian, Internal Jugular, or Brachial Vein

Equipment

1. A 3 F or 5 F balloon-tipped bipolar pacing catheter with syringe for balloon inflation.
2. Pulse generator and connecting cable.
3. Electrically safe ECG machine with adaptor to connect distal catheter electrode to V lead.
4. Equipment for percutaneous catheter sheath insertion (cutdown equipment may be necessary for insertion via the brachial vein).

5. Sterile drapes, gown, gloves, hair covers, masks, povidone–iodine solution, and material for cleansing insertion site.

Technique

1. Prepare the insertion site with povidone–iodine solution and drape in sterile manner.
2. Infiltrate the skin with 1% lidocaine without epinephrine if the patient is awake.
3. Test the balloon on the catheter tip before insertion.
4. Attach the limb leads of an electrically safe ECG machine to the patient.
5. After the vein has been entered, either with a percutaneous catheter-sheath system or via cutdown, insert the catheter into the vein.
6. When the catheter tip is in the area of the high right atrium, attach the V lead of the ECG machine to the distal electrode terminal of the catheter and inflate the balloon with the recommended inflation volume

(usually 1.5 mL). (Using surface markers, one can predetermine the length of catheter that must be inserted to reach the right atrium, as described in Chapter 11.)

7. Request the patient to inhale deeply; quickly advance the catheter an additional 5–8 cm. Follow the intracavitary ECG recorded from the catheter tip to determine the catheter location.

8. Deflate the balloon when the catheter passes across the tricuspid valve into the right ventricle as indicated by a large QRS complex.

9. Insert the catheter further until ST elevation is seen on the ECG, indicating that the catheter tip is against the right ventricular endocardium. (If the catheter passes into the pulmonary artery instead, the QRS amplitude will diminish.)

10. Disconnect the V lead from the pacemaker catheter and attach the connecting cable from the pulse generator to the electrode terminals.

11. Document ventricular capture by the pacemaker and the pacing threshold while recording a surface ECG (as previously described).

12. Set the generator output two or three times above threshold in the demand mode and at the desired rate.

13. If a percutaneous catheter sheath without infusion sidearm was used for insertion, withdraw it from the skin onto the proximal catheter.

14. Suture the catheter in place. (Looping the catheter near the insertion site and tying that in place as well may prevent catheter dislodgement if the proximal catheter is pulled.) Cover the insertion site with povidone–iodine ointment and a sterile dressing.

15. Obtain a chest x-ray film (include a lateral view if possible) to observe catheter position and to detect the presence of pneumothorax or other complications related to the catheter insertion.

16. Immobilize the arm if the catheter was inserted via the brachial vein.

Blind Catheter Insertion From the Femoral Vein

Equipment

1. A 5 F balloon-tipped bipolar pacing catheter with syringe for balloon inflation, or a regular 6 F or 7 F pacing catheter. The distal 10 cm of either catheter should be preformed into a "J" configuration.

2. A sheath of suitable size for percutaneous introduction of the catheter.

3. Other equipment the same as for subclavian, internal jugular, or brachial vein insertion.

Technique

1. Generally the right femoral vein is used. Shave the groin and cleanse the insertion site with povidone–iodine solution and drape in a sterile manner.

2. Infiltrate the skin with 1% lidocaine without epinephrine if the patient is awake.

3. If a balloon-tipped catheter is used, the balloon should be tested prior to insertion.

4. Attach the limb leads of an electrically safe ECG machine to the patient.

5. Insert the catheter through the sheath into the vein.

6. If a balloon-tipped catheter is used, inflate the balloon after the catheter has been inserted approximately 15 cm into the vein. Attach the V lead from the ECG machine to the distal electrode terminal.

7. Continue to advance the catheter, maintaining the rotation of the catheter so that when the catheter is in the right atrium, the tip points toward the tricuspid valve and the right ventricle. Use surface markers as previously described to determine the catheter length that must be inserted to reach the right atrium. Also follow the intracavitary ECG recorded from the catheter tip to determine the catheter tip location.

8. If using a balloon catheter, deflate the balloon as soon as the catheter passes through the tricuspid valve. Continue inserting the catheter until ST segment elevation is seen on the ECG recorded from the catheter tip, indicating that the tip is against the right ventricular endocardium.

9. Once the catheter is in place in the right ventricle, follow the technique described under "Blind Catheter Insertion from Subclavian, Internal Jugular, or Brachial Vein".

Insertion of a Transmyocardial (Transthoracic) Pacing Stylet

Equipment

1. A transmyocardial pacing stylet.

2. A 6 inch (15.2 cm) 18-gauge thin-wall cannula with blunt end and an inner obturator with trocar point (supplied with stylet).

3. An adaptor to attach the proximal end of the stylet to a pulse generator.

4. Pulse generator and connecting cable.

5. Povidone–iodine solution and material for cleansing the insertion site. The area of insertion should be draped in a sterile manner, and the operator should wear gloves. Ideally, sterile gowns, hair covers, and masks should also be worn.

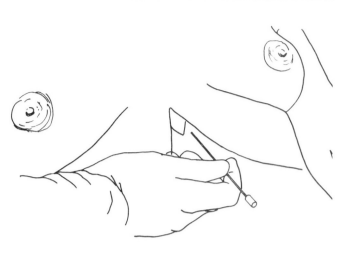

Figure 2. Subxiphoid approach for insertion of transmyocardial pacing stylet.

Technique (Figure 2)

1. The subxiphoid approach should be used to lessen the risk of inadvertent lung puncture. The skin around the area of the xiphoid should be cleansed with povidone–iodine solution and draped in a sterile manner.
2. Insert the placement needle below the xiphoid tip and about 1 cm to the patient's left. Direct the needle cephalad at an angle of 20° to 30° with the frontal plane.
3. Once the needle is inserted, remove the inner trocar and attach a syringe to the end of the needle. If blood does not appear with aspiration, slowly withdraw the needle until blood appears. If no blood is obtained, withdraw the needle, reinsert the inner trocar, and attempt the needle placement again.
4. Once the ventricular chamber has been entered, introduce the pacing stylet through the needle. Insert the pacing stylet to the depth indicated by a marker on the proximal end of the wire, indicating that the curve of the pacing stylet has reformed inside the ventricle.
5. Remove the needle while maintaining the position of the stylet to the ventricle. Do not withdraw the pacing stylet back through the placement needle.
6. Slide the electrical adaptor over the proximal end of the pacing stylet and attach the leads to the external pulse generator.
7. If ventricular capture is not evident on the surface ECG with the pacer generator on, gently manipulate the stylet until ventricular capture is seen. Exercise caution with manipulation so that the stylet is not dislodged from the ventricular cavity.
8. Secure the pacing stylet by suturing it to the skin of the chest wall.

9. If the ventricular cavity cannot be entered from the subxiphoid approach, the needle may be inserted in the fourth or fifth intercostal space adjacent to the left sternal edge to avoid both the lung and the internal mammary artery, which lies one to two fingers' breadths from the sternal edge. The cardiac apex is still another approach, but the risk of pneumothorax is significantly increased.
10. As soon as possible, chest x-ray film should be obtained to document the position of the catheter and the absence of a pneumothorax.

Complications of Cardiac Pacing

Thrombophlebitis and Pulmonary Emboli

Thrombophlebitis is rare, except following brachial vein insertions. In addition, some investigators report a low incidence of femoral vein thrombosis when that route is used for prolonged cardiac pacing. However, phlebitis and/or thrombosis of any vein may develop after a catheter is inserted.[10,25-27] Pulmonary embolism from a temporary transvenous pacemaker is rare.

Sepsis

Local infection at the insertion site and/or bacteremia are uncommon but may follow insertion of a pacing catheter under emergency conditions with less than optimal asepsis and may follow frequent manipulations to reposition the catheter. Since bipolar catheters require less manipulation after the initial insertion, the incidence of sepsis with bipolar catheters is less compared to unipolar catheters. The incidence of local and systemic infection increases the longer the pacing catheter is left in place. Care of the insertion site, as for any intravascular catheter, must be performed.

Perforation of the Right Ventricle[30-34]

Perforation of the right ventricle is uncommon and usually without sequelae. It may be recognized by loss of pacing (capture); synchronous diaphragmatic, intercostal, or abdominal contraction at the same rate as the pacemaker; or the development of a pericardial friction rub. Electrocardiographic changes suggestive of electrode perforation include a change in the frontal plane vector of the pacemaker artifact and a change in the QRS complex from the usual left bundle branch block pattern of a right ventricular endocardial pacemaker to a right bundle branch block pattern. The latter is due either to pacing the left ventricular epicardium from a catheter free in the pericardial space or pacing the left ventricular endocardium by a pacemaker that has perforated the intraventricular septum. When the ECG is recorded from a pacemaker wire (as described above) which has perforated the right ventricle, the QRS complex, ST segment, and T wave will resemble a V_3 or V_4 lead (Figure 3). Cardiac tamponade following perforation of the right ventricle is rare; usually the only treatment required is to withdraw the catheter into the right ventricle until normal sensing and capture reappear. Myocardial perforation is more common with stiffer catheters and when the catheter is inserted from the arm or femoral vein. Bipolar catheters may have a higher incidence of perforation compared to unipolar catheters.

Diaphragmatic Stimulation

Although it may indicate myocardial perforation, diaphragmatic stimulation may also occur without perforation. If the catheter is directed posteriorly in a large right ventricle that rests on the hemidiaphragm, the heart and the hemidiaphragm may be paced simultaneously. If the catheter becomes dislodged into the superior vena cava, cardiac pacing will cease but the right phrenic nerve may be stimulated and cause diaphragmatic contraction.[26]

Pacemaker Generator Failure

Pacemaker generator failure includes failure of sensing, oversensing, and failure of pacing.

Failure of sensing of a demand pacemaker is most commonly due to a low amplitude QRS signal, especially when using a bipolar catheter. The signal may be increased by either repositioning the catheter to obtain a larger bipolar signal or by converting to a unipolar system.[35] Loss of sensing also may be caused by a failing battery or by setting the sensitivity control of the generator too high.

Oversensing may be due to undesirable signals originating either within the body or from extraneous sources. Signals originating within the body may come from skeletal muscle contractions, large P or T waves, or from the pacemaker system itself (precipitated by a loose connection or intermittent separation of a fractured wire). Extraneous sources may include electromagnetic fields, stray electrical currents, and manipulation of the connecting cable.

Failure of pacing with loss of pacing artifact is due either to fracture of the catheter or failure of the

EPICARDIAL ELECTROGRAM

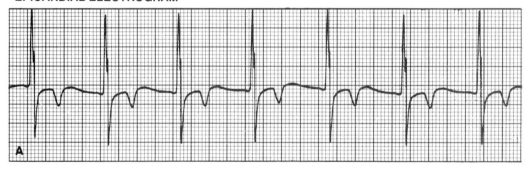

INTRACARDIAC ELECTROGRAM

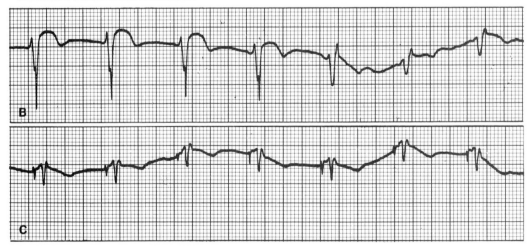

Figure 3. Perforation of right ventricle with pacing catheter. The ECG is recorded from catheter tip. Upper tracing (A) resembles V_3 lead and is recorded from myocardium before catheter is withdrawn. In middle tracing (B) electrogram with ST segment elevation is recorded as catheter is withdrawn to endocardial position; as catheter is withdrawn further into right ventricular cavity, ST segment elevation decreases. In bottom tracing (C) a typical right atrial electrogram is recorded with catheter tip in right atrium.

generator. The continuity of the catheter may be determined by recording an ECG connecting the V lead to each electrode terminal in turn. If an ECG can be recorded through the lead, the wire is intact. A straight line indicates wire disruption, and AC interference indicates a partial break in the wire.

Failure of pacing with persistence of the pacing artifact (spike) indicates malposition of the catheter or excessive threshold (exit block), battery depletion such that enough current is present to generate a pacing artifact but not enough to depolarize the heart, or a break in the electrode insulation that diverts the current and reduces the output of the catheter tip. If exit block occurs, catecholamine infusion may be useful to increase cardiac excitability and restore capture until the catheter can be repositioned.[36] Conversion from a bipolar to a unipolar system may also restore capture.[35]

Cardiac Arrhythmias

Ventricular arrhythmias may occur during both insertion and subsequent pacing. The catheter may induce arrhythmias by irritating the endocardium, especially if the catheter is not fixed in one place within the right ventricle, or by competition. Competition occurs when either a fixed-mode pacemaker is used or the demand mode is malfunctioning such that there is a dissociation between the pacemaker rhythm and the spontaneous rhythm. Both endocardial irritation and competition may induce ventricular fibrillation, especially in an ischemic heart characterized by a lowered fibrillation threshold. The risk of pacemaker-induced arrhythmias is also increased in the presence of metabolic acidosis, hypoxemia, excessive sympathetic activity or catecholamines, and digitalis excess.[12]

Pacemaker-Induced Heart Sounds

The pacemaker may induce a presystolic click (probably related to diaphragmatic or intercostal muscle stimulation), systolic clicks and murmurs related to movement of the catheter within the right ventricle, and catheter-induced tricuspid insufficiency. Friction rubs may be produced either by contact of the catheter with the endocardium or following myocardial perforation.[31,37-42]

Knotting of the Catheter

The flexible pacing catheter may knot upon itself or around other intracardiac catheters.[43,44]

ST and T Wave Abnormalities Following Cessation of Pacing

T wave inversion and ST segment depression may occur on the unpaced electrocardiogram subsequent to ventricular pacing and persist for a variable length of time after termination of pacing. The magnitude of the T wave inversion is related to the amount of electrical

power used for ventricular pacing; the time required for reversion to normal is related to the duration of pacing.[45]

Electrical Hazards[6,9,46]

Microcurrents (those that cannot be perceived if applied to the skin) can cause ventricular fibrillation if applied to a pacemaker catheter. All hospital personnel must be trained to prevent contact between the catheter terminals and conductive surfaces, and all electrical equipment used on patients with external pacemakers must be electrically safe. The following specific precautions must be taken:

1. Use only battery-operated pacemakers.
2. Leakage current of an ECG unit that is connected to the catheter terminals should not exceed 10 μA. When an ECG unit is connected to the catheter terminals, no other line-operated equipment should contact the patient, and the patient should be isolated from ground.
3. Handle catheter terminals carefully, wear rubber gloves when touching the exposed terminals, and keep liquids or conductive materials away from the terminals.
4. If a pacemaker is not attached to the catheter terminals, carefully insulate and cover the terminals so that they cannot contact liquids or conductive materials.
5. Push the catheter terminals all the way into the pacemaker connectors and secure them.
6. To prevent short-circuiting the pacemaker's output or completing a path for leakage current, place the entire pacemaker and its terminals inside a rubber surgical glove.
7. Since extension cables and their added length and connectors increase the risk of microshock and fibrillation, connections between catheters and extension cables must be secure and well insulated. If alligator clips are used, make certain that the connections between the alligator clip and the pacemaker electrode terminal are covered.
8. Do not replace external pacemaker batteries while the pacemaker is in use on a patient, except when the pacemaker circuitry provides for brief continued pacing during battery change. Since a low-impedance pathway between the battery terminals of an external pacemaker to its output terminals may exist, contact with the battery terminals may be just as hazardous to the patient as contact with the pacing catheter terminals themselves. If battery replacement is necessary while the pacing catheter is connected, extreme care should be taken to avoid contacting the pacemaker battery terminals with the hands or any conductive objects. Wear rubber gloves. It is better to disconnect the catheter from the pacemaker, taking care to avoid contacting the catheter terminals, and then replace the battery.

The pacemaker may be susceptible to outside interference, especially with a unipolar wire, since this serves as an antenna. Electrocardiographic telemetry units are usually safe. To check for safety, monitor the ECG and place the transmitter in normal proximity to the pacemaker; if the performance is normal on all modes of operation, the transmitter is probably safe. Electrosurgical units usually inhibit a demand pacemaker. Since the ECG cannot be viewed with the electrosurgical unit activated, the pulse or heart sounds should be monitored during this time. Physiologic monitors or other line-operated equipment may have electrical current leakage which can interfere with pacemaker function. The ECG should be monitored when a line-operated device is connected to the patient. Since microwave blood warmers or ovens and diathermy units can inhibit a pacemaker within 10 feet, patients must avoid close contact with such units.[6,9]

Part II: Pericardiocentesis

Pericardiocentesis or needle aspiration of fluid from the pericardium is indicated to 1) obtain fluid for diagnostic study, 2) obtain information regarding the physiological mechanism of venous pressure elevation, and 3) relieve cardiac tamponade.[47] In this section, the pathophysiology of cardiac tamponade, the clinical diagnosis of tamponade, and the technique of pericardiocentesis will be described.

Anatomy of the Pericardium[48]

The pericardium encloses the heart and the first few centimeters of the great vessels in a serous sac lined by mesothelial cells. The visceral pericardium is closely applied to the heart surface as the epicardium and is reflected at or near the sites of attachment of the great vessels to form the parietal pericardium. The base is attached to the tendinous and muscular portion of the left hemidiaphragm. In front, except where the pericardium is attached superiorly to the manubrium and inferiorly to the xiphoid process by pericardial-sternal ligaments, the percardium is separated from the anterior wall of the thorax by the lungs and pleura. A small area of the parietal pericardium, variable in size but usually corresponding with the left half of the lower portion of the body of the sternum and the medial ends of the cartilages of the fourth and fifth ribs on the left, is not covered by lung or pleura and comes into direct relationship with the chest wall.

The pericardial sac normally contains up to 50 mL fluid that has the same composition as serum. In the adipose tissue beneath the visceral pericardium and on the mediastinal aspect of the parietal pericardium are located arteries, veins, lymphatics, and nerves. The pericardium reacts to injury by exuding fluid, fibrin, or cells.

Cardiac Tamponade

Pathophysiology

Cardiac tamponade is impairment of ventricular diastolic filling as a consequence of increased pressure caused by accumulation of fluid within the pericardial sac.[49-52] Tamponade is most commonly related to one of three causes: 1) trauma, which may be direct or indirect, penetrating or nonpenetrating; 2) infection; and 3) neoplastic disease.[53] Myocardial rupture following acute myocardial infarction, uremia, and collagen-vascular diseases are also important causes of tamponade. However, iatrogenic cardiac tamponade may follow cardiac surgery, CPR, perforation of the heart by vascular catheter or transvenous pacemaker, or it may be due to radiation or drug reactions, such as to hydralazine or procainamide.[54]

As fluid is added to the pericardial space, the rate of rise of the pressure within the pericardial space depends on several factors. These include the compliance of the pericardium, the volume and rapidity of fluid accumulation, the blood volume, and the size of the heart.[49-51] The intrapericardial pressure remains relatively unchanged until a certain volume within the pericardial sac is exceeded, and pressure rapidly rises (Figure 4). With acute increases in fluid, as little as 200 mL may produce a marked rise in intrapericardial pressure. This explains why the removal of only small amounts of fluid may be

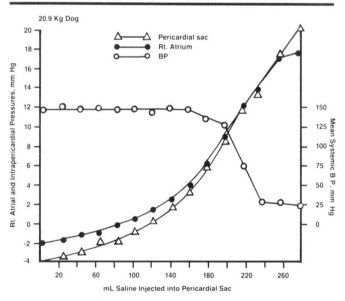

Figure 4. Production of cardiac tamponade by serial injections of saline solution into pericardial sac of anesthetized dog. As more than 160 mL saline is injected into the pericardial sac, right atrial and intrapericardial pressures rise more steeply and blood pressure (BP) falls more abruptly. Blood pressure falls to shock levels as intrapericardial pressure exceeds 14 mmHg. (Adapted from "Pericardial Diseases", in Fowler NO (ed): *Cardiac Diagnosis and Treatment,* ed 2. Hagerstown, Md, Harper & Row Publishers Inc, 1976, p 863. Used by permission.)

followed by a dramatic decrease in intrapericardial pressure and improvement of the patient. However, with slow accumulation of pericardial fluid over weeks or months, there is a gradual stretching of the pericardium with an increase in its compliance. More than 2 L of fluid may then accumulate without a severe rise in intrapericardial pressure.

As the steep portion of the pressure volume curve is reached, intrapericardial pressure rises and ventricular diastolic filling is impaired. Since right ventricular diastolic filling depends on the gradient between venous pressure and right ventricular diastolic pressure, venous pressure initially rises to maintain this gradient. But since increased pericardial tension inhibits filling throughout the cardiac cycle, the early rapid filling during early diastole is abolished. As intrapericardial pressure rises further, venous pressure can no longer increase sufficiently to maintain diastolic filling, and cardiac stroke volume falls. Reflex tachycardia may initially maintain cardiac output; augmented sympathetic tone also increases myocardial contractility and ejection fraction to maintain stroke volume. As cardiac output continues to fall, systemic vascular resistance increases to maintain blood pressure at the expense of further depressing stroke volume. Finally, as intrapericardial pressure rises further, systemic arterial blood pressure can no longer be maintained, and a shock-like state ensues.[49] At this point, Beck's triad of hypotension, increased venous pressure, and a small quiet heart may be fulfilled.[55] Cardiac arrest is then imminent.

Hypovolemia may mask the usual clinical manifestations of cardiac tamponade. In fact, the dynamics of tamponade become apparent in some patients only after volume administration. Although hypervolemia usually accentuates the clinical manifestations of tamponade, cardiac dynamics are favored by the increase in ventricular filling pressure which accompanies hypervolemia and which results in an increase in stroke volume.[47]

Clinical Manifestations[47,49-53]

Elevation of the central venous pressure is virtually always present in cardiac tamponade since the earliest compensatory mechanism to increased intrapericardial pressure is generally a rise in central venous pressure. In addition, since intrapericardial pressure remains elevated throughout diastole, early rapid ventricular filling is inhibited, and both the Y descent in the venous pulse and the early diastolic filling dip in the ventricles are curtailed (Figure 5).

With cardiac tamponade, all intracardiac pressures are equal to intrapericardial pressure during diastole; cardiac catheterization reveals equilibrium of central venous, right atrial, left atrial, right ventricular diastolic, left ventricular diastolic, and pulmonary artery occlusive pressures (PAOP's). In the presence of superimposed left

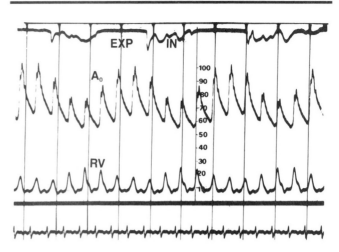

Figure 5. Pressures in patient with cardiac tamponade. From top: respirations, aortic (Ao) pressure, right ventricular (RV) pressure, pressure baseline, and ECG. Note pulsus paradoxus (25 mmHg). The RV pressure pulse is abnormal and displays small amplitude and increased diastolic pressure. There is no early diastolic dip. EXP = expiration; IN = inspiration. (Adapted from Shabetai R, et al: The hemodynamics of cardiac tamponade and constrictive pericarditis. *Am J Cardiol* 26:481, 1970. Used by permission.)

ventricular dysfunction, left ventricular diastolic, left atrial, and PAO pressures will be higher than right atrial pressures, and PAOP's will be higher than right atrial and right ventricular diastolic pressures, but right atrial and right ventricular diastolic pressures are still equal to pericardial pressure. In the absence of left ventricular dysfunction and in the presence of equilibration of all diastolic pressures, the elevation of the left ventricular diastolic pressures is not due to left ventricular failure but to the normal left ventricular pressure plus the addition of the pericardial pressure.

Pulsus paradoxus, which is defined as a greater than 10-mmHg decline (Figure 5) in systolic arterial pressure with normal inspiration, is usually present with tamponade. However, considerable effusion may exist without pulsus paradoxus, especially if such effusion complicates left ventricular dysfunction manifested by high left ventricular diastolic pressure.[56,57] The term "pulsus paradoxus" is a misnomer and somewhat misleading in that the decrease in arterial pressure during inspiration is merely an exaggeration of a normal phenomenon. Without tamponade there is a normal inspiratory decline in systolic pressure of less than 10 mmHg that is due both to the transmission of the inspiratory decline in intrathoracic pressure to the heart and aorta and to the delay in transit through the lungs of the normal inspiratory increase of right ventricular stroke volume. In the presence of cardiac tamponade, there is a normal decrease in intrapericardial pressure with inspiration and a normal increase in right ventricular filling. However, because of competition of the ventricles for space within the distended and restricted pericardial sac and a shift of the ventricular septum to the left, there is selective impairment of left ventricular filling and a decrease in left ventricular stroke volume. There is also increased capacity of the pulmonary veins since there is a greater fall in pulmonary venous pressure than intrapericardial pressure; this also leads to reduced left ventricular filling.

Finally, the normal decrease in intrathoracic pressure decreases aortic systolic pressure as it normally does in the absence of tamponade. A direct arterial pressure tracing during normal inspiration may show much more pressure variation than is appreciated at the bedside with cuff measurement. Therefore, intraarterial systolic pressure measurements should be recorded for accurate documentation of pulsus paradoxus if it is not apparent using cuff measurements. Pulsus paradoxus may be difficult to detect in the presence of cardiac arrhythmias, rapid erratic respiratory patterns, and severe hypotension. In addition, several clinical conditions may produce this condition in the absence of cardiac tamponade. Pulsus paradoxus may be present in obstructive airway disease and may be due to either primary impairment of left ventricular filling with inspiration or increased inspiratory filling of the right ventricle with exaggerated inspiratory decrease in left ventricular filling, or it may be merely an exaggerated fall in arterial pressure due to the fall in intrathoracic pressure during inspiration. Since the blood flow velocity in the aorta, stroke volume, and pulse amplitude do not decline in this situation, the latter explanation is the most likely.

Pulsus paradoxus may also occur in restrictive cardiomyopathy and constrictive pericarditis. This sign may be present in pulmonary embolism and right ventricular failure and is probably due to inhibition of normal inspiratory increase in venous return. Hypovolemia may be associated with pulsus paradoxus and is probably due to the restricted intrapulmonary blood volume with an exaggerated decrease in left ventricular filling because of the sponging action on intrapulmonary capillaries with inspiration. This leads to a fall in stroke volume and arterial pressure.[58] Finally, mechanical ventilation, particularly in the presence of hypovolemia, causes fluctuation of the arterial pressure curve similar to pulsus paradoxus.

Echocardiography may be used not only to document the presence of a pericardial effusion but also to show evidence of cardiac tamponade.[59-62] In the presence of tamponade, there is right ventricular compression as evidenced by a markedly reduced end-expiratory end-diastolic dimension due to a sudden increase in anterior motion (toward the right rather than the left ventricular cavity) of the interventricular septum. Right ventricular compression disappears following pericardiocentesis

and is not present with pericardial effusion without tamponade.

As tamponade becomes severe with a decrease in stroke volume and a rise in systemic vascular resistance, there is a fall in systolic pressure, a rise in diastolic pressure, and a narrowing of the arterial pulse pressure. However, hypotension in the presence of tamponade is usually a late finding.

The ECG often shows low voltage and nonspecific ST–T wave abnormalities. Electrical alternans, a beat-to-beat change in the axis of the electrocardiogram, which is due to a swinging motion of the heart within the pericardial effusion, may be present. Total alternans, which involves the P wave as well as the QRS, may be more specific for pericardial effusion.[63] Electromechanical dissociation may also be a manifestation of cardiac tamponade.

Treatment[47,49-52,64]

The specific therapy for cardiac tamponade is drainage of the pericardial fluid. However, until drainage can be performed, or if it is unsuccessful, the following measures may be helpful.

Volume infusion has been shown to increase stroke volume in cardiac tamponade by its effect on increasing ventricular filling pressure. Rapid intravenous administration of fluid (preferably whole blood, plasma, or colloid solutions, although saline may be effective initially) will often provide hemodynamic support for the patient with acute tamponade. The first 500 mL of fluid should be given over a 10-minute period, to be followed by 100 to 500 mL/hr thereafter, according to the response of the patient to the initial volume load. The administration of fluid volume is especially important when pericardiocentesis cannot be performed immediately or is unsuccessful.[65]

Isoproterenol increases heart rate and myocardial contractility and, therefore, stroke volume and lowers systemic vascular resistance. These effects combine to increase cardiac output in the presence of cardiac tamponade. Finally, recent studies have shown that, if ventricular filling pressure is maintained, arterial or generalized vasodilators may increase forward stroke volume. Norepinephrine and pure alpha-adrenergic agonists increase systemic vascular resistance and will further depress stroke volume. Digitalis also does not increase stroke volume in tamponade, presumably because of its effect of increasing afterload. Therefore, norepinephrine, alpha-adrenergic agents, and digitalis should be avoided in acute cardiac tamponade.

Description of Pericardiocentesis

Needle pericardiocentesis is indicated when cardiac tamponade represents an immediate threat to life or when it is progressive and produces increasingly severe hemodynamic impairment. In general, it should be performed in any patient with acute tamponade in whom systolic pressure has fallen more than 30 mmHg from the patient's normal level and in whom emergency surgery cannot be accomplished immediately. Specific indications for emergency pericardiocentesis include respiratory distress, progressive hypotension with jugular venous distension, and other signs of circulatory compromise in patients with pericardial effusion.

However, open drainage is safer and more effective. Procedures include subxiphoid pericardiostomy, which not only allows for drainage of pericardial fluid but also provides a biopsy specimen that is especially necessary for the diagnosis of granulomatous and lymphomatous invasion of the pericardium; parietal pericardiectomy (pericardial window) via a left thoracotomy, which provides for continuing drainage of fluid and thereby prevents recurrence; and finally, a visceral pericardiectomy, which is necessary for effusive constrictive pericarditis and constrictive pericarditis.[48,66]

Needle pericardiocentesis should be performed only by a skilled and experienced physician. One must be sure that large amounts of pericardial fluid are present. This may require echocardiography. The patient's ECG should be continuously monitored, and ideally, invasive hemodynamic monitoring should be employed as well. Full resuscitative equipment, as well as personnel experienced in its use, must be available. Atropine may be used as a premedication to avoid the occasional hypotensive vasovagal reaction that follows puncture of the pericardium.[47]

There are three approaches that may be used. The subxiphoid approach is preferred because it avoids the pleura and the coronary vessels. If this approach is unsuccessful, the needle may be inserted in the fifth intercostal space adjacent to the left side of the sternum where the pericardium is not normally covered by lung. (The presence of chronic obstructive pulmonary disease may be an exception!) The needle may also be inserted at the cardiac apex, but there is a greater danger of producing a pneumothorax with this approach. The latter two approaches also involve the risk of lacerating the left anterior descending coronary artery.

Ideally, the ECG V lead should be connected to the needle with a sterile alligator clip, taking care to assure that the system is properly grounded. If ST segment elevation occurs as the needle is advanced, ventricular contact is suggested; if PR segment elevation occurs, atrial contact is suggested. Elevation of both ST and PR segments may also indicate pericardial contact with no intervening fluid within the pericardial sac. However, these are signs indicating need for withdrawal of the needle. Other signs of epicardial contact include atrial and ventricular arrhythmias and atrioventricular conduction abnormalities. Monitoring the ECG from the pericardiocentesis needle may prevent entry of the needle into the pericardium where there is no cushioning layer of fluid present. It also immediately signals entry of the needle into the myocardium, allowing the operator to withdraw the needle and avoid myocardial and/or coronary artery laceration. If blood or fluid is obtained without the appearance of ST or PR segment shift or cardiac arrhythmias, this is an indication that the fluid was obtained from the pericardial sac rather than the cardiac chamber. However, in the presence of myocardial scarring due to old transmural infarction or infiltrative myocardial disease, the needle may enter an electrically silent area of the myocardium and not produce PR or ST segment elevations or cardiac arrhythmias.[67-69]

If V-lead monitoring from the pericardiocentesis needle is not feasible, or if immediate pericardiocentesis is necessary to sustain life of the patient, an alternate approach is to use a 20-gauge spinal needle as an exploring needle over which a 14-gauge needle has been placed. Once the pericardial space is entered with a spinal needle, the large-bore needle is advanced over the spinal needle into the pericardial space and the spinal needle is removed.[70]

Equipment Required

1. A short-bevel large-bore needle at least 16-gauge and 9 cm long.
2. A 30- or 50-mL syringe.
3. Sterile alligator connector to ECG V lead.
4. A 20-gauge spinal needle if V-lead monitoring is not used.
5. Povidone–iodine solution for skin preparation.
6. Syringe with small-bore needle and 1% lidocaine without epinephrine for local anesthetic.
7. Sterile gloves and sterile drapes; ideally, sterile gowns, hair covers, and face masks should be worn.

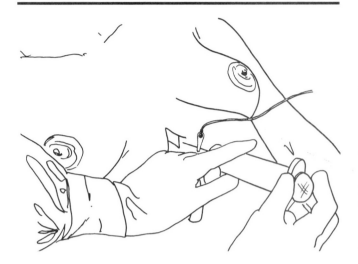

Figure 6.   Subxiphoid approach for pericardiocentesis.

Technique (see Figure 6)

1. Have the patient in a supine position or the upper torso elevated 20° to 30°.
2. Prepare the area around the xiphoid with povidone–iodine solution.
3. If the patient is conscious or responsive to pain, infiltrate the skin and subcutaneous tissues to the left of the xiphoid with 1% lidocaine without epinephrine to a depth of 1.5–2 inches (3.8–5.0 cm).
4. Locate the insertion site below the tip of the xiphoid and 1 cm to the patient's left. A small skin incision with a scalpel blade will facilitate entry of the large-bore needle.
5. Attach the large-bore needle to the syringe and connect the alligator clamp with ECG V lead to the needle. Insert the large-bore needle attached to the syringe at a 20° to 30° angle with the frontal plane. Aspiration should be continuous. As the needle is advanced beneath the skin, the resistance of the taut pericardium may be felt, and entry into the pericardial space may produce a distinct "giving" sensation. Contact of the needle against the epicardium may be accompanied by a scratching sensation, or by PR or ST segment elevation if the ECG V lead is connected to the pericardiocentesis needle as described above.
6. If grossly bloody fluid is obtained, it should not clot if from the pericardial space. In addition, a drop of bloody fluid on a gauze pad should spread out as a homogenous deep red spot if it is blood; but if it is bloody pericardial fluid, it should separate with a central deep red spot and a peripheral halo which is much less bloody.[71]

It may be advantageous to insert a catheter into the pericardial space. This avoids the potential epicardial or coronary artery injury that might be produced by the sharp tip of a needle. It also allows for continuous drainage of fluid from the pericardial space. A catheter may be inserted either by passing it directly through the pericardiocentesis needle and then withdrawing the needle or by advancing a flexible-tipped wire through the needle, removing the needle, and then advancing a catheter over the wire. Use of the wire allows a much larger catheter to be passed into the pericardial space than can be inserted through a needle.[72-74]

Hazards[53,64,66,75,76]

Significant risks accompany pericardiocentesis. Cardiac arrhythmias, including ventricular fibrillation and asystole, may occur; puncture or laceration of the cardiac chambers or the coronary arteries are possibilities; air may be inadvertently injected into the cardiac chambers when the intention was to inject air into the pericardial sac, and either hemothorax or pneumothorax, or both, may occur. Hemorrhage from myocardial or coronary artery puncture or laceration following pericardiocentesis may in itself produce cardiac tamponade, especially in the patient with thrombocytopenia or if thrombolytic therapy has been employed.

Part III: Intracardiac Injections

An intracardiac injection may be used to administer epinephrine for treatment of ventricular fibrillation, asystole, or electromechanical dissociation during ACLS when an IV or endotracheal route is not available.[77-79] There are anecdotal data which suggest that intracardiac epinephrine may have been effective in restoring cardiac contractions in asystole or electromechanical dissociation when IV epinephrine was ineffective. Whether it was the needle stick or the drug itself that proved effective has not been resolved. Nevertheless, IV and endotracheal routes should always be used initially. Nonetheless, this procedure can be associated with substantial morbidity and should be avoided unless no other route is available for the administration of epinephrine.[80]

Equipment Needed

Equipment for intracardiac injections should include the following:

1. Povidone–iodine solution for skin sterilization.
2. An 18-gauge 3½-inch (8.9-cm) needle attached to a syringe filled with the drug to be injected.
3. Sterile gloves to be worn for optimal asepsis.

Injection Sites

As with pericardiocentesis, the subxiphoid approach is preferred. If this approach is unsuccessful, the needle may be inserted in the fifth left intercostal space, at the edge of the sternum to avoid the internal mammary artery.

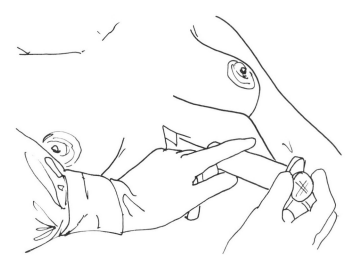

Figure 7. Subxiphoid approach for intracardiac injection.

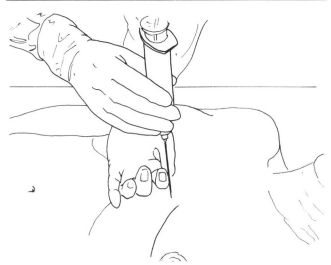

Figure 8. Left parasternal approach in fifth intercostal space for intracardiac injection.

Technique

The steps in the process of intracardiac injections are as follows:

1. Have the patient in a supine position.
2. Cleanse the area of insertion with povidone–iodine solution.
3. Insert the needle at a 20° to 30° angle with the frontal plane below the tip and 1 cm to the (patient's) left of the xiphoid (see Figure 7).
4. Maintain suction on the syringe and stop once blood appears. If no blood appears when the needle is fully advanced, continue maintaining suction and slowly withdraw the needle. If no blood appears, withdraw the needle altogether and repeat the attempt.
5. If the left parasternal approach is used, insert the needle in the fifth left intercostal space at the sternal edge with the needle perpendicular to the frontal plane (Figure 8).

Complications

The major hazard of an intracardiac injection is the need to interrupt CPR during the period of injection. Although uncommon, the following complications may follow intracardiac injections: pneumothorax, pneumopericardium, hemopericardium (with or without tamponade), myocardial laceration, coronary artery laceration, internal mammary artery laceration, and intramyocardial injection.[77-79]

Part IV: Tension Pneumothorax

Intrapleural pressure is normally subatmospheric throughout the respiratory cycle. Because of elastic recoil of the lung, the intraalveolar pressure is at all times greater than intrapleural pressure; therefore, transpulmonary pressure, which is alveolar pressure minus intrapleural pressure, is always positive.[81,82] The transpulmonary pressure gradient is markedly increased during coughing, breathing against an airway obstruction, and with positive-pressure ventilation.

If a break occurs in the alveolopleural barrier, there is entry of air into the pleural space, and the elasticity of the lung causes it to collapse. This condition is called a pneumothorax. As long as the transpulmonary gradient is maintained, the air leak will continue. Lung collapse ceases when either the communication is sealed or intraalveolar and intrapleural pressures become equal.[81-84]

Etiology of Pneumothorax

The etiology of pneumothorax may be classified into four groups.[85]

Group 1: Alveoli become overdistended and rupture. As long as there is a pressure gradient between alveoli and the connective tissue surrounding them, air extravasates and travels toward the hilum in the perivascular and peribronchial spaces.[86,87] This produces pneumomediastinum, which distends and may tear the friable mediastinal pleura, allowing air to enter the pleural space and resulting in a pneumothorax. Air may also extend from the mediastinum into the neck, into the retroperitoneal and free peritoneal spaces, and to the opposite pleural space. Once extravasation of air begins, a minimal pressure gradient is required for the process to continue.

Group 2: The fascial planes of the neck are injured by being either incised at operation or lacerated by trauma, allowing entry of air into the mediastinum, producing mediastinal emphysema. If there is subsequent tearing of the mediastinal pleura, this condition will lead to pneumothorax. If inspiration is obstructed in this situation, mediastinal pressure becomes markedly lower than atmospheric pressure, allowing air to be forced into the pretrachial fascia, producing pneumomediastinum. During exhalation, the inlet may be closed, entrapping the air. This raises the pressure within the mediastinum, which tears the mediastinal pleura and causes a pneumothorax.

Group 3: There is a direct connection of the distal airway to the pleural space, i.e., a bronchopleural fistula. High airway pressure either from positive-pressure ventilation or coughing may cause rupture of a bleb on the surface of the lung. Fractured ribs caused by non-penetrating injuries to the chest wall may puncture both the parietal and visceral pleura and tear the underlying lung, or a needle introduced through the chest wall into the pleural space may tear the lung; the tear may be inapparent until positive pressure is applied to the airway. Each of these produces a pneumothorax.

Group 4: In this category, there is a break in the parietal pleura, which connects the pleural space with an extrathoracic source of air, producing pneumothorax. Causes include traumatic esophageal pleural fistulas, emergency tracheostomy, thoracotomy, diaphragmatic tears (both traumatic and during abdominal operations), or a needle in the pleural space which is open to air, such as during thoracentesis.

Causes, Manifestations, and Emergency Treatment of Tension Pneumothorax

Air under pressure in the pleural space is referred to as a tension pneumothorax. A pneumothorax may be converted to a tension pneumothorax if there is a ball-valve mechanism at the site of the leak which permits air to enter but not leave the pleural space; at each inspiration the volume of gas in the pleural space increases, and the pressure becomes markedly elevated during exhalation.[81,84,88] If positive pressure is applied to the airway such as during positive-pressure ventilation or coughing,[86,89] intraalveolar pressure becomes markedly elevated, air leak increases, and there follows a rapid accumulation of air under pressure in the pleural space.[89]

Direct causes of a tension pneumothorax include barotrauma from positive-pressure ventilation alone (especially with PEEP) and with endobronchial intubation;

malfunctioning exhalation valves on bag–valve–mask units,[90,91] ventilators, or anesthesia machines,[92] especially with preexisting chronic obstructive pulmonary disease, acute necrotizing pneumonitis, or pulmonary infarction.[93-97] Tension pneumothorax has also been reported following fiberoptic bronchoscopy with closed lung biopsy[98] and with pneumoperitoneum.[99,100]

Tension pneumothorax is characterized by ipsilateral collapse of the lung with compression of the mediastinal structures and the contralateral lung. Venous return is inhibited both by the increased intrathoracic pressure and by the displacement of the mediastinum and heart with kinking of the venae cavae. This leads to a decrease in cardiac output which ultimately may lead to cardiovascular collapse.[83,84,89,101]

Clinical Manifestations

In this syndrome, the spontaneously breathing patient experiences dyspnea and may complain of chest pain. Examination reveals tachypnea, tachycardia, and distended neck veins with florid facies. The patient may be hypertensive initially, with hypotension a later finding. Compared to the contralateral side, the hemithorax under tension may be more prominent and hyperresonant with diminished breath sounds; wheezing may be audible.[83] The trachea may be deviated to the contralateral side. However, significant tension pneumothorax may be present without these typical physical findings.

In the patient being treated with positive-pressure ventilation, there is an increase in peak pressure needed to deliver the tidal volume due to increased pleural pressure; there is a diminution of expiratory volume due to the air leak from the lungs. There may be increased end-expiratory pressure even with the discontinuation of PEEP.[89,102]

If a pulmonary artery catheter is in position, a sudden increase in pulmonary artery pressure will be noted, presumably due to both the compressive effect of the pneumothorax and hypoxic pulmonary arterial vasoconstriction.[103] The electrocardiogram may show a rightward shift in the mean frontal axis, a diminution in precordial voltage, and precordial T wave inversion.[101] Hypoxemia, caused both by intrapulmonary shunting and decreased cardiac output, will be present.

A chest x-ray film will show the ipsilateral lung totally collapsed toward the hilum.[83,84] However, there may be a localized tension pneumothorax with various degrees of lung collapse if there is coexistent pulmonary or pleural disease. The trachea and the heart are usually displaced to the contralateral side while on the ipsilateral side the intercostal spaces are widened and the diaphragm is pushed downward. It may be inverted if the pneumothorax occurs on the left side, but this effect is prevented on the right side by the liver.

Treatment

Since a tension pneumothorax may produce cardiovascular collapse and cardiac arrest, emergency relief of pressure must be accomplished as soon as the clinical diagnosis is apparent. This may allow little time for x-ray film confirmation. A diagnostic needle tap with a large-bore needle should be performed in the second or third anterior intercostal space. Since the internal mammary artery parallels the sternum approximately one or two finger's breadths from its edge, the needle must be inserted in the midclavicular line to avoid serious bleeding from these vessels.[104] In addition, the needle should be inserted over the top of a rib to avoid the intercostal artery and vein that run on the lower border of each rib.[104]

A moistened glass syringe may be attached to the needle that is inserted into the chest; if there is air under tension, the plunger will be pushed back. Another technique is to attach one end of IV tubing to the needle and place the other end under water in a container on the floor. If there is air under tension in the chest, it will be seen bubbling from the tubing under the water. However, in the presence of cardiovascular collapse from a tension pneumothorax, simply inserting a catheter-over-needle device into the chest, removing the needle, and leaving the catheter open to the air is appropriate. Air escaping through the needle with a hissing noise is proof of tension pneumothorax. Although this maneuver may produce a pneumothorax in itself, an external open pneumothorax is less lethal than an internal closed valve-like tension pneumothorax. With open pneumothorax, positive-pressure ventilation or spontaneous exhalation against resistance can reexpand the lung.

Equipment Needed: 1) Povidone–iodine solution for skin preparation. 2) A 14-gauge catheter-over-needle device.

Technique:

1. Cleanse the overlying skin with povidone–iodine solution.
2. Insert the 14-gauge catheter-over-needle device into the second intercostal space in the midclavicular line just above the top of the third rib.
3. Entry into the pleural space and confirmation of air under tension will be evident by hearing the escape of air through the open needle.
4. Remove the needle and leave the catheter in the pleural space open to atmospheric air.
5. As soon as available, tube thoracostomy with underwater seal drainage should be performed for definitive treatment.

Complications of Treatment: The most common complication is due to misdiagnosis. If a pneumothorax is present but not under tension, inserting the needle will convert it from closed pneumothorax to an open pneumothorax. If there is no pneumothorax, insertion of a needle open to atmosphere will produce a pneumothorax. This can be easily treated with a tube thoracostomy.

Insertion of either a steel needle or a Teflon catheter may lacerate the lung and produce significant pulmonary injury or hemothorax.[105] If the needle is inserted adjacent to the sternum, the internal mammary artery may be punctured; if the needle is inserted at the lower margin of the rib, the intercostal vessels may be lacerated. Either event may lead to significant hemothorax.

References

1. Zoll PM: Resuscitation of the heart in ventricular standstill by external electrical stimulation. *N Engl J Med* 247:768-771, 1952.
2. Zoll PM, Zoll RH, Falk RH, et al: External non-invasive temporary cardiac pacing: Clinical trials. *Circulation* F1:937-944, 1985.
3. Thevenet A, Hodges PC, Lillehei CW: The use of myocardial electrode inserted percutaneously for control of complete atrioventricular block by an artificial pacemaker. *Dis Chest* 34:621-631, 1958.
4. Roe BB: Intractable Stokes-Adams disease. A method of emergency management. *Am Heart J* 69:470-472, 1965.
5. Kodjababian GH, Gray RE, Keenan RL, et al: Percutaneous implantation of cardiac pacemaker electrodes. *Am J Cardiol* 19:372-376, 1967.
6. Evaluation: External pacemakers. *Health Devices* 3:75-96, 1974.
7. Lown B, Kosowsky BD: Artificial cardiac pacemakers. *N Engl J Med* 283:907-916, 971-977, 1023-1031, 1970.
8. Solomon N, Escher DJW: A rapid method for insertion of the pacemaker catheter electrode. *Am Heart J* 66:717-718, 1963.
9. Preston TA: A new temporary pacing catheter with improved sensing and safety characteristics. *Am Heart J* 88:289-293, 1974.
10. Escher DJW, Furman S, Solomon N: Transvenous emergency cardiac pacing. *Ann NY Acad Sci* 167:583-596, 1969.
11. Hartzler GO, Maloney JD, Curtis JJ, et al: Hemodynamic benefits of atrioventricular sequential pacing after cardiac surgery. *Am J Cardiol* 40:232-236, 1977.
12. Resnekow L, Lipp H: Pacemaking and acute myocardial infarction. *Prog Cardiovasc Dis* 14:475-499, 1972.
13. Hindman MC, Wagner GS, Jaro M, et al: The clinical significance of bundle branch block complicating acute myocardial infarction. 1. Clinical characteristics, hospital mortality, and one-year follow-up. 2. Indications for temporary and permanent pacemaker insertion. *Circulation* 58:689-699, 1978.
14. Mullins CB, Atkins JM: Prognosis and management of ventricular conduction blocks in acute myocardial infarction. *Mod Concepts Cardiovasc Dis* 45:129-133, 1976.
15. Jacobson CB, Lester RM, Scheinman MM: Management of acute bundle branch block and bradyarrhythmias. *Med Clin North Am* 63:93-112, 1979.
16. Preston TA: The use of pacemaking for the treatment of acute arrhythmias. *Heart Lung* 6:249-255, 1977.
17. Haft JI: Treatment of arrhythmias by intracardiac electric stimulation. *Prog Cardiovasc Dis* 16:539-568, 1974.
18. Waldo AL, MacLean WAH, Karp RB, et al: Entrainment and interruption of atrial flutter with atrial pacing. Studies in man following open heart surgery. *Circulation* 56:737-745, 1977.
19. Barold SS, Linhart JW: Recent advances in the treatment of ectopic tachycardias by electrical pacing. *Am J Cardiol* 25:698-706, 1970.
20. Haft JI, Kosowsky BD, Lau SH, et al: Termination of atrial flutter by rapid electrical pacing of the atrium. *Am J Cardiol* 20:239-244, 1967.
21. Pittman DE, Makar JS, Kooros KS, et al: Rapid atrial stimulation: Successful method of conversion of atrial flutter and atrial tachycardia. *Am J Cardiol* 32:700-706, 1973.
22. Lister JW, Gosselin AJ, Nathan DA, et al: Rapid atrial stimulation in the treatment of supraventricular tachycardia. *Chest* 63:995-1001, 1973.

23. Massumi RA, Kistin AD, Tawakkol AA: Termination of reciprocating tachycardia by atrial stimulation. *Circulation* 36:637-643, 1967.

24. Lister JW, Cohen LS, Bernstein WH, et al: Treatment of supraventricular tachycardias by rapid atrial stimulation. *Circulation* 38:1004-1059, 1968.

25. Cheng FI: Percutaneous transfemoral venous cardiac pacing. A simple and practical method. *Chest* 60:73-78, 1971.

26. Furman S, Escher DJW: Temporary transvenous pacing. *Principles and Techniques of Cardiac Pacing.* New York, Harper & Row Publishers Inc, 1970, pp 62-112.

27. Meister SG, Banka VS, Helfant RH: Transfemoral pacing with balloon-tipped catheters. *JAMA* 225:712-714, 1973.

28. Schnitzler RN, Caracta AR, Damato AN: "Floating" catheter for temporary transvenous pacing. *Am J Cardiol* 31:351-354, 1973.

29. Bing OH, McDowell JW, Hantman J, et al: Pacemaker placement by electrocardiographic monitoring. *N Engl J Med* 287:651, 1972.

30. Birch LM, Berger M, Thomas PA: Synchronous diaphragmatic contraction. A complication of transvenous cardiac pacing. *Am J Cardiol* 21:88-90, 1968.

31. Glassman RD, Noble RJ, Tavel ME, et al: Pacemaker-induced endocardial friction rub. *Am J Cardiol* 40:811-814, 1977.

32. Bernstein V, Roten CE, Peretz DI: Permanent pacemakers: 8-year follow-up study. Incidence and management of congestive cardiac failure and perforations. *Ann Intern Med* 74:361-369, 1971.

33. Drozd P, Escher DJW, Furman S: Pacing by a bipolar transvenous "semifloating" elecath electrode. *Circulation* 40 (supp 3):III-73, 1969.

34. Nathan DA, Center S, Pina RE, et al: Perforation during indwelling catheter pacing. *Circulation* 33:128-130, 1966.

35. Coder DM: Temporary cardiac pacing in a community practice. *IMJ* 153:27-30, 1978.

36. Barold SS: Modern concepts of cardiac pacing. *Heart Lung* 2:238-252, 1973.

37. Nachnani GH, Gooch AS, Hsu I: Systolic murmurs induced by pacemaker catheters. *Arch Intern Med* 124:202-205, 1969.

38. Kluge WF: Pacemaker sound and its origin. *Am J Cardiol* 25:362-366, 1970.

39. Kramer DH, Moss AJ, Shah PM: Mechanisms and significance of pacemaker-induced extracardiac sound. *Am J Cardiol* 25:367-371, 1970.

40. Korn M, Schoenfeld CD, Ghahramani A, et al: The pacemaker sound. *Am J Med* 49:451-458, 1970.

41. Pupillo GA, Talley RC, Linhart JW: "Pacemaker heart sound" caused by diaphragmatic contractions. *Am Heart J* 82:711-712, 1971.

42. Cheng TO, Ertem G, Vera Z: Heart sounds in patients with cardiac pacemakers. *Chest* 62:66-70, 1972.

43. Kimball JT, Killip T: A simple bedside method for transvenous intracardiac pacing. *Am Heart J* 70:35-39, 1965.

44. Boal BH, Keller BD, Ascheim RS, et al: Complications of intracardiac electrical pacing — knotting together of temporary and permanent electrodes. *N Engl J Med* 280:650-651, 1969.

45. Chatterjee K, Harris A, Davies G, et al: Electrocardiographic changes subsequent to artificial ventricular depolarization. *Br Heart J* 31:770-779, 1969.

46. Anand RK, Smith SA, Starobin OE: A safe approach to pacing during coronary angiography. *N Engl J Med* 288:1395-1396, 1973.

47. Hancock EW: Management of pericardial disease. *Mod Concepts Cardiovasc Dis* 48:1-6, 1979.

48. Roberts WC, Spray TL: Pericardial heart disease: A study of its causes, consequences, and morphologic features, in Spodick D (ed): *Pericardial Diseases.* Cardiovascular Clinics, vol 7, No. 3. Philadelphia, FA Davis Co, 1976, pp 11-65.

49. Fowler NO: Physiology of cardiac tamponade and pulsus paradoxus. II. Physiological, circulatory, and pharmacological responses in cardiac tamponade. *Mod Concepts Cardiovasc Dis* 47:115-118, 1978.

50. Shabetai R: The pathophysiology of cardiac tamponade and constriction, in Spodick D (ed): *Pericardial Diseases.* Cardiovascular Clinics, vol 7, No. 3. Philadelphia, FA Davis Co, 1976, pp 67-89.

51. Shabeta R, Fowler NO, Guntheroth WG: The hemodynamics of cardiac tamponade and constrictive pericarditis. *Am J Cardiol* 26:480-489, 1970.

52. Fowler NO: Physiology of cardiac tamponade and pulsus paradoxus. I. Mechanisms of pulsus paradoxus in cardiac tamponade. *Mod Concepts Cardiovasc Dis* 47:109-113, 1978.

53. Fowler NO: The recognition and management of pericardial disease and its complications, in Hurst JW, Logue RB, Schlant RC, et al (eds): *The Heart, Arteries and Veins.* New York, McGraw-Hill Book Co Inc, 1978, pp 1640-1659.

54. Spodick DH: The pericardium: Structure, function, and disease spectrum, in Spodick DH (ed): *Pericardial Diseases.* Cardiovascular Clinics, vol 7, No. 3. Philadelphia, FA Davis Co, 1976, pp 1-10.

55. Beck CS: Two cardiac compression triads. *JAMA* 104:714-716, 1935.

56. Reddy PS, Curtiss EI, O'Toole JD, et al: Cardiac tamponade: Hemodynamic observations in man. *Circulation* 58:265-272, 1978.

57. Shabetai R: The pericardium: An essay on some recent developments. *Am J Cardiol* 42:1036-1043, 1978.

58. Massumi RA, Mason DT, Vera Z, et al: Reversed pulsus paradoxus. *N Engl J Med* 289:1272-1275, 1973.

59. Cosio FG, Martinez JP, Serrano CM, et al: Abnormal septal motion in cardiac tamponade with pulsus paradoxus. Echocardiographic and hemodynamic observations. *Chest* 71:787, 1977.

60. Settle HP, Adolph RJ, Fowler NO, et al: Echocardiographic study of cardiac tamponade. *Circulation* 56:951-959, 1977.

61. Schiller NB, Botvinick EH: Right ventricular compression as a sign of cardiac tamponade. An analysis of echocardiographic ventricular dimensions and their clinical implications. *Circulation* 56:774-779, 1977.

62. Armstrong WF, Schilt BF, Helper DJ, et al: Diastolic collapse of the right ventricle with cardiac tamponade: An echocardiographic study. *Circulation* 65:1491, 1982.

63. Usher BW, Popp RL: Electrical alternans: Mechanism in pericardial effusion. *Am Heart J* 83:459-463, 1972.

64. Pories WJ, Gaudiani VA: Cardiac tamponade. *Surg Clin North Am* 55:573-589, 1975.

65. Cooper FW Jr, Stead EA Jr, Warren JV: Beneficial effect of intravenous infusions in acute pericardial tamponade. *Ann Surg* 120:822-825, 1944.

66. Kilpatrick ZM, Chapman CB: On pericardiocentesis. *Am J Cardiol* 16:722-728, 1965.

67. Bishop LH Jr, Estes EH Jr, McIntosh HD: The electrocardiogram as a safeguard in pericardiocentesis. *JAMA* 162:264-265, 1956.

68. Sobol SM, Thomas HM Jr, Evans RW: Myocardial laceration not demonstrated by continuous electrocardiographic monitoring occuring during pericardiocentesis. *N Engl J Med* 292:1222-1223, 1975.

69. Kerber RE, Ridges JD, Harrison DC: Electrocardiographic indications of atrial puncture during pericardiocentesis. *N Engl J Med* 282:1142-1143, 1970.

70. Moncure AC, McEnany MT: Cardiovascular emergencies, in Wilkins EW Jr (ed): *Textbook of Emergency Medicine.* Baltimore, Williams & Wilkins Co, 1978, pp 377-399.

71. Hancock EW: Cardiac tamponade. *Med Clin North Am* 63:223-237, 1979.

72. Glancy DL, Richter MA: Catheter drainage of the pericardial space. *Cathet Cardiovasc Diagn* 1:311-315, 1975.

73. Owens WC, Schaefer RA, Rahimtoola SH: Pericardiocentesis: Insertion of a pericardial catheter. *Cathet Cardiovasc Diagn* 1:317-321, 1975.

74. Wei JY, Taylor GJ, Achuff SC: Recurrent cardiac tamponade and large pericardial effusions: Management with an indwelling pericardial catheter. *Am J Cardiol* 42:281-282, 1978.

75. Krikorian JG, Hancock EW: Pericardiocentesis. *Am J Med* 65:808-814, 1978.

76. Wong B, Murphy J, Chang CJ, et al: The risk of pericardiocentesis. *Am J Cardiol* 44:1110-1114, 1979.

77. Amey BD, Harrison EE, Straub EJ, et al: Paramedic use of intracardiac medications in prehospital sudden cardiac death. *JACEP* 7:130-134, 1978.

78. McSwain NE Jr: Intracardiac injections of medication, editorial. *JACEP* 7:170-171, 1978.

79. Davidson R, Barresi V, Parker M, et al: Intracardiac injections during cardiopulmonary resuscitation, a low-risk procedure, abstracted. *Crit Care Med* 7:126, 1979.

80. Hasegawa EA: The endotracheal administration of drugs. *Heart Lung* 15:60-63, 1986.

81. Killen DA, Gobbel WG: *Spontaneous Pneumothorax.* Boston, Little Brown & Co, 1968.

82. Comroe JH: *Physiology of Respiration.* Chicago, Yearbook Medical Publishers, 1979, p 102.
83. Teplick SK, Clark RE: Various faces of tension pneumothorax. *Postgrad Med* 56:87-92, 1974.
84. Fraser RG, Pare JA: *Diagnosis of Diseases of the Chest.* Philadelphia, WB Saunders Co, 1977, vol 1, ed 2, pp 598-600.
85. Martin JT, Patrick RT: Pneumothorax: Its significance to the anesthesiologist. *Anesth Analg* 39:420-429, 1960.
86. Macklin CC: Transport of air along sheaths f pulmonic blood vessels from alveoli to mediastinum; clinical implications. *Arch Intern Med* 64:913-926, 1939.
87. Macklin MT, Macklin CC: Malignant interstitial emphysema of the lungs and mediastinum as an important occult complication in many respiratory diseases and other conditions: An interpretation of the clinical literature in the light of laboratory experiment. *Medicine* 23:281-358, 1944.
88. Scoggin CH, Sahn SA, Petty TL: Status asthmaticus. A nine-year experience. *JAMA* 238:1158-11162, 1977.
89. Safar P: Blunt chest injuries, in Weil MH, Henning RJ (eds): *Handbook of Critical Care Medicine.* New York, EM Books, 1979, pp 93-103.
90. Klick JM, Bushnell LS, Bancroft ML: Barotrauma, a potential hazard of manual resuscitators. *Anesthesiology* 49:363-365, 1978.
91. Wisborg K, Jacobsen E: Functional disorders of Ruben and Ambu-E valves after dismantling and cleaning. *Anesthesiology* 42:633-634, 1975.
92. Dean HN, Parsons DE, Raphaely RC: Case report: Bilateral tension pneumothorax from mechanical failure of anesthesia machine due to misplaced expiratory valve. *Anesth Analg* 50:195-198, 1971.
93. Mundth ED, Foley FD, Austen WG: Pneumothorax as a complication of pulmonary infarct in patients on positive pressure respiratory assistance. *J Thorac Cardiovasc Surg* 50:555-560, 1965.
94. Rohlfing BM, Webb WR, Schlobohm RM: Ventilator-related extra-alveolar air in adults. *Radiology* 121:25-31, 1976.
95. Kumar A, Pontoppidan H, Falke KJ, et al: Pulmonary barotrauma during mechanical ventilation. *Crit Care Med* 1:181-186, 1973.
96. Zwillich CW, Pierson DJ, Creagh CE, et al: Complications of assisted ventilation. A prospective study of 354 consecutive episodes. *Am J Med* 57:161-170, 1974.
97. Powner DJ, Snyder JV, Morris CW, et al: Retroperitoneal air dissection associated with mechanical ventilation. *Chest* 69:739-742, 1976.
98. Hazards of fiberoptic bronchoscopy, editorial. *Br Med J* 1:212-213, 1979.
99. Stutz FH: Bilateral tension pneumothorax after pneumoperitoneum: A case report. *Milit Med* 136:894-895, 1971.
100. Nayak IN, Lawrence D: Tension pneumothorax from a perforated gastric ulcer. *Br J Surg* 63:245-247, 1976.
101. Netter FH: Respiratory system. The Ciba Collection of Medical Illustrations. Summit, NJ, Ciba, 1979, vol 7, pp 243-244.
102. Estafanous FG, Viljoen JF, Barsoum KN: Diagnosis of pneumothorax complicating mechanical ventilation. *Anesth Analg* 54:730-735, 1975.
103. McLoud TC, Barash PG, Ravin CE, et al: Elevation of pulmonary artery pressure as a sign of pulmonary barotrauma (pneumothorax). *Crit Care Med* 6:81-84,1978.
104. Grant JCB: *An Atlas of Anatomy,* ed 6. Baltimore, Williams & Wilkins Co, 1972.
105. Hansbrough JF, Chandler JF: Lung laceration following catheter insertion into the chest for pneumothorax. *Emer Med Ser* 8:48, 1979.

Credit is given to Peter Miniscalco for artwork and photography.

Postresuscitation Management

Chapter 14

There is no simple overall prescription for the management of the patient in the postresuscitation period. The causes of cardiopulmonary arrest are multiple and varied, and the range of results of resuscitation wide. The goal of this chapter is to provide information that can be used to continue to support physiologic systems after a spontaneous pulse has returned and to determine possible etiologies of the arrest.

Postresuscitation management for the two extremes of resuscitation results will be discussed. At one extreme is the situation in which the patient is awake, responsive, and breathing spontaneously. At the other is the situation in which single- or multiple-system failure requiring supplemental or total support is still present.

The Two Extremes of Resuscitation Results

Maximal Response to Resuscitation

The patient is awake, responsive, and breathing spontaneously. The resuscitation team should accomplish the following:

a. Apply ECG monitor leads.
b. Provide supplemental oxygen with nasal prongs and humidifier or face mask and nebulizer.
c. Start an intravenous (IV) infusion with 5% dextrose in water. If the arrest rhythm was ventricular fibrillation (VF) or ventricular tachycardia (VT), inject a bolus of lidocaine and follow with a lidocaine infusion. If the heart rate is below 50 beats/min, consider the use of IV atropine if hemodynamics are still not optimal and morphine if the patient is in pain (see Chapter 7).
d. Seek the precipitating cause of the cardiac arrest.
e. Assess the hemodynamic status; auscultate the heart and lung fields.
f. Review vital signs and urine output.
g. Determine whether the patient is a candidate for continuing aggressive care.
h. Review a 12-lead ECG and portable anteroposterior chest film.
i. Review arterial blood gases and pH, serum electrolytes including magnesium and calcium (ionized), and previous as well as current drug therapy.
j. Transfer the patient to a special care unit for monitoring, observation, and further therapeutic interventions.
k. Assess for the possibility of myocardial injury.
l. If pulmonary congestion or pulmonary edema is visible on the chest x-ray film, it is advisable to insert a pulmonary artery catheter to distinguish between cardiogenic and noncardiogenic pulmonary edema (see "Cardiovascular System"). Diuretics, inotropes, and/or vasodilators may be indicated if congestive heart failure is present. Supraventricular tachycardia may often require cardioversion or treatment with antiarrhythmic drugs, especially if it is associated with hemodynamic instability.

Single or Multiple System Failure Requiring Supplemental or Total Support

The patient is intubated, and spontaneous breathing may be absent or present. The patient may:

a. Have required a prolonged period of external chest compression,
b. Have received multiple drugs,
c. Be in coma or show decreased responsiveness,
d. Be hemodynamically unstable.

Unless the cardiac arrest occurred in a special care unit, arrangements should be made immediately to transfer the patient to a special care unit. When the arrest occurs out of the hospital, transportation should proceed as outlined in Chapter 1. When in the hospital, transfer to the special care unit requires the assistance of at least three clinical personnel. In addition to the physical handling of the patient, each of the three assumes specific responsibilities to 1) support ventilation and provide oxygenation with a manual resuscitator and oxygen system (bag–valve or other type), 2) monitor ECG, carotid pulse, and blood pressure and initiate external chest compression if an arrest occurs en route to the special care unit, and 3) regulate the intravenous therapy being delivered.

Prior to transportation to the special care unit, the IV fluid lifeline should be secured in good position. The ECG leads should be connected to a portable monitor–defibrillator for continuous ECG monitoring by the ACLS provider who has that responsibility.

During transportation, the monitor–defibrillator should go with the patient, as should a full E cylinder of oxygen with suitable connections to a bag–valve (with reservoir) system. Appropriate drugs (which include epinephrine, lidocaine, atropine, and additional IV fluid) should be readily available.

There are special carts that can accommodate all of these functions. Ideally, in each hospital there is at least one such dedicated cart.

Chapter 14

Management in the Special Care Unit

The systems approach discussed here is designed for the first 72 hours after cardiac arrest.

Respiratory System

Observe the patient for spontaneous breathing; if present, look for evidence of flail chest, which may have been caused by external chest compression.

Auscultation

Auscultate to ascertain that breath sounds are bilateral and equal. Unilateral breath sounds on the right are suggestive of intubation of the right main-stem bronchus by an endotracheal tube that has been advanced too far into the airway. Unilateral breath sounds are also consistent with a pneumothorax.

Air, blood, or fluid in the pleural space as well as the collapse of the lung due to obstruction of the airway may also account for absence of transmitted breath sounds. Râles are due to fluid in the airway caused by secretions, aspiration of gastric contents (noncardiogenic pulmonary edema), or pulmonary edema precipitated by heart failure.

Chest X-ray

The position of the endotracheal tube (the tip should be level with the arch of the aorta) and the position of the central venous catheter, if one has been placed, should be checked. Current x-ray films should always be compared with previous films, if available. Attention should be paid to lung fields, vascular pattern, height of diaphragms, cardiac silhouette, pleural spaces, and ribs. Fractured ribs may have perforated the pleura and lung during external chest compression and produced a pneumothorax. Decubitus films should be obtained if pleural fluid is suspected. Always request bilateral decubitus films even if only unilateral fluid is suspected. If fluid is present in the pleural space, the lung field is obscured partially when the lateral decubitus film is obtained. When the patient is turned to the other decubitus position, the fluid in the pleural space drains by gravity into the retrocardiac space, and pathology in the lung field can be identified more readily.

Mechanical Ventilation

A volume-limited ventilator should be used to accommodate the following:

1. Full-Time Mechanical Ventilation: Options for assist-control or intermittent mandatory ventilation (IMV) should be available.

2. Tidal Volume: An adequate tidal volume in milliliters can be estimated by multiplying the patient's ideal body weight in kilograms by 10.[1] Lung volumes are related to ideal, not absolute, weight.

3. Inspiratory–Expiratory Ratio (I:E): This is an expression of the ratio of duration of inspiration to the duration of expiration; it should be 1:2 or 1:1.5. The longer exhalation time may facilitate venous return during positive-pressure mechanical ventilation and assure completion of exhalation when airway resistance is increased.

4. Respiratory Rate: An initial respiratory rate or frequency ("f") of 10–12 times/min is recommended.

5. Pressure Limit: This level should be set at 10 cmH_2O higher than the pressure generated by the delivered tidal volume. Excessively high pressures must be avoided so that the risks of barotrauma, including pneumothorax, may be reduced.

6. Oxygen (F_IO_2): The fractional inspired oxygen (F_IO_2) should be 1.0 (i.e., inspired O_2 percent = 100%) initially. The starting F_IO_2 should be high since there is no indication of the degree of hypoxemia. Making a guess and starting at lower F_IO_2 could be lethal.

7. Sensitivity: A 2 cmH_2O sensitivity setting (setting for assist-control) is recommended. This setting dictates the inspiratory effort required by the patient to initiate the next mechanical ventilation. There should be no attempt to change the sensitivity as a means of controlling the patient's respiratory rate. If the IMV mode is selected, sensitivity is set to maximum or "least sensitive" or bypassed by the IMV circuitry.

8. Humidifier Temperature: A midrange humidifier temperature setting is recommended, or if a thermometer is in circuit and is close to the endotracheal tube, a temperature of 97°F or 36°C (just below body temperature) should be prescribed.

9. Positive End-Expiratory Pressure (PEEP): A positive end-expiratory pressure of 5 cmH_2O maintains functional residual capacity and prevents alveolar collapse.[2] Therapeutic PEEP above 5 cmH_2O may be required.[3]

Suction

The endotracheal tube, trachea, and major bronchi should be suctioned every 1–2 hours. If pulmonary edema is present, it may be necessary to suction more frequently. If the F_IO_2 is less than 1.0, it should be increased to 1.0 prior to suctioning. Each suctioning episode should not exceed 15 seconds, and the patient should be reoxygenated between each episode. Because the patient is ventilated with PEEP, it is simpler to reoxygenate the patient using the mechanical ventilator rather than a manual resuscitator bag. However, a manual resuscitator bag with reservoir and a PEEP valve attached to the expiratory port must be available at all times at the bedside. The PEEP valve attached to the resuscitator bag should provide the same quantity of PEEP as that provided by the ventilator. If the tracheal aspirate is thick, humidification needs to be reassessed. If the humidifier is at the correct temperature, nebulized half-normal saline should be delivered for 10 min/hr or an ultrasonic device added.

The tracheal aspirate should be sent to the laboratory for Gram's stain, culture, and sensitivity. If the patient is, or becomes, febrile and a pneumonic infiltrate is seen on chest x-ray film, appropriate antibiotic therapy can be started without delay.

Volume and Pressure in Endotracheal Tube Cuff

This volume and pressure should be measured and charted every 4 hours. Be certain that the endotracheal tube is of optimum size and has a high-compliance, low-pressure cuff.[4] As long as there is no leak between the cuff and the tracheal wall, the cuff volume will probably remain reasonably constant. If the cuff is intact and increasing volumes are required to prevent a leak, malacia of the trachea is developing. Increases in cuff volume can result in an increase in cuff pressure and damage to the wall of the trachea. Normal arteriolar or proximal capillary hydrostatic pressure is approximately 40 cm H_2O. As the endotracheal tube cuff pressure exceeds 40 cm H_2O, blood flow in the tracheal wall circulation adjacent to the cuff will be impaired; the result is necrosis, malacia, or stenosis of the tracheal wall. If systemic mean blood pressure is decreased, arteriolar pressure will be decreased and less cuff pressure, theoretically, will be required to impair tracheal circulation.

Expensive apparatus is not necessary to measure intracuff pressure. Simply attach one side of a three-way stopcock to the valve of the pilot tube of the endotracheal tube, and another side of the stopcock to the mercury column of a sphygmomanometer (an aneroid manometer is equally good), and measure the pressure directly. Remove the three-way stopcock after use to prevent air leak from the cuff of the endotracheal tube. Routine deflation of the cuff is not necessary, but should an attempt be made to deflate the cuff, the hypopharynx should be suctioned first.

Arterial Blood

A sample should be collected and analyzed 20 minutes following initiation of alteration in the level of mechanical ventilation. This is the time required to reach a steady state in ventilation and $PaCO_2$. This sample can be obtained from the radial or femoral artery by trained members of a special care unit team. The radial artery usually can be palpated unless the patient has poor peripheral circulation, i.e., shock.

About 2–3 mL of arterial blood should be collected anaerobically in a heparinized syringe, the needle removed, and the syringe hub covered with a small rubber cap. Excess heparin in the syringe will adversely affect pH determination. The syringe should be placed in a bag of crushed ice and the sample transported rapidly to the laboratory for measurement of PaO_2, $PaCO_2$, and pH.

The $PaCO_2$ and pH are examined in order to assess ventilation and acid–base balance.

Decreased $PaCO_2$: If $PaCO_2$ is less than 35 mmHg and pH more than 7.45, the patient is hyperventilated and the respiratory frequency or IMV rate of the ventilator should be reduced. Blood gases should then be re-measured after 20 minutes. A blood sample should be sent to the chemistry laboratory to recheck the serum potassium level. Respiratory alkalosis results in a re-duced serum potassium; if digitalis has been prescribed, the combination of digitalis and hypokalemia can result in arrhythmias. A $PaCO_2$ of less than 36 mmHg and a pH of less than 7.36 constitute a hyperventilatory response to a metabolic acidosis. If possible, treat the underlying cause of the metabolic acidosis and remeasure the arterial blood gases. Continue the steps until the $PaCO_2$ and pH are within normal limits.

Increased $PaCO_2$: If the $PaCO_2$ is more than 44 mmHg and the pH is less than 7.35, the condition is hypoventilation. Increase the frequency of IMV, and after 20 minutes remeasure the arterial blood gases. If the response is minimal, an incorrect tidal volume may have been selected. Increase tidal volume by 100 mL and repeat arterial blood gases. Monitor adjustments of changes in 1) respiratory frequency and 2) tidal volume. Further adjustments of respiratory frequency may have to be made subsequently.

If the $PaCO_2$ is more than 45 mmHg and the pH is normal, the patient may have chronic obstructive pulmo-nary disease (COPD). Under these circumstances the ventilator settings should not be adjusted as the patient probably has chronic CO_2 retention with compensatory retention of bicarbonate.

Hypoventilation may be a physiologic response to a metabolic alkalosis secondary to, for example, loop diuretics or nasogastric suctioning. Review the chart to see if diuretics have been given; also observe the intake and output chart to assess nasogastric suction and urine volumes. Metabolic alkalosis usually is associated with hypokalemia; therefore, the serum potassium should be rechecked. The hypokalemia of metabolic alkalosis is due to a shift of potassium from extracellular to intra-cellular fluid and excretion of potassium by the kidney in an attempt to retain hydrogen ions.

Metabolic alkalosis and hypokalemia can usually be corrected with potassium chloride. Ten to 15 milli-equivalents (mEq) of potassium chloride per hour can be infused through a central vein. No more than 10 mEq/hr should be infused through a peripheral vein. After three sequential doses, serum potassium and acid–base balance are reassessed. If the potassium is still below normal and the metabolic alkalosis is still present, further potassium chloride should be prescribed in the same manner as before. If, after the first additional sequential dose has been given, the serum potassium remains low, a lower replacement schedule should be used so that no more than 200 mEq is administered in a 24-hour period. Intravenous potassium is contraindicated in patients in oliguric renal failure. If the serum potassium has returned to normal and a significant metabolic alkalosis that impairs function (e.g., causes respiratory depression) still persists, the condition can be corrected with acetazolamide.

If renal function is intact, acetazolamide (Diamox), 250–500 mg, can be administered IV. Bicarbonate reabsorption occurs in the proximal tubule of the nephron. Initially, sodium is reabsorbed and hydrogen is secreted into the lumen and combined with the bicarbonate to form carbonic acid. The carbonic acid dissociates and the CO_2 enters the tubular cell and forms carbonic acid; it dissociates to hydrogen ions and bicarbonate. Hydrogen is secreted into the tubule in exchange for sodium, and bicarbonate is retained. In the tubule cell the reaction $CO_2 + H_2O = H_2CO_3$ is rate-dependent on carbonic anhydrase. Acetazolamide inhibits the action of carbonic anhydrase and prevents the conservation of bicarbonate by the proximal tubule.

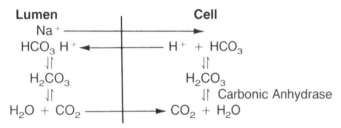

Arterial Oxygen Tension (PaO₂). The inspired oxygen concentration is reduced using the "rule of seven" to give a PaO_2 of 100 mmHg. One atmosphere of 100% oxygen (minus $PaCO_2$ and water vapor) is approximately equal to 700 mmHg (at sea level). Therefore, 1% oxygen is approximately equal to 7 mmHg.

Rule of seven: To provide a PaO_2 of 100 mmHg:

$$\frac{\text{Reported } PaO_2 - 100}{7}$$

Example: If $PaO_2 = 380$ mmHg on $F_IO_2 = 0.90$,

$$\frac{380 - 100}{7} = \frac{280}{7} = 40\%$$

i.e., 40% of the oxygen is unnecessary.

Reduce O_2 concentration by 40% from 90% to 50%:

$$F_IO_2 = 0.90 \text{ to } 0.50.$$

Titrate back F_IO_2 and repeat arterial blood gases after 20 minutes. Further adjustments can be made using the rule of seven, and subsequently, a PaO_2 of 75–80 mmHg can be achieved. This technique takes away guesswork and prevents undershooting PaO_2 if F_IO_2 is reduced indiscriminately.

If the PaO_2 is less than 350 mmHg when F_IO_2 equals 0.90, a significant intrapulmonary shunt exists and PEEP must be increased from prophylactic levels to therapeutic levels[3] and/or cardiac output must be improved. Decisions can be made only after measurement of intrapulmonary shunt and cardiac index (see "Cardiovascular System").

Definition of Intrapulmonary Shunt: In the normal lung, there is relative matching between ventilation and circulation. If alveoli cease to function, collapse, or fill with fluid but the adjacent circulation continues, venous blood flowing through that portion of the lung is not oxygenated. This is termed intrapulmonary shunting. If hemodynamics remain unchanged as intrapulmonary shunting increases, arterial oxygen tension decreases. The percent of intrapulmonary shunt is defined as that percent of right ventricular output that perfuses nonfunctioning alveoli.

Measurement of Intrapulmonary Shunt: This measurement has customarily been made with the patient breathing 100% oxygen.[5] Because 100% oxygen results in absorptive atelectasis, evidence indicates that this technique provides inaccurate information and the measured shunt is, in fact, higher than the true shunt.[6] To overcome this problem, the intrapulmonary shunt is measured with the patient breathing a lower F_IO_2 (0.3–0.6) when possible. If the patient has chronic obstructive lung disease, measurement of intrapulmonary shunt at $F_IO_2 = 1.0$ is probably better. This eliminates confusion due to ventilation:perfusion inequality, which, in COPD, becomes evident at an F_IO_2 less than 1.0. To perform the measurement the patient is left undisturbed for a period of 20 minutes, at which time an arterial and a mixed venous sample of blood are collected. A mixed venous blood sample can be collected from either a central venous catheter, if the tip of the catheter is in the right atrium, or the distal port of a pulmonary artery catheter. The latter provides a more accurate mixed venous sample. Arterial and venous oxygen tensions are assessed and arterial and venous oxygen contents are either measured with an oximeter or calculated using an oxygen dissociation graph. Measurement of hemoglobin is also required if an oximeter is not available.

To calculate intrapulmonary shunt, see "Glossary". Normal intrapulmonary shunt ($\dot{Q}_s/\dot{Q}_t$) is up to 5% of cardiac output.

Causes of increased $\dot{Q}_s/\dot{Q}_t$ in patients in the early postresuscitation period include

1. cardiogenic pulmonary edema,
2. aspiration pneumonitis,
3. nonaspiration pneumonitis,
4. pulmonary bone marrow emboli from trauma to the sternum during CPR,
5. Adult Respiratory Distress Syndrome (ARDS), particularly associated with sepsis,
6. atelectasis,
7. contributory causes of the arrest, e.g., thermal injuries, toxic chemicals, etc.

As $\dot{Q}_s/\dot{Q}_t$ increases, PaO_2 decreases. Initial therapy to decrease $\dot{Q}_s/\dot{Q}_t$ and increase PaO_2 should be through the use of therapeutic PEEP.

Application of Therapeutic PEEP

Positive end-expiratory pressure should be increased in increments of 2.5–5.0 cmH$_2$O. If the ventilator is set in the assist-control mode, with each change in PEEP the sensitivity of the ventilator may have to be readjusted. With each incremental increase in PEEP, a check should be made of vital signs, particularly systemic blood pressure. The use of intraarterial pressure monitoring is essential since readings are continuously displayed and acute changes are easily appreciated. Arterial blood gases should be reassessed 20 minutes after PEEP levels have been changed. PEEP may decrease $\dot{Q}_s/\dot{Q}_t$ and simultaneously decrease cardiac output, but it has been shown in some patients that PEEP may decrease $\dot{Q}_s/\dot{Q}_t$ and increase cardiac output.[7] An assessment of these changes can be made only by sequential measurement of both $\dot{Q}_s/\dot{Q}_t$ and cardiac output.

The objective of optimal PEEP is to reduce the intrapulmonary shunt. Since cardiac output may also be decreased, fluid administration or vasoactive drugs may be required to restore cardiac output. If the pulmonary artery occlusive pressure (PAOP) is grossly elevated, fluid infusion may be contraindicated and diuretics, vasodilators (nitroglycerin and nitroprusside), or inotropes (dobutamine and amrinone) may be necessary. Calcium appears to have only a transient effect in augmenting cardiac output and offers little assistance in this setting. If IMV rather than the assist-control mode is used, less depression of cardiac output may be produced by therapeutic PEEP but only if the patient has some spontaneous ventilation. The improvement in cardiac output with IMV is due to a reduction in intrathoracic pressure on inspiration and an increase in venous return.

Intermittent Mandatory Ventilation (IMV)[8]

If the patient initially is spontaneously breathing or starts to show signs of assisting the ventilator (assist light illuminated), or is fully responsive, he or she may be switched from the assist-control mode of ventilation to IMV. This mode allows the patient to breathe spontaneously while the machine continues to deliver a preset number of breaths per minute. The advantage of the use of the IMV system is that during spontaneous ventilations, transpulmonary pressure decreases; with assist-control ventilation, transpulmonary pressure increases and barotrauma and decreased cardiac output are potential hazards. The IMV rate is initially set at the same respiratory rate as the assist-control mode and is slowly reduced if the arterial blood gas levels (particularly $PaCO_2$ and pH) remain satisfactory until it is minimal (2 per minute). When the IMV rate is minimal, the spontaneous respiratory rate is not markedly elevated, and the arterial blood gases are satisfactory ($PaCO_2$ and pH within normal limits, PaO_2 equal or close to 100 mmHg with a low F_IO_2 and PEEP 5 cmH$_2$O), discontinuation of mechanical ventilation can be considered. Oxygen and humidity are delivered via a T piece. If arterial blood gases remain acceptable and the patient is responsive enough to protect his or her own airway, the endotracheal tube may be removed and the patient oxygenated with a face mask and nebulized oxygen.

If PaO_2 and pH are within normal limits and PaO_2 is about 100 mmHg but only with a high F_IO_2 or on therapeutic levels of PEEP, the patient should be left to breathe spontaneously with therapeutic PEEP. This is termed continuous positive airway pressure, or CPAP. As arterial oxygen tension improves, PEEP can be reduced in small steps, sequentially following the arterial oxygen tension. When the PEEP level reaches 5 cmH$_2$O, as indicated above, the possibility of extubation may be entertained.

High-Frequency Positive-Pressure Jet Ventilation (HFPPJV)

Transtracheal jet ventilation, described in Chapter 3 as an emergency ventilatory technique, has now evolved into a sophisticated procedure for total and prolonged ventilatory support termed "high-frequency positive-pressure jet ventilation".

Oxygen and air at 50 psi are passed through an oxygen blender to a high-frequency jet ventilator (HFJV). The ventilator operates using either a fluidic or electronic system. The gas mixture leaves the HFJV and terminates in the jet port of a jet endotracheal tube. The jet endotracheal tube has a T piece attached to the 15-mm connector. Ambient pressure gas from the flow meter of the oxygen blender moves through a reservoir bag and corrugated wide-bore tubing to one arm of the T piece. This system delivers the gas that is entrained during HFPPJV. The other arm of the T piece is attached to corrugated tubing and is the exhalation limb of the system. It terminates in a PEEP valve. Currently, the tendency is to use HFPPJV at rates of 100–150 per minute. The I:E ratio is normally 1:2. Adjustment of the driving pressure will alter carbon dioxide washout and $PaCO_2$. Adjusting the F_IO_2 on the oxygen blender and varying the level of PEEP will alter PaO_2.

Because of the low tidal volumes and negligible internal compliance, high peak pressures are not generated during inspiration. Hence, HFPPJV does not promote impedance of venous return and cardiac output. In the post-cardiac-arrest period this is of major importance. The absence of high peak pressure also reduces the hazard of barotrauma to the lungs and the propensity to develop a pneumothorax if rib fractures occurred as a result of external cardiac compression.

HFPPJV does not interfere with spontaneous ventilation which occurs simultaneously with jet ventilation. The reduction in transthoracic pressure further promotes venous return and cardiac output.

Cardiovascular System

The cardiovascular system should be assessed from the eye grounds to the peripheral pulses in the hands and feet. Careful auscultation of the heart and lungs should be carried out with documentation of normal and abnormal findings. The character of the neck veins in patients who do not have intracardiac catheters is recorded. The complete cardiovascular examination and the documentation of findings, both normal and abnormal, constitutes a baseline for continuing comparison during the ensuing days.

A clinical assessment of the cardiovascular system will include a review of:

1. Vital signs, blood pressure, pulse for rate and rhythm, and urine output;
2. A 12-lead ECG;
3. Chest x-ray film (if not previously reviewed) for evaluation of cardiac silhouette and evidence of pulmonary edema;
4. Serum electrolytes, including Mg and Ca (ionized), serum protein, and albumin;
5. Serial ECG's and cardiac enzymes;
6. Current and previous therapy;
7. Specific procedures as indicated, e.g., echocardiographic assessment for presence of pericardial fluid.

If the patient is hemodynamically unstable, blood pressure decreased, pulse rate increased, and urine output decreased, it is necessary to assess both circulating fluid status and ventricular function. The assessment of circulating or intravascular fluid requires information about hydrostatic and oncotic pressures. Hydrostatic pressure measurements of the pulmonary circulation are obtained with a pulmonary artery flow-directed catheter. Central venous pressures correlate with right ventricular function but should not be used to determine left ventricular function in critically ill patients.[9,10]

When the pulmonary artery catheter is in the "occluded position", the pressure recorded reflects left atrial pressure. (See Figure 19, Chapter 12.) In turn, left atrial pressure reflects left ventricular end-diastolic pressure and end-diastolic volume in the absence of mitral valvular disease. Unfortunately, when the PAOP exceeds 15 mmHg, the 95% confidence limit of predicting left atrial pressure is at least $\pm$ 5 mmHg.[11] Hemodynamic status is assessed using the combination of systemic and pulmonary vascular pressures as well as cardiac output. Cardiac output is measured most easily using a pulmonary artery flow-directed catheter with a thermistor probe. For techniques of insertion of a pulmonary artery flow-directed catheter, see Chapter 12.

Oscilloscopic Patterns and Pressures

The proximal and distal ports of a pulmonary artery flow-directed catheter, when attached through a transducer to a monitor, provide information about waveform and pressure. The proximal port is used to record the right atrial waveform and pressure. The right atrial waveform has oscillations of narrow amplitude with normal pressures up to 8 mmHg. The distal port is used to obtain samples of mixed venous blood, to record right ventricular pressures during passage of the catheter, and to indicate pulmonary artery pressure (PAP) and PAOP when the catheter is positioned correctly. The pulmonary artery and right ventricular tracings have a similar systolic configuration with almost identical pressures in the absence of pulmonic valvular or outflow obstruction. The pulmonary artery diastolic pressure is generally higher than the right ventricular diastolic pressure, which is 0–8 mmHg. The pulmonary occlusive pressure is a tracing of low amplitude. The mean occlusive pressure is most usually recorded and is normally up to 5 mmHg lower than the pulmonary artery diastolic pressure (see "Glossary"). When pulmonary artery hypertension is present but left heart pressures are normal, the pulmonary artery diastolic and PAOP difference may be far greater than 5 mmHg.

When a patient is mechanically ventilated, the positive pressure affects the tracing and pressure readings. The application of positive end-expiratory pressure will increase the PAOP above left atrial pressure.[12] Each 5 mmHg increase in PEEP may increase PAOP by 1 mmHg. However, the change in PAOP with PEEP will depend on the compliance of the lung: Greater changes will be produced in the compliant than the noncompliant lung. Further, during mechanical ventilation, the PAOP will vary with the pattern of ventilation and will be higher during the inspiratory phase than during the expiratory phase. Therefore, the measurements, to be consistent and comparable, should always be made during the expiratory phase and from a paper recording of the waveform tracing.

Frequent recordings of pulmonary artery pressures and PAOP's allow immediate decisions to be made with respect to fluid intake, diuretics, and other therapy. In the event that the catheter no longer can be floated into the occluded position, pulmonary artery diastolic pressures can be used to estimate the PAOP (if the pulmonary artery diastolic pressures have been adequately recorded and the pulmonary artery diastolic and PAO pressure difference is known).[13]

A PAOP less than 5 mmHg is consistent with hypovolemia. A PAOP above 17 mmHg usually is consistent with pulmonary vascular congestion; and above 24 mmHg, with pulmonary edema. However, when pulmonary edema develops without a markedly elevated occlusive pressure, an abnormality in the plasma oncotic pressure needs to be considered.

Cardiac Output

If a triple-lumen pulmonary artery flow-directed catheter is inserted, the proximal port can be used to inject dye and the cardiac output measured using the dye dilution method. Alternatively, if a quadruple-lumen catheter is inserted, the proximal port is used to inject saline while the fourth lumen carries the thermistor probe or temperature sensor. The manufacture of small, lightweight, and easily portable cardiac output computers permits cardiac outputs to be measured simply and accurately using the thermodilution technique. Once the quadruple-lumen catheter has been inserted and is in the correct position, trained members of the special care unit team can measure cardiac output at prescribed intervals. The patient's hemodynamic data can be assessed and compared with previous readings. The data will indicate the changes produced by therapy such as fluids and drugs. The changes in cardiac output coupled with changes in PAOP allow the team leader to assess changes in cardiac function and effectively optimize cardiac output with appropriate therapy (see Chapters 2 and 12).

Measured and Derived Data

Measurement of systemic blood pressure, pulse rate, cardiac output, pulmonary artery and occlusive pressures, and knowledge of the patient's height and weight or calculated surface area programmed into a calculator can provide the following: cardiac index, stroke index, left ventricular stroke work, systemic or peripheral vascular resistance, right ventricular stroke work, and pulmonary vascular resistance. If a sample of mixed venous blood from the distal port and a sample of arterial blood are drawn simultaneously, arterial–mixed-venous oxygen content difference [$C(a-v)O_2$] can be measured and intrapulmonary shunt and oxygen consumption calculated. (See "Glossary".)

It has been observed that following an acute myocardial infarction, optimum cardiac output is obtained with PAOP's higher than those required in normal hearts.[14] However, as PAOP is adjusted, cardiac output measurements should be followed in order not to overshoot and result in adverse effects. The object is to derive a Starling's Curve and optimize cardiac output.

The ongoing assessment of cardiac output, PAOP, and systemic vascular resistance will provide the basis for fluid therapy, diuretic therapy, and other complex interventions aimed at adjusting ventricular preload, afterload, and contractility. (See Chapters 2 and 12.) Again, repeat assessment of these parameters should be made after fluids and drugs have been administered. (See Appendix 1.)

Pacing

Artificial cardiac pacing using a temporary transvenous pacemaker may be indicated in symptomatic second- or third-degree AV block after an acute myocardial infarction or in symptomatic drug-resistant arrhythmias such as sinus bradycardia and sinus arrest (see Chapters 2 and 13). Once in position, the pacing wire can be attached to a demand-type pacemaker which functions only when the R-R intervals of the natural rhythm exceed a preset limit.

Pulmonary Edema

In the lungs the vascular bed includes pulmonary capillaries, and the ventilation system consists of the alveolar walls. Interposed between these two is the interstitial space. The alveolar wall is made up of a number of cells, among which is the Type II pneumocyte that produces surfactant. Pulmonary lymphatics are found away from the functioning units of the lung and closer to the bronchioles. Excess liquid from the vascular compartment, the interstitial space, or the alveolar compartment drains into the profuse network of pulmonary lymphatics.

Chemical substances required for normal tissue function, such as H_2O, Na^+ ion, Cl^- ion, glucose, etc., diffuse out of the capillaries with ease because of their small molecular size whereas albumin, because of its large molecular size, passes in minimal quantities. In all tissues, this constant exchange of fluid occurs across the whole length of the capillary bed.

Four factors govern the normal movement of fluid into and out of the capillary:

Inside the vessel:
1. Capillary hydrostatic pressure pushes fluid out of the capillary.
2. Plasma colloid osmotic pressure (COP) by osmosis moves fluid into the capillary.

Outside of the vessel:
1. Interstitial fluid hydrostatic pressure pushes fluid into the capillary.
2. Interstitial colloid osmotic pressure by osmosis moves fluid out of the capillary.

In the lung the interstitial pressure is less than atmospheric pressure. Hence, there are three pressures moving fluid out and one pressure exerting an inward influence. The high plasma osmotic pressure versus the low pulmonary capillary hydrostatic pressure results in a tendency to pull fluid from the interstitial space and keep it dry.

The subatmospheric interstitial pressure pulls the alveolar epithelium toward the capillary endothelium, tending to obliterate the interstitial space. The obliteration of the interstitial space promotes rapid gas exchange.

The low pulmonary capillary hydrostatic pressure and the high plasma osmotic pressure allow a considerable margin for increase in hydrostatic pressure before the hydrostatic pressure exceeds the oncotic pressure and pulmonary edema occurs. This condition is a reality and provides a safety valve that reduces the likelihood of pulmonary edema, as follows: pulmonary capillary hydrostatic pressure, 7 mmHg; plasma osmotic pressure, 25 mmHg; this results in a margin of 18 mmHg.

In the generation of pulmonary edema, fluid initially accumulates in the interstitial space. This space expands to accommodate fluid and can become several times its original volume. Simultaneously, pulmonary lymphatic drainage increases in an attempt to reduce the alveolar edema. When the interstitial space can no longer accommodate more fluid and lymphatic drainage is at a maximum, alveolar flooding or alveolar edema occurs.

The presence of râles on auscultation is the common clinical hallmark of alveolar edema, and characteristic infiltrates due to the presence of interstitial and alveolar fluid may be documented by chest x-ray film.

Etiology of Pulmonary Edema: Causes of pulmonary edema include

1. increased hydrostatic pressure in the pulmonary capillary bed,
2. decreased plasma colloid osmotic pressure,
3. pulmonary lymphatic obstruction, and
4. increased permeability of the pulmonary capillary endothelium.

Plasma Colloid Osmotic Pressure (COP): Plasma colloid osmotic pressure in normal subjects is 25 ± 2 mmHg. When plasma colloid osmotic pressure exceeds capillary hydrostatic pressure by only 4 mmHg or less, alveolar edema occurs.[15] If the osmotic pressure is less than 25 mmHg, alveolar edema occurs at a lower hydrostatic pressure.[16] Osmotic pressure is reduced when plasma proteins and, particularly, albumin levels are reduced. There is a significant correlation between low osmotic pressure and mortality in patients in special care units,[15] though currently there is no evidence that infusion of albumin at regular intervals to increase the osmotic pressure will change mortality rate. Such studies are awaited. However, it may be prudent to infuse albumin when COP is less than 17 mmHg.

Pulmonary edema that develops in the patient after a cardiac arrest may not be based on left ventricular failure but may be due to a decrease in osmotic pressure or to a change in permeability of the pulmonary vascular bed. The precipitating factor could be aspiration of gastric fluid of low pH during resuscitation. Noncardiogenic pulmonary edema (NCPE) is diagnosed by measuring PAOP, cardiac index, and COP. In the face of a normal PAOP, if serum albumin is not grossly decreased, the colloid osmotic pressure will significantly exceed the PAOP. Under these circumstances, pulmonary edema cannot be precipitated on the basis of cardiac failure and is not due to a significant reduction in colloid osmotic pressure but is probably associated with changes in capillary permeability. However, cardiogenic and noncardiogenic pulmonary edema and left ventricular failure and aspiration may occur concurrently, in which case each component may have to be treated separately. The patient may need therapy immediately! (See Appendix 2.)

Therapy for Pulmonary Edema: All forms of pulmonary edema result in intrapulmonary shunting and hypoxemia. For the post-cardiac-arrest patient who is intubated, primary therapy consists of mechanical ventilation and PEEP. The latter is increased progressively until the optimum PEEP is found.[3]

Although mechanical ventilation and PEEP improve oxygenation by reducing intraalveolar edema and increasing functional residual capacity (FRC), this form of treatment does not reverse the pathologic cause of the pulmonary edema.

Whether or not PEEP is initiated, additional therapy may be indicated. For cardiogenic pulmonary edema, therapy includes diuretics, vasodilators and inotropes (see Chapter 8); in NCPE, however, diuretics in the face of a normal PAOP will only result in acute hypovolemia. If a low COP is contributory to pulmonary edema, albumin (25 g) should be infused every 6 or 8 hours. Failure to differentiate between cardiogenic and noncardiogenic pulmonary edema and to understand the mechanism of noncardiogenic pulmonary edema may result in a totally inappropriate therapeutic response.

Other Cardiovascular Considerations

In treating an unstable cardiovascular system and maintaining adequate fluids in the circulatory bed, it must be remembered that blood contains red cells that are the primary conveyors of oxygen to the tissues.

Hence, it is necessary to maintain the hemoglobin level between 10 and 12 g/100 mL in these patients to provide adequate oxygen for the myocardium and other organs.

While recurrent arrhythmias are a relatively uncommon cause of hospital death following resuscitation,[17] an important exception is the patient with ventricular fibrillation caused by acute myocardial infarction. Recurrent episodes of ventricular tachycardia and fibrillation may be frequent in the first few hours after resuscitation in patients with acute infarction, and such patients require intensive rhythm observation and treatment.

Renal System

Following resuscitation from cardiopulmonary arrest, urine output may be decreased or absent. Sterile catheterization with closed drainage allows urine output to be measured and charted on an hourly basis and individual "spot" samples to be specifically analyzed. In assessing urine output, the following information must be considered:

1. Fluid intake.
2. Fluid output: nasogastric suction, diarrhea, vomitus, etc.; sensible and insensible loss, as well as urine output.

Assessment of the renal system must include measurement of the following:

1. Serum electrolytes.
2. Serum urea nitrogen and creatinine.
3. Serum protein and albumin.
4. Serum osmolality.
5. Urine electrolytes, urea nitrogen, creatinine.
6. Urine osmolality.

An assessment of urine electrolytes should never be made immediately following the administration of diuretics. A minimum interval of 12 hours, and preferably 24 hours, should elapse between diuretic administration and collection of urine for electrolytes.

Acute renal failure (ARF) is defined as a rapid deterioration of renal function with accumulation of nitrogen waste products in the blood. In addition to renal causes, acute renal failure may be prerenal (PR) or postrenal in origin.

The major causes of prerenal failure are hypovolemia, both absolute and/or relative, and reduced cardiac output. These two states can be assessed after the measurement of PAOP and cardiac output. If present, these situations should be corrected. However, with a failing heart, improvement in cardiac output may not be possible. Postrenal causes include obstruction of the urethra, bladder neck, and ureters. The former two can be excluded by placement of a Foley catheter.

Renal causes originate from ischemic disorders, nephrotoxins (which include antibiotics), and diseases of glomeruli and other small blood vessels. After prerenal and postrenal causes have been excluded, examination of the urine significantly assists the diagnosis of acute renal failure of renal origin.

Urine Volume:[18] Oliguric renal failure is defined as a urine output less than 400 mL/24 hr. In 20% of patients with acute renal failure, the urine volume may be as high as 2 L/24 hr (nonoliguric renal failure). However, BUN and creatinine continue to rise.

Urine Sediment:[18] Renal tubular cells, tubular cell casts, a few red and white cells, and proteinuria are compatible with acute renal failure. Tubular cell casts are usually absent in prerenal and postrenal failure.

Urine Sodium:[18] In prerenal failure, the urine sodium is less than 10 mEq/L. This is consistent with volume depletion, during which the kidney becomes avid in its protection against additional salt loss, while in acute renal failure, the urine sodium usually is greater than 20 mEq/L.

Urine Osmolality:[18] In prerenal failure, the urine osmolality usually is more than 100 mOsm above plasma osmolality. In acute renal failure, urine osmolality usually equals or is less than plasma osmolality.

Urine:Plasma Creatinine Ratios:

> PR> 14:1
> ARF< 14:1

Urine:Plasma Urea Ratios:

> PR> 14:1
> ARF< 14:1

Renal Failure Index:

$$= \frac{\text{Urine Na}}{\text{U/P Creatinine Ratio}}$$

Fractional Excretion of Filtered Sodium (FE$_{Na}$)

$$FE_{Na} = \frac{\text{U/P Na Ratio}}{\text{U/P Creatinine Ratio}} \times 100$$

The BUN:creatinine ratio is considerably in excess of 20:1 in prerenal causes such as blood in the gastrointestinal tract or extensive catabolism, e.g., fever or trauma. In uncomplicated acute renal failure, the BUN:creatinine ratio does not usually exceed the range of 10:1 to 15:1. Unfortunately, some patients with either prerenal or acute renal failure have indices at variance with those set out above. In these patients, the renal failure index or the FE$_{Na}$ are the best urinary indices for determining whether PR or ARF is the presenting clinical entity:[19]

Prerenal (PR):Renal failure index < 1.0 and FE$_{Na}$ < 1.0.

Acute renal failure:Renal failure index > 1.0 and FE$_{Na}$ >1.0.

Prerenal causes sometimes can be superimposed on renal causes.

In oliguric renal failure, potassium should not be added to the IV infusion unless serum potassium is below the lower limit of the normal range; the infusion of sodium should be governed by urine losses and plasma levels. Calcium replacement should be controlled by plasma calcium levels.

Intravenous Alimentation

Calories are essential and are best provided in the form of carbohydrates. It was previously believed that protein restriction should be maximum in patients with acute renal failure, but current evidence indicates that the infusion of essential amino acids promotes the early reversal of acute renal failure and a progressive reduction in creatinine and BUN.[20] The eight essential amino acids in required daily amounts are contained in 250 mL of a 5.1% commercial solution (Nephramine). The 250 mL contain 12.80 g essential amino acids and 1.46 g nitrogen. The solution is diluted with 500 mL of 70% dextose solution, providing 1,190 calories. Alternate solutions containing mixtures of essential and nonessential amino acids have not been demonstrated to be superior in patients with renal failure.[21] The primary goal is to keep protein content reduced prior to dialysis while energy source is maintained at 35 kcal/kg/day. The total fluid volume of 750 mL equals (for a febrile patient) or is only slightly in excess of (for a nonfebrile patient) the insensible fluid loss in those patients who are mechanically ventilated. The fluid must be infused through a central venous line which was not and will not be used for any other IV injectate. After starting therapy, if evidence of hyperglycemia is found (initially, blood sugar estimates should be made every 6 hours), insulin should be added to the therapeutic regimen. In the patient who is oliguric in spite of normal cardiac index and blood pressures, the use of increasing doses of IV furosemide (up to 1 g total dose) may convert oliguric renal failure to the more easily treated polyuric or normal volume renal failure.

Dialysis

Early dialysis is now the treatment of choice for patients with acute renal failure. Dialysis may be either peritoneal or by hemodialysis. Venovenous hemodialysis can be performed using subclavian catheters[22] and may make unnecessary the surgical placement of an arterial–venous shunt. These double lumen catheters more commonly inserted into the subclavian vein allow for repeated dialysis as required. They should be changed weekly as there is risk of infection and thrombosis; the catheters should be replaced in the contralateral vein. Catheter insertion is performed using the Seldinger technique, using a flexible guidewire. Catheter patency is maintained by heparin flush every 12 hours with 2,000–3,000 units of heparin.

Gastrointestinal System (GI)

If bowel sounds are absent, a nasogastric tube should be inserted and its position ascertained when the next chest x-ray is obtained. All nasogastric suction should be charted and included in the total intake and output chart. Because of the high incidence of stress ulceration and GI bleeding in critically ill patients, prophylactic antacid should be administered every hour to increase the pH of gastric contents. Therapy with an H_2 blocking agent, which inhibits gastric acid secretion and maintains an increased gastric pH, may contribute to the prevention of gastrointestinal bleeding.

Determining the Etiology of Cardiac Arrest

In the postresuscitation period diagnostic testing should be carried out to better determine the etiology of the cardiac arrest: a) acute infarction, b) transient ischemia, c) severe left ventricular dysfunction due to past myocardial infarction or fibrosis, and d) metabolic causes.

Acute Myocardial Infarction and Sudden Arrhythmic Death

Only 25% of patients develop clear evidence for acute myocardial infarction after resuscitation from ventricular fibrillation. The diagnosis may be difficult to make with assurance and is primarily based on serial ECG findings.[23,24] High levels of creatine kinase activity are common following resuscitation. This elevation is presumably due to skeletal muscle trauma secondary to chest compression during CPR and to cardiac muscle ischemia during arrest and attempted resuscitation. There is a coincident elevation in the MB (myocardial) fraction, making the level of MB activity an inaccurate indicator of acute myocardial necrosis. Yet, the importance of recognizing whether ventricular fibrillation was the result of acute infarction is of paramount importance, both for assigning and for selecting a course of subsequent therapy. In follow-up studies of patients who have been resuscitated from out-of-hospital cardiac arrest, the development of new Q waves on serial ECG's is associated with only a 5% recurrence rate of cardiac arrest over the next 12 months.[25] On the other hand, patients who show less specific electrocardiographic findings of ischemia or injury, or who develop only enzyme evidence compatible with infarction or simply resuscitative efforts are at substantially higher risk for a recurrent episode of cardiac arrest (20–30%) during the next two years.[26]

These findings suggest that when ventricular fibrillation occurs because of acute myocardial infarction it is the result of transient electrical instability due to acute thrombosis and myocardial necrosis. When ventricular fibrillation is due to other causes, however, these initial precipitating factors and their associated risk for cardiac arrest persist after resuscitation. This latter group of patients requires further diagnostic testing to better elucidate the cause of fibrillation and to guide therapy.

Metabolic Abnormalities

If serial ECG's have failed to demonstrate evidence for acute infarction (new Q waves), other assessments of cardiac anatomy and function will be necessary to help determine the cause of cardiac arrest. Metabolic causes should also be considered. The most common include the recent initiation of antiarrhythmic drug treatment and hypokalemia. The overall incidence of proarrhythmia effects, including ventricular fibrillation, following antiarrhythmic drug treatment has been reported to be 5–15%.[27] Prolongation of the QT interval is often noted, and ventricular fibrillation may be initiated by *torsade de points.*[28] Electrophysiologic testing may help to confirm the diagnosis. Unlike the majority of patients resuscitated from primary ventricular fibrillation (not associated with acute infarction) in whom programmed electrical stimulation of the right ventricle induces ventricular tachycardia/fibrillation, most patients with cardiac arrest secondary to antiarrhythmic drug reaction or hypokalemia fail to have meaningful arrhythmias reproducibly evoked by programmed stimulation when tested in a drug-free state.[29] Thirty percent of patients resuscitated from out-of-hospital cardiac arrest have evidence of hypokalemia on admission to the hospital.[30] It is often difficult to determine whether this finding is due to sodium bicarbonate administration during resuscitation, secondary to exogenous administration or high levels of endogenous circulating catecholamines, or instead, the result of a true metabolic abnormality which may have been the cause of ventricular fibrillation. The diagnosis is usually made by excluding other causes. The lack of evidence of ischemia or underlying structural heart disease combined with the inability to initiate sustained ventricular arrhythmias by programmed electrical stimulation of the right ventricle provides strong secondary evidence for hypokalemia-induced cardiac arrest in such patients.

Other less frequent metabolic abnormalities include hypomagnesemia, hypothermia, and toxic reactions to phenothiazines, tricyclic antidepressants, and cocaine.

Structural Heart Disease Other Than Acute Ischemic Infarction

Exercise testing, echocardiography, radionuclide ventriculography, and cardiac catheterization are helpful in evaluating transient ischemia or underlying structural heart disease as possible causes of cardiac arrest. Large hypokinetic or akinetic ventricular segments identified by echocardiography or radionuclide ventriculography plus a severely depressed ejection fraction are often the first clues that myocardial scarring is the primary substrate for ventricular fibrillation. Most of these patients have inducible ventricular tachycardia/fibrillation with electrophysiologic testing, and the response can be a useful guide to assessing the efficacy of antiarrhythmic drug therapy. These patients commonly have repetitive ventricular ectopy recorded during ambulatory monitoring, and thus, the response to antiarrhythmic drug therapy can also be determined with serial Holter recordings, with a 70% reduction in the total number of PVC's and total suppression of runs of 3 or more repetitive beats constituting a success. The best test (programmed stimulation or prolonged monitoring) for assigning effective therapy aimed at preventing a recurrent episode of cardiac arrest has not yet been clarified.[31] The tests appear complementary in detecting arrhythmias and adequate therapeutic responses.

Transient Ischemia

Patients who experience chest pain or who were engaged in exertion immediately prior to arrest should be suspected of having transient ischemia as an etiology. Noninvasive studies and cardiac catheterization in such patients often demonstrate preservation of left ventricular contractility and the presence of one or more high-grade coronary stenoses. Treadmill exercise testing may evoke chest pain, ST segment depression, and/or Thallium myocardial perfusion defects. Programmed electrical stimulation may fail to elicit ventricular tachycardia in such patients, suggesting that fibrillation is possible only during ischemia.[32] These patients seem ideally suited for coronary bypass surgery although the benefit of such an approach has yet to be rigorously studied.

Perhaps the most difficult patient in whom to select therapy is one with evidence of both myocardial scarring and clinically evident ischemia or silent but extensive underlying coronary artery disease. Most of these patients have inducible arrhythmias with electrophysiologic testing. The role of coronary bypass surgery as a single treatment in this setting is unclear. Also, it is unusual for such patients to have only monomorphic ventricular tachycardia induced with programmed stimulation, and thus, they are far from ideal candidates for simultaneous endocardial resection or ablation procedures at the time of surgery. Consequently, coronary bypass surgery, antiarrhythmic drugs, and implantable defibrillators are often all prescribed — pointing out our as yet uninformed approach to the management of such patients.

Therapeutic Means to Prevent Sudden Arrhythmic Death

Reduction of Risk Factors

Among the many risk factors for coronary heart disease and sudden arrhythmic death, cessation of cigarette smoking has been shown to reduce the incidence of ventricular fibrillation. It is clear that even after adjusting for other major risk factors of coronary heart disease, cessation of smoking is an important therapeutic approach in preventing sudden arrhythmic death.[33]

Emergency Cardiac Care

To date, the most effective measure in preventing sudden arrhythmic death has been the widespread out-of-hospital implementation of emergency cardiac care. The treatment of cardiac arrest is obviously not an ideal means for containing the problem of sudden arrhythmic death. However, until the population at risk can be accurately identified and effectively treated, efforts to further improve the treatment delivered should continue in this important approach.

Coronary Artery Bypass Grafting

Coronary artery bypass grafting in selected patients with ischemic heart disease has been shown to improve survival rates in patients with chronic stable angina and also in patients resuscitated from ventricular fibrillation, largely through a reduction in the rate of sudden arrhythmic death.[34,35] This is not evident in patients who have moderate or severe angina combined with three-vessel coronary disease and impaired left ventricular function. Survival is also improved in patients with severe stenosis of the left main coronary artery, although this abnormality is an infrequent finding in victims of sudden arrhythmic death.[36,37]

Pharmacologic Therapy

Beta-Adrenergic Agents

Several studies have demonstrated a reduction in mortality, primarily fewer sudden arrhythmic deaths, in patients receiving beta-blockers following acute myocardial infarction.[38-42] However, the impact of prescribing beta-blocker treatment to patients with a recent infarction will have little effect on the overall incidence of sudden arrhythmic death. Only 10–15% of victims have a history of acute infarction occurring within the 2 years prior to sudden arrhythmic death.[39,43] Secondly, the blanket administration of beta-blockers to all patients recovering from myocardial infarction is an undirected approach to the problem. For every 100 patients treated, only 3 or 4 derive any benefit from treatment. The remainder are left to bear the costs and side effects of such a treatment strategy.

Antiarrhythmic Agents

Antiarrhythmic drugs have been demonstrated to be effective in suppressing ectopic ventricular beats, as well as episodes of recurrent ventricular tachycardia.[44-47] These agents have not as yet been shown to be effective in preventing sudden arrhythmic death in unselected patients. It is also important to note that all antiarrhythmic drugs have potential proarrhythmic effects and may even cause ventricular fibrillation.[29] Although antiarrhythmic drug therapy seems on the surface to be a rational approach to the problem of sudden arrhythmic death, there is as yet but meager evidence to support the use of these drugs as a general approach to all patients with arrhythmias. The available results, however, do favor long-term use of antiarrhythmic drugs in patients with symptomatic sustained ventricular tachycardia or a history of resuscitation from ventricular fibrillation. The results of small, randomized trials in patients with otherwise asymptomatic arrhythmias have as yet failed to demonstrate a major benefit of such therapy on subsequent survival. In addition, the use of antiarrhythmic drugs in an empirical manner can be hazardous.[45,48-57] Large clinical trials are being conducted in an effort to determine whether these agents can prevent sudden arrhythmic death in unselected patients with ischemic heart disease and asymptomatic arrhythmias.[58] The results of these studies will be important in determining the relative importance of each of the above treatment strategies.

Electrical Therapy

Programmed ventricular electrical stimulation appears to be of most benefit in assessing and treating patients with sustained ventricular tachycardia and fibrillation and is not as helpful in patients with less serious forms of ventricular arrhythmia.[59]

Implantable defibrillators are a recent approach to the management of the patient at high risk to develop sudden arrhythmic death.[60,61] To date, these devices have been used primarily in patients previously resuscitated from ventricular fibrillation or tachycardia and in whom pharmacologic or surgical therapy appears to be either an imperfect or an unsatisfactory approach to the prevention of recurrent episodes of cardiac arrest. Such a strategy is obviously limited, and the devices are in their technological infancy. Candidates must be identified as being at high risk for development of cardiac arrest, be suitable candidates for the invasive procedure required for placement of the electrodes, and also be amenable to the frequent follow-up required for testing and servicing the device.

Automatic external defibrillators are an even newer adjunct to the treatment regimen for preventing sudden arrhythmic death. Like all regimens, they require identification of the appropriate patient, and in addition, a household member or coworker must be taught how to use the device.[62,63] On the other hand, these devices are a noninvasive approach and may therefore be a suitable solution for the patient at intermediate risk of developing cardiac arrest or may serve as a secondary measure after surgical or pharmacologic approaches have been taken for the patient.

Cerebral Resuscitation

Magnitude of the Problem

Cerebral damage is a major contributing factor in a high percent of inhospital deaths following successful cardiac resuscitation, and a significant proportion of the survivors suffer severe neurologic deficits.[64]

The initial neurologic findings can be used to predict the likelihood of full neurologic recovery.[65] The first assessment of pupillary response, eye movements, motor response, and blood glucose level provides useful prognostic information (Table 1). Most patients who ultimately recover full neurologic function awaken and improve dramatically in the first 48 hours following resuscitation. If the patient remains totally unresponsive, with no evidence of either cognitive or motor recovery after 3 days, the chance of regaining meaningful cerebral function is almost nil.[64,66] The measurement of the level of cerebrospinal fluid CK-BB enzyme can also be useful in assessing prognosis in these comatose patients. It is best done at 48–72 hours after the arrest. Levels of 25 IU or more have been uniformly associated with severe residual neurologic deficits.[67,68] Patients who do not recover and who manifest severe cerebral dysfunction usually succumb to pneumonia or multisystem failure within 1–2 weeks following resuscitation. The postresuscitation patient with severe cerebral dysfunction almost never meets the criteria for brain death as brain stem function is almost always spared.

Research into the mechanisms of cerebral injury as well as possible methods of preservation has greatly accelerated in the past few years but has yet to provide a technique or a drug whose efficacy is sufficiently proven to warrant a recommendation for its routine use in the postresuscitation setting. The search for therapeutic measures is aimed in two major directions: 1) improving cerebral perfusion during CPR to minimize the period of absent or low cerebral blood flow and 2) ameliorating the injurious changes that occur at the time of reperfusion and reoxygenation of the brain that lead to the "postresuscitation syndrome".

Neurologic, Neuropathologic, and Biochemical Consequences of Cardiac Arrest

Arrest of the cerebral circulation produces a progression of symptoms, including fixation of the eyes, blurring of vision, narrowing of the visual fields, loss of consciousness, and finally, convulsions.[69] Loss of consciousness occurs within 5–11 seconds and coincides with the appearance of slow wave activity on the electroencephalogram (EEG). Neurologic outcomes following arrest vary widely. Following mild-to-moderate ischemia, outcomes range from transient confusion and amnesia to permanent focal neurologic deficits.[70] More severe, prolonged ischemia is associated with a vegetative state or brain death. The most vulnerable areas of the central nervous system are the cerebral cortex (layers 3, 5, 6), the hippocampi, the cerebellum (Purkinje cell layer), the basal ganglia, and the thalamus.

Cerebral oxygen stores become depleted within 15 seconds of total circulatory arrest, and cerebral energy charge as well as cerebral glucose stores are virtually exhausted within 5 minutes.[71] When oxygen is depleted, anaerobic glycolysis continues while glucose and/or glycogen are available, resulting in the production of lactic acid sufficient to reduce intracellular pH from 7.0 to approximately 6.4 if normoglycemia is present prior to arrest. Lactate production is greater, and tissue pH lower, if hyperglycemia is present at the time of arrest; similarly, less lactate is produced if hypoglycemia is present.

Energy-requiring reactions, such as the sodium–potassium pump, cease, and the extracellular potassium concentration rises.[72] When extracellular K^+ concentration reaches 10–15 μmol/ml, a sudden influx of Ca^{++} into neurons occurs, presumably because voltage-dependent Ca^{++} gates are opened.[73] Free fatty acids are released from membrane lipids, perhaps triggered by depletion of high-energy phosphates and influx of Ca^{++}. Other consequences of uncontrolled Ca^{++} influx and a resultant high intracellular Ca^{++} concentration include proteolysis, disassembly of microtubules, and protein phosphorylation. Ischemia, particularly in

Table 1. Initial Neurologic Assessment

Motor Function Points	Pupil Response Points	Eye Movements Points	Blood Glucose Level Points
0 Absent	0 Absent	0 Absent	0 ⩾ 300 mg%
1 Extensor Posturing	3 Present	1 Present	1 < 300 mg%
2 Flexor Posturing			
3 Nonposturing			
4 Withdrawal or Localizing			

Total Score	Likelihood of Awakening
0–2	5%
3,4	25%
5–7	75%
8,9	95%

Modified from Longsreth.[61] Used with permission.

association with hyperglycemia, leads to swelling of astrocytes. This occurs primarily because of an extracellular-to-intracellular translocation of fluid with little net accumulation of water content; however, severe ischemia may be associated with a net gain in tissue water content.[71]

When flow is restored, an initial reactive hyperemia is followed by a prolonged period during which cerebral blood flow and metabolism are markedly reduced.[74] Reperfusion failure occurs in four stages: 1) multifocal no-reflow;[75] 2) transient global hyperemia;[76] 3) prolonged global hypoperfusion;[76] and 4) the period in which either recovery takes place, hypoperfusion persists, or flow decreases to zero with resultant brain death. Reactivity of the cerebral vessels to CO_2 and changes in perfusion pressure is markedly attenuated.[77] Elevations in intracranial pressure (ICP) are not common but ICP that is initially normal following resuscitation may later increase.[78]

The specific biochemical events leading to neuronal damage are incompletely understood. While the events occurring during ischemia trigger cell damage, the reactions that ultimately lead to cell destruction are probably those associated with reperfusion. Such reactions include alterations in protein metabolism (disaggregation of polyribosomes, delayed recovery of protein synthesis), peroxidation of structural lipids secondary to release of free radical compounds, and mitochondrial dysfunction perhaps secondary to persistent acidosis and/or intracellular Ca^{++} accumulation.[71]

Therapeutic Measures

Measures for Improving Cerebral Blood Flow During CPR

Numerous studies have documented the relatively low cardiac output and organ blood flow values obtainable with external chest compression.[79-81] While open-chest massage may be associated with higher blood flows,[80-82] the technique has limited application as it requires special training and equipment. The best way to provide optimal cerebral blood flow is to rapidly restore spontaneous circulation (e.g., by early defibrillation).

In the past several years a number of investigators have examined methods and pharmacologic agents that might improve organ blood flow during CPR. Many of these studies have centered around variations in the techniques of external chest compression and ventilation. Chandra and colleagues[83] demonstrated that at least in some individuals blood flow during CPR did not result from direct compression of the cardiac ventricles as proposed by Kouwenhoven, et al.,[84] but instead resulted from the increase in intrathoracic pressure caused by external chest compression. Because of the presence of valves in the jugular venous system the increased pressure is transmitted unequally to the carotid arteries and jugular veins, allowing forward flow to the head.[85] Following this, a number of alternative techniques of CPR were introduced, all with the goal of producing further increases in intrathoracic pressure and thus improving cardiac output and organ blood flow.[83,86-89] However, these alternative methods have not been adopted for use during CPR in humans. Some methods increase carotid flow but decrease cerebral blood flow (e.g., volume loading),[90] others increase carotid blood flow at the expense of myocardial flow,[91] and still others have been shown not to result in improved survival or neurologic outcome following cardiopulmonary arrest (e.g., interposed abdominal compression).[92]

Of the pharmacologic agents employed during resuscitation, epinephrine is the one that results in an improvement in both cerebral and myocardial blood flow.[93-95]

Measures Used in the Postresuscitation Period

The therapeutic measures that have been examined for their efficacy in the postresuscitation period are myriad, and only those that have been extensively examined and/or look promising at the present time will be mentioned.

The foundation of postresuscitation care resides in continuous observation, monitoring, and provision of supportive care. Such support must include maintenance of adequate oxygenation and systemic blood pressure and may necessitate endotracheal intubation and mechanical ventilation as well as support of the circulation with pharmacologic agents. Of prime importance in cerebral preservation is the maintenance of an adequate cerebral perfusion pressure (CPP). As mentioned earlier, following an episode of global ischemia a short period of cerebral hyperperfusion is followed by hypoperfusion which lasts many hours. Any reduction of CPP will contribute to a further decrease in cerebral blood flow. Since CPP is equal to the difference between systemic mean arterial pressure (MAP) and intracranial pressure (ICP) the maintenance of a normal CPP depends on the avoidance of systemic hypotension and the control of elevated ICP.

A number of studies have demonstrated that neurologic outcome following global ischemia is improved if systemic blood pressure is maintained within the normal range during the postischemic period.[96-98] In fact, a short period of mild hypertension may be of value; but severe, prolonged, or repeated hypertension is associated with a poor neurologic outcome.[98] If ICP is increased, it should be controlled by elevation of the head 15–20 degrees, administration of diuretics, and hyperventilation. Muscle paralysis and mechanical ventilation per se do not improve neurologic outcome.[99] However, hyperventilation can be used to control increased ICP if needed.

It should be remembered that hypocapnia decreases ICP by producing cerebral vasoconstriction and reducing cerebral blood volume. Whether this is efficacious in a postarrest patient whose cerebral blood flow may already be low is something that must be decided on an individual patient basis. Todd and associates found that cats made hypocapnic ($PaCO_2 = 15-20$ mmHg) following cardiac resuscitation had improved cerebral vessel CO_2 responsiveness, no difference in CBF or EEG, and lower ICP than cats that were slightly hypercarbic ($PaCO_2 = 40-45$ mmHg).[100] They suggested that the improvement in cerebrovascular responsiveness may have been a result of higher pH values in the cerebral tissue of the hypocapnic animals. The value of hyperventilation in post-cardiac-arrest cerebral resuscitation is, however, as yet unproven. The major advantage of controlled ventilation may be the provision of adequate oxygenation and the prevention of hypercarbia.

Conditions that increase the brain's oxygen requirement ($CMRO_2$), such as seizure activity and hyperthermia, must be treated vigorously. It is particularly deleterious for these conditions to persist at a time when the delivery of oxygen to the brain may be suboptimal because of hypoperfusion.

Among the pharmacologic agents investigated for their possible efficacy in cerebral preservation, the ones that until recently looked most promising were the barbiturates. Improved neurologic outcome in dogs receiving barbiturates prior to global ischemia[101] and in monkeys given barbiturates after global ischemia[102] were not obtained when the studies were repeated.[103,104] Although the result of a clinical feasibility trial using thiopental for patients who suffered circulatory arrest for 5 minutes or longer and who remained comatose for 10 minutes following the restoration of adequate spontaneous circulation and oxygenation looked promising,[105] the results from a multi-institutional study failed to show a difference in neurologic outcome between the controls and the patients treated with thiopental.[106]

Promising results, with improved cerebral blood flow and neurologic outcome, have been obtained in laboratory animals given calcium channel blockers prior to[107,108] or immediately following global brain ischemia.[109-113] Some studies, however, have failed to demonstrate improvements in blood flow[114,115] or in neurologic outcome.[115,116] Others have noted that even when early neurologic recovery is good following calcium-blocking therapy neurologic status may deteriorate at 16–18 hours postresuscitation.[117] It was theorized that this deterioration might result from peroxidative tissue injury at the time of reperfusion. Whether calcium channel blockers will prove to be efficacious in humans following cardiac arrest and, if so, whether they work primarily by improving flow, by ameliorating the cascade of cellular events initiated by intracellular calcium accummulation,[118] or by a combination of effects remains to be investigated.

Other pharmacologic agents that have been or are being investigated for their possible efficacy in this role include prostaglandin inhibitors, phenytoin, benzodiazepines, etomidate, and deferoxamine. At present no single therapeutic measure clearly emerges as the best method for cerebral resuscitation following cardiac arrest. Perhaps optimum results will be obtained only when a multifaceted approach[119,120] is used in which good postresuscitation intensive care is combined with several specific measures designed to preserve neuronal function.

Glossary

Gas Phase Symbols

F: Fractional concentration of a gas

P: Pressure

I: Inspired

A: Alveolar

BP: Barometric pressure = 760 mmHg sea level (use 747 for convenient calculations)

VP H_2O: Vapor pressure of water. In the respiratory tract, at 37°C, the vapor pressure is 47 mmHg

T: Tidal

D: Dead space or wasted ventilation

f: Respiratory frequency per minute

Blood Phase Symbols

Q: Blood flow, Q_S: Shunt flow, Q_T: Total flow (Q_T = cardiac output)

P: Pressure

S: Saturation in the blood phase: Hb fully saturated at PaO_2 150 mmHG

a: Arterial

c: Pulmonary end capillary

v: Venous; $\bar{v}$ = mixed venous

C: Content

Examples:

Sum of physically dissolved oxygen in plasma = partial pressure of oxygen × solubility coefficient (0.0031 mL/mmHg/100 mL blood) plus the oxygen chemically combined with the hemoglobin = Hb × % S × 1.34 (1.34 is mL of oxygen combined with 1 g Hb when Hb is fully saturated).

CaO_2 = O_2 content in arterial blood

$C\bar{v}O_2$ = O_2 content in mixed venous blood

$PaCO_2$ = arterial carbon dioxide pressure

$C(a-\bar{v})O_2$ = arterio-mixed venous oxygen content difference

PcO_2 = pulmonary end-capillary oxygen pressure; therefore $PcO_2 = PAO_2$

To calculate PAO_2, use the following formula:
$$PAO_2 = F_IO_2 \times (BP-47)-PACO_2$$

Since the $PACO_2$ is difficult to measure and approximates the easily measurable $PaCO_2$, the formula is altered to read:
$$PAO_2 = F_IO_2 \times (747-47) - PaCO_2$$

At any altitude the current barometric pressure must be known, e.g., 5200 ft = 630 mmHg.

To calculate the intrapulmonary shunt, use the shunt equation:

$$\frac{Q_S}{Q_T}\% = \frac{Cc\,O_2 - CaO_2}{Cc\,O_2 - C\bar{v}O_2} \times 100$$

If $PaO_2 > 150$ mmHg:

$$\frac{Q_S}{Q_T}\% = \frac{P(A\text{-}a)\,O_2 \times 0.0031}{P(A\text{-}a)\,O_2 \times 0.0031 + C(a\text{-}\bar{v})\,O_2} \times 100$$

Example: $PaO_2 = 350$ mmHg; $P\bar{v}O_2 = 40$ mmHg;
Hb = 15 g; $S\bar{v}O_2 = 75\%$.
$PaCO_2 = 45$ mmHg

$$\frac{Q_S}{Q_T}\% = \frac{[[(700 - 45) - 350] \times 0.0031]}{\cfrac{[[(700 - 45) - 350] \times 0.0031]}{+ [(350 \times 0.0031) + (15 \times 1.34)]}}$$
$$\frac{}{- [(40 \times 0.0031) + (15 \times 1.34 \times 0.75)]} \times 100$$

$$= \frac{(305 \times 0.0031)}{(305 \times 0.0031) + (21.185 - 15.199)} \times 100$$

$$= \frac{0.9455}{6.9315} \times 100$$

$$= 13.6$$

If $PaO_2 < 150$ mmHg, use the regular shunt equation:

$$\frac{Q_S}{Q_T}\% = \frac{CcO_2 - CaO_2}{CcO_2 - C\bar{v}O_2} \times 100$$

Example: $PaO_2 = 75$ mmHg, $SaO_2 = 95\%$;
$PaCO_2 = 50$ mmHg, Hb = 12 g
$P\bar{v}O_2 = 35$ mmHg, $S\bar{v}O_2 = 66.5\%$

$$\frac{Q_S}{Q_T} = \frac{[(PaO_2 \times 0.0031) + (Hb \times 1.34 \times 1.0)]}{[(PaO_2 \times 0.0031) + (Hb \times 1.34 \times 1.0)]}$$
$$\frac{- [(PaO_2 \times 0.0031) + (Hb \times 1.34 \times SaO_2)]}{- [(PVO_2 \times 0.0031) + (Hb \times 1.34 \times SvO_2)]} \times 100$$

$$= \frac{[(700 - 50) \times 0.0031 + (12 \times 1.34)]}{[(700 - 50) \times 0.0031 + (12 \times 1.34)]}$$
$$\frac{- [(75 \times 0.0031) + (12 \times 1.34 \times 0.95)]}{- [(35 \times 0.0031) + (12 \times 1.34 \times 0.665)]} \times 100$$

$$= \frac{18.0950 - 15.5085}{18.0950 - 10.8017} \times 100 \quad = 35$$

RAP: Right atrial pressure: 0 to 8 mmHg

RVP: Right ventricular pressure: $\dfrac{28 \text{ to } 30 \text{ mmHg}}{0 \text{ to } 8}$

PAP: Pulmonary artery pressure: $\dfrac{28 \text{ to } 30 \text{ mmHg}}{10 \text{ to } 12}$

PAOP: Pulmonary artery occlusive pressure (mean): 5 to 12 mmHg

LAP: Left atrial pressure

MAP: Mean systemic arterial pressure =
Diastolic $+ \left(\dfrac{\text{systolic} - \text{diastolic}}{3}\right)$

CO: Cardiac output

CI: Cardiac index:
$$\frac{CO}{\text{Body surface area}} = 3.0 \pm 0.5 \text{ L/min/M}^2$$

SVI: Stroke volume index:
$$\frac{CI}{\text{Heart rate}} = 40 \pm 7 \text{ mL/beat/M}^2$$

LVSWI: Left ventricular stroke work index
$$= (MAP - PAOP) \times SVI \times 0.0136$$
$$= 43 - 56 \text{ g M/M}^2$$

Work performed by the left ventricle to pump the stroke volume against the aortic pressure/M^2

SVRI: Systemic vascular resistance index
$$= \frac{(MAP - RAP) \times 80}{CI}$$
$$= 1300 - 2900 \text{ dyne/sec/cm}^{-5}/\text{M}^2$$
Impedance to left ventricular output /M^2

RVSWI: Right ventricular stroke work index
$$= (\overline{PA} - RAP) \times SVI \times 0.0136$$
$$= 6 - 10 \text{ g M/M}^2$$

Work performed by the right ventricle to pump the stroke volume to the pulmonary artery pressure/M$_2$

PVRI: Pulmonary vascular resistance index
$$= \frac{(\overline{PA} - PAOP) \times 80}{CI}$$
$$= 100 - 240 \text{ dyne/sec/cm}^{-5}/\text{M}^2$$

Appendix I: Correlation of Pulmonary Artery Pressure, Pulmonary Artery Occlusive Pressure (PAOP), and Cardiac Index (CI)

Pulmonary Artery Pressure	Pulmonary Artery Occlusive Pressure	CI	Probable Etiology
N or ↓	↓	↓	Hypovolemia
N or ↑	↑	↓	Left ventricular failure (with large V waves in PAOP, consider acute MR or VSD)
N or ↑	N or ↑	↓	Cardiac tamponade (CVP = PAP = PAOP). Right ventricular infarct (CVP inappropriately ↑ for PAOP)
↑	N or ↓	↓	Pulmonary embolus
↑	N	N	COPD
N	N	↑	Hyperdynamic state (e.g., thyrotoxicosis)
N or ↑	↓	↑	Gram-negative sepsis

Note: N = normal   ↑ = elevated   ↓ = low
This is a highly simplified table intended to assist thought about etiologic processes in hemodynamic monitoring.

Appendix 2: Types of Pulmonary Edema

Types

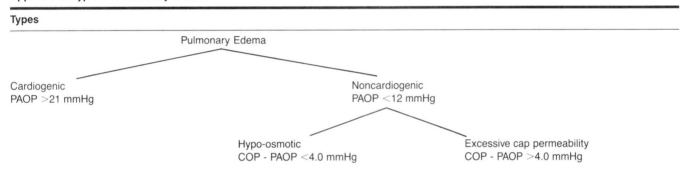

Cardiogenic pulmonary edema can occur with a PAOP <21 mmHg if the COP <25 mmHg.

Etiologies

Cardiogenic	Hypo-osmotic	↑ CAP Permeability
Left ventricular failure	(Effect 1° due to ↓ albumin)	Aspiration
Pump failure	Failure to make albumin:	HCl, H₂O (fresh and salt)
Mitral regurgitation	Starvation	Noxious gases
Ventricular septal defect	Liver disease	(SO₂, N₂O, NH₃, Cl₂)
Fluid overload	Losses of albumin:	Thermal injuries
Mitral stenosis	Renal	Oxygen toxicity
Severe hypertension	GI	Pulmonary fat emboli
Neurogenic	Acute pancreatitis	Shock lung syndrome
High altitude	Peritonitis	Gram-negative sepsis
	Ascites	

References

1. Pontoppidan H, Hedley-Whyte J, Bendixen HH, et al: Ventilation and oxygen requirements during prolonged artificial ventilation in patients with respiratory failure. *N Engl J Med* 273:401-409, 1965.
2. Dammann JF, McAslan TC: PEEP: Its use in young patients with apparently normal lungs. *Crit Care Med* 7:14-19, 1979.
3. Gallagher TJ, Civetta JM, Kirby RR: Terminology update: Optimal PEEP. *Crit Care Med* 6:323-326,1978.
4. Cooper JD, Grillo HC: Analysis of problems related to cuffs on intratracheal tubes. *Chest* 62 (suppl):21S-27S, 1972.
5. Bendixen HH, Egbert LD, Hedley-Whyte J, et al: *Respiratory Care.* St. Louis, CV Mosby, 1965.
6. Reines HD, Civetta JM: The inaccuracy of using 100% oxygen to determine intrapulmonary shunt in spite of PEEP. *Crit Care Med* 7:301-303, 1979.
7. Sladen A, Sweatman A, Klain M: Computerized physiologic profiles of cardiorespiratory responses to PEEP challenge as an index of prognosis. *Intensive Care Med* 3:117, 1977.
8. Downs JB, Klein EF Jr, Desautels D, et al: Intermittent mandatory ventilation: A new approach to weaning patients from mechanical ventilators. *Chest* 63:331-335, 1973.
9. Forrester JS, Diamond G, McHugh TJ, et al: Filling pressures in the right and left sides of the heart in acute myocardial infarction: A reappraisal of central-venous-pressure monitoring. *N Engl J Med* 285:190-193, 1971.

10. Civetta JM, Gabel JC: Flow directed-pulmonary artery catheterization in surgical patients: Indications and modifications of technique. *Ann Surg* 176:753-756, 1972.

11. Walston A II, Kendal ME: Comparison of pulmonary wedge and left atrial pressure in man. *Am Heart J* 86:159-164, 1973.

12. Lozman J, Powers SR Jr, Older T, et al: Correlation of pulmonary wedge and left atrial pressures. A study in the patient receiving positive end expiratory pressure ventilation. *Arch Surg* 109:270-277, 1974.

13. Fisher ML, DeFelice CE, Parisi AF: Assessing left ventricular filling pressure with flow-directed (Swan-Ganz) catheters: Detection of sudden changes in patients with left ventricular dysfunction. *Chest* 68:542-547, 1975.

14. Crexells C, Chatterjee K, Forrester JS, et al: Optimal level of filling pressure in the left side of the heart in acute myocardial infarction. *N Engl J Med* 289:1263-1266, 1973.

15. Rackow EC, Fein IA, Leppo J: Colloid osmotic pressure as a prognostic indicator of pulmonary edema and mortality in the critically ill. *Chest* 72:709-713, 1977.

16. Weil MH, Henning RJ, Morissette M, et al: Relationship between colloid osmotic pressure and pulmonary artery wedge pressure in patients with acute cardiorespiratory failure. *Am J Med* 64:643-650, 1978.

17. Thompson RG, Hallstrom AP, Cobb LA: Bystander-initiated cardiopulmonary resuscitation in the management of ventricular fibrillation. *Ann Intern Med* 90:737-740, 1979.

18. Schrier RW: *Renal and Electrolyte Disorders*. Boston, Little, Brown, and Co, 1976.

19. Miller TR, Anderson RJ, Linas SL, et al: Urinary diagnostic indices in acute renal failure. A prospective study. *Ann Intern Med* 89:47-50, 1978.

20. Abel RM, Beck CH Jr, Abbott WM, et al: Improved survival after treatment with intravenous essential L-amino acids and glucose: Results of a prospective, double-blind study. *N Engl J Med* 288:695-699, 1973.

21. Mirtallo JM, Schneider PJ, Mavko K, et al: A comparison of essential and general amino acid infusions in the nutritional support of patients with compromised renal function. *J Parenter Enter Nutr* 6:109-113, 1982.

22. Uldall PR, Dyck RF, Woods F, et al: A subclavian cannula for temporary access for hemodyalysis or plasma pheresis. *Dial Trans* 8:963, 1979.

23. Baum RS, Alvarez H, Cobb LA: Survival after resuscitation from out-of-hospital ventricular fibrillation. *Circulation* 50:1231-1235, 1974.

24. Cobb LA, Werner JA: Predictors and prevention of sudden cardiac death, in Hurst JW (ed): *The Heart*. New York, McGraw Hill, pp. 538-546, 1982.

25. Schaffer WA, Cobb LA: Recurrent ventricular fibrillation and modes of death in survivors of out-of-hospital ventricular fibrillation. *N Engl J Med* 293:259-262, 1975.

26. Cobb LA, Hallstrom AP, Weaver WD, Copass MK, Hedgecock M, Haynes RE: Prognostic factors in patients resuscitated from sudden cardiac death, in Wilhelmsen L, Hjalmarsen M, Longren, Sonar AB (eds): *Acute and Longterm Management of Myocardial Ischemia*. Molndal, Sweden, 1978, pp 106-113.

27. Velebit V, Podrid P, Lown B, Cohen BH, Grayboys TB: Aggravation and provocation of ventricular arrhythmias by antiarrhythmic drugs. *Circulation* 65:886-893, 1982.

28. Smith WM, Gallagher JJ: "Les torsades des pointes:" an unusual ventricular arrhythmia. *Ann Intern Med* 93:578-584, 1980.

29. Ruskin JN, McGovern B, Garan H, DiMarco JP, Kelley E: Anti-arrhythmic drugs: The possible cause of out-of-hospital cardiac arrest. *N Engl J Med* 309:1302-1306, 1983.

30. Thompson RG, Cobb LA: Hypokalemia after rsuscitation from out-of-hospital ventricular fibrillation. *JAMA* 248:2860-2863, 1982.

31. Anderson JL, Mason JW: Testing the efficacy of antiarrhythmic drugs. *N Engl J Med* 315:391-393, 1986.

32. Morady F, Scheinman MM, Hess DS, Sung RJ, Shen E, Shapiro W: Electrophysiologic testing in the management of survivors of out-of-hospital cardiac arrest. *Am J Cardiol* 51:85-89, 1983.

33. Hallstrom AP, Cobb LA, Ray R: Smoking as a risk factor for recurrence of sudden cardiac arrest. *N Engl J Med* 314:271-275, 1986.

34. European coronary study group: Long-term results of prospective randomised study of coronary artery bypass surgery and stable angina pectoris. *Lancet* 2:1173-1180, 1982.

35. Cobb LA, Hallstrom AP, Weaver WD, Trobaugh GB, Greene HL: Considerations under long-term management of survivors of cardiac arrest. *Ann NY Acad Sci* 432:247-257, 1984.

36. Takaro T, Hultgren HN, Lipton MJ, Detre KM, Participants in the Study Group: The VA cooperative randomized study of surgery for coronary arterial occlusive disease: II. Subgroup with significant left main lesions. *Circulation* 54(suppl III):107-117, 1976.

37. Weaver WD, Lorch GL, Alvarez HA, Cobb LA: Angiographic findings and indicators in patients resuscitated from sudden cardiac death. *Circulation* 54:895-900, 1976.

38. The Norwegian Multicenter Study Group: Timolol-induced reduction in mortality and reinfarction in patients surviving acute myocardial infarction. *N Engl J Med* 304:801-807, 1981.

39. Improvement in prognosis of myocardial infarction by long-term beta-adrenoreceptor blockade using Practolol. A multi-center international study. *Br Med J* 3:735-740, 1975.

40. Wilhelmsson C, Vedin JA, Wilhelmsen L, Tibbin G, Werko L: Reduction of sudden death after myocardial infarction by treatment with alprenolol: preliminary results. *Lancet* 2:1157-1160, 1974.

41. Hjalmarson A, Elmfeldt D, Herlitz J, Holmberg S, Malek I, Nyberg G, Ryden L, Swedberg K, Vedin A, Waagstein F, Waldenstrom A, Waldenstrom J, Wedel H, Wilhelmsen L, Wilhelmsson C: Effect on mortality of metoprolol in acute myocardial infarction. A double-blind randomised trial. *Lancet* 2:823-827, 1981.

42. β-Blocker Heart Attack Trial Research Group: A randomized trial of propranolol in patients with acute myocardial infarction. *JAMA* 247:1707-1714, 1982.

43. Friedman GD, Klatsky AL, Siegelaub AB: Predictors of sudden cardiac death. *Circulation* 52(suppl III):164-169, AHA monograph #47, 1975.

44. Josephson ME, Horowitz LN: Electrophysiologic approach to the therapy of a recurrent sustained ventricular tachycardia. *Am J Cardiol* 43:631-642, 1979.

45. Ruskin JN, DiMarco JP, Garan H: Out-of-hospital cardiac arrest: Electrophysiologic observations and selections of long-term anti-arrhythmic therapy. *N Engl J Med* 303:607-613, 1980.

46. Swerdlow CD, Gong G, Echt DS, et al: Clinical factors predicting successful electrophysiologic-pharmacologic study in patients with ventricular tachycardia. *J Am Coll Cardiol* 1:409-416, 1983.

47. Mason JW, Swerdlow CD, Winkle RA, Griffin JC, Ross DL, Keffe DL, Clusin WT: Programmed ventricular stimulation predicting vulnerability of ventricular arrhythmias and their response to anti-arrhythmic therapy. *Am Heart J* 103:633-637, 1982.

48. Mason JW, Winkle RA: Accuracy of the ventricular tachycardia-induction study for predicting the long-term efficacy and inefficacy of antiarrhythmic drugs. *N Engl J Med* 303:1073-1077, 1980.

49. Lown B: Sudden cardiac death: the major challenge confronting contemporary cardiology. *Am J Cardiol* 43:313-328, 1979.

50. Myerberg RJ, Briese FW, Conde C, Mallon SM, Liberthson R, Castellanos A: Long-term antiarrhythmic therapy in survivors of prehospital cardiac arrest. Initial 18 months' experience. *JAMA* 238:2621-2624, 1977.

51. Impact Research Group: International mexiletine and placebo antiarrhythmic coronary trial: I. Report on arrhythmia and other findings. *J Am Coll Cardiol* 4:1148-1163, 1984.

52. Collaborative Group: Phenytoin after recovery from myocardial infarction: Controlled trial in 568 patients. *Lancet* 2:1055-1057, 1971.

53. Peter T; Ross D, Duffield A, et al: Effect on survival after myocardial infarction of long-term treatment with phenytoin. *Br Heart J* 40:1356-1360, 1978.

54. Ryden L, Arnman K, Conradson TB, et al: Prophylaxis of ventricular tachyarrhythmias with intravenous and oral tocainide in patients with and recovering from acute myocardial infarction. *Am Heart J* 100:1006-1012, 1980.

55. Bastain BC: A prospective randomized trial of tocainide in patients following myocardial infarction. *Am Heart J* 100:1017-1022, 1980.

56. Chamberlain DA, Jewitt DE, Julian DB, et al: Oral mexiletine in high-risk patients after myocardial infarction. *Lancet* 2:1324-1327, 1980.

57. Van Durme JP: Chronic antidysrhythmic treatment after myocardial infarction. Design of the Ghent-Rotterdam aprindine study, in Boissel JP, Klimt CR (eds): *Multi-Center Controlled Trials: Principles and Problems*. Paris, Editions INSERM, 43-48, 1977.

58. The CAPS Investigators: The Cardiac Arrhythmia Pilot Study. *Am J Cardiol* 57:91-95, 1986.

59. Schoenfeld MH, McGovern B, Garan H, Kelly E, Grant G, Ruskin JN: Determinants of the outcome of electrophysiolgic study in patients with ventricular tachyarrhythmias. *J Am Coll Cardiol* 6:298-306, 1985.

60. Mirowski M: The automatic implantable cardioverter-defibrillator: An overview. *J Am Coll Cardiol* 6:461-466, 1985.

61. Mirowski M, Reid PR, Winkle RA, Mower MM, Watkins, L, Jr, Stinson EB, Griffith LSC, Kallman CH, Weisfeldt M: Mortality in patients with implanted automatic defibrillators. *Ann Int Med* 98:585-588, 1983.

62. Cummins RO, Eisenberg MS, Stults KR: Automatic external defibrillators; clinical issues for cardiology. *Circulation* 73:381-385, 1986.

63. Weaver WD, Hill D, Bolles J, Hallstrom AP, Cobb LA: Training family of victims at risk for cardiac arrest in the use of an automatic external defibrillator, abstracted. *Circulation* 72(supp III):III-9, 1985.

64. Levy DE, Bates D, Caronna JJ, et al: Prognosis in nontraumatic coma. Ann Int Med 94:293-301, 1981.

65. Longstreth WT, Jr, Diehr P, Inui TS: Predication of awakening after out-of-hospital cardiac arrest. *N Engl J Med* 308:1378-1382, 1983.

66. Longstreth WT, Jr, Inui TS, Cobb LA, Copass MK: Neurologic recovery after out-of-hospital cardiac arrest. *Ann Intern Med* 98:588-592, 1983.

67. Longstreth WT Jr, Blayson KJ, Chandler WL, Sumi SM: Cerebrospinal fluid creatine kinase activity and neurologic recovery after cardiac arrest. *Neurology* 34:834-837, 1984.

68. Kjekshus JK, Vaagenes P, Hetland O: Assessment of cerebral injury with spinal-fluid creatine kinase (CSF-K) in patients after cardiac resuscitation. *Scand J Clin Lab Invest* 40:437-444, 1980.

69. Rossen R, Kabat H, Anderson JP: Acute arrest of cerebral circulation in man. *Arch Neurol Psychiat* 50:510-528, 1943.

70. Caronna JJ, Finklestein S: Neurological syndromes after cardiac arrest. *Stroke* 9:517-520, 1978.

71. Siesjo BK, Wieloch T: Cerebral metabolism in ischaemia: Neurochemical basis for therapy. *Br J Anaesth* 57:47-62, 1985.

72. Astrup J, Symon L, Branston NM, Lassen NA: Cortical evoked potential and extracellular K+ and H+ at critical levels of brain ischemia. *Stroke* 8:51-57, 1977.

73. Harris RJ, Symon J, Branston NM, Bayham M: Changes in extracellular calcium activity in cerebral ischemia. *J Cereb Blood Flow Metab* 1:203-209, 1981.

74. Miller CL, Lampard DG, Alexander K, Brown WA: Local cerebral blood flow following transient cerebral ischemia. I. Onset of impaired reperfusion within the first hour following global ischemia. *Stroke* 11:534-541, 1980.

75. Ames A III, Wright RL, Kowada M, et al: Cerebral ischemia: II. The no-reflow phenomenon. *Am J Pathol* 52:437-453, 1968.

76. Synder JV, Nemoto EM, Carrol Safar P: Global ischemia in dogs: intracranial pressures, brain blood flow and metabolism. *Stroke* 6:21-27, 1975.

77. Nemoto EM, Synder JV, Carroll RG. Morita H: Global ischemia in dogs: Cerebrovascular CO2 reactivity and autoregulation. *Stroke* 6:425-431, 1975.

78. Senter HJ, Wolf A, Wagner FC Jr: Intracranial pressure in nontraumatic ischemic and hypoxic cerebral insults. *J Neurosurg* 54:489-493, 1981.

79. Wilder RJ, Weir D, Rush BF, Ravitch MM: Methods of coordinating ventilation and closed chest cardiac massage in the dog. *Surgery* 53:186-194, 1963.

80. Del Guercio LRM, Feins NR, Cohn JD, et al: Comparison of blood flow during external and internal cardiac massage in man. *Circulation* 31(suppl I):171-180, 1965.

81. Weiser FM, Adler LN, Kuhn LA: Hemodynamic effects of closed and open chest cardiac resuscitation in normal dogs and those with acute myocardial infarction. *Am J Cardiol* 10:555-561, 1962.

82. Bircher N, Safar P: Cerebral preservation during cardiopulmonary resuscitation. *Crit Care Med* 13:185-190, 1985.

83. Chandra N, Rudikoff M, Weisfeldt ML: Simultaneous chest compression and ventilation at high airway pressure during cardiopulmonary resuscitation. *Lancet* 1:175-178, 1980.

84. Kouwenhoven WB, Jude JR, Knickerbocker GG: Closed chest cardiac massage. *JAMA* 173:1064-1067, 1960.

85. Niemann JT, Rosborough JP, Hausknecht M, et al: Pressure-synchronized cineangiography during experimental cardiopulmonary resuscitation. *Circulation* 64:985-991, 1981.

86. Niemann JT, Rosborough JP, Ung S, Criley JM: Hemodynamic effects of continuous abdominal binding during cardiac arrest and resuscitation. *Am J Cardiol* 53:269-274, 1984.

87. Ralston SH, Babbs CF, Niebauer MJ: Cardiopulmonary resuscitation with interposed abdominal compression in dogs. *Anesth Analg* 61:645-651, 1982.

88. Warren ET, Pass HI, Crawford FA Jr.: External cardiopulmonary resuscitation augmented by the military antishock trousers. Am *Surgeon* 49:651-654, 1983.

89. Maier GW, Tyson GS Jr, Olsen CO, et al: The physiology of external cardiac massage: High-impulse cardiopulmonary resuscitation. *Circulation* 70:86-101, 1984.

90. Ditchey RV, Lindenfeld J: Potential adverse effects of volume loading on perfusion of vital organs during closed-chest resuscitation. *Circulation* 69:181-189, 1984.

91. Sanders AB, Ewy GA, Alferness CA, et al: Failure of one method of simultaneous chest compression, ventilation and abdominal binding during CPR. *Crit Care Med* 10:509-513, 1982.

92. Mateer Jr, Stueven HA, Thompson BM, et al: Interposed abdominal compression CPR versus standard CPR in prehospital cardiopulmonary arrest: preliminary results. *Ann Emerg Med* 13:764-766, 1984.

93. Holmes HR, Babbs CF, Voorhees WD, et al: Influence of adrenergic drugs upon vital organ perfusion during CPR. *Crit Care Med* 8:137-140, 1980.

94. Michael JR, Guerci AD, Koehler RC et al: Mechanisms by which epinephrine augments cerebral and myocardial perfusion during cardiopulmonary resuscitation in dogs. *Circulation* 69:822-835, 1984.

95. Ralston SH, Voorhees WD, Babbs CF: Intrapulmonary epinephrine during prolonged cardiopulmonary resuscitation: Improved regional blood flow and resuscitation in dogs. *Ann Emerg Med* 13:79-86, 1984.

96. Cantu RC, Ames A III, Dixon J, Di Giacinto G: Reversibility of experimental cerebrovascular obstruction induced by complete ischemia. *J Neurosurg* 31:429-431, 1969.

97. Fischer EG, Ames A: Studies on mechanisms of impairment of cerebral circulation following ischemia: Effects of hemodilution and perfusion pressure. *Stroke* 3:538-542, 1972.

98. Bleyaert AL, Sands PA, Safar P, et al: Augmentation of postischemic brain damage by severe intermittent hypertension. *Crit Care Med* 8:41-47, 1980.

99. Gisvold SE, Safar P, Rao G, et al: Prolonged immobilization and controlled ventilation do not improve outcome after global brain ischemia in monkeys. *Crit Care Med* 12:171-179, 1984.

100. Todd MM, Tommasino C, Shapiro HM: Cerebrovascular effects of prolonged hypocarbia and hypercarbia after experimental global ischemia in cats. *Crit Care Med* 13:720-723, 1985.

101. Goldstein A Jr., Wells BA, Keats AS: Increased tolerance to cerebral anoxia by pentobarbital. *Arch Int Pharmacodyn* 161:138-143, 1966.

102. Bleyaert AL, Neomoto EM, Safar P, et al: Thiopental amelioration of brain damage after global ischemia in monkeys. *Anesthesiology* 49:390-398, 1978.

103. Steen PA, Milde JH, Michenfelder JD: No barbiturate protection in a dog model of complete cerebral ischemia. *Ann Neurol* 5:343-349, 1979.

104. Gisvold SE, Safar P, Hendrickx HHL, et al: Thiopental treatment after global brain ischemia in pigtailed monkeys. *Anesthesiology* 60:88-96, 1984.

105. Breivik H, Safar P, Sands P, et al: Clinical feasibility trials of barbiturate therapy after cardiac arrest. *Crit Care Med* 6:228-244, 1978.

106. Brain Resuscitation Clinical Trial I Study Group: Randomized clinical study of thiopental loading in comatose survivors of cardiac arrest. *N Engl J Med* 314:397-403, 1986.

107. Steen PA, Newberg LA, Milde JH, Michenfelder JD: Nimodipine improves cerebral blood flow and neurologic recovery after complete cerebral ischemia in the dog. *J Cereb Blood Flow Metab* 3:38-43, 1983.

108. Mabe H, Nagai, H, Takagi T, et al: Effect of nimodipine on cerebral functional and metabolic recovery following ischemia in the rat brain. *Stroke* 17:501-505, 1986.

109. Winegar CP, Henderson O, White BC, et al: Early amelioration of neurologic deficit by lidoflazine after fifteen minutes of cardiopulmonary arrest in dogs. *Ann Emerg Med* 12:471-477, 1983.

110. Vaagenes P, Cantadore R, Safar P, et al: Amelioration of brain damage by lidoflazine after prolonged ventricular fibrillation cardiac arrest in dogs. *Crit Care Med* 12:846-855, 1984.
111. Edmonds HL, Wauquier A, Melis W, et al: Improved short-term neurological recovery with flunarizine in a canine model of cardiac arrest. *Am J Emerg Med* 3:150-155, 1985.
112. Steen PA, Gisvold SE, Milde JH, et al: Nimodipine improves outcome when given after complete cerebral ischemia in primates. *Anesthesiology* 62:406-414, 1985.
113. Milde LN, Milde JH, Michenfelder JD: Delayed treatment with nimodipine improves cerebral blood flow after complete cerebral ischemia in the dog. *J Cereb Blood Flow Metab* 6:332-337, 1986.
114. Dean JM, Hoehner PJ, Rogers MC, Traystman RJ: Effect of lidoflazine on cerebral blood flow following twelve minutes total cerebral ischemia. *Stroke* 15:531-535, 1984.
115. Newberg LA, Steen PA, Milde JH, Michenfelder JD: Failure of flunarizine to improve cerebral blood flow or neurologic recovery in a canine model of complete ischemia. *Stroke* 15:666-671, 1984.
116. Steen PA, Newberg LA, Milde JH, Michenfelder JD: Cerebral blood flow and neurologic outcome when nimodipine is given after complete cerebral ischemia in the dog. *J Cereb Flow Metab* 4:82-87, 1984.
117. White BC, Aust SD, Afors KE, Aronson LD: Brain injury by ischemic anoxia: Hypothesis extension — A tale of two ions? *Ann Emerg Med* 13:862-867, 1984.
118. Schanne FAX, Kane AB, Young EE, Farber JL: Calcium dependence of toxic cell death: A final common pathway. *Science* 206:700-702, 1979.
119. Gisvold SE, Safar P, Rao G, et al: Multifaceted therapy after global brain ischemia in monkeys. *Stroke* 15:803-812, 1984.
120. Safar P: Recent advances in cardiopulmonary cerebral resuscitation: A review. *Ann Emerg Med* 13:856-862, 1984.

Special Resuscitation Situations

Chapter 15

Special resuscitation situations are cardiopulmonary arrests or other life-threatening emergencies that require modification or extension of conventional life support techniques. Examples include near drowning, hypothermia, trauma, electrical shock, and cardiac arrest in the pregnant patient. Although there are many important aspects in the management of patients in these situations, the primary focus of this chapter will be on the most severely stricken patient who has developed, or is in imminent danger of developing, cardiopulmonary arrest.

Drowning and Near Drowning

Drowning is defined as death due to submersion (and usually suffocation) in water or other fluid media. Near drowning is the term used when recovery, at least temporarily, occurs following submersion injury. Drowning and near drowning episodes may occur with or without aspiration, the latter usually due to prolonged laryngospasm during submersion. Ten to 15% of drownings occur without aspiration of water or gastric contents.[1] Other terms used to describe clinical phenomena associated with drowning episodes include the immersion syndrome (sudden death triggered by vagally induced arrhythmias) following submersion in cold water and delayed or secondary drowning, defined as a near drowning episode followed by the recurrence of respiratory symptoms 3–4 hours or less after the initial episode.[2]

Incidence

There are over 80,000 near drowning incidents in the United States per year.[3] Drowning is the third leading cause of accidental death and claims approximately 9,000 lives per year. The peak incidence is in teenagers and in children under the age of 4 years.

Pathophysiology

The major physiological consequences of near drowning are hypoxia, acidosis, and pulmonary edema.[4] Hypoxia results from the lack of air exchange and from the damage caused by the inhalation of fluid. There is often, initially, a combined respiratory and metabolic acidosis. By the time the victim reaches the hospital emergency department, the respiratory acidosis is usually corrected but the metabolic acidosis, due to hypoperfusion and the build-up of lactic acid, remains.

Pulmonary edema occurs in up to 75% of near drowning cases. Aspiration of hypertonic seawater (approximately 3% sodium chloride) is associated with a shift of intravascular fluid into the alveoli. Fresh water aspiration causes pulmonary edema by injuring the alveolar capillary membrane and removing surfactant, allowing protein-rich plasma to enter the alveolar space.

Significant electrolyte abnormalities are usually not present in near drowning. The hematocrit is typically normal, although hemolysis can occur (especially with fresh water near drowning). Renal failure may occur due to hypotension, lactic acidosis, or myoglobinuria.

Drowning may be associated with other injuries, such as spinal cord damage (diving), air embolism (SCUBA diving), or hypothermia; and it may occur as a complication of alcohol or other drug ingestion, hypoglycemia, or seizures.

Treatment of Near Drowning

Initial Field Resuscitation

The victim must be reached and removed from the water by rescuers. It is essential that rescuers exercise caution and take steps to ensure their own safety while retrieving the victim.

Effective respiratory support of the victim should be the primary goal of the initial rescue effort. Mouth-to-mouth ventilation should be started just as soon as the rescuer can safely apply the technique. It is sometimes possible to initiate rescue breathing before the victim is physically removed from the water. Attempts to drain water from the breathing passages by any means other than postural drainage or suction are not necessary or advisable and may increase the risk of vomiting and aspiration.[5] Any particulate foreign matter that is obstructing the upper airway (such as seaweed or sand) and can be extracted easily from the victim's mouth by the rescuer should be removed. If there is evidence of particulate foreign matter obstruction of the airway (either by visual inspection of the mouth or by the rescuer finding that the lungs cannot be adequately inflated with rescue breathing), the Heimlich maneuver (subdiaphragmatic abdominal thrusts) should be used. If rescue breathing fails to revive the victim, the Heimlich maneuver may be performed on the grounds that a particulate foreign matter obstruction may have been overlooked.

In controlled studies of near drowning using experimental animals, pulmonary function, arterial blood gases, and clinical outcome are not influenced by the use of the Heimlich maneuver.[5] Accordingly, the Heimlich maneuver is not recommended for the initial management of near drowning victims when there is no evidence of particulate foreign matter airway obstruction because it may induce vomiting and aspiration. Also, the Heimlich maneuver should not be used to deliberately induce vomiting on the grounds that it will "prevent vomiting later."

As soon as the victim is removed from the water onto a hard flat surface, the rescuer should check carefully for the victim's carotid pulse, which may be difficult to detect because of vasoconstriction or depression of the cardiac output in the victim. If there is no pulse, chest compressions should be started.

Advanced Life Support Measures

The initial goal of advanced life support management should be the improvement and optimization of ventilation beyond that provided with basic life support measures. Advanced life support providers should establish an adequate protected airway in the victim as soon as possible, preferably with an endotracheal tube. Until the airway can be protected, the chin-lift or jaw-thrust, without head-tilt, is the best way to maintain a patent upper airway. The head-tilt is not recommended, unless it is essential for ventilation, because of the frequent association of cervical spine injuries with near drowning.

Patients should receive oxygen in as high a concentration as possible through a non-rebreathing mask. Suction must be used as indicated to remove secretions. Positive-pressure ventilation with continuous positive airway pressure (CPAP) or positive end expiration pressure (PEEP) is indicated and, if available, should be used by rescuers if they are trained and experienced in such techniques.

If there is suspicion that the victim suffered a neck injury (usually associated with a diving injury or fall), the cervical spine must be protected by the rescuers, using manual head and neck support, a cervical collar, a backboard, or their equivalent. Nasotracheal intubation or an emergency cricothyroidotomy may be preferable to orotracheal intubation in such cases. Bronchospasm should be managed with inhaled terbutaline or isoetharine, or with intravenous aminophylline. These agents are not available on prehospital life support units in most EMS systems; such drugs are usually given after the patient is brought to the hospital emergency unit.

Intravenous lactated Ringer's solution or normal saline should be started at a keep-open rate (or faster if there is obvious evidence of hypovolemia, such as hypotension due to severe blood loss due to an injury sustained in a diving accident). The cardiac rhythm should be monitored continuously because hypoxia and acidosis may cause arrhythmias. The safety or efficacy of sodium bicarbonate in the near drowning victim is unknown; routine use of this agent for the near drowning victim is not recommended.

Initial laboratory tests should include serial blood gases, hematocrit, white blood cell count, electrolytes, and blood urea nitrogen. If the victim is unresponsive, a nasogastric tube should be inserted to decompress the stomach (preferably after the airway is protected with an endotracheal tube) and urine output should be monitored with a Foley catheter. An electrocardiogram is especially important in elderly patients or in patients with underlying heart disease to detect myocardial ischemia, infarction, or arrhythmia.

Since the core temperature may be lowered during cold water immersion, prehospital rescuers should use blankets to maintain the patient's temperature during transportation. The core temperature should be checked and, if abnormal, monitored continuously after arrival at the hospital while the victim is rewarmed. The rapid development of hypothemia during immersion (especially in cold fresh water) protects cerebral function during the period of anoxia. Children have survived without neurological impairment following up to 40 minutes in cold water submersion.[6]

All victims of near drowning, no matter how mild the episode appears to have been, should be brought to the hospital for evaluation and observation. Patients who go on to develop delayed symptoms (secondary drowning) display signs of respiratory distress usually within the first four hours.[2] These patients should be admitted to the hosptal for further observation and treatment.

Prognosis

The prognosis of near drowning victims who require CPR is directly related to the level of consciousness within the first hour of successful resuscitation. Virtually all patients who are initially aware will survive with excellent neurological recovery.[7] Patients who are initially unresponsive have a survival rate of 82%, but only half of the survivors become neurologically normal.[7,8] The key to success is the provision of early, effective ventilatory support.

Cardiac Arrest Due to Physical Trauma

Cardiac arrest due to major blunt or penetrating trauma is managed differently than the routine cardiac arrest that is not accompanied by hypovolemia, tension pneumothorax, or cardiac tamponade. Initial management is the same (the ABC's of resuscitation), with maintenance of the airway (using the jaw-thrust without head-tilt because of the high frequency of concomitant neck injuries), rescue breathing, and support of circulation (chest compressions). Patients who are still breathing but unresponsive and who require respiratory support are, preferably, intubated nasotracheally. Apneic patients should be intubated orotracheally if it can be accomplished without excessive movement of the cervical spine; if not, a cricothyrotomy may be necessary.[9] If a cricothyrotomy cannot be performed rapidly and safely due to lack of proper equipment or personnel experienced in the technique, an esophageal obturator airway may provide an alternative method of airway management.

Tension pneumothorax should be suspected in any trauma victim; the resuscitation team should carefully check for the presence of unequal breath sounds in the right and left chest and for a tracheal shift. If there is any evidence of tension pneumothorax, a diagnostic pleural aspiration should be performed. A large-bore (#14 or #16 gauge) needle or intracath attached to a syringe should be inserted into the second or third intercostal space in the mid-clavicular line anteriorly. If a tension pneumothorax is present, the high intrathoracic pressure will usually push the needle plunger out toward the end of the syringe. An acceptable alternative procedure initially, and the definitive procedure if pneumothorax is confirmed by the needle aspiration, is insertion of a chest tube.

At least two large-bore intravenous lines should be inserted, preferably in different extremities. Intravenous crystalloid fluid (normal saline or lactated Ringer's) should be infused rapidly as needed to maintain arterial pressure and perfusion, on the assumption that hypotension is due to hypovolemia unless there is evidence to the contrary in a severely injured accident victim. Pneumatic antishock trousers may be of limited assistance temporarily by increasing peripheral vascular resistance and by stabilizing long bone fractures in the lower extremities.

Extensive, time-consuming care of trauma victims in the field is usually not warranted. However, there is evidence that the initiation of basic and advanced life support by paramedics for trauma cardiac arrest victims may improve survival.[10] The final decision whether to "load and go" or to begin definitive care prior to transport must be based on the unique characteristics of each incident. Patients should be brought to the nearest trauma care facility which best meets their medical needs, as defined by the regional emergency medical services and trauma care system plan. Criteria for such decision-making are delineated as part of the Advanced Trauma Life Support Standards.[9]

In the emergency department, chest trauma victims who have a palpable blood pressure should be resuscitated with volume and, when indicated, tube thoracostomy, pericardiocentesis, and exploratory thoracotomy. Autotransfusion should be used if available, or the patient should receive type-specific or O-negative blood if more than 2–3 L of crystalloid fluid have been required.

Closed chest compressions are ineffective in most patients with cardiac arrest due to trauma. In the emergency department, patients with penetrating chest trauma and cardiac arrest should have an immediate thoracotomy performed by a physician skilled in this technique to allow for open cardiac massage and decompression of cardiac tamponade, if present.[11-13] If severe hypovolemia is present, the thoracic aorta can be temporarily cross-clamped to control subdiaphragmatic bleeding. The pulmonary hilum can be unilaterally cross-clamped to prevent air embolism and to control hemorrhage in patients with injury to hilar structures.

Blunt trauma victims who are initially found by prehospital providers to be in cardiac arrest or in whom the systolic pressure cannot be maintained above 60 mmHg despite aggressive volume resuscitation rarely survive.[12,14] Some trauma care specialists have argued that many of these patients should not receive emergency thoracotomy because it is unlikely to alter outcome and, thus, adds additional needless expense for the family and survivors.[12,14]

A patient with a massive head injury due to either blunt or penetrating trauma is also generally considered a poor candidate for emergency department thoracotomy.[15] Although survival is low, selected patients with cardiac arrest due to penetrating injury below the diaphragm may benefit from emergency thoracotomy and aortic cross-clamping.[13]

Many patients who survive cardiac arrest and emergency thoracotomy make a full neurological recovery.[15] Return of consciousness within the first 12 hours is the best predictor of a favorable outcome.

Accidental Electrocution

The frequency of accidental death by electrocution is about 0.54 per 100,000 population per year in the United States.[16] Generated electricity accounts for over 90% of the deaths. Half of the deaths are due to contact with low voltage (below 1,000 volts). Low-voltage deaths are equally common in the home and in the workplace; such deaths are more frequent in the summer and early fall. The majority (86%) of high-voltage deaths occur on the job, and there is no seasonal preponderance.

Pathophysiology of Injury Due to Electrical Current

The danger of cardiac arrest is related principally to the magnitude and duration of the electrical current.[17] The voltage of the electrical source and the electrical resistance of the body tissues through which the electricity passes are only important in that they determine the magnitude of the current flow. Alternating current at 60 Hertz (the frequency used by power companies) is generally more dangerous to humans than direct current at any given voltage because it is more likely to induce ventricular fibrillation.

When a low-current intensity (1 milliampere, or mA) is applied from the body surface, there is little danger of harm and the electrical current is usually felt as a tingling sensation in the area of contact. Progressively higher currents cause increasingly unpleasant and painful sensations. At approximately 10 mA, tetanic muscular contractions may occur, which may make it difficult or impossible for a hand grasping an energized object to let go. The current at which it is not possible to release an energized wire, the "let go current", varies considerably from person to person within the range of 5–30 mA.[18] By 40–50 mA, the tetanic contractions may involve all muscles, including the diaphragm and the intercostals, causing respiratory arrest until the current flow stops. With short duration contact at this current level, normal respiration usually resumes immediately after the current flow ceases. Longer contact can cause prolonged apnea with resultant hypoxemia, tissue hypoxia, secondary cardiac arrest, and death.

Higher currents (100 mA to several amperes), even of brief duration, can directly induce ventricular fibrillation. Brief duration shocks at or just above 10 A may result in a current flow of sufficient strength that the heart holds its contraction in systole until release of the current. This is thought to protect against or reverse ventricular fibrillation in some circumstances. Defibrillators used in resuscitation deliver current in this range.

Higher current flow (several tens of amperes) may cause prolonged respiratory arrest.[19] Massive currents of several hundred amperes can induce both respiratory arrest and cardiac arrhythmia, including ventricular fibrillation. Rarely, the victim of such a massive electrical shock may not lose consciousness immediately. Electrical power linemen receiving such injuries have even been reported to climb down the utility pole before collapsing in cardiac arrest, presumably due to a ventricular arrhythmia.[17]

The passage of current through body tissue generates heat and may produce injury similar to that of a burn and a crush injury.[20] Current often flows along nerves and blood vessels where there is disruption of the vascular endothelium and thrombosis. The resultant thermal injury may be of sufficient severity to require debridement, escharotomy, fasciotomy, or amputation.[20]

Secondary injuries, caused when the victim is thrown by contact with an electrical source, may include cervical spine or other bony fractures, closed head injury, and peripheral nerve damage. Myoglobinuria may occur due to muscle injury.

Lightning

Lightning acts as a massive DC countershock, depolarizing the entire myocardium at once, following which the heart's normal rhythm may resume.[21] In one published series,[22] death occurred in 30% of 66 victims struck by lightning. The patients who died were those who suffered an immediate cardiac arrest. Respiratory arrest often lasts longer than asystole and the victim may die from hypoxia if CPR is not started promptly. Patients who do not arrest immediately have an excellent chance of recovery.

Management of the Victim of Severe Electrical Shock

The rescuer must be certain that the current is off before attempting to touch the victim or move the victim from the electrical source. If possible, the current should be switched off at its source. Alternatively, the rescuer may have to separate the victim from the current using a rubber object or other nonconductive material such as dry nonmetallic rope or wood.[23] Rescuers should not touch a victim who is still in contact with an active current source without the protection of nonconductive material. If unconscious, the victim should be assessed for the presence of adequate breathing and circulation. Rescue breathing and chest compressions should be started when indicated, taking care to protect the cervical spine from further motion or injury if there is any likelihood that the victim was thrown or suffered a fall. In such a case the chin-lift or jaw-thrust, without head-tilt, should be used to open the airway. A cervical collar or its equivalent should be used if available. Any obvious orthopedic injury should be immobilized.

When a power lineman on a utility pole is electrocuted, rescue breathing can often be initiated by rescuers on the pole, with chest compressions if needed as soon as the victim can be lowered to the ground. Even if there is no loss of consciousness, a victim of high-voltage electrical shock should receive cardiac monitoring and transport to the hospital because of the danger of delayed cardiac arrest from a life-threatening arrhythmia.

Since virtually all victims of lightning injury who do not go into immediate cardiac arrest survive,[22] when multiple victims are simultaneously struck by lightning, individuals who appear clinically dead immediately following the strike should be treated before other victims showing signs of life.[22,23] Most patients who are successfully resuscitated from cardiac arrest due to lightning or other high-voltage electrical shock injury will have return of spontaneous respirations within 30 minutes.[24] Complete recovery has been reported after resuscitation of up to several hours in occasional patients. Therefore, the victim of cardiac arrest due to electrical shock may warrant prolonged aggressive efforts in certain circumstances. The decision to terminate resuscitation should be made by a physician well versed in the treatment of electrical injuries based on all the factors unique to the specific incident.

When significant crush or burn injury is suspected, intravenous fluids (lactated Ringer's or normal saline) should be given at a rate sufficient to maintain the urine output at 50–100 mL/hr to minimize the likelihood of renal shutdown due to myoglobinuria and/or dehydration from third space fluid losses. Mannitol (25 g initially, followed by 12.5 g every hour for 6 hours) should be given if myoglobinuria is present. Surgical consultation for local debridement and full-thickness exploration should be obtained.

Accidental Hypothermia

Hypothermia is defined as a core body temperature below 35° C. Because many standard medical thermometers do not read below 34.4° C, clinical hypothermia can be easily overlooked. Most clinically significant episodes of hypothermia result from an accidental fall in core body temperature due to injury, immersion in cold water, or prolonged exposure to a cold environment. The very young and the very old are the most susceptible to hypothermia.[25-27] Infants lose the same amount of heat per unit of body surface area as adults but cannot produce as much heat as adults; infants also have a larger body surface area relative to total body mass than adults. Older individuals have a lower metabolic rate than the young, making it difficult for them to maintain a normal body temperature when subjected to an ambient temperature below 18° C.

Alcohol ingestion increases the risk of hypothermia by causing cutaneous vasodilation, impairment of the shivering mechanism, hypothalamic dysfunction, and a lack of awareness of the environment.[28,29] Other medical conditions commonly associated with the development of accidental hypothermia include drug ingestion (especially barbiturates or phenothiazines), diabetes (especially in the presence of hypoglycemia), hypothyroidism, hypopituitarism, hypoadrenalism, anorexia nervosa, head injury, and sepsis.[6] Immersion in cold water, as in near drowning, can cool the body temperature much more rapidly than exposure to cold air because the thermal conductivity of water is 32 times greater than that of air.[30] Hypothermia can occur in previously healthy individuals (such as cross-country skiers or hikers) who become injured and are exposed to the cold for prolonged periods.

Clinical Features

The most important clinical effect of a lowered core body temperature is a gradual and progressive decline in basal metabolic rate and oxygen consumption.[27,30] Mild hypothermia (above 30° C) results in shivering, loss of fine motor coordination, and lethargy.[27,30,31] Below 30° C the pupils are usually dilated and there is hyporeflexia.

Reflex vasoconstriction helps to preserve the core temperature but makes detection of the pulse and blood pressure difficult. The hypothermic patient may appear clinically dead but may still be viable with proper diagnosis and aggressive management. Fully successful clinical recovery has occurred in a patient with an initial core temperature as low as 17° C.[30] The only way to establish the potential viability of the hypothermic patient is to attempt resuscitation and active rewarming.

Hemodynamically, mild hypothermia causes a rise in pulse rate, blood pressure, peripheral vascular resistance, central venous pressure, and cardiac output. Moderate-to-severe hypothermia (below 30° C) causes bradycardia, arrhythmias (atrial fibrillation is common but virtually any atrial, junctional, or ventricular arrythmia can occur), hypotension, and a fall in cardiac output. The risk of ventricular fibrillation or asystole, the usual final event leading to death, increases as the temperature drops below 28° C. The J wave (Osborn wave), which is most prominent in leads V3 or V4 (Figure 1), occurs in 80% of hypothermia patients and increases in size with decreasing core body temperature.[32]

Oxygenation and acid–base balance are altered by hypothermia. Mild hypothermia initially causes hyperventilation. As the core temperature decreases there is respiratory depression with anoxia and carbon dioxide

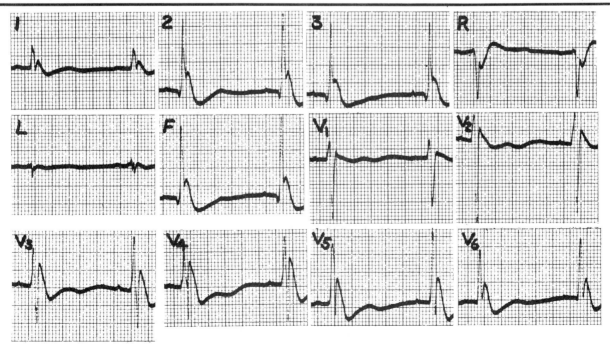

Figure 1.   Typical J wave (Osborn wave) seen in hypothermia. (From Marriott HJ: *Practical Electrocardiography*, ed 6. Baltimore, Williams and Wilkins Co, 1977, p 466.)

retention.[27] A combined respiratory and metabolic acidosis may occur due to hypoventilation, carbon dioxide retention, reduced hepatic metabolism of organic acid due to decreased perfusion of the liver, poor peripheral perfusion, and increased lactic acid production from poor perfusion of skeletal muscle and shivering.[27,31] There is controversy about whether arterial blood gases should be corrected for temperature in the hypothermic patient.[33,34]

Hypothermia affects the function of all organic systems.[30] It inhibits the release of antidiuretic hormone and decreases oxidative renal tubular activity, causing diuresis and volume depletion.[35] The hematocrit is elevated due to dehydration and splenic contraction.[30] Plasma viscosity increases significantly below 27° C.[30] Insulin release and the peripheral utilization of glucose are inhibited during hypothermia, causing hyperglycemia, which reverts with rewarming and usually does not require treatment with insulin.[36]

General Principles of Treatment

Early recognition of hypothermia is essential. Health care providers in the field and in the emergency department must maintain a high index of suspicion in any patient with an altered level of consciousness who has been subjected to even a modestly cool environment. A thermometer capable of registering a temperature of 30° C or less is essential in all emergency treatment facilities.

Because the cold heart is irritable and susceptible to serious arrhythmia, care should be taken to move the patient gently during transportation or during transfer of the patient from a litter to a hospital bed. The patient should be monitored continuously, and equipment for resuscitation (including a defibrillator) should be immediately available. Routine laboratory evaluation usually includes arterial blood gases, a complete blood count, prothrombin time, partial thromboplastin time, glucose, electrolytes, blood urea nitrogen, serum creatinine, amylase, liver function tests, electrocardiogram, chest x-ray, and urinalysis.

The hypothermic heart is usually unresponsive to cardioactive drugs, pacemaker stimulation, and defibrillation.[14,15] Nonessential interventions should generally be avoided until the core temperature is increased above 30° C. However, indicated and necessary procedures should not be withheld. For example, endotracheal intubation of the severely hypothermic patient may be needed to protect the airway, to correct hypoxemia and hypercarbia, and to deliver warm humidified oxygen. There is little evidence that intubation is likely to precipitate ventricular fibrillation in this setting as long as the patient is adequately ventilated (usually with a bag–valve–mask device) and the respiratory acidosis is corrected by hyperventilation prior to attempting intubation.[39]

The effect of most drugs and hormones is diminished during hypothermia. In addition, metabolism of drugs and hormones is usually reduced, causing accumulation in the body and potential toxicity during rewarming if repeated doses have been administered. Nonessential drugs and hormones should generally be avoided until the temperature is corrected to above 30° C. Indicated and necessary drugs should not be withheld, although they may need to be given in reduced doses, at less frequent intervals, or both. Hypoglycemia should be treated with glucose. Hyperglycemia during hypothermia will often correct spontaneously with rewarming; the use of insulin may be necessary in specific cases, but there is a hazard of inducing hypoglycemia as the body temperature is corrected.[30] Volume depletion should be corrected.

Field Management

Once hypothermia is suspected, every effort should be made to minimize further heat loss, to begin the rewarming process, and to cautiously transport the patient to an appropriate advanced life support treatment facility. If possible, wet garments should be removed and replaced with dry (preferably warm) garments.[30] Blankets and/or an insulated sleeping bag may be used to retain body heat. A normothermic rescuer may lie alongside the victim underneath the covers to assist in rewarming. If available, airway rewarming with warm humidified oxygen should be used because it can improve the patient's heat balance by as much as 23 kcal/hour.[40]

In-Hospital Management

Mild Hypothermia (30° C or above)

Patients with mild hypothermia generally have a good prognosis regardless of the rewarming method used.[30,31] External rewarming is most appropriate, either passively by using blankets and allowing the patient's own metabolism slowly to restore normothermia, or actively by using electric blankets, hot water bottles, or warm baths. Though effective, warm baths have the disadvantage of not allowing the cardiac rhythm to be monitored, creating a potential serious hazard if an arrhythmia develops. If hypothermia has developed over a prolonged period of time, the core temperature should probably be restored gradually (at a rate of 0.5–1.0° C per hour).

Moderate-to-Severe Hypothermia (below 30° C)

Rewarming is not the mirror image of the cooling process, especially for patients who have developed moderate-to-severe degrees of hypothermia over a prolonged period of time. In such patients, attempts at rewarming by application of external heat (such as immersion of the patient in a warm water bath) is hazardous because sudden peripheral vasodilation will cause perfusion of vascular beds containing cold, lactic-acid-rich blood. Return of this blood into the central core may cause a temporary paradoxical "afterdrop" in core temperature and pH, increasing the likelihood of ventricular fibrillation.[30] For this reason, patients with moderate-to-severe hypothermia should generally be treated with core rewarming. The most popular current techniques include administration of warmed (43° C) intravenous fluids through a central line; warm (42°–46° C) humidified oxygen (most effective via endotracheal tube); peritoneal lavage using a fluid temperature of 43° C; and mediastinal irrigation and cardiopulmonary bypass (usually reserved for moderate-to-severe hypothermia complicated by cardiac arrest).

Hypothermia-Induced Cardiac Arrest

Treatment of a patient in cardiac arrest due to hypothermia is different from the treatment of a normothermic patient in cardiac arrest. The most common cardiac rhythms in hypothermia-induced arrest are ventricular fibrillation and asystole. However, the fibrillating hypothermic heart is often resistant to defibrillation until the core temperature is raised, and the temperature at which the heart will respond to defibrillation is variable. In general, defibrillation should be attempted as soon as possible. If unsuccessful, CPR should be continued and aggressive attempts should be made to rapidly rewarm the core, using a combination of techniques, with repeated attempts at defibrillation periodically as the core temperature increases. There are conflicting reports about the efficacy of bretylium tosylate in this setting.[41]

The patient should be intubated as soon as possible and should be ventilated with warmed, humidified oxygen. Open chest cardiac massage may be indicated since the ventricles may be stiff when there is severe hypothermia, and irrigation of the pericardial sac can be performed using warmed sterile fluids.[42] Peritoneal lavage[43] and cardiopulmonary bypass[42] have been used successfully to treat patients with hypothermia-induced cardiac arrest.

How long should attempts at resuscitation be continued? In general, children or young adults who develop cardiac arrest due to a sudden severe drop in core temperature (as in cold water immersion) should be treated aggressively, since survival without neurological impairment may be possible. A common problem is how to manage the unwitnessed cardiac arrest victim who is found in a cool or cold environment. The victim could have arrested due to hypothermia or the cold body temperature could be due to death. The clinical maxim that patients who appear dead after prolonged exposure to cold temperature should not be considered dead until they have been restored to near normal core temperature and remain unresponsive to resuscitation[43] cannot be applied literally in all cases. Instead, the decision to terminate resuscitation must be individualized by the physician in charge based on the unique circumstances of each incident.

Pregnancy

The dramatic alterations in maternal cardiovascular physiology induced by pregnancy make cardiopulmonary resuscitation of expectant mothers unique. During pregnancy, maternal blood volume and cardiac output increase by up to 150% of nonpregnant levels and uterine blood flow increases from 2% before pregnancy to between 20 and 30% during the last trimester of pregnancy to accommodate the needs of the fetus.[44,45] In order to permit this marked but essential increase in flow, the uteroplacental vascular bed must be maximally dilated. In addition, when the mother is supine, the gravid uterus may compress the iliac vessels, the inferior vena cava, and the abdominal aorta, resulting in hypotension and as much as a 25% reduction in cardiac output.[46]

Management of Cardiac Arrest During Pregnancy

When cardiac arrest occurs in a pregnant woman before the 24th week of gestation (the putative onset of fetal viability), the rescuer's primary concern should be directed towards saving the mother, whose chances of survival are far better than those of the fetus. Conventional therapy and procedures applicable to any arrest situation should be utilized as indicated and appropriate.

Beyond the 24th week of gestation, the rescuer must consider the life of the potentially viable fetus as well as that of the mother. Precipitating events for cardiac arrest include arrhythmia, congestive heart failure, myocardial infarction, iatrogenic hypermagnesemia, or intracranial hemorrhage in a toxemic patient. Spontaneous bleeding, including intrahepatic bleeding, may occur, resulting in hypovolemia.

Most of the standard resuscitation procedures can and should be applied without modification. For example, if ventricular fibrillation is present, it should be treated with defibrillation according to the ventricular fibrillation algorithm.[45,47] Closed-chest compressions and support of ventilation may be done conventionally. To obviate the effects of the gravid uterus on venous return, a wedge, such as a pillow or similar device, should be placed under the right abdominal flank and hip to gently push the uterus to the left side of the abdomen.[45]

Lidocaine crosses the placenta. However, when used in standard doses, there appears to be little effect on the fetus.[48] The use of vasopressors such as epinephrine, norephinephrine, and dopamine should be avoided if possible since they induce uteroplacental vasoconstriction, especially when hypoxemia and/or hypotension is present, which may endanger the life of the fetus.[44,45]

If 5–10 minutes of standard CPR, leftward displacement of the gravid uterus, airway management, fluid volume restoration, and defibrillation (if indicated) fail to restore effective circulatory function, an attempt to evaluate fetal viability via external monitoring or real-time ultrasound, though difficult, may be useful in deciding if and when open-chest heart massage and/or caesarean section is required. In addition, pharmacological treatment of the infant *in utero* may be necessary.[45] If standard measures are not successful within 15 minutes of the onset of arrest, thoracotomy and open-chest cardiac massage should be performed if the fetus is still viable.[45] If there is no return of spontaneous effective maternal circulation or there is evidence of fetal distress after 5 minutes of CPR with open-chest cardiac massage, some have recommended that caesarean section be performed immediately.[45]

Complications from Cardiopulmonary Resuscitation

Maternal complications that can occur when CPR is performed during pregnancy include laceration of the liver, uterine rupture, hemothorax, and hemopericardium.[45] Fetal complications include cardiac arrhythmia or standstill from material defibrillation and drug therapy, central nervous system toxicity from antiarrhythmic drugs, and altered uteroplacental perfusion from maternal hypoxemia, acidosis, and vasoconstriction. A neonatologist is an essential member of the resuscitation team for a pregnant patient.

References

1. Modell JH: Drowning versus near-drowning: A discussion of definitions. *Crit Care Med* 9:351-352, 1981.
2. Pratt FD, Haynes BE: Incidence of "secondary drowning" after saltwater submersion. *Ann Emerg Med* 15:1084-1087, 1986.
3. Baker SP, O'Neill B, Karpf RD: *The Injury Fact Book.* Lexington, Ma, DC Heath and Co, 1984, pp 154-155.
4. Redding JS: Drowning and near-drowning. *Postgrad Med* 74:85-97, 1983.
5. Ornato JP: The resuscitation of near-drowning victims. *JAMA* 256:75-77, 1986.
6. Siebke H, Rod T, Breivik H, et al: Survival after 40 minutes of submersion without cerebral sequela. *Lancet* 1:1275-1277, 1975.
7. Conn AW, Barker GA: Fresh water drowning and near-drowning — an update. *Can Anaesth Soc J* 31:s38-s44, 1984.
8. Modell JH, Graves SA, Kuck EJ: Near-drowning: Correlation of level of consciousness and survival. *Can Anaesth Soc J* 27:211-215, 1980.
9. *Advanced Trauma Life Support Instructor's Manual.* American College of Surgeon's Committee on Trauma.
10. Harnar TJ, Oreskovich MR, Copass MK, et al: Role of emergency thoracotomy in the resuscitation of moribund trauma victims. *Am J Surg* 142:96-99, 1981.
11. Hoffman JR: Emergency department thoracotomy. *Ann Emerg Med* 10:175-178, 1981.
12. Bodai BI, Smith JP, Ward RE, et al: Emergency thoracotomy in the management of trauma. *JAMA* 249:1891-1896, 1983.
13. Baker CC, Thomas AN, Trunkey DD: The role of emergency room thoracotomy in trauma. *J Trauma* 20:848-855, 1980.
14. Flynn TC, Ward RE, Miller PW: Emergency department thoracotomy. *Ann Emerg Med* 11:413-416, 1982.
15. Baker CC, Caronna JJ, Trunkey DD: Neurologic outcome after emergency room thoracotomy for trauma. *Am J Surgery* 139:677-681, 1980.
16. Wright RK, Davis JH: The investigation of electrical deaths: A report of 220 fatalities. *J Forensic Science* 25:514-521, 1980.
17. Knickerbocker GG: Factors affecting resuscitation from electric shock, in *Proceedings of the National Conference on Standards for Cardiopulmonary Resuscitation (CPR) and Emergency Cardiac Care* (ECC). Dallas, American Heart Association, 1975, pp 73-85.
18. Bernstein T: Effects of electricity and lightning on man and animals. *J Forensic Sci* 18:3-11, 1973.
19. Hodgkin BC, Langworty O, Kouwenhoven WB: Effect on breathing of an electric shock applied to the extremities. *IEEE Trans: Power Apparatus and Systems* PAS-92 4:1388-1391, 1973.
20. Rouse RG, Dimick AR: The treatment of electrical injury compared to burn injury: A review of pathophysiology and comparison of patient management protocols. *J Trauma* 18:43-47, 1978.
21. Golde RH, Lee WR: Death by lightning. *Proc Inst Electric Eng* 123:1163-1180, 1976.
22. Cooper MA: Lightning injuries: Prognostic signs for death. *Ann Emerg Med* 9:134-138, 1980.
23. Kobernick M: Electrical injuries: Pathophysiology and emergency management. *Ann Emerg Med* 11:633-638, 1983.
24. Dixon GF: The evaluation and management of electrical injuries. *Crit Care Med* 11:384-387, 1983.
25. Fox RH, Woodward PM, Exton-Smith AN, et al: Body temperature in the elderly: A national study of physiological, social, and environmental conditions. *Br Med J* 1:200-206, 1973.
26. Goldman A, Exton-Smith AN, Francis G, et al: A pilot study of low body temperatures in old people admitted to hospital. *J Roy Coll Physicians Lond* 11:291-306, 1977.
27. Edlich RF, Silloway KA, Feldman PS, et al: Cold injuries and disorders. *Current Concepts Trauma Care* 4-11, 1986.
28. Weyman AE, Greenbaum DM, Grace WJ: Accidental hypothermia in an alcoholic population. *Am J Med* 56:13-21, 1974.
29. White JD: Hypothermia: The Bellvue experience. *Ann Emerg Med* 11:417-424, 1982.
30. Reuler JB: Hypothermia: Pathophysiology, clinical settings, and management. *Ann Intern Med* 89:519-527, 1978.
31. Harnett RM, Pruitt JR, Sias FR: A review of the literature concerning resuscitation from hypothermia: I and II. *Aviat Space Environ Med* 54:425-434, 487-295, 1983.
32. Okada M, Nishimura F, Yoshino H, et al: The J wave in accidental hypothermia. *J Electrocardiol* 16:23-28, 1983.
33. Wears RL: Blood gases in hypothermia, letter. *JACEP* 8:247, 1979.
34. Ream AK, Reitz BA, Silverberg G: Temperature correction of pCO_2 and pH in estimating the acid base status: An example of the emperor's new clothes? *Anesthesiology* 56:41-44, 1982.
35. Segar WE: Effect of hypothermia on tubular transport mechanisms. *Am J Physiol* 195:91-96, 1958.
36. Curry DL, Curry KP: Hypothermia and insulin secretion. *Endocrinology* 87:750-755, 1970.
37. Towne WD, Geiss WP, Yanes HO, et al: Intractable ventricular fibrillation associated with profound accidental hypothermia — Successful treatment with partial cardiopulmonary bypass. *N Engl J Med* 287:1135-1136, 1972.
38. Truscott DG, Firor WB, Clein LJ: Accidental profound hypothermia: Successful resuscitation by core rewarming and assisted circulation. *Arch Surg* 106:216-218, 1973.
39. Gillen JP, Vogel MFX, Holterman JJ, et al: Ventricular fibrillation during orotracheal intubation of hypothermic dogs. *Ann Emerg Med* 15:412-416, 1986.
40. Shanks CA, Marsh HM: Simple core rewarming in accidental hypothermia. *Brit J Anaesth* 45:522-525, 1973.
41. Elenbaas RM, Mattson K, Cole H, et al: Bretylium in hypothermia-induced ventricular fibrillation in dogs. *Ann Emerg Med* 13:994-999, 1984.
42. Althaus U, Aeberhard P, Schupbach P, et al: Management of profound accidental hypothermia with cardiorespiratory arrest. *Ann Surg* 195:492-495, 1982.
43. Southwick FS, Dalglish PH Jr: Recovery after prolonged asystolic cardiac arrest in profound hypothermia. *JAMA* 243:1250-1253, 1980.
44. Sullivan JM, Ramanathan KB: Management of medical problems in pregnancy — Severe cardiac disease. *N Engl J Med* 313:304-309, 1985.
45. Lee RV, Rodgers BD, White LM, et al: Cardiopulmonary resuscitation of pregnant women. *Am J Med* 81:311-318, 1986.
46. Kerr MG: The mechanical effects of the gravid uterus in late pregnancy. *J Obstet Gynaecol Br Commonw* 72:513-529, 1965.
47. Curry JJ, Quintana FJ: Myocardial infarction with ventricular fibrillation during pregnancy treated by direct current defibrillation with fetal survival. *Chest* 58:82-84, 1970.
48. Rotmensch HH, Elkayam U, Frishman W: Antiarrhythmic drug therapy during pregnancy. *Ann Intern Med* 98:487-497, 1983.

Putting It All Together: Resuscitation of the Patient

Chapter 16

Resuscitation is a team effort that must be efficient and organized. The primary goals of the resuscitation team are:

1. To reestablish the patient's spontaneous effective circulation and respiration and
2. To preserve function in the patient's vital organs during resuscitation.

This chapter will integrate the ACLS knowledge and skills into an organized, effective resuscitation plan.

Principles of Management (Table 1)

The ACLS Team

Whether resuscitation is performed in or out of the hospital, an effective ACLS team is composed of a team leader and one or more team members who can assume well-defined roles. There must be one person in control, i.e, the team leader, who is responsible for directing and coordinating the team's actions. Team members are responsible for carrying out the assignments of the team leader.

ACLS Team Leader

The team leader's responsibilities include:

1. The supervision and direction of team members,
2. Patient assessment, and
3. Problem-solving.

The ACLS team leader must be a highly proficient ACLS provider. An effective team leader must have good leadership skills and be able to think and convey a sense of order in an emergency environment. If a qualified physician is present, he or she should direct the resuscitation. If the team leader is not a physician (but rather, e.g., the paramedic in a field resuscitation), he or she must be authorized to perform this role and must stay within the bounds of the emergency care system procedures and protocols. When required, nonphysician team leaders must seek direction from physicians (e.g., base station physicians) or other authorized personnel (e.g., base station nurses).

The team leader must be clearly identified to the other members of the team and should be the only person to give orders. This does not mean that suggestions from other team members are precluded. Such suggestions may be extremely valuable in helping the leader decide on the most appropriate course of action. However, all final decisions are made by the team leader.

The team leader must look at the "big picture" and not focus on isolated problems to the exclusion of events that are occurring "globally". The ACLS algorithms provide a framework for dealing with life-threatening cardiorespiratory emergencies in a logical sequence. The algorithms are not appropriate for every unique clinical circumstance, and the team leader must adapt them and the general ACLS principles when necessary. However, staying with the algorithms, when appropriate, can improve the team's operating efficiency. For example, when the team leader calls out the diagnosis of the cardiac rhythm, team members can anticipate interventions and orders that will likely follow according to the ACLS algorithms.

Supervision of team members includes ensuring that correct CPR and ACLS are performed. The team leader must decide when to start and when to stop CPR. He or she must be sure that the pulse is checked following each defibrillation. The team leader must be in a position to continually review the adequacy of ventilation, the hand position for CPR, the depth of cardiac compressions, and the proper rate and sequence of CPR. If the team leader is not satisfied with the quality of any procedure being performed by any other team members, he or she must convey these concerns to the other providers and ascertain that appropriate corrective action is taken. He or she must also assure that interruptions for intubation, defibrillation, or moving the patient do not exceed 30 seconds (5 seconds for assessment of spontaneous breathing and pulse) and that airway adjuncts are used properly. The team leader is also responsible for the safety of all members on the resuscitation team, especially when procedures such as defibrillation are being performed.

The team leader is responsible for patient assessment, including obtaining the patient's history, resuscitation status, physical findings, and cardiac rhythm. The team leader is also responsible for ensuring that the patient's regular physician and family are informed and involved in critical decisions as early as possible during resuscitation. When the patient does not respond to treatment, the team leader is responsible, if he or she is a physician, for deciding when to terminate resuscitative efforts. When the team leader is not a physician, local protocols and legislation determine who is empowered to make this decision.

Table 1. Principles for the Management of Cardiac Arrest. Note: Many of these activities will be enacted simultaneously. Their order in this table does not mandate their exact sequence of occurrence in the code setting.

Priorities	Equipment from cart	Intervention
1. Recognition of arrest		1. Initiate CPR and call for help.
2. Arrival of resuscitation team, emergency cart, monitor–defibrillator	2a. Cardiac board b. Mouth-to-mask or bag–valve–mask unit with O$_2$ tubing c. Oral airway d. (oxygen and regulator if not already at bedside)	2a. Place patient on cardiac board. b. Ventilate with 100% O$_2$ with oral airway and mouth-to-mask or bag–valve–mask device. c. Continue chest compressions.
3. Identification of team leader		3a. Assess patient. b. Direct and supervise team members. c. Solve problems. d. Obtain patient history and information about events leading up to the code.
4. Rhythm diagnosis	4. Cardiac monitor with quick-look paddles — defibrillator (limb leads, ECG machine — 12 lead)	4a. Apply quick-look paddles first. b. Limb leads, but do not interrupt CPR.
5. Prompt defibrillation if indicated		5. Use correct algorithm.
6. Venous access	6a. Peripheral or central IV materials b. IV tubing, infusion fluid	6a. Peripheral: antecubital. b. Central: internal jugular, or subclavian.
7. Drug administration	7. Drugs as ordered (and in anticipation, based on algorithms) for bolus and continuous infusion	7a. Use correct algorithm. b. Bolus or infusion.
8. Intubation	8a. Suction equipment b. Laryngoscope c. Endotracheal tube and other intubation equipment d. Stethoscope	8a. Connect suction equipment. b. Intubate patient (interrupt CPR no more than 30 seconds). c. Check tube position (listen for bilateral breath sounds). d. Hyperventilate, and oxygenate.
9. Ongoing assessment of the patient's response to therapy during resuscitation		9. Assess frequently: a. pulse generated with CPR (IS THERE A PULSE?); b. adequacy of artificial ventilation; c. spontaneous pulse after any intervention/rhythm change (IS THERE A PULSE?); d. spontaneous breathing with return of pulse (IS THERE BREATHING?); e. blood pressure, if pulse is present; f. decision to stop, if no response to therapy.
10. Documentation	10. Resuscitation record	10. Accurately record events while resuscitation is in progress.
11. Drawing arterial and venous blood specimens	11. Arterial puncture and venipuncture equipment	11a. Draw specimens. b. Treat as needed, based on results.
12. Controlling or limiting crowd		12. Dismiss those not required for bedside tasks.

Problem-solving includes recognizing and determining the cause of equipment malfunction, making certain that therapy is administered correctly whenever the outcome of an intervention is other than expected, and determining the cause of abnormal laboratory results. For example, rather than merely ordering repeated countershocks or drugs when defibrillation is unsuccessful, the team leader should consider whether an underlying reason for resistance to therapy is present. Are ventilation and oxygenation adequate? Is the endotracheal tube correctly positioned? Are breath sounds equal bilaterally? Is there a pulse with CPR? Is paddle position correct? Has the proper conductive material been used?

Additional Members of the ACLS Team

The team leader is responsible for delegating duties to other resuscitation team members. The number of tasks and roles assigned to each member will vary, depending on the team size, skills and qualifications of team members and the needs of the patient. Primary roles performed by ACLS team members may include:

1. Airway management (ventilation, oxygenation, intubation, suctioning),
2. External chest compressions,
3. Use of "quick-look" paddles and defibrillation,
4. Establishment of IV access and administration of drugs ordered by the team leader,
5. Placement of ECG chest or limb leads and operation of the ECG machine,
6. Patient assessment,
7. Cardiac rhythm analysis, and
8. Communicating with a base station physician, including sending ECG telemetry during field resuscitation.

Support roles performed by ACLS team members may include:

1. Management of supplies for resuscitation (e.g., dispensing medications and supplies from the crash cart);
2. Assistance with procedures (airway management, defibrillation, IV line placement, ECG monitoring);
3. Documentation of the resuscitation record (keeping track of the sequence of interventions, noting the time when medications are administered, reminding the team leader when a drug is to be repeated, and reporting blood work results to the team leader);
4. Liaison functions (obtaining pertinent patient history, inquiring about resuscitation status, communicating with the family, and notifying the attending physician);
5. Crowd control.

It is vital that all team members maintain clear communication and an awareness of what other team members are doing. By working together and anticipating orders according to the ACLS algorithms, team members maximize the chances for successful resuscitation.

In the hospital setting, there is seldom a problem in quickly assembling several qualified team members to assist in a cardiac resuscitation. In fact, if a general call for assistance (such as an overhead page with a designated signal) is made, too many rescuers may respond for the team to function efficiently. In the out-of-hospital arrest environment, though, the opposite problem may exist. There may be only one or two other providers on the scene to assist the team leader. The speed and efficiency of the team are usually optimal when several (three to five) providers can work together.

Priorities

The factors that most affect the chances for successful resuscitation, listed in order of their usual importance, are:

1. Rapid defibrillation for VF or pulseless VT;
2. Continued effective CPR with the establishment of a secure airway (preferably endotracheal tube) and the administration of 100% oxygen;
3. Epinephrine, given repeatedly and in a dosage adequate to maintain coronary and cerebral perfusion.

When several qualified rescuers are present, a number of priorities may be addressed simultaneously.

An initial step in assessing the patient is to establish that a cardiac arrest has indeed occurred. If CPR is ongoing when the team (and the team leader) arrive on the scene, the team leader may wish to interrupt CPR momentarily to verify pulselessness. If no pulse is present, CPR should be resumed and the adequacy of ventilations and compressions should be immediately evaluated. The team leader should observe the chest to confirm that there is adequate rise and fall with ventilations. Breath sounds should be checked in several lung fields bilaterally. In addition, the team leader should ensure that a good pulse is generated with chest compressions and that such compressions are being performed with appropriate technique.

As soon as a monitor–defibrillator is available, the patient's rhythm must be identified. If the rhythm is ventricular fibrillation (VF) or ventricular tachycardia (VT) and the pulse is absent, the patient should be defibrillated immediately. This step should precede CPR if a monitor–defibrillator is immediately available. The team leader must always be certain that all members of the team are clear (standing back) before the patient is countershocked.

As soon as possible, the team leader must attempt to determine the etiology of the arrest. Potential precipitating factors include electrolyte abnormalities (especially potassium and calcium), acidosis, hypoxemia, tension pneumothorax, cardiac tamponade, and hypovolemia. If any correctable factors can be identified, corrective action should be taken. This is particularly important when electromechanical dissociation is present; in the absence of correcting such an abnormality, there is little chance for patient survival.

The team leader must determine who will intubate the patient and must ensure that excessive time is not spent in the process. After intubation the team leader must assess the adequacy of ventilation and check for equal bilateral breath sounds. The team leader should select the site for placement of the IV or central line.

Constant vigilance must be maintained by the team leader while CPR is performed. The adequacy of ventilation may change, e.g., the endotracheal tube may be pushed down the right main stem bronchus or it may become dislodged. A pneumothorax may develop. The quality of chest compressions may deteriorate.

Arterial blood gases may be measured during some in-hospital resuscitations where results can be available rapidly. Because venous capacitance vessels quickly distend during CPR and arteries are underfilled, especially below the diaphragm, it is easy to draw blood mistakenly from a vein instead of an artery. Once it is certain that arterial blood has been collected, the PaO_2 and $PaCO_2$ should be checked. The PaO_2 should ideally be greater than 100 mmHg, and the $PaCO_2$ should be less than 40 mmHg. If the PaO_2 is low, the leader must ascertain that 100% oxygen is indeed being administered. If the $PaCO_2$ is greater than 40 mmHg, the adequacy of ventilation must be checked; bilateral equal breath sounds should be confirmed. If breath sounds are unequal, the endotracheal tube may need to be repositioned. If this maneuver does not restore equal breath sounds, a pneumothorax should be suspected; if present, it should be relieved with aspiration and/or chest tube insertion. If the $PaCO_2$ is high and there are adequate bilateral breath sounds, the tidal volume and ventilatory rate should be increased. After the PaO_2 and $PaCO_2$ have been checked, the arterial pH should be noted. This measure is more difficult to use because arterial values do not reflect the severity of the mixed venous or tissue pH disturbance. When significant arterial acidosis is present, efforts should first be made to increase ventilation to lower $PaCO_2$, which will correct arterial, venous, and tissue acidosis. Bicarbonate may exacerbate venous and tissue acidosis by producing CO_2. Thus, its use is not recommended unless hyperkalemia and/or preexisting acidosis is present.

The team leader must be ever observant. Though the algorithms provide a good "cookbook," the team leader must remain a "thinking cook."

Management of Cardiac Arrest

Ventricular Fibrillation and Pulseless Ventricular Tachycardia (Figure 1)

Survival from VF or VT demands rapid, early electrical countershock. **As soon as a monitor–defibrillator is available, CPR should be interrupted and "quick-look" paddles or pads should be applied to determine the rhythm.** If a monitor defibrillator is available when the patient arrests, the rhythm should be checked immediately (rather than starting CPR if only one rescuer is present). If an automatic defibrillator is available, it should be applied.

If VF or VT is confirmed, immediate defibrillation with 200 J is recommended. If the victim remains pulseless and VF or ventricular tachycardia persists, defibrillation with 200–300 J followed by 360 J should be used (see Chapter 6). To simplify defibrillation, facilitate use of automatic and semi-automatic devices, and avoid the delays inherent in synchronization, VT without a pulse should be treated the same as VF (see Figure 1).

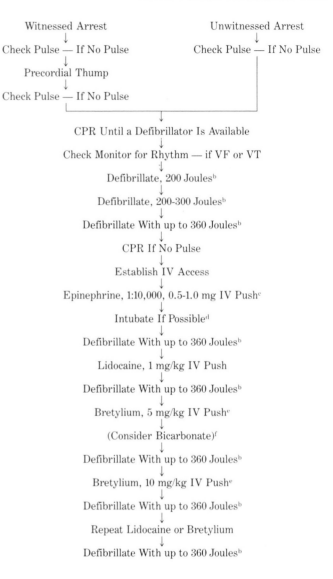

Figure 1. Ventricular fibrillation (and pulseless ventricular tachycardia).[a] This sequence was developed to assist in teaching how to treat a broad range of patients with ventricular fibrillation (VF) or pulseless ventricular tachycardia (VT). Some patients may require care not specified herein. This algorithm should not be construed as prohibiting such flexibility. Flow of algorithm presumes that VF is continuing. CPR indicates cardiopulmonary resuscitation.

[a]Pulseless VT should be treated identically to VF.

[b]Check pulse and rhythm after each shock. If VF recurs after transiently converting (rather than persists without ever converting), use whatever energy level has previously been successful for defibrillation.

[c]Epinephrine should be repeated every five minutes.

[d]Intubation is preferable. If it can be accompanied simultaneously with other techniques, then the earlier the better. However, defibrillation and epinephrine are more important initially if the patient can be ventilated without intubation.

[e]Some may prefer repeated doses of lidocaine, which may be given in 0.5-mg/kg boluses every eight minutes to a total dose of 3 mg/kg.

[f]Value of sodium bicarbonate is questionable during cardiac arrest, and it is not recommended for routine cardiac arrest sequence. Consideration of its use in a dose of 1 mEq/kg is appropriate at this point. Half of original dose may be repeated every ten minutes if it is used.

If a monitor–defibrillator is not initially available and the arrest has been witnessed, a solitary precordial thump is recommended for the pulseless victim. Because the amount of energy needed to convert VF rapidly increases with time, a thump is likely to be successful only if it is delivered soon after the patient collapses. If asystole is present, a precordial thump may, rarely, cause a rhythm to resume. The rescuer should not be concerned about inducing a less optimal rhythm in a pulseless victim. However, the precordial thump is not indicated in a patient with a pulse unless a defibrillator is available to treat VF should it occur. The importance of early definitive care also guides the logic for the use of a defibrillator when no monitor is available. In a pulseless patient (whether the arrest is witnessed or not), blind defibrillation (without documentation of the rhythm) initially with 200 J and, subsequently, if no pulse returns, with 200–300 and 360 J, is recommended.

If a defibrillator is not immediately available or if defibrillation and/or the precordial thump have been unsuccessful, initiate CPR to support ventilation and circulation. **Supplemental oxygen at a concentration of 100% should be administered. Thereafter, placement of an IV line and intubation assume primary importance.** Following medications, administration of a 50-ml bolus of IV fluid and elevation of the arm are recommended to enhance delivery of drugs to the central circulation. As soon as the IV line has been secured, **0.5–1.0 mg of epinephrine should be administered and repeated at least every 5 minutes.** In the event that intubation is accomplished prior to placement of an IV line, epinephrine 1.0 mg in appropriate 10 ml dilution can be administered by the endotracheal route.

Once ventilation and circulation are optimized, defibrillation should be reattempted with 360 J. If unsuccessful, therapy with an antiarrhythmic agent should be instituted. Although neither lidocaine nor bretylium consistently affect the defibrillation threshold (the energy required to successfully terminate VF), both raise the VF threshold (the energy required to induce VF). Since immediate and unrecognized recurrence of VF may be responsible for some of the apparent failures of defibrillation, either drug might be helpful in interrupting persistent VF. Although both drugs are associated with a nearly identical success rate in clinical studies, most healthcare providers are more familiar with lidocaine and there is less toxicity associated with it. As a result, lidocaine is now recommended as the agent of choice treating refractory VF. **Lidocaine should be given in a dose of 1 mg/kg, followed by a repeat defibrillation at 360 J.** Subsequent treatment may include repeated doses of lidocaine 0.5 mg/kg or bretylium 5 mg/kg followed by 10 mg/kg. If VF or VT persist, CPR should be continued for 1–2 minutes after each drug dose to allow the drug to reach the central circulation prior to defibrillation (360 J).

Additional information concerning the patient may be available which may indicate that interventions other than those included in this sequence are appropriate. Such interventions should be applied if there is an appropriate indication and justification. If resuscitative efforts are not initially successful, a central line should be placed to ensure better delivery of therapeutic agents to the central circulation.

Asystole

The prognosis for patients with asystole is poor. Generally, patients with asystole have end-stage cardiac function or have had a prolonged arrest and are not resuscitatable. On occasion, asystole may be preceded by progressive conduction system dysfunction and bradycardia. Such patients may be salvageable if appropriate interventions are made before asystole develops. Because of the poor prognosis associated with asystole and the possibility that VF (which is potentially treatable by defibrillation) may masquerade as asystole, **the diagnosis of asystole should be confirmed in at least two lead configurations.** If the team leader has any doubt about whether the rhythm is asystole or fine VF, the rhythm should be treated as though it were VF.

If Rhythm Is Unclear and Possibly Ventricular Fibrillation, Defibrillate as for VF. If Asystole is Present[a]
↓
Continue CPR
↓
Establish IV Access
↓
Epinephrine, 1:10,000, 0.5 - 1.0 mg IV Push[b]
↓
Intubate When Possible[c]
↓
Atropine, 1.0 mg IV Push (Repeated in 5 min)
↓
(Consider Bicarbonate)[d]
↓
Consider Pacing

Figure 2.   Asystole (cardiac standstill). This sequence was developed to assist in teaching how to treat a broad range of patients with asystole. Some patients may require care not specified herein. This algorithm should not be construed to prohibit such flexibility. Flow of algorithm presumes asystole is continuing. VF indicates ventricular fibrillation; IV, intravenous.

[a]Asystole should be confirmed in two leads.

[b]Epinephrine should be repeated every five minutes.

[c]Intubation is preferable; if it can be accomplished simultaneously with other techniques, then the earlier the better. However, cardiopulmonary resuscitation (CPR) and use of epinephrine are more important initially if patient can be ventilated without intubation. (Endotracheal epinephrine may be used.)

[d]Value of sodium bicarbonate is questionable during cardiac arrest, and it is not recommended for the routine cardiac arrest sequence. Consideration of its use in a dose of 1 mEq/kg is appropriate at this point. Half of original dose may be repeated every ten minutes if it is used.

If asystole is confirmed, CPR must be continued to support ventilatory and circulatory function. **Supplemental oxygen at an inspired concentration of 100% should be administered. The patient should be intubated, and a large-bore peripheral IV line should be started in the antecubital fossa.** As soon as the IV line has been secured, **0.5–1.0 mg of epinephrine should be administered and repeated at least every 5 minutes.** Following medications, administration of a 50-ml bolus of IV fluid and elevation of the arm are recommended to enhance delivery of drugs to the central circulation. If the patient is successfully intubated prior to placement of an IV line, epinephrine can be administered by the endotracheal route.

Atropine has been shown to be useful in some patients with asystole because this rhythm can result from increased parasympathetic tone.

Additional information concerning the patient may be available which may indicate that interventions other than those included in this sequence are appropriate. Such interventions should be applied if there is an appropriate indication and justification. If resuscitative efforts are not initially successful, a central line should be placed to ensure better delivery of therapeutic agents to the central circulation.

Electromechanical Dissociation (Figure 3)

The prognosis for patients with electromechanical dissociation (EMD) is invariably poor unless an underlying cause can be identified and corrected. Accordingly, **the highest priority is to maintain the patient while searching for a correctable etiology.** The most common correctable causes of EMD are hypovolemia, cardiac tamponade, tension pneumothorax, hypoxemia, and acidosis. Other less correctable causes include massive myocardial damage from infarction, prolonged ischemia during resuscitation, and pulmonary embolism. Patients with profound shock of any cause or kind (including anaphylactic, septic, neurogenic, and hypovolemic) may initially present with EMD.

It is helpful to check the neck veins or to note whether there is brisk backflow of blood when a central venous line is inserted in a patient with EMD. Most normovolemic patients with cardiac arrest not due to external physical trauma have an elevated venous volume and pressure during CPR; hence, the neck veins should be distended in the supine position, and blood usually returns freely when a central line is inserted. When EMD is present and neck vein distention is absent or there is no brisk backflow during central IV line insertion, hypovolemia should be suspected. When the victim of obvious external physical trauma is in cardiac arrest, massive bleeding (external or internal) should be assumed. If the neck veins are prominent in such a patient or if there is brisk backflow from a central IV line, tension pneumothorax or pericardial tamponade should be suspected.

Continue CPR
↓
Establish IV Access
↓
Epinephrine, 1:10,000, 0.5 - 1.0 mg IV Push[a]
↓
Intubate When Possible[b]
↓
(Consider Bicarbonate)[c]
↓
Consider Hypovolemia,
Cardiac Tamponade,
Tension Pneumothorax,
Hypoxemia,
Acidosis,
Pulmonary Embolism

Figure 3. Electromechanical dissociation. This sequence was developed to assist in teaching how to treat a broad range of patients with electromechanical dissociation. Some patients may require care not specified herein. This algorithm should not be construed to prohibit such flexibility. Flow of algorithm presumes that electromechanical dissociation is continuing. CPR indicates cardiopulmonary resuscitation; IV, intravenous.

[a]Epinephrine should be repeated every five minutes.

[b]Intubation is preferable. If it can be accomplished simultaneously with other techniques, then the earlier the better. However, epinephrine is more important initially if the patient can be ventilated without intubation.

[c]Value of sodium bicarbonate is questionable during cardiac arrest, and it is not recommended for routine cardiac arrest sequence. Consideration of its use in a dose of 1 mEq/kg is appropriate at this point. Half of original dose may be repeated every ten minutes if it is used.

If acute hypovolemia is present (e.g., secondary to massive bleeding), volume should be given. Tension pneumothorax should be treated by needle aspiration and/or chest tube insertion. Cardiac tamponade should be treated by pericardiocentesis followed by thoracotomy when indicated. Hypoxemia is treated by improving oxygenation and ventilation; acidosis, by improving CPR technique and hyperventilating the patient.

General treatment of EMD includes **CPR to support ventilation and circulation, supplemental oxygen at a concentration of 100%, and intubation. A large-bore peripheral IV line should be started, preferably in the antecubital fossa.** As soon as the IV line has been secured, **0.5–1.0 mg of epinephrine should be administered and repeated at least every 5 minutes.** Following medications, administration of a 50-ml bolus of IV fluid and elevation of the arm are recommended to enhance delivery of drugs to the central circulation. If the patient is successfully intubated prior to placement of an IV line, epinephrine can be administered by the endotracheal route.

If bradycardia is present with EMD, atropine may be administered in an attempt to induce cardioacceleration (see Figure 5).

Additional information concerning the patient may be available which may indicate that interventions other than those included in this sequence are appropriate. Such interventions should be applied if there is an appropriate indication and justification. If resuscitative efforts are not initially successful, a central line should be placed to ensure better delivery of therapeutic agents to the central circulation.

Immediate Postresuscitation Care

Critical decisions need to be made during the early postresuscitation period. **The airway must be supported continuously, and adequate perfusion must be maintained. Supplemental oxygen at a concentration of 100% is essential until direct measurement of arterial oxygen (PaO$_2$) indicates otherwise.** The patient may require intubation if not done previously. Steps to prevent aspiration (positioning) in the unintubated patient are essential. Arterial blood gases should be used to guide proper ventilatory support once the patient is in a hospital environment.

When resuscitative efforts are prolonged, hypotension is common following return of spontaneous circulation. Waiting a few minutes to allow blood pressure to rise is frequently the most prudent course of action. **Should hypotension persist, dopamine at the lowest dose that permits an "adequate" blood pressure is the agent of choice.** Arterial systolic pressure should be titrated to at least 90 mmHg if possible without exacerbating ischemia or inducing arrhythmias in order to assure adequate cerebral perfusion.

If either lidocaine or bretylium appeared to be effective during resuscitation, it should be continued. If these drugs are administered as a bolus during the arrest, additional bolus doses may be needed to maintain adequate blood levels until a steady-state concentration can be achieved by continuous IV infusion. Generally, these agents are continued for at least 24 hours.

Underlying abnormalities that may have led to the arrest should be actively sought and corrected. Common abnormalities that may require correction after the arrest include electrolyte imbalances (especially hypokalemia), hypoxemia, and acidosis. Arterial acidosis may paradoxically worsen in the period immediately after restoration of perfusion due to "wash out" of carbon dioxide and lactate from reperfused vascular beds. If adequate circulation is reestablished and ventilation is supported, the acidosis will frequently be self-limiting.

Additional information concerning the patient may be available which may indicate that interventions other than those included in this sequence are appropriate. Such interventions are not precluded.

Management of Life-Threatening Arrhythmias Without Cardiac Arrest

Sustained Ventricular Tachycardia With a Pulse (Figure 4)

The symptomatic patient with VT requires emergency treatment. Cardioversion is the treatment of choice. In general, the rhythm is responsive to low levels of electrical energy. If the patient is severely ill (e.g., hypotensive), **a large-bore peripheral IV line should be placed, and the patient should be cardioverted immediately,** starting at an energy level of 50 J. **When**

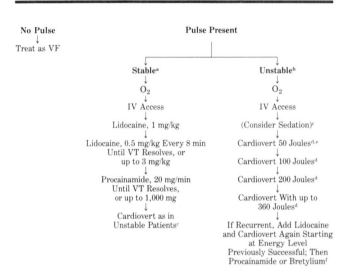

Figure 4. Sustained ventricular tachycardia (VT). This sequence was developed to assist in teaching how to treat a broad range of patients with sustained VT. Some patients may require care not specified herein. This algorithm should not be construed as prohibiting such flexibility. Flow of algorithm presumes that VT is continuing. VF indicates ventricular fibrillation.

[a]If patient becomes unstable (see footnote b for definition) at any time, move to "Unstable" arm of algorithm.

[b]Unstable indicates symptoms (e.g., chest pain or dyspnea), hypotension (systolic blood pressure <90 mmHg), congestive heart failure, ischemia, or infarction.

[c]Sedation should be considered for all patients, including those defined in footnote b as unstable, except those who are hemodynamically unstable (e.g., hypotensive, in pulmonary edema, or unconscious).

[d]If hypotension, pulmonary edema, or unconsciousness is present, unsynchronized cardioversion should be done to avoid delay associated with synchronization.

[e]In the absence of hypotension, pulmonary edema, or unconsciousness, a precordial thump may be employed prior to cardioversion.

[f]Once VT has resolved, begin intravenous (IV) infusion of antiarrhythmic agent that has aided resolution of VT. If hypotension, pulmonary edema, or unconsciousness is present, use lidocaine if cardioversion alone is unsuccessful, followed by bretylium. In all other patients, recommended order of therapy is lidocaine, procainamide, and then bretylium.

patients are severely ill, excessive time should not be spent attempting to synchronize the cardioversion since such efforts can be difficult and time consuming.

If the patient is less severely ill, following initiation of oxygen therapy and placement of an IV line, time may be taken to administer a short-acting amnestic sedative and to synchronize the cardioversion. Cardioversion with 50 J will usually successfully convert VT so that higher energies (100, 200, and 360 J) are rarely necessary. Recurrent episodes are by far more common than resistant episodes, emphasizing the need for prompt institution of antiarrhythmic therapy as soon as conversion occurs. Careful monitoring of the cardiac rhythm is essential to ensure that recurrent tachycardia is not attributed to resistance to cardioversion. Lidocaine is the pharmacological agent of choice, followed by procainamide and bretylium (see Figure 4).

For patients with VT who are hemodynamically stable and asymptomatic, a trial of pharmacological therapy is warranted. Lidocaine is the drug of choice. Several doses of the drug may be given until the tachycardia resolves or a total of 3 mg/kg has been administered. If lidocaine does not convert the rhythm, procainamide can be tried. Intravenous loading of this drug is accomplished at a rate of 20 mg/min until a total dose of up to 1000 mg has been given or until the tachycardia resolves. This may be followed by a continuous infusion at 1–4 mg/min. If the arrhythmia is resistant to both agents or if the patient becomes unstable in any way, cardioversion should be attempted.

Using verapamil to treat an asymptomatic patient with a wide-complex tachycardia on the assumption that the rhythm must be supraventricular because the patient is hemodynamically stable is dangerous and may lead to a disastrous result if the rhythm turns out to be VT. Criteria for differentiating between ventricular and supraventricular tachycardia have previously been discussed in Chapter 5. If the diagnosis of a wide-complex tachycardia remains in question, it should be presumed to be ventricular in origin and treated accordingly.

The variant of VT known as torsade de pointes is a paroxysmal tachycardia that is generally best treated by overdrive electrical pacing (atrial pacing is preferred). Cardioversion, lidocaine, magnesium, and isoproterenol also have been used successfully. It is important to search for an underlying cause (hypokalemia, use of quinidine or procainamide, tricyclic antidepressant overdose, etc.) and to institute corrective measures if possible.

Additional information concerning the patient may be available which may indicate that interventions other than those included in this sequence are appropriate. Such interventions are not precluded.

Bradycardia
(Heart rate <60 beats/min) (Figure 5)

Bradycardia rarely requires emergency treatment in and of itself. Treatment is needed only when bradycardia is associated with symptoms (e.g., chest pain, dyspnea, lightheadedness, hypotension, or ventricular ectopy). Supplemental oxygen should be used if available. When emergency treatment is required, atropine in a dose of 0.5 mg is the drug of choice (see Figure 5). Doses lower than 0.5 mg may paradoxically exacerbate bradycardia. On the other hand, higher doses may induce excessive cardioacceleration with adverse effects, especially in patients with ischemic heart disease. Atropine may be repeated as needed to a total dose of 2.0 mg. In general, the placement of a temporary pacemaker is preferable to the administration of multiple doses of atropine. Patients with Type II second- or third-degree AV block will generally require temporary demand pacing even if they respond to atropine.

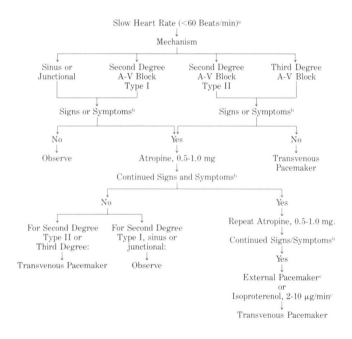

Figure 5. Bradycardia. This sequence was developed to assist in teaching how to treat a broad range of patients with bradycardia. Some patients may require care not specified herein. This algorithm should not be construed to prohibit such flexibility. AV indicates atrioventricular.

[a]A solitary chest thump or cough may stimulate cardiac electrical activity and result in improved cardiac output and may be used at this point.

[b]Hypotension (blood pressure <90 mmHg), premature ventricular contractions, altered mental status or symptoms (e.g., chest pain or dyspnea), ischemia, or infarction.

[c]Temporizing therapy.

Should a patient not respond to atropine and continue to require treatment, isoproterenol may be used if pacing is not immediately available. In general, low doses (2–10 μg/min) of this drug suffice. Isoproterenol must be infused cautiously since it may induce or exacerbate myocardial ischemia. As **temporary external pacing** becomes more widely available, it **will likely replace isoproterenol** (and even atropine) for the emergency treatment of bradycardia. Both are temporizing measures and should be followed by the placement of a temporary transvenous pacemaker.

Additional information concerning the patient may be available which may indicate that interventions other than those included in this sequence are appropriate. Such interventions are not precluded.

Suppression of Ventricular Ectopy (Figure 6)

Prophylactic lidocaine should be given to all patients with definite acute myocardial infarction even if ventricular ectopy is not present. Dosage regimens are given in Chapter 7. In other circumstances, when suppression of ventricular ectopy is required (e.g., patients with unstable angina having frequent PVC's or couplets), **the treatment of choice is also lidocaine after contributing factors such as hypoxemia, acidosis, alkalosis, electrolyte imbalance, digitalis (or other drug) intoxication, and bradycardia have been appropriately managed.** An initial 1-mg/kg bolus is given, and a continuous infusion at 2 mg/min should be started. This is followed by additional 0.5-mg/kg boluses as required for arrhythmia control. These boluses may be given every 2–10 minutes up to 3 mg/kg, or until ectopy is adequately suppressed. The IV infusion may be titrated upward as needed. In general, the more lidocaine needed initially to suppress ventricular ectopy, the higher the maintenance dose of the infusion. Subsequent dosage should be guided as indicated in Chapter 7.

If adequate suppression of ventricular ectopy is not achieved with lidocaine or if the drug is not well tolerated, procainamide may be tried. To avoid hypotension, procainamide must be infused slowly (no faster than 20 mg/min) when given by IV infusion. A loading dose sufficient to suppress the ectopy or up to a maximum of 1000 mg may be given, followed by a continuous maintenance infusion of 1–4 mg/min.

If adequate suppression is not achieved with procainamide, bretylium may be used in a dose of 5–10

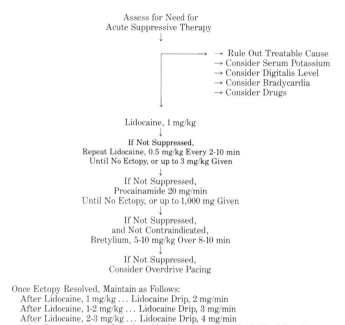

Once Ectopy Resolved, Maintain as Follows:
After Lidocaine, 1 mg/kg ... Lidocaine Drip, 2 mg/min
After Lidocaine, 1-2 mg/kg ... Lidocaine Drip, 3 mg/min
After Lidocaine, 2-3 mg/kg ... Lidocaine Drip, 4 mg/min
After Procainamide ... Procainamide drip, 1-4 mg/min (Check Blood Level)
After Bretylium .... Bretylium Drip, 2 mg/min

Figure 6. Ventricular ectopy: acute suppressive therapy. This sequence was developed to assist in teaching how to treat a broad range of patients with ventricular ectopy. Some patients may require therapy not specified herein. This algorithm should not be construed as prohibiting such flexibility.

mg/kg. The agent should be diluted in normal saline at least 4 to 1 and infused slowly over 8–10 minutes to avoid severe hypotension, nausea, and vomiting. If successful, additional doses may be given every few hours as needed or a continuous maintenance infusion can be started at 1–2 mg/min.

If serious ventricular arrhythmias persist despite the use of all of these agents, additional measures such as overdrive pacing or a trial with other less commonly used antiarrhythmic drugs may be considered.

Additional information concerning the patient may be available which may indicate that interventions other than those included in this sequence are appropriate. Such interventions are not precluded.

Supraventricular Tachycardia (Figure 7)

Supraventricular tachycardia **requires emergency treatment when it:**

1. **Causes or exacerbates cardiovascular dysfunction** (e.g., induces or exacerbates chest pain, dyspnea, other signs of ischemia, hypotension, or congestive heart failure) or
2. **Occurs in a setting where deleterious effects due to the tachycardia are likely** (e.g., patients with acute ischemic heart disease such as acute myocardial infarction).

In such emergency situations, **synchronized cardioversion is the treatment of choice** unless sinus tachycardia is present or cardioversion is contraindicated (e.g., in the presence of digitalis intoxication). Suggested energies for the initial attempt at cardioversion are

1. Atrial flutter: 25 J
2. Paroxysmal supraventricular tachycardia (PSVT): 75–100 J
3. Atrial fibrillation: 100 J

Supplemental oxygen should be administered. An IV line should always be in place prior to cardioversion so that if a more malignant ventricular arrhythmia or bradycardia results from the procedure it can be treated immediately. If time permits, a short-acting sedative should be given to reduce the discomfort associated with the procedure. During the time the patient is sedated, close observation and maintenance of the airway is essential to prevent aspiration and to ensure adequate ventilation if oversedation occurs. Proper synchronization of the cardioversion is essential to minimize the chance that a malignant ventricular arrhythmia will be induced. If synchronization cannot be accomplished, unsynchronized cardioversion would be indicated only for the most dire of clinical circumstances, e.g., severe and very marked hypotension or severe ischemia.

If the initial attempt at cardioversion does not result in at least transient conversion of the rhythm disturbance, additional attempts at higher energies are warranted. In general, no more than 200 J are needed to convert atrial flutter whereas atrial fibrillation and PSVT may occasionally require as much as 360 J. **When transient reversion is followed by recurrence of the rhythm disturbance, further attempts at cardioversion are not warranted** until additional therapy is administered to prevent recurrence.

Coincident with emergency treatment, **attempts should be made to identify and correct any underlying abnormalities that may have led to the tachycardia.** Unless this is done, control of the rhythm disturbance is unlikely. Congestive heart failure, hypoxemia, electrolyte disturbances, and acid–base abnormalities are extremely common precipitating causes of supraventricular rhythm disturbances. If emergency cardioversion is unsuccessful and/or the rhythm disturbance recurs, one should consider administering IV medications in an attempt to control the ventricular response to the tachycardia. Commonly used agents include digitalis, verapamil, or beta blockers. Under certain circumstances IV procainamide may also be used to terminate the rhythm disturbance.

In the case of **a more stable patient with supraventricular tachycardia,** a less urgent approach to treatment is reasonable. **Vagal maneuvers** may be helpful in differentiating between the various types of supraventricular tachyarrhythmias and/or in converting patients with PSVT. The most commonly employed vagal maneuvers are carotid massage (unless cerebrovascular disease or a carotid bruit is present), the Valsalva maneuver, head-down tilt with deep inspiration, and/or activation of the "diving reflex" by ice water facial immersion (unless ischemic heart disease is suspected). Vagal maneuvers should be performed only by individuals trained in their proper use. Patients should be

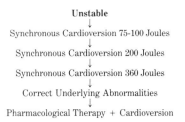

Unstable
↓
Synchronous Cardioversion 75-100 Joules
↓
Synchronous Cardioversion 200 Joules
↓
Synchronous Cardioversion 360 Joules
↓
Correct Underlying Abnormalities
↓
Pharmacological Therapy + Cardioversion

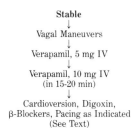

Stable
↓
Vagal Maneuvers
↓
Verapamil, 5 mg IV
↓
Verapamil, 10 mg IV
(in 15-20 min)
↓
Cardioversion, Digoxin,
β-Blockers, Pacing as Indicated
(See Text)

Figure 7. Paroxysmal supraventricular tachycardia (PSVT). This sequence was developed to assist in teaching how to treat a broad range of patients with sustained PSVT. Some patients may require care not specified herein. This algorithm should not be construed as prohibiting such flexibility. Flow of algorithm presumes PSVT is continuing.

If conversion occurs but PSVT recurs, repeated electrical cardioversion is *not* indicated. Sedation should be used as time permits.

electrocardiographically monitored during the procedure, and an IV line should already be in place to provide access for treatment should bradycardia occur.

If vagal maneuvers are unsuccessful, pharmacological treatment may be required. **Verapamil is generally the drug of choice for the treatment of PSVT.** Contraindications to the use of verapamil include a history of severe bradycardia, hypotension, congestive heart failure, or concomitant acute use of IV beta blockers. The usual dose of verapamil is 5 mg given IV. A repeat dose of 10 mg can be given in 15–30 minutes if the initial dose is unsuccessful. If hypotension occurs, it may often be reversed by slow IV infusion of 0.5–1.0 g of calcium chloride. Other approaches include the use of digitalis IV or orally, beta blockers, diltiazem, or Type 1 antiarrhythmic agents.

Medical therapy is similar for **atrial flutter** in the patient who is hemodynamically stable. Digitalis or verapamil are most often tried first in an attempt to slow the ventricular response. Beta blockers or Type 1 antiarrhythmic agents may then be added. Atrial flutter will often convert to sinus rhythm or atrial fibrillation when the ventricular response slows.

Patients with **atrial fibrillation** who are hemodynamically stable rarely convert to sinus rhythm in response to vagal maneuvers or verapamil. Approaches to the stable patient revolve around the slowing of the ventricular response. Verapamil, digitalis, and beta blockers may all be used either alone or in combination for this purpose. However, one should not administer IV verapamil and propranolol near to each other in time, since this combination may result in a potentially dangerous slowing of the ventricular response. Either may exacerbate heart failure.

In general, reducing the ventricular response to 100 beats/min or less improves hemodynamic performance and serves as an excellent measure of the adequacy of therapy. On the other hand, attempts to slow a rapid ventricular rate that is physiological (e.g., in response to an underlying abnormality) are doomed to failure unless the underlying cause has been corrected. Once the ventricular response has been slowed, Type 1 antiarrhythmic agents may be added to the regimen in an attempt to convert atrial fibrillation to sinus rhythm. The success of such an approach depends on the duration of atrial fibrillation, the left atrial chamber size, and whether the precipitating cause of the rhythm disturbance can be corrected.

When a wide-complex tachycardia is present and one is certain that it is not ventricular in origin or due to preexcitation, the treatment approach is the same as for a narrow-complex supraventricular tachycardia. However, **should there be any doubt about the etiology of a wide-complex tachycardia, one must presume the rhythm to be VT or due to preexcitation** and treat accordingly, even if the patient is not in cardiovascular collapse.

The choice of treatment for a patient with supraventricular tachycardia in the prehospital setting depends on the severity of the hemodynamic compromise, the patient's underlying disease, the skill and training of the emergency care providers, and the estimated time of transport to the nearest appropriate emergency care facility. In general, field cardioversion is best avoided if transport time to the hospital is expected to be short, unless the patient is hemodynamically severely compromised or symptomatic. If time permits, prehospital providers should consult with their base station physician and/or nurse in making such decisions.

Additional information concerning the patient may be available which may indicate that interventions other than those included in this sequence are appropriate. Such interventions are not precluded.

Organizational Aspects of Cardiopulmonary Resuscitation

The basic components of a comprehensive response to in-hospital cardiopulmonary resuscitation include 1) administrative coordination, 2) communication, 3) equipment, 4) a record of resuscitation, 5) training, and 6) personnel. For prehospital cardiac arrest, additional components are required, including 1) public training in CPR and the "signals and actions for survival", 2) use of the universal 911 telephone number for emergency help, 3) an efficient dispatch center, 4) a first response team, ideally one trained to perform CPR and defibrillate, and 5) an ACLS team that can continue patient care and transport the patient to the hospital.

Administrative Coordination

Regardless of the clinical setting, an administrative organization must be in place to coordinate the overall program. In a hospital, a CPR or resuscitation committee should be composed of hospital personnel who, by virtue of their training, interest, and responsibility, represent the disciplines necessary for successful resuscitation. These disciplines most commonly include anesthesiology, cardiology, critical care medicine, emergency medicine, surgery, primary care medicine, nursing (both clinical and administrative), respiratory therapy, and hospital administration. Pediatrics and obstetrics should also be represented if the institution provides services to populations cared for by these specialties. All clinical members of the committee should be trained in CPR and ACLS.

For the outpatient setting, the structure is likely to be different, but there must be strong medical control in the form of a designated physician (medical director) who directs the medical care provided by any and all personnel involved in the EMS system or unit. In many states this is mandated by law.

The functions of the resuscitation committee and/or medical director should be as follows:

1. Develop a resuscitation policy statement and formalize a plan. The plan should detail operation of the program and have staff and administrative approval. It should be detailed in writing.
2. Establish a process to identify patients who are not candidates for resuscitation — especially relevant for the in-hospital setting.
3. Determine the qualifications and assess the competence of personnel involved in resuscitation (including certification according to state and/or local regulations and laws).
4. Define protocols that allow nonphysicians to function in extended roles as appropriate (e.g., to permit endotracheal intubation, defibrillation, or to administer emergency IV drugs). In addition, the scope and limits of such activities should be defined in detail.
5. Design, implement, and evaluate basic and advanced resuscitation training programs and assure that an on-going quality assurance program is in place.
6. Plan a communication (alert) system that permits rapid and effective initiation of resuscitation.
7. Plan and designate which personnel will respond to any given resuscitation emergency and who will be responsible for transport of the equipment.
8. Standardize necessary equipment and plan its location, maintenance, and restocking.
9. Develop and implement a resuscitation record.
10. Provide on-going monitoring of the operation of the program, evaluation of and feedback on performance, and review of resuscitation records to assure the quality of resuscitation.

Communication

Following cardiac arrest, the sooner CPR and ACLS are provided to restore spontaneous respiration and circulation, the greater the chance of survival. The resuscitation team must reach the scene of an arrest in the shortest possible time. Each system must develop a method of communication that meets its special needs for both notification of the emergency and dispatch of the appropriate personnel and equipment. In the hospital, a priority signal (letters or numbers) should be established for dialing the switchboard operator or paging center. In the community the use of the universal 911 number (for all emergencies) that can connect the caller to the appropriate medical dispatcher is recommended. If 911 is not available, a single, easily identifiable number should be used for all emergencies.

Equipment

In each resuscitation unit, resuscitation equipment, including drugs and the resuscitation record, is usually stored in an emergency cart or box. For ACLS to be initiated promptly, the equipment must reach the arrest scene rapidly. It must be strategically located, and there must be an effective plan for getting the equipment promptly to the resuscitation site.

The placement of each piece of equipment should be standardized so that it is stored in the same place in each cart or box. This greatly facilitates locating equipment when in an unfamiliar setting.

Recommendations for equipment and drugs to be stocked are listed in Table 2. If the monitor–defibrillator is separate from the other equipment, a designated person must be assigned to bring it to the scene of the arrest.

To guarantee that drugs will be available when needed, they should be stored together in a sealed tray or cart. Ideally, there should be an exchange mechanism so that once a seal is broken, the entire tray is returned to be restocked and resealed. Drugs for bolus administration are best supplied in single-dose, prefilled syringes instead of multi-dose vials. Whenever possible, drugs for continuous infusion should also be supplied in premixed containers.

It may be helpful to store equipment for specific tasks together. Thus, bags or containers may be organized, according to sequence of use, in three groups: 1) equipment needed initially (face mask with one-way valve, oxygen inlet); 2) secondary airway equipment (suction catheters, bag–valve–mask device), and 3) intubation equipment. In contrast, some organizations may prefer to store all respiratory equipment in an organized fashion in one single area.

Equipment for peripheral and central venous cannulation may be stored in separate containers or drawers. While it may not be practical to store IV equipment and fluids together, they should at least be organized and readily accessible.

Equipment for field use must be lightweight, durable, and stored efficiently in kits or tackle boxes that can be brought to the scene and set up quickly. The same general principles noted above apply in organizing such kits.

Record of Resuscitation

The resuscitation (code) record is an essential component of any resuscitation effort. From it, one should be able accurately to reconstruct the sequence of events that occurred during the code with correlation of interventions and responses. In addition, the code record provides documentation of the CPR and ACLS that were performed during resuscitation. Such documentation allows the evaluation of appropriateness of care and

Table 2. Equipment for Adult Resuscitations. Organize in sequence of use. A group may be placed in a clear bag, container, or specific area of a cart and sealed.

A. AIRWAY

Group I: Initial
Oral and nasal airways (large, medium, and small adult)
Face mask with one-way valve and oxygen inlet
O_2 connector to O_2 source and flow meter, O_2 tubing

Group II: Secondary
Tonsil tip and straight suction catheter
Wall outlet suction unit
Bag–valve–mask unit with O_2 reservoir

Group III: Intubation
Laryngoscope handle
Curved and straight adult blades
Endotracheal tubes with low-pressure cuffs, sizes 7, 8, 9
Stylet
Lubricating jelly and/or anesthetic jelly (water soluble)
10-mL syringe
Stethoscope
Optional
McGill forceps
Topical anesthetic spray

B. VENOUS ACCESS

Group IV: Peripheral
Alcohol or iodophor prep sponge
IV catheter (catheter-over-needle, 5–5.5 cm) 14 gauge (1 or more), 16 gauge (1 or more), 18 gauge (1 or more)
IV tubing — minidrip administration set (1 or more), stopcock (1 or more), IV extension set (1 or more)
5% dextrose/water 500 mL
2″ × 2″ sterile gauze sponges
1″ adhesive tape
Tourniquet

Group V: Central
Sterile drapes and gloves (masks, haircovers, sterile gown)
Iodophor prep solution
4″ × 4″ sterile gauze sponges
10-mL nonluerlock syringe
18 gauge thin-wall, 6-cm-long needle
0.035 guidewire, at least 35 cm long
16 gauge 15- to 20-cm-long catheter
Suture material: 2-0 silk on curved needle, needle holder, scissors
IV tubing: minidrip administration set (1), stopcock (1), IV extension set (1)
5% dextrose/water 500 mL
Dressing material: iodophor or antibiotic ointment, gauze sponges, adhesive tape

C. ADDITIONAL EQUIPMENT

IV Equipment/fluids
5% dextrose/water 250 mL (4)
5% dextrose/water 500 mL (2)
Normal saline 1000 mL (2)
Lactated Ringer's 1000 mL (2)
IV microdrip infusion pump tubing (4)
IV microdrip administration set (2)
IV maxidrip administration set (2)
IV extension set (2)
Blood administration set (2)
Blood pump
Armboard
Needles of various sizes — 21 and 22 gauge, 3.5–4 cm; 22 gauge, 8.75 cm intracardiac
Syringes, various sizes, including one 50-mL glass syringe
Arterial blood gas sampling kits
16 gauge CVP catheter, 0.035 guidewire, 18 gauge thin-wall needle (2)
16 gauge, 5 cm catheter-over-needle (4)
18 gauge, 5 cm catheter-over-needle (4)
Introducer sheath — 8 French with high flow side arm (2)
Vascular cutdown tray
Alcohol or iodophor prep sponges
Iodophor or antibiotic ointment
Medication labels

Nasogastric Intubation (all together in a plastic bag)
Nasogastric tube
Lubricating jelly
Catheter tip syringe
1″ tape

Additional endotracheal tubes, sizes 7, 8, 9
4 × 4″ sterile gauze sponges
Sterile gloves, drapes, masks, haircovers, sterile gowns
Cardiac arrest board

D. OPTIONAL EQUIPMENT
CVP manometer
Chest tubes
Chest drainage system, Heimlich valve
Emergency medication drug calculation sheets
O_2 cylinder and portable suction machine
External pacemaker
Percutaneous transvenous pacemaker
Transthoracic pacemaker
Pacemaker generator
Pericardiocentesis tray
Cricothyrotomy kit (scalpel and size 5 tracheostomy tube)

enables the prospective collection of data for measuring the outcome and the effects of training. The code record should include the following:

1. Patient demographics
2. Whether the arrest was respiratory or cardio-respiratory, witnessed or unwitnessed
3. Times of the arrest, the initiation of CPR, and the initiation of ACLS (to assist in determining arrest time before CPR, CPR and ACLS times, and total resuscitation time)
4. Drug therapy (including doses and routes of administration)
5. Sequential cardiac rhythms (with a mechanism to allow correlation of ECG tracings with patient status, therapy, and responses to therapy)
6. Countershocks administered (including energy level)
7. Presence of spontaneous pulse
8. Special procedures
9. Vital signs and response to the above interventions
10. Patient status and disposition at the end of the arrest.

Retrospective evaluation of resuscitation attempts is an effective method for upgrading the performance of CPR and ACLS. However, for such evaluation, an accurate log of each resuscitation experience must be kept. Review of these records will suggest modifications in procedures and provide information for improving training programs.

Monitoring and evaluating prehospital cardiac arrest management must be done under the supervision of the medical director. It must include the following:

1. A coordinated and standardized recordkeeping system for the prehospital incident. This record becomes part of the hospital record, and copies should be retained in a data collection center and in the files of the medical director for the EMS system.
2. Review of all calls and all therapy provided for its consistency with established treatment protocols.
3. Capability for physician monitoring of all medical emergency calls, from the time the 911 operator receives the call to the time responsibility for the patient's medical care is transferred to a physician within the fixed facility.
4. Formal procedures for correcting and disciplining either personnel or agencies that improperly deviate from treatment protocols.

Training

All physicians, nurses, and other healthcare personnel who have direct patient contact should be trained and certified in CPR. All physicians, nurses, and other healthcare personnel whose daily responsibilites require proficiency in acute cardiac care (such as emergency and critical care personnel, paramedics, etc.) should also be trained and should maintain proficiency in ACLS.

Neonatal Resuscitation

Chapter 17

The ideal environment for neonatal resuscitation is the delivery room or the neonatal intensive care unit. In these settings, problems can be anticipated, and trained personnel as well as appropriate equipment are always available. Resuscitation in the delivery room is dealt with in a separate course; delivery-room and neonatal-intensive-care personnel should take that course.

Unfortunately, many deliveries occur outside the delivery room — in the home, en route to the hospital, or in the emergency department, where conditions may be less than optimal. This chapter offers a practical approach to resuscitation of the newborn in the peripartum period in the emergency room or other non-optimal setting, using AHA standards.[1]

Marked changes occur in the cardiovascular and respiratory systems at the moment of birth. The former undergoes a rapid transition from the fetal to the postpartum circulation. The respiratory system, which is essentially nonfunctional *in utero,* must suddenly initiate and maintain the respiratory process. When prepartum events cause asphyxia, they preclude a smooth postpartum transition. The aim of the resuscitative process is restoration of normal cardiopulmonary function.

The vast majority (approximately 80%) of newborn infants require no resuscitation beyond maintenance of temperature and suctioning of the airway. Of the small number who require further intervention, most will respond to a high oxygen environment and bag–mask ventilation. A small number of severely asphyxiated infants require chest compression; and an even smaller number, resuscitative medications. In approaching newborn resuscitation, an inverted pyramid represents the relative frequencies of performance of the various resuscitative steps (Figure 1). Resuscitation should proceed in a stepwise fashion, with *reassessment* prior to each step, so that complications from unnecessarily aggressive intervention may be avoided.

Triage

Since best results are obtained in the most ideal environment, every effort should be made to delay the birth of an infant at high risk until the mother can be transported to a delivery room. Prehospital delays as well as stops in the emergency room or admitting office are inappropriate.

Preparation

Most resuscitations of neonates in the emergency department occur without prior notice. The resuscitative process can, however, be facilitated by preparing equipment and training personnel in advance, by obtaining a brief history, and by assigning personnel prior to, or immediately upon, admission to the emergency room.

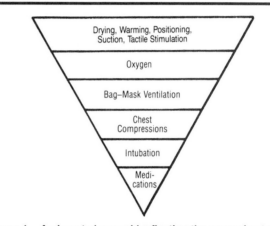

Figure 1. An inverted pyramid reflecting the approximate relative frequency of neonatal resuscitative efforts. Note that a majority of infants respond to simple measures. Most infants that require chest compression will usually require intubation and these efforts are often performed simultaneously.

Advance

Every emergency department should maintain an easily accessible neonatal resuscitation tray that is periodically checked and replenished. The tray should contain proper equipment (Table 1), as well as charts listing the correct medication dosages for neonates of various weights (Table 2). Unless equipment is meticulously organized and readily available in the emergency department, even the most sophisticated personnel will find it difficult to perform a successful neonatal resuscitation.

Table 1. Resuscitation Equipment for the Emergency Room

A. Items that should be readily accessible
Radiant warmer
Suction with manometer
Resuscitation bag (250-750 mL)
Face masks (newborn & premature size)
Laryngoscope with extra battery and bulb
Laryngoscope blades (straight 0 & 1)
Oral airways
Shoulder roll
Tape (½ or ¾ inch)
Scissors
Oxygen tubing
Gloves
Medications
    Epinephrine 1:10,000
    Sodium bicarbonate 4.2%*
    Volume expander
B. Items that should be on newborn resuscitation tray
Bulb syringe
DeLee suction trap with 10 Fr. catheter
Endotracheal tubes (2.5, 3.0, 3.5, and 4.0)
Suction catheters (5 F & two 8 F taped to ET tubes)
Endotracheal tube stylet
Umbilical catheter (5 Fr)
Syringe (10 mL & 20 mL)
Three-way stopcock
Feeding tube (5 & 8 F)
Towels
OB kit/cord cutting materials
Naloxone

*If the adult 8.4% solution is the only one available, it should be diluted 1:1 with sterile water.

Table 2. Neonatal Resusci-Card

Ventilation Rate:	40–60 minute
Compression Rate:	120/minute
Medications:	Heart rate <80/minute despite adequate ventilations with 100% O_2 and chest compressions

MEDICATION	CONCENTRATION	DOSE
Epinephrine	1:10,000 (0.1 mg/mL)	0.01-0.03 mg/kg
Sodium Bicarbonate	0.5 mEq/mL	2 mEq/kg

WEIGHT	EPINEPHRINE Total mL	BICARBONATE Total mL	ET/SUCTION CATHETER	LARYNG BLADE
1 kg	0.1–0.3 mL	4 mL	2.5/5 Fr	0
2 kg	0.2–0.6 mL	8 mL	3.0/8 Fr	0
3 kg	0.3–0.9 mL	12 mL	3.5/8 Fr	0–1

Immediate

As soon as it is evident that a neonatal resuscitation may be necessary, a pre-arranged plan for assigning personnel according to levels of competence should be put into action. There is usually little time for an in-depth history, but often a brief history reveals key information that may alter the course of the resuscitation. For example, if there is a history of particulate meconium in the amniotic fluid, the resuscitation team must be prepared to suction the trachea under direct vision; if the labor is premature, one can anticipate a probable resuscitation; and if twins are expected, the team must be prepared to resuscitate two infants.

When a newborn has been resuscitated prior to arrival at the hospital, special problems include hypothermia and difficulty in maintaining vascular access and airway control during transport. Preparation for receiving the newborn in the emergency room should be similar to preparation for a full resuscitation, and on arrival, the newborn should be carefully evaluated.

Resuscitation Procedure

The Environment

All newborns have difficulty tolerating a cold environment.[2] Asphyxiated infants are particularly at risk, and recovery from acidosis is delayed by hypothermia.[3] Hypothermia may be a special problem for the infant born outside the hospital. Heat loss may be prevented by 1) placing the infant under a preheated warmer and 2) quickly drying the infant of amniotic fluid. A radiant warmer should be switched on as soon as it is known that a neonatal resuscitation may be necessary. Other ways of warming the infant, if a radiant warmer is not available, include using warm towels and placing the naked infant against the body of the mother, with covers over both.

Positioning

The newborn should be placed on his/her back in a slight Trendelenburg (head down) position with the neck slightly extended. A 1-inch thickness of blanket or towel placed under the infant's shoulders is helpful in maintaining head position. If copious secretions are present, the infant's head should be turned to the side.

Suctioning

To assure an open airway, first the mouth and then the nose should be suctioned. In the emergency room there is frequently insufficient time to adequately adjust the wall suction; in this setting, therefore, manual bulb suction or a DeLee suction trap with a 10 F catheter is preferred. If a mechanical suction apparatus with an 8 or 10 F suction catheter is used, pressure should not exceed −100 mmHg (−136 cm H_2O). Deep suctioning of the oropharynx may produce a vagal response and cause bradycardia and/or apnea.[4] Suctioning should therefore continue for no longer than 10 seconds at a time, and heart rate should be continuously monitored (see "Heart Rate", below). In order to minimize hypoxia, time should be allowed between suctionings for the lungs to be ventilated, spontaneously or with assistance, with 100% oxygen.

Meconium aspiration is a major cause of neonatal death and morbidity, and its prevention deserves special attention.[5] If meconium is not adequately removed from the airway, a high percent (60%) of infants with thick meconium in the amniotic fluid will aspirate this fluid at the initiation of respiration. Some of these newborns (approximately 20%) will develop complications following meconium aspiration, including respiratory distress, aspiration pneumonia, and pneumothorax.[6] To prevent aspiration, infants born with particulate meconium staining require thorough hypopharyngeal suctioning before initiation of respiration and, therefore, before completion of the delivery.[7] Suctioning is ideally performed after the head, but not the rest of the body, is delivered. If the hypopharynx has not been cleared of meconium before the onset of respiration, as is likely to happen with a precipitous delivery in the emergency room, the trachea should be intubated to remove as much of the meconium as possible from the lower airway.[8] As meconium is viscous, suction should be applied directly to the endotracheal tube, using the full caliber of the tube to evacuate the thick, tenacious material. Suction catheters inserted through the endotracheal tube are inadequate. The evacuation can be performed with an intervening mask, or by a regulated wall suction device. As suction is applied directly to the endotracheal tube, the tube is slowly withdrawn. It is imperative that an intervening mask be used to prevent cross infection — in both directions.[9] To facilitate the use of wall suction, the suction control port, removed from a suction catheter, can be attached directly to the endotracheal tube.[10] If meconium is removed via the endotracheal tube, the infant should be reintubated and suctioned again to remove as much meconium as possible. The presence of watery or thin meconium does not require routine endotracheal intubation.

Tactile Stimulation

Drying and suctioning produce enough stimulation to induce effective respirations in most infants. Two additional safe methods of providing tactile stimulation are 1) slapping or flicking the soles of the feet, and 2) rubbing the infant's back. More vigorous methods of stimulation should be avoided. If the infant fails to establish spontaneous and effective respirations following a brief period of stimulation, positive-pressure ventilation is required.

Assessment

If the infant is born in the emergency room, the assessment is performed after clearing the airway and stimulating the infant. If, however, the delivery takes place before arrival in the emergency room, the assessment should be performed immediately after placing the infant in a warmed environment.

Respiratory Effort

Breathing rate and depth should increase immediately with *brief* stimulation; time should not be taken to stimulate the infant more than twice.

If the respiratory response is appropriate, the heart rate is evaluated next. If the respiratory response is inappropriate (shallow, slow, or absent respirations), positive-pressure ventilations should be started immediately. Continued tactile stimulation of an apneic infant which will delay the onset of assisted, needed ventilations is not indicated.

Heart Rate

The heart rate is a critical determinant of the resuscitation sequence and may be evaluated by 1) listening to the apical beat with a stethoscope, 2) feeling the pulse by lightly grasping the base of the umbilical cord, or 3) feeling the brachial or femoral pulse. A cardiotachometer monitoring system can also be used but takes time to set up.

The presence of respirations does not guarantee an adequate pulse rate. Shallow respirations may primarily ventilate airway dead space and thus provide inadequate alveolar ventilation.

If the heart rate is >100 beats/min and spontaneous respirations are present, the assessment is continued. If the heart rate is <100 beats/min, positive-pressure ventilations should be started immediately.

Color

An infant may occasionally be cyanotic despite adequate ventilations and a heart rate >100 beats/min. If central cyanosis is present in an infant with spontaneous respirations and an adequate heart rate, free-flow oxygen should be given until the cause can be further evaluated. Oxygen therapy is unnecessary for infants with peripheral cyanosis (blue extremities only), a condition common in the first few minutes of life and due to sluggish peripheral circulation.

The Apgar Score

The Apgar scoring system (Table 3) has been widely used as an indicator of the need for resuscitation at birth. Five objective signs are evaluated, and the total score is noted at 1 minute and at 5 minutes after the complete birth of the infant. If the 5-minute Apgar score is less than 7, additional scores are obtained every 5 minutes for a total of 20 minutes. The need for resuscitation can, however, be more rapidly assessed by evaluating the

Table 3. Apgar Scoring

Sign	0	1	2
Heart rate	Absent	Slow (<100/min)	>100/min
Respirations	Absent	Slow, irregular	Good, crying
Muscle tone	Limp	Some flexion	Active motion
Reflex irritability (catheter in nares)	No response	Grimace	Cough or sneeze
Color	Blue or pale	Pink body with blue extremities	Completely pink

heart rate, respiratory activity, and *color* than by the total Apgar score. Since even a short delay in initiating resuscitation may result in a long delay in establishing spontaneous and regular respirations, resuscitation should be started immediately when indicated by inadequate respirations and/or heart rate. It should not be delayed for obtaining the one-minute score.

Ventilation

The vast majority of infants who require ventilatory support may be adequately ventilated using a bag and mask. Indications for positive-pressure ventilation include 1) apnea, 2) heart rate less than 100 beats/min, and 3) persistent central cyanosis in a maximal oxygen environment.

An assisted ventilatory rate of 40-60 breaths/min should provide adequate ventilation. Tidal volumes in newborn and, especially, preterm infants are small. To minimize the chance of possible iatrogenic complications, it is best to begin bag–mask ventilations with small volumes, increasing rapidly, though in small increments, until an adequate tidal volume is achieved. It is imperative to maintain a tight face mask seal for adequate ventilations. In most infants, initial lung inflation requires pressures of 30–40 cmH$_2$O, and in some, pressures as high as 60 cm may be needed; less pressure is usually required for succeeding breaths. Signs of adequate ventilation include bilateral expansion of the lungs as judged by chest wall motion and auscultation of breath sounds. Inability to inflate the lungs adequately requires further suctioning and repositioning of the head and face mask. If these maneuvers fail to provide adequate

ventilation, immediate laryngoscopic examination of the upper airway and intubation of the trachea is required. Bag and mask ventilation may produce gastric distention requiring periodic decompression. If bag–mask positive-pressure ventilations are required for longer than approximately 2 minutes, an orogastric tube should be inserted into the stomach and left in place during ventilations.

After adequate ventilation has been established for 15–30 seconds, subsequent steps depend on the heart rate. If the heart rate is >100 beats/min and spontaneous respirations are present, positive-pressure ventilation may be discontinued. Gentle tactile stimulation, such as rubbing the baby's skin, may help to maintain spontaneous breathing. If there are no spontaneous respirations, assisted ventilation must be continued.

If, despite adequate ventilations, the heart rate is <60 beats/min or 60–80 beats/min and not rapidly increasing, positive-pressure-assisted ventilations should be continued and chest compressions initiated.

Ventilation Bags

Self-Inflating Bag (Figure 2): The self-inflating bag, because of its elasticity, refills independent of gas flow. The most widely used bags of this type have an intake valve at one end to allow rapid reinflation. This valve, essential to the self-inflating feature, dilutes oxygen directed into the bag with air drawn in through the valve. To deliver high concentrations of oxygen with a self-inflating bag requires the use of an attached oxygen reservoir. In addition, oxygen cannot be given passively via the mask with many self-inflating bags.

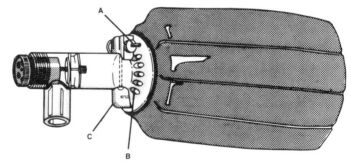

Figure 2. Two types of self-inflating resuscitation bags. Right: Non-reservoir-type bag with gas intake (A), air intake valve (B), and pressure limiting assembly (C). Below: Reservoir-type bag with gas intake (A), intake valve (B), pressure-limiting assembly (C), and gas reservoir (D).

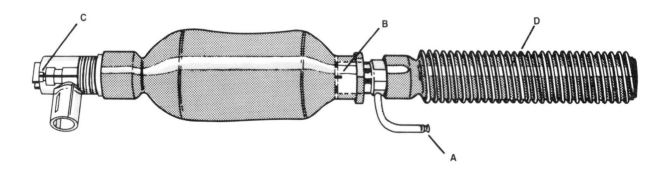

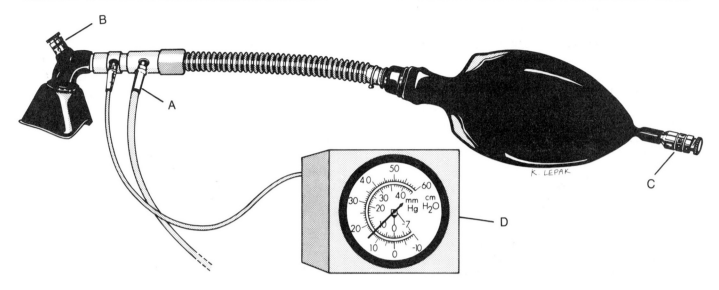

Figure 3. Anesthesia bag with gas intake line (A), controlled exit valve (B), bag exit valve (C), and in-line pressure manometer (D).

Many of the self-inflating bags are equipped with a pressure-limited pop-off valve that is usually preset at 30–35 cmH$_2$O. Since the first breaths of a neonate's nonaerated lung may require higher pressures, this feature may prevent initial effective inflation unless the pop-off valve is occluded. Self-inflating bags that have a device to bypass the pop-off valve and an in-line manometer are preferred. Bag volumes should not exceed 750 mL; larger bags make it difficult to accurately provide the small tidal volumes (6 to 8 mL/kg) that infants require.

Anesthesia Bag (Figure 3): The anesthesia bag inflates only when air or oxygen from a compressed gas source is forced into it. It requires a well-modulated flow of gas into the inlet port, correct adjustment of the flow control valve, and careful attention to a tight seal at the face mask. Since an anesthesia bag can deliver very high pressures, a port with an attached pressure gauge must be present to monitor peak ventilatory pressures. The anesthesia bag requires more training in its proper use than a self-inflating bag.

Face Masks

Face masks have either cushioned or noncushioned rims and are round or anatomically shaped. Anatomically shaped masks are designed to fit the contours of the infant's face and have a low dead space (<5 ml). The anatomical shape and cushioned rim provide the greatest chance for making a tight seal, and they help avoid malpositioning the mask. A correctly positioned mask should cover the infant's nose and mouth but not the eyes. Face masks fitting preterm, term, and large newborns should be available on the neonatal resuscitation tray.

Endotracheal Intubation

Endotracheal intubation is indicated 1) when bag–mask ventilation is ineffective, 2) when tracheal suctioning is required, especially for thick meconium, and 3) when prolonged positive-pressure ventilation is necessary.

The supplies and equipment for endotracheal intubation should be kept together and readily available on the neonatal resuscitation tray. Sterile, disposable tubes of nonirritating material should be used. Those designated IT (implantation tested) or Z79 meet the required standards. Tubes with a uniform internal diameter are preferred to those that are tapered. Most endotracheal tubes intended for neonatal use have a black line — vocal cord line — near the tip. If this guide is placed at the cord level, the tip of the tube is likely to be above the carina. The endotracheal tube size required is related to the infant's weight (Table 2).

The position of the endotracheal tube may be checked 1) by observing for symmetrical chest wall motion and listening for equal breath sounds, especially at the apices, and noting the absence of breath sounds over the stomach, and 2) if the tube is to remain in place following the resuscitation, a chest roentgenogram.

Chest Compressions

Asphyxia causes tissue hypoxia, acidosis, poor myocardial contractility, bradycardia, and eventually, cardiac arrest. This critical state can often be avoided by prompt and effective ventilation and oxygenation. Chest compressions should be performed if the heart rate is <60 beats/min or 60–80 beats/min and not rapidly increasing despite adequate ventilation with 100% oxygen for 15-30 seconds.

There are two techniques for performing chest compressions in the neonate and small infant. One[11] employs both thumbs placed on the lower third of the sternum, with the fingers encircling the torso and supporting the back (Figure 4). The thumbs should be positioned side-by-side on the sternum just below a line between the two nipples. In the very small infant the thumbs may have to be superimposed. The xiphoid portion of the sternum should not be compressed because of potential damage to abdominal organs.

If the infant is large or the resuscitator's hands are too small to encircle the chest, two-finger compression with the ring and middle fingers on the sternum one finger's breadth below the nipple line, but being careful not to compress the xiphoid, is applied. The sternum is compressed to a depth of ½″ to ¾″ at a rate of 120 times/ min. The compression phase should be smooth, not jerky, and equal in time to the relaxation phase. The thumbs or fingers should not be lifted off the sternum during the relaxation phase. The pulse rate should be checked periodically and chest compressions discontinued when the spontaneous heart rate reaches 80 beats/min or greater. Compressions should always be accompanied by positive-pressure ventilations with 100% oxygen at a rate of 40–60 per min.

Medications and Fluids

Myocardial dysfunction and shock in the neonatal period are usually the result of profound hypoxia. Medications should be administered if, despite adequate ventilation with 100% oxygen and chest compression, the heart rate remains <80 beats/min.

There is no current evidence that two previously recommended drugs, atropine and calcium, are useful in the acute phase of neonatal resuscitation. Sodium bicarbonate may be useful in a prolonged resuscitation to help correct metabolic acidosis,[12] but should not be used in brief arrests or episodes of bradycardia.[13-17] In the absence of adequate ventilation, sodium bicarbonate will not improve blood pH. Hypoxemia and acidosis may be best corrected with adequate oxygenation and ventilation.

Routes of Administration

The umbilical vein is preferred for vascular access during neonatal resuscitation because the vessel is easily located and cannulated, but the catheter is usually withdrawn at the end of the resuscitation to minimize the danger of infection or portal vein thrombosis.

The cord is trimmed with a scalpel blade 1 cm above the skin attachment and held firmly to prevent bleeding. The umbilical vein is recognized as a thin-walled single vessel, in contrast to the arteries, which are paired, thicker walled, and often constricted. The vein lumen is larger than that of the artery, so the vessel that continues to bleed after the cord is cut is usually the vein. A 5.0 F umbilical catheter with a radiopaque marker, attached to a three-way stopcock and filled with saline, is inserted so that the tip is just below the skin and there is free flow of blood; the catheter is inserted a short distance to avoid inadvertent infusion of hypertonic solutions into the liver. A wedged hepatic position is recognized by failure of free blood return. If this occurs, the catheter should be withdrawn to a position where blood can be freely aspirated.

Vascular access via other routes may also be obtained. Cannulating the umbilical artery is more time consuming and difficult, but it is useful for monitoring blood pressure, blood gases, and acid–base balance. Fluids and most medications may be given via this route. Peripheral veins in the extremities and scalp are difficult to access in neonates during a resuscitation.

When venous access is not readily available, the endotracheal tube is the most easily accessible route for delivery of epinephrine[18,19] and should eliminate the need for intracardiac injections. Since the optimal dose for the endotracheal route is currently not certain,[20] the intravenous dose is recommended.[21,22] It is advisable to dilute the medication in 1–2 ml of normal saline and to deliver it via a feeding tube passed into the endotracheal tube so that the medication is delivered into the trachea.

Epinephrine

Epinephrine is an endogenous catecholamine with potent α- and β-adrenergic-stimulating properties; in the cardiac arrest setting, α-adrenergic-medicated vasoconstriction may be the more important action.[23] Vasoconstriction elevates the perfusion pressure during chest compression, increases coronary blood flow, and enhances delivery of oxygen to the heart. Additionally, epinephrine improves myocardial contraction, stimulates spontaneous contractions, and increases heart rate.

Indications: Asystole or spontaneous heart rate <80 beats/min despite adequate ventilation with 100% oxygen and chest compressions for 30 seconds.

Dose: 0.01–0.03 mg/kg (0.1–0.3 mL/kg of the 1:10,000 solution). May be repeated every 5 minutes if required.

Route: Intravenously or via endotracheal tube and diluted 1 to 1 with normal saline or sterile water.

Volume Expanders

Volume expanders are indicated in the presence of hypovolemia, which should be suspected in any infant who requires resuscitation.

Indications: Evidence of acute bleeding from the fetal-maternal unit with 1) pallor that persists after oxygenation, 2) faint pulses with a good heart rate, and 3) poor response to resuscitation with adequate ventilation.

Dose: 1) 10 mL/kg O-negative blood cross matched with the mother's blood; 2) 10 mL/kg 5% albumin/saline solution or other plasma substitute; or 3) 10 mL/kg normal saline or Ringer's lactate. Volume expanders are given over 5–10 minutes.

Route: Intravenously.

Dopamine

Indications: Dopamine is indicated in the treatment of hypotension and/or poor peripheral perfusion in the pediatric patient in whom a stable rhythm is present or has been restored. Low doses (1-5 μg/kg/min) enhance renal and splanchnic blood flow.

Dose: Dopamine has a short plasma half-life and must be delivered by a constant infusion pump. Infusions can be prepared according to Table 5.1. Another method is to add 60 mg of dopamine into 100 mL of diluent, resulting in a final concentration of 600 μg/mL. Infusions of 1 mL/kg/hr of this mixture deliver 10 μg/kg/min, a reasonable starting dose for the child with shock. The infusion can then be adjusted as indicated by improvement in the patient's perfusion or blood pressure. Infusion rates above 20 μg/kg/min produce predominant vasoconstrictive effects without any further inotropic effect and should be used with caution.

Naloxone Hydrochloride

Naloxone hydrochloride is a narcotic antagonist without direct respiratory effects.

Indications: For the reversal of respiratory depression in the neonate induced by a variety of narcotics given to the mother within 4 hours of delivery. Prompt and adequate ventilatory assistance should always precede the administration of naloxone. Since the duration of action of narcotics may exceed that of naloxone, continued surveillance of the infant is necessary. Naloxone can induce a withdrawal reaction in an infant of a narcotic-addicted mother and should be used with caution if this condition is suspected.

Dose: 0.01–0.05 mg/kg (0.5 mL/kg–2.5 mL/kg) of the solution (*Narcan*, 0.02 mg/mL). The initial dose should be repeated every 2–3 minutes as needed.

Route: Intravenously, via the endotracheal tube or, if perfusion is adequate, subcutaneously or intramuscularly.

Postresuscitation Care

Some emergency departments, especially those located in rural areas, may receive infants born outside the hospital who have already been resuscitated. An infant who has been resuscitated prior to arrival at the hospital should be assumed to be at risk of having an airway problem. Some of the more common complications in the postresuscitation phase include dislodgement or endobronchial placement of the endotracheal tube during transport, endotracheal tube occlusion by mucus or meconium, and pneumothorax. The latter can be especially difficult to diagnose by auscultation, since breath sounds in the neonate may be transmitted. A diagnosis of pneumothorax should be considered in a newborn who deteriorates after an initial response or who fails to respond to resuscitative efforts.

Communication with a neonatal intensive care unit should be established as soon as it is known that there is a potential neonatal resuscitation. Postresuscitation care, while still in the emergency room, may include determination of arterial blood gases, correction of documented metabolic acidosis, treatment of hypotension with volume expanders and/or inotropic agents, and treatment of seizures, hypoglycemia, and hypocalcemia. A chest roentgenogram may help to rule out a pneumothorax and demonstrate the location of the endotracheal tube.

After a successful resuscitation the infant should be monitored closely by trained observers in an intensive care area.

References

1. Standards and Guidelines for Cardiopulmonary Resuscitation (CPR) and Emergency Cardiac Care (ECC). *JAMA* 255:2969,1986.
2. Scopes JW, Ahmed I: Range of critical temperatures in sick and premature newborn babies. *Arch Dis Child* 41:417, 1966.
3. Adamsons K Jr, Gandy GM, Jeames LS: The influence of thermal factors upon oxygen consumption of the newborn human infant. *J Pediatr* 66:495, 1965.
4. Cordero L Jr, Hon EH: Neonatal bradycardia following nasopharyngeal suction. *J Pediatr* 78:441, 1971.
5. Carson BS, Losey RW, Bowes WAJ, et al: Combined obstetric and pediatric approach to prevent meconium aspiration syndrome. *Am J Obstet Gynecol* 126:712, 1976.
6. Fox WW, Gutsche BB, DeVore JS: A delivery room approach to the meconium aspiration syndrome. *Clin Pediatr* 16:325, 1977.
7. Gregory GA, Gooding CA, Phibbs RH, et al: Meconium aspiration in infants — A prospective study. *J Pediatr* 85:848, 1974.
8. Ting P, Brady JP: Tracheal suction in meconium aspiration syndrome. *Am J Obstet Gynecol* 122:767, 1975.
9. Ballard JL, Musial MJ, Myers MG: Hazards of delivery room resuscitation using oral methods of endotracheal suctioning. *Pediatr Infect Dis* 5:198, 1986.
10. Eisner P: Suctioning meconium from the trachea: A new solution to an old problem. *Pediatrics* 78:713, 1986.
11. Todres ID, Rogers MC: Methods of external cardiac massage in the newborn infant. *J Pediatr* 86:781, 1975.

12. Bishop RL, Weisfeldt ML: Sodium bicarbonate administration during cardiac arrest: Effect on arterial pH, PCO₂ and osmolality. *JAMA* 235:506, 1976.

13. Ostrea EM Jr, Odell GB: The influence of bicarbonate administration on blood pH in a "closed system": Clinical implications. *J Pediatr* 80:671, 1972.

14. Simmons MA, Adock, EW, Bard, H, et al: Hypernatremia and intracranial hemorrhage in neonates. *N Engl J Med* 291:6, 1974.

15. Finberg L: The relationship of intravenous infusions and intracranial hemorrhage — A commentary. *Pediatrics* 91:777, 1977.

16. Papile L, Burstein J, Burstein R, et al: Relationship of intravenous sodium bicarbonate infusions and cerebral intraventricular hemorrhage. *J Pediatr* 93:834, 1978.

17. Graf H, Leach W, Arieff AI: Evidence for a detrimental effect of bicarbonate therapy on hypoxic lactic acidosis. *Science* 227:754, 1985.

18. Greenberg MI, Roberts JR, Baskin SI, et al: The use of endotracheal medication for cardiac arrest. *Top Emerg Med* 1(2):29, 1979.

19. Ward JT Jr: Endotracheal drug therapy. *Am J Emerg Med* 1:71, 1983.

20. Lindemann R: Endotracheal administration of epinephrine during cardiopulmonary resuscitation. *Am J Dis Child* 136:753, 1982.

21. Roberts JR, Greenburg MI, Knaub MA, et al: Comparison of the pharmacological effects of epinephrine administered by the intravenous and endotracheal routes. *JACEP* 7:260, 1978.

22. Roberts JR, Greenburg MI, Knaub MA, et al: Blood levels following intravenous and endotracheal epinephrine administration. *JACEP* 8:53, 1979.

23. Zaritsky A, Chernow B: Use of catecholamines in pediatrics. *J Pediatr* 105:341, 1985.

Resuscitation of Infants and Children

Chapter 18

In contrast to adults, cardiopulmonary arrest in infants and children is rarely a sudden, primarily cardiac, event. Instead, it is usually the end result of a progressive deterioration in respiratory and circulatory function whose final common pathway, regardless of the underlying disease, is cardiopulmonary failure (Figure 1). Survival from cardiac arrest in infants and children is low,[1,2] and of those who do survive, many are neurologically impaired.[3] Cardiac arrest can, however, often be prevented if the clinician recognizes the symptoms of respiratory failure and/or shock and promptly initiates therapy.

Assessment of Respiratory Failure and Shock

Respiratory failure is a clinical state characterized by inadequate elimination of carbon dioxide and/or inadequate oxygenation of the blood.[4] This may be secondary to intrinsic lung or airway disease, or due to inadequate respiratory effort (e.g., the patient with apnea or shallow respiration from intracranial pathology). The terms "shock" and "respiratory failure" are used differently in pediatrics than in adult medicine. Shock is a clinical state characterized by inadequate delivery of oxygen and substrates to meet the metabolic demands of the tissues.[5-7] It may occur with a normal, increased, or most frequently, decreased cardiac output. Shock may be further classified as a compensated or decompensated condition. In compensated shock, blood pressure remains normal; decompensated shock is characterized by hypotension and often, by a low cardiac output.

As with shock, respiratory failure is often preceded by a "compensated" state in which the patient, through increased effort, is able to maintain adequate gas exchange at the expense of an increase in the work of breathing. This compensated state is characterized by the use of accessory muscles of respiration, inspiratory retractions, tachypnea, and tachycardia.

Although respiratory failure and shock may begin as clinically distinct syndromes, they progress to an indistinguishable state of cardiopulmonary failure, caused by insufficient oxygen delivery to tissues and reduced clearance of metabolites, in the final moments before arrest.

Assessment of Respiratory Performance

Signs of impending respiratory arrest include:
1) increased respiratory rate, effort, and/or diminished

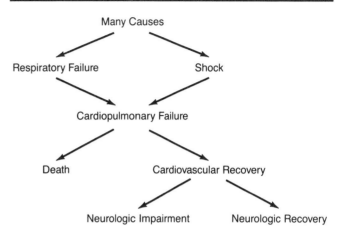

Figure 1. Pathway of various disease states leading to cardiopulmonary failure in infants and children.

inspiratory breath sounds, 2) diminished level of consciousness or response to pain, 3) poor skeletal muscle tone, or 4) cyanosis.

Normal ventilation is accomplished with minimal work. The normal respiratory rate decreases with age: it is around 40 breaths/min in the newborn, approximately 24 breaths/min in the 1-year-old child and approximately 18 breaths/min in the 18 year old. Tidal volume (the volume of each breath) remains fairly constant throughout life at approximately 6–8 mL/kg and is assessed by auscultation over the lungs, the quality of air movement, and adequacy of chest-wall excursion.

Abnormal respirations are classified as too fast (tachypnea), too slow (bradypnea), absent (apnea), and/or associated with an increased work of breathing. Minute ventilation, the product of tidal volume and respiratory rate, may be low (hypoventilation) because each breath is shallow, or because too few breaths are taken each minute. The work of breathing may be increased because of airway obstruction, pulmonary parenchymal disease, or a chest-wall disorder.

Respiratory Rate

Tachypnea is often the first manifestation of respiratory distress in infants. Tachypnea without respiratory distress ("quiet tachypnea") commonly results from an attempt to maintain normal pH in nonpulmonary diseases.

Bradypnea in an acutely ill infant or child is an ominous sign. Causes include fatigue, hypothermia, and central nervous system depression. Fatigue needs to be especially emphasized. An infant breathing at a rate of 80 breaths/min with increased respiratory effort will likely tire; a decreasing respiratory rate in a child with tachypnea is not necessarily a sign of improvement!

Respiratory Mechanics

Increased work of breathing, as evidenced by retractions with flaring of the alae nasae, may be seen in pulmonary problems ranging from airway obstruction to alveolar disease. Head bobbing with each breath is often an indication of impending respiratory failure. Extreme inspiratory efforts draw the chest in while thrusting the abdomen out, causing "see-saw" or rocky respirations.

As work of breathing increases, a greater proportion of cardiac output must be delivered to the respiratory muscles, which in turn produce more carbon dioxide. Respiratory acidosis is followed by metabolic acidosis when the work of breathing exceeds the ability to provide adequate tissue oxygenation. Tracheal intubation and mechanical ventilation are then necessary to treat decompensated respiratory failure.

Stridor (an inspiratory high pitched sound) is a sign of upper airway obstruction from the supraglottic space to the lower trachea. Some causes of upper airway obstruction include: 1) congenital abnormalities, such as vocal cord paralysis, airway tumor, or cyst, 2) infections, such as epiglottitis or croup, and 3) aspiration of a foreign body.

Prolonged expiration, usually accompanied by wheezing, is a sign of bronchial and bronchiolar obstruction, and is often caused by bronchiolitis or asthma.

Grunting is caused by premature glottic closure accompanying active chest wall contraction during early expiration. Infants grunt to increase airway pressure, thereby preserving or increasing functional residual capacity in diseases that cause accumulation of interstitial or alveolar fluid (e.g., pulmonary edema, pneumonia, atelectasis, and adult respiratory distress syndrome).

Cyanosis

Cyanosis is a fairly late and inconstant sign of respiratory failure and is best seen in the mucus membranes of the mouth and nail beds; cyanosis of the extremities alone (peripheral cyanosis) is more likely due to circulatory failure (shock) than to pulmonary failure. Arterial blood oxygen tension should be measured whenever a question of serious respiratory impairment exists, even in the absence of cyanosis.

Assessment of Cardiovascular Performance

Organ perfusion is in part dependent on cardiac output (heart rate × stroke volume) and perfusion pressure. Blood pressure is the product of cardiac output and peripheral resistance. Of these variables, heart rate and blood pressure can be measured easily; cardiac output and peripheral vascular resistance must be qualitatively assessed by examination of pulses and evaluation of tissue perfusion.

Although shock is often associated with a low cardiac output, septic and anaphylactic shock may be characterized by an increase in cardiac output and a low vascular resistance.[8] The patient then has the appearance of being well perfused with bounding pulses and a wide pulse pressure. Despite this appearance, the patient's metabolic demand may be increased in excess of the increase in oxygen delivery, and there is often a mismatch between tissue flow and metabolic demand ("distributive shock"). This form of shock may be quite subtle, and a high index of suspicion is required. Attention to the assessment signs discussed below and analysis of arterial blood gases should lead to the correct diagnosis.

Heart Rate

Normal heart rates of infants and children are given in Table 1. Sinus tachycardia is a common response to stress and may be due to anxiety, fever, hypoxia, hypercapnia or hypovolemia. The presence of tachycardia necessitates further evaluation to determine the underlying cause. When tachycardia fails to compensate adequately, hypoxia and hypercapnia with acidosis develop, and bradycardia ensues. Bradycardia in a distressed child is an ominous sign of impending cardiac arrest.

Blood Pressure

Normal blood pressure is maintained as long as the circulation compensates adequately with vasoconstriction, tachycardia, and increased cardiac contractility. When compensation fails, hypotension occurs. Hypotension is a late and often sudden sign of cardiovascular decompensation in infants and children. Even mild hypotension is therefore serious and must be treated quickly and vigorously, since cardiopulmonary arrest is often close at hand. An observed fall of 10 mmHg in systolic pressure, especially when accompanied by an

Table 1. Heart Rates in Normal Children

Age	Range	Mean
Newborn to 3 mo	85–205	140
3 mo to 2 yr	100–190	130
2 yr to 10 yr	60–140	80
>10 yr	50–100	75

increased heart rate, should prompt careful serial evaluations for other signs of shock. Normal blood pressure values for age are given in Figure 2. The lower limit of systolic blood pressure has been approximated by the formula 70 + (2 × age in years).

Peripheral Circulation

Since sinus tachycardia is nonspecific, and hypotension is a late sign of shock, the diagnosis of early shock depends on clinical assessment of stroke volume and peripheral vascular resistance. This is best assessed by

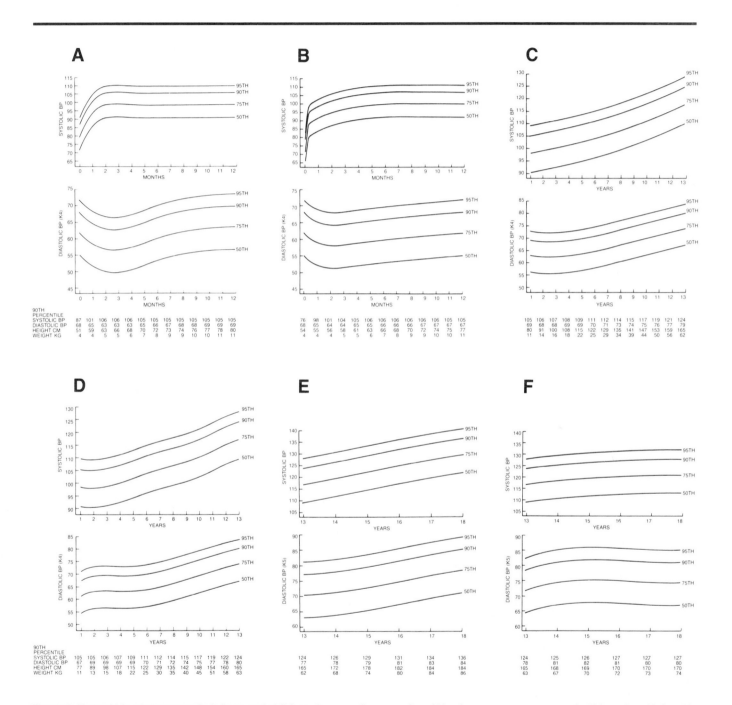

Figure 2. Normal blood pressures in infants and children. Age-specific percentiles of blood pressure measurements in A) boys from birth to 12 months, B) girls from birth to 12 months, C) boys from 1 to 13 years, D) girls from 1 to 13 years, E) boys from 13 to 18 years, and F) girls from 13 to 18 years. Korotkoff Phase IV used for diastolic blood pressure in A–D; Korotkoff Phase V in E and F. (From Report of the Second Task Force on Blood Pressure Control in Children—1987. *Pediatrics* 79:1, 1987. Reproduced by permission of *Pediatrics*.)

evaluating the presence and volume of peripheral pulses and adequacy of end-organ perfusion.

The carotid, axillary, brachial, radial, femoral, dorsalis pedis, and posterior tibial pulses are readily palpable in healthy infants and children. A discrepancy in volume between central and peripheral pulses may be due to vasoconstriction associated with hypothermia, or may be an early sign of diminished stroke volume. The palpable pulse is related to the pulse pressure (difference between systolic and diastolic pressure); as shock progresses, the pulse pressure narrows making the pulse "thready" and finally impalpable. Loss of central pulses is a premorbid sign. As previously noted, septic shock, in contrast to low-output shock, is often characterized by a wide pulse pressure and bounding pulses.

End-Organ Perfusion

Decreased perfusion of the *skin* is an early sign of shock. Normally, the hands and feet are warm, dry, and pink to the distal phalanx. As cardiac output decreases, the line of demarcation between warmth and coolness ascends toward the trunk. Slow capillary refilling (>2 seconds) after blanching is evidence of low cardiac output. In testing for capillary refill, the extremity should be lifted slightly above the level of the heart.

In children with sudden onset of *brain* ischemia, few signs of neurologic compromise precede loss of consciousness.[4] Muscular tone is lost and generalized convulsions and pupillary dilatation may occur. When hypoperfusion occurs somewhat more gradually, as in shock, symptoms are more insidious. An alteration of consciousness occurs, with confusion and lethargy. An alternating picture of agitation and lethargy is often seen, with the child quiet when undisturbed and combatative when procedures are attempted. Infants may be irritable and have a fretful look, weak cry, and wrinkled brow. After 2 months of age, an infant should normally focus on his or her parent's face. Failure to recognize parents may be an early, ominous sign of cortical hypoperfusion or cerebral dysfunction. This may only be obvious to the parents, who may not be able to describe the problem any better than "there's something wrong."

More profound hypoperfusion induces still greater changes in the level of consciousness. The child may cease to respond to verbal stimuli and, in deeper coma, may only respond to painful stimuli. Deep tendon reflexes may be depressed, pupils may be small but reactive, and a crescendo–decrescendo breathing pattern (Cheyne-Stokes) may be apparent. Hypotonia and intermittent flexor or extensor posturing may occur with prolonged cerebral hypoperfusion or extreme hypoxemia ($PaO_2 < 30$ mmHg).

Urinary output is directly proportional to glomerular filtration rate and *renal* blood flow. The rate of urinary flow is a good indicator of therapeutic progress. Normal urine output is 1–2 mL/kg/hr; a flow of less than 1 mL/kg/hr, in the absence of renal disease, is a sign of poor perfusion. An indwelling urinary catheter facilitates accurate determination of urine flow.

Rapid Cardiopulmonary Assessment
(Table 2)

Recognition of the physiologically unstable infant or child is a difficult, but critical, clinical challenge that can be made by physical examination alone. Simple laboratory tests are useful to confirm its presence and determine its severity but are not essential to make the diagnosis. Every clinician working with sick children should be able to diagnose pulmonary and circulatory failure and impending cardiopulmonary arrest based on a rapid cardiopulmonary assessment. The main goal of this assessment is to answer the question, "Does this child have pulmonary or circulatory failure that may lead to arrest?" The assessment should take less than half a minute to complete and is designed to evaluate pulmonary and cardiovascular integrity and its effect on target organs. Table 3 lists signs or historical facts that, if

Table 2. Rapid Cardiopulmonary Assessment

Respiratory Assessment	Cardiovascular Assessment
Airway Patency	*Circulation*
Breathing	Heart Rate
Rate	Blood Pressure
Air Entry	Peripheral Pulses
Chest rise	Present/absent
Breath sounds	Volume
Stridor	Skin Perfusion
Wheezing	Capillary refill time
Mechanics	Temperature
Retractions	Color
Grunting	Mottling
Color	CNS Perfusion
	Recognition of parents
	Reaction to pain
	Muscle tone
	Pupil size

Table 3. Selected Conditions Requiring a Rapid Cardiopulmonary Assessment

Any of the following:

___ Respiratory rate > 60
___ Heart rate > 180 (under 5 years)
            > 150 (over 5 years)
___ Respiratory distress
___ Trauma
___ Burns
___ Cyanosis
___ Failure to recognize parents
___ Diminished level of consciousness
___ Seizures
___ Fever with petechiae
___ Admission to an ICU

present, place the child in a high-risk group and should prompt a rapid cardiopulmonary assessment. Examination of the ill infant or child is not complete following the initial rapid cardiopulmonary assessment. These patients are often in a dynamic state, and repeated assessments are necessary.

Management of Respiratory Failure and Shock

Airway and Breathing

The goals of airway management are to anticipate and recognize respiratory problems and support or supplant those functions that are compromised or lost. In an emergency, initiation of some or all of the steps of emergency airway management is not dependent on diagnosing the cause of the respiratory dysfunction.

The airway in a child differs from that in an adult in several important ways.[10] The upper airway is more flexible and smaller, the tongue is relatively larger, the glottic opening is higher, and the smallest diameter is at the cricoid cartilage rather than the cords. The lower airways are small and the supporting cartilage not well developed; therefore, the airways are easily obstructed. The pediatric patient is further compromised by a high metabolic rate (oxygen consumption is 6–8 mL/kg/min in a child compared to 3–4 mL/kg/min in an adult), and hypoxemia therefore occurs rapidly with onset of apnea or inadequate alveolar ventilation.

A child with signs of acute respiratory distress should be immediately provided with humidified oxygen in the highest concentration available. Since anxiety adds to the child's oxygen consumption and may increase the respiratory distress, children who are alert should be allowed to remain with their parents and should be introduced to airway equipment slowly and gently. If a child is somnolent or unconscious, the airway may be obstructed by a combination of flexion of the head and flaccidity of the jaw and tongue, the latter falling against the posterior pharynx. Noninvasive methods of opening the airway should precede the use of adjuncts. Suctioning secretions from the oro- and nasopharynx may be necessary and sufficient to achieve a clear airway.

If despite a patent airway and administration of oxygen, ventilation is inadequate, as judged by insufficient chest movement and inadequate breath sounds, assisted ventilation must be provided.

Oxygen Delivery Systems

Nasal cannulae are unsuitable for children in an emergency since the inspired oxygen concentration cannot be controlled and humidification cannot be provided.

Nasal catheter use is discouraged since it has no advantage over the nasal cannula and may cause hemorrhage from trauma, or gastric distension.

An oxygen tent is a clear plastic shell that envelopes the entire child. If an $FiO_2 > 30\%$ is needed, a tent is not satisfactory.

Oxygen masks are often not tolerated by infants, but the soft vinyl pediatric mask may be accepted by children.

A face tent (or shield) is a high-flow soft plastic "bucket" which is often better tolerated by children than a mask. An oxygen concentration equal to that of the gas source can be delivered if a high flow (10–15 L/min) is provided, although stable concentrations in excess of 40% FiO_2 are not reliable.

An oxygen hood is a clear Plexiglas dome that encompasses the patient's head. It is well-tolerated by infants, allows easy access to the chest, trunk, and extremities, and allows control of oxygen concentration, temperature, and humidity. A gas inflow rate of $\geqslant$ 10–15 L/min will maintain approximately the same oxygen concentration within the hood as the gas source. As a rule, the hood is not large enough to be used with children over 1 year of age.

Airways

An oropharyngeal airway is useful in maintaining airway patency in an unconscious infant or child but may stimulate retching and vomiting in a conscious one. A range of sizes is available for children of all ages. The proper size may be estimated by placing the airway next to the face so that the flange is at the level of the central incisors and the bite block segment is parallel to the hard palate; the tip of the airway should be at the angle of the jaw.

A nasopharyngeal airway is better tolerated by conscious patients than an oropharyngeal airway. It is available in a variety of sizes (French 12–36); a 12 F airway (approximately the size of a 3.0 mm ET tube) will generally fit the nasopharynx of a term infant. The outside diameter should not be so large as to cause sustained blanching of the alae nasae. The proper length is estimated by measuring from the tip of the nose to the tragus of the ear (the cartilaginous area anterior to the external auditory canal). Small diameter airways may become obstructed by mucus, blood, vomitus, or the soft tissues of the pharynx.

Ventilation Systems

Assisted ventilation must not await placement of an endotracheal tube. In the vast majority of respiratory emergencies, infants and children can be successfully ventilated with a bag–valve–mask device, even when airway obstruction from conditions such as epiglottitis produces respiratory failure.

Face masks are available in a variety of sizes. The proper mask size should provide an air tight seal on the face and should extend from the bridge of the nose to the cleft of the chin, enveloping the nose and mouth but avoiding compression of the eyes. Failure to obtain a tight mask fit results in a lowered inspired oxygen concentration during spontaneous respiration, and precludes adequate assisted or controlled ventilation. The mask may be held on the face with a one-handed head-tilt/chin-lift maneuver. In infants and small children, the 4th and 5th fingers are hooked behind the angle of the jaw and lifted upwards, while the base of the 3rd finger supports the jaw. Caution is used to avoid compression of the submental triangle, which can result in airway obstruction. A two-person procedure, with one holding the mask to the face and the second ventilating, may be more effective maintaining a tight mask fit.

During mask ventilation, the degree of head extension required to open the airway varies. Infants and toddlers are best maintained in a neutral sniffing position without hyperextension of the head. The rescuer may have to move the head gently through a range of extension to find the optimal position; hyperextension is avoided since it can produce airway obstruction. Gastric distension can be minimized in unconscious infants and children by the applications of gentle cricoid pressure (Sellick maneuver). Excessive pressure must be avoided since it may produce tracheal compression in infants. The maneuver is performed by a second rescuer using one fingertip in infants, and the thumb and index finger in children.

Bag–Valve Devices: Self-inflating bag–valve ventilating devices are available in a variety of sizes for infants and children. Selecting an appropriately sized bag–valve device is necessary so that a sense of the patient's lung compliance is conveyed to the operator. In infants a bag volume of 250–750 mL should be used, since larger bags make it difficult to regulate the small tidal volumes. A bag–valve device should be equipped with an oxygen reservoir to deliver the highest possible oxygen concentration. Oxygen concentrations of 60–95% can be provided by a reservoir-equipped bag–valve device with a 10- to 15-L/min oxygen inflow.

Many bags are equipped with a pressure-limited pop-off valve set at 35–40 cmH$_2$O. Devices used for resuscitation should either have no pop-off valve, or one that is easily occluded, since pressures required for ventilation during CPR may exceed the pop-off limit. Ventilation pressures can best be monitored by having a manometer in line with the bag–valve device.

Bag–valve devices with a fish mouth or leaf flap operated outlet valve (e.g., the Laerdal bag) may be used to provide supplemental oxygen to an older child during spontaneous ventilation if a tight mask seal or endotracheal tube is in place. These valves open during inspiration allowing the child to inspire the gas mixture contained in the bag. Infants, however, cannot sustain the increased work of breathing required to open the outlet valve, and respiratory insufficiency may result. Bag–valve devices with spring-loaded disk or ball-operated outlet valves (e.g., Ambu) will not open during patient inspiration; gas is only delivered when the bag is compressed. Thus, many bag–valve devices are not useful as sources of supplemental oxygen, and none

are recommended for this purpose in infants.

Endotracheal Airway: When prolonged ventilation is required, or when adequate ventilation cannot be achieved with a mask attached to a bag–valve device, the face mask is replaced with an endotracheal tube.

Cuffed endotracheal tubes are indicated only in children over the age of 8 years; in children less than 8 years, the circular narrowing at the level of the cricoid cartilage serves as a functional cuff. A properly selected uncuffed tube will allow a minimal air leak at the cricoid ring; absence of an air leak indicates that excessive pressure is likely at the level of the cricoid cartilage.

Recommended tube sizes are given in Table 4. Several methods and formulas have been developed for estimating correct tube size. In one such formula, used for children > 1 year of age, the internal diameter (i.d.) in millimeters may be approximated as follows:

$$\text{i.d.} = (16 + \text{pt's age in years})/4$$

Simple visual estimation can be made by choosing an endotracheal tube with an outside diameter approximating the diameter of the child's little finger.

Adult and pediatric laryngoscopy handles are interchangeable and differ only in diameter. Blades may be curved or straight, and several sizes are available (Table 4). A straight blade is preferred in infants, since it provides greater displacement of the tongue into the floor of the mouth and better visualization of the relatively cephalad and anterior glottis.

Proper positioning of the tube must be confirmed by 1) observing symmetrical chest movement, 2) auscultating equal breath sounds over the lateral chest wall bilaterally, 3) noting absence of breath sounds over the stomach, and 4) observing condensation in the endotracheal tube during expiration.

Circulation Support

Vascular Access

Establishing vascular access for infusion of medications and fluids, and for obtaining blood specimens for laboratory examination is a crucial step in pediatric advanced life support. The intratracheal route is an alternative for the administration of some medications (see below), but intravenous or intraosseous access is mandatory for infusion of fluids. In the course of cardiopulmonary resuscitation, large volumes of fluid can be inadvertently given which may cause postresuscitative complications. In order to avoid this hazard, infusion pumps should be used for all vascular infusions in infants and children except when large volumes are deliberately given as part of the resuscitative effort. If infusion pumps are not available, mini-drips should be used and the infusion rate carefully regulated.

Table 4. Guidelines for Face Mask, Laryngoscope, and Tracheal Tube Sizes.

Patient Age	Face Mask	Laryngoscope	ID (mm)	Endotracheal Tube Size Length (cm): Midtrachea to Teeth	Suction Catheter (Fr)
Premature infant	0 Rendell-Baker 1 Vital Signs	Miller 0*	2.5, 3.0 Uncuffed	8	5 or 6
Term infant	1 Rendell-Baker 2 Vital Signs	Miller 0 or 1* Wis-Hipple 1 Robertshaw 0	3.0, 3.5 Uncuffed	10	6
6 months			3.5, 4.0 Uncuffed	12	8
1 year	2 Rendell-Baker	Wis-Hipple 1½ Robertshaw 1	4.0, 4.5 Uncuffed	12	8
2 years	3 Vital Signs	Miller 2 Flagg 2	4.5 Uncuffed	14	8
4 years	3 Rendell-Baker		5.0 Uncuffed	16	10
6 years	4 Vital Signs		5.5 Uncuffed	16	10
8 years	Small Trimar	Miller 2 MacIntosh 2	6.0 Cuffed or Uncuffed	18	10
10 years			6.5 Cuffed or Uncuffed	18	12
12 years	Ohio 2 or 3 5 Vital Signs	MacIntosh 3	7.0 Cuffed	20	12
Adolescent	Ohio 3 or 4	MacIntosh 3 Miller 3	7.0, 8.0 Cuffed	22	12

*Oxyscope modifications are available for Miller 0 and 1 blades. They may reduce the likelihood of hypoxemia during laryngoscopy in infants.

Venous Cannulation: During cardiopulmonary resuscitation, the largest and most easily accessible vein that does not require interruption of resuscitation is the preferred access site.

Central cannulation allows the use of a larger cannula and is a more direct route for drug administration than peripheral cannulation. Central access can be obtained via the femoral, internal jugular, external jugular, and in older children, the subclavian veins. The femoral vein is often used because it is relatively easily cannulated without interfering with the resuscitative effort. It may be wise to use a longer catheter for femoral catheterizations, which usually can be directed into the thorax without difficulty.

Peripheral venipuncture can be performed in veins of the scalp, arm, hand, leg, and foot. It has the disadvantage of small vessel size and distance from the central circulation.

Intraosseous Cannulation: In emergency situations, rapid vascular access is often difficult,[12,13] and intraosseous administration of fluids and medications has long been known to be a safe and effective alternate

procedure for children under six years of age.[14,15] Catecholamines,[16] whole blood, calcium, antibiotics, digitalis, heparin, lidocaine, atropine, and sodium bicarbonate have been successfully infused by the intraosseous route. Intraosseous fluid and drug administration therefore appears to be a valuable and safe technique in the treatment of critically ill infants and children and should be considered as a temporary measure during emergencies when other vascular sites are not immediately available.

Technique: The use of bone marrow needles and trephins is emphasized in the literature, but a standard 16- or 18-gauge hypodermic or spinal needle with a stylette can be inserted into the anterior surface of the tibial bone 1–3 cm below the tibial tuberosity. The needle should be directed perpendicularly or slightly inferiorly in order to avoid the epiphyseal plate. Berg[16] points out that the infusion will be successful if the needle is clearly in the marrow as evidenced by 1) lack of resistance after the needle passes through the bony cortex, 2) the needle standing upright without support, 3) the ability to aspirate bone marrow into a syringe connected to the needle, and 4) free flow of an infusion without significant subcutaneous infiltration. If the needle becomes obstructed with bone or marrow, it can be replaced with a second needle passed through the same cannulation site.

Priorities in Venous Access: Because vascular access may be extremely difficult in infants and children, a protocol is needed for the administration of drugs and fluids during resuscitation[17] (Figure 3). Medications, i.e., epinephrine, atropine, lidocaine and naloxone should be administered via the endotracheal tube, while vascular access is being sought. In children under 6 years of age, an intraosseous cannula should be immediately placed, and used for volume expansion and additional medications, should they become necessary. In older children, a cutdown of the saphenous vein or percutaneous central access should be obtained, the choice depending on the skill of the rescuers. Of the central venous access sites, the femoral is probably the safest and easiest to cannulate.

Arterial Cannulation: Arterial cannulation allows direct blood pressure measurement and easy blood sampling for oxygen and acid–base analysis. Indwelling arterial catheters can be placed percutaneously in the radial, dorsalis pedis, posterior tibial arteries, and femoral artery. Temporal artery cannulation is associated with severe complications, probably caused by emboli to the internal carotid circulation, and is best avoided.[18,19]

All indwelling arterial catheters have a risk of localized or generalized infection, air or particulate embolization, inadvertent injection of a sclerosing solution, and thrombosis of the artery. Predisposing factors for occlusion of the radial artery are: 1) age of the patient (66% in children younger than 5 years of age vs. 34.4% in those more than 5 years of age), 2) insertion technique (70% by cutdown vs. 31% by the percutaneous technique), and 3) duration of cannulation (71.4% in those longer than 4 days vs. 43.6% in those less than 4 days).[20] A modified Allen test, to assess the adequacy of collateral circulation from the ulnar artery, must be performed before radial artery cannulation.

Volume Expansion

In the treatment of shock, the type of fluid used for initial volume expansion is controversial. Crystalloid solutions, such as lactated Ringer's solution and normal saline are inexpensive, readily available, free from reactions, and they effectively expand the interstitial water space and correct sodium deficits, but are not efficient in expanding circulating volume. Ringer's lactate may be preferred since it avoids hyperchloremic acidosis that may result from the infusion of large volumes of sodium chloride. Dextrose-containing solutions are best not given unless hypoglycemia is documented; iatrogenic hyperglycemia may induce an osmotic diuresis. Colloids, such as 5% albumin, fresh frozen plasma, blood, and the synthetic colloids (Hetastarch, Dextran 40, Dextran 60), are much more effective in rapidly expanding the

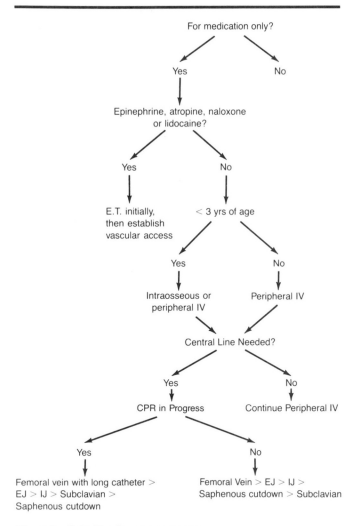

Figure 3. Priorities in venous access.

intravascular compartment. Two disadvantages are potential adverse reactions and higher cost. In traumatic shock, blood should be given as soon as it is available. Blood administration may also be helpful in septic and other forms of shock, but is not a first line volume expander in these settings.

An underlying principle of volume expansion is to give a volume bolus as rapidly as possible, reassess the patient, and then give additional boluses with frequent reassessment. In the patient with hypovolemic shock, 20 mL/kg of crystalloid solution is given, the child is reassessed, and if perfusion is still diminished, an additional 20 mL/kg of volume is given. Subsequent volume, either colloid or crystalloid, is given as needed. The child with hypovolemic shock often requires at least 40–60 mL/kg in the first hour of resuscitation and, occasionally, up to 100–200 mL/kg may be needed. In septic shock, 60–80 mL/kg is often required in the first hour. The key to successful fluid therapy is infusion of a sufficient amount of fluid based on frequent patient assessment.

Pharmacologic Support

Acute

General Guidelines: During cardiac arrest, intravenous drug delivery is preferred, but since it may be difficult to achieve, the endotracheal route can be used to deliver atropine, epinephrine, and lidocaine.[21] Optimal endotracheal doses for pediatric patients are not known. Although studies suggest that a larger dose must be given endotracheally than intravenously to produce the same hemodynamic effects,[22,23] in the absence of data in children, at least the same dose given intravenously is recommended for endotracheal administration. Medications must be injected as deeply as possible into the tracheobronchial tree in order to be absorbed, and should therefore be diluted in 1–2 mL of normal saline and injected through a catheter passed beyond the endotracheal tube tip, followed by several positive-pressure ventilations.

Central venous administration of medications during external chest compressions provides more rapid onset and higher peak concentrations than peripheral venous injections and is therefore the preferred route. Medications, including catecholamines,[16] are well absorbed from the bone marrow; intraosseous injections can therefore be considered equivalent to intravenous injections and are preferable to the endotracheal route.

Oxygen: Oxygen should be administered in all arrest situations, in any condition in which hypoxemias is suspected, and in any condition of respiratory difficulty that may lead to cardiac arrest (e.g., severe asthma, croup, epiglottitis, foreign body obstruction). Oxygen should not be withheld in an emergency, even if the measured arterial oxygen tension is high, since oxygen delivery to tissues may still be compromised by a low cardiac output.

Dose: The highest available oxygen concentration should be used.

Epinephrine: The most common rhythm disturbances in pediatric arrest patients are asystole and bradycardia, often associated with absent pulses (i.e., electromechanical dissociation). In these settings, epinephrine may generate electrical and mechanical activity of the heart.

Dose: 0.01 mg/kg of 1:10,000 solution (0.1 mL/kg) given via IV, ET, or intraosseous route. Dose may be repeated at 5-minute intervals.

Sodium Bicarbonate: Since respiratory failure is the major cause of cardiac arrest in pediatric patients, prompt and efficient ventilation is essential for management of both acidemia and hypoxemia of arrest. Treatment of the metabolic component of acidosis includes hyperventilation to reduce partial pressure of CO_2 and, if necessary, $NaHCO_3$ infusion. Administration of this medication results in the production of carbon dioxide which, since it crosses cell membranes more rapidly than bicarbonate, can transiently worsen intracellular acidosis[24] and result in impaired myocardial performance.[25,26] In view of these potential toxicities, sodium bicarbonate is not indicated in mild-to-moderate metabolic acidosis, especially when due to inadequate circulating volume; the acidosis will resolve with ventilation and volume replacement. In severe acidosis (pH < 7.20) use of bicarbonate is controversial. It is unclear whether data in adults are applicable in children.

Dose: 1 mEq/kg via IV or intraosseous route. Further doses of sodium bicarbonate should be based on measurements of arterial pH and $PaCO_2$. When these measurements are not available, subsequent doses of sodium bicarbonate (0.5 mEq/kg) may be given every 10 minutes of continued cardiac arrest.

Atropine: Atropine is used to treat bradycardia accompanied by poor perfusion or hypotension, to diminish the vagally mediated bradycardia accompanying intubation attempts, and in the uncommon event of symptomatic bradycardia with atrioventricular block. Low doses of atropine may be accompanied by paradoxical bradycardia in infants; therefore, a minimum dose of 0.1 mg should be used. When used to block vagal-induced bradycardia during intubation, it is important to recognize that atropine may also mask hypoxemia-induced bradycardia.

Dose: It is important to give a vagolytic dose — 0.02 mg/kg via IV, ET, or intraosseous route, with a minimum dose of 0.1 mg and a maximum dose of 1.0 mg. Atropine may be repeated in 5-minute intervals to maximum dose of 1.0 mg in a child and 2.0 mg in an adolescent.

Glucose: During cardiac resuscitation of an infant or child, a rapid bedside glucose test should be obtained and glucose administered if hypoglycemia is present. It may also be indicated in infants and children who fail to respond to the usual resuscitation measures.

Dose: 0.5–1.0 g/kg IV in a solution of D25W (2–4 mL/kg). Since glucose is supplied as D50W, it must be diluted 1:1 with sterile water.

Calcium Chloride: Based on recent evidence, there is no support for the use of calcium in asystole or in electromechanical dissociation. Calcium is indicated only when hypocalcemia has been documented or is suspected, and should be considered in the treatment of hyperkalemia, hypermagnesemia, and following calcium channel blocker overdose.

Dose: Calcium is available in three different salts; calcium chloride is the recommended form since it delivers ionized calcium directly, whereas the gluconate and gluceptate salts must be first hepatically metabolized.

The currently recommended dose of 5–7 mg/kg of elemental calcium IV or intraosseous route is based on its safe use in anesthetized patients. Calcium chloride is a 10% solution (100 mg/mL of the calcium salt) that contains 1.36 mEq of elemental calcium per milliliter (27.2 mg/mL of elemental calcium). Therefore, 0.2–0.25

mL/kg of calcium chloride will deliver 5–7 mg/kg of elemental calcium. Since repeated doses of calcium increase the risk of morbidity, it is recommended that the initial dose be repeated only one time in 10 minutes and that further doses be based on measured calcium deficiency. Rates of 2–20 μg/kg/min have been effective.

Stabilization

The following medications may be used to help stabilize a child in whom blood pressure, or perfusion, remain unstable following fluid administration for shock, or in the postresuscitation phase. Preferably these medications should be infused into a central or secure peripheral IV, and they should not be mixed with sodium bicarbonate or other alkaline solutions which will inactivate them.

Catecholamines may be diluted in a number of intravenous solutions: D5W, D10W , D5W ½ NS, D5NS, or Ringer's lactate for continuous infusion. In the postarrest setting, the infusion should be given rapidly (10–20 mL/hr) until an effect is achieved (i.e., an increase in heart rate or blood pressure); the rate is then decreased to the desired dose. Failure to initially increase the infusion rate may significantly delay delivery of medication until the dead space in the intravenous tubing and catheter are filled at the slow infusion rates used in children. All of the catecholamines are rapidly metabolized, so decreasing the infusion rate as soon as a physiologic effect is seen prevents toxicity.

Isoproterenol: Isoproterenol may be used to treat hemodynamically significant bradycardia due to heart block resistant to atropine, or recurring shortly after an atropine dose. Isoproterenol may be used to increase the heart rate (if it is < 80 beats/min) in the infant with poor perfusion, even if the measured blood pressure is normal. Epinephrine infusion, however, is preferable in this setting since it does not cause as large a fall in diastolic blood pressure. Isoproterenol potentially compromises coronary perfusion since it has no alpha-adrenergic effects and decreases diastolic blood pressure. Furthermore, isoproterenol increases myocardial oxygen demand by increasing myocardial contractility and heart rate. The latter causes further diminution in coronary perfusion by decreasing diastolic filling time. Therefore, isoproterenol should be used only for the treatment of bradycardia, and the infusion should not be advanced beyond that needed to increase the heart rate.

Dose: Isoproterenol must be administered by a constant infusion pump. The infusion is prepared as per Table 5. Start with 1 ml/kg/hr to deliver 0.1 μg/kg/min. Rates up to 1.0 μg/kg/min have been effective. Adjust to the patient's clinical response, with tachycardia acting as the major limiting factor.

Dopamine: Dopamine is indicated for the treatment of hypotension and/or poor peripheral perfusion in the pediatric patient in whom a stable rhythm is present or has been restored. Dopamine may produce tachycardia, excessive increases in blood pressure, and arrhythmias. High infusion rates may produce extremity ischemia.

Dose: Dopamine must be delivered by a constant infusion pump. Infusions can be prepared according to Table 5. The infusion is adjusted according to clinical response. Infusion rates above 20 μg/kg/min produce predominant vasoconstrictive effects without any further inotropic effect and should be used with caution. If further inotropic effect is needed, epinephrine with its direct alpha- and beta-adrenergic effects is preferable.

Dobutamine: Dobutamine is indicated for the treatment of hypotension and/or poor perfusion in the postresuscitation phase. It has less peripheral vascular action than dopamine; the latter may therefore be preferred in the hypotensive patient. Dobutamine may produce tachycardia, and/or tachyarrhythmia. Nausea, vomiting, hypertension, and hypotension are less frequent side effects.

Dose: Dobutamine must be infused by a constant infusion pump. Infusions can be prepared according to Table 5. Begin the infusion at 5–10 mL/hr (5–10 μg /kg/min) and adjust according to clinical response; infusion rates over 20 μg/kg/min, if needed, suggest that a more potent agent, such as epinephrine, should be used.

Epinephrine Infusion: Epinephrine is a very potent catecholamine which is indicated in patients with hypotensive shock, or who are hemodynamically unstable. Epinephrine can cause ventricular ectopy as well as supraventricular and ventricular tachycardia. High infusion rates (> 0.5–0.6 μg/kg/min) can produce profound vasoconstriction, which may compromise extremity and skin blood flow.

Dose: Epinephrine infusions are prepared according to Table 5. Begin the infusion at 1–2 mL/hr (0.1–0.2 μg/kg/min) and adjust every 5 minutes until the desired clinical effect is achieved. Rates up to 10 mL/hr (1 μg/kg/min) may be used with caution.

Table 5. Preparation of Catecholamine Infusions in Children

Isoproterenol Epinephrine	0.6 × body weight (in kg) is the mg dose added to make 100 mL	Then 1 mL/hr delivers 0.1 μg/kg/min
Dopamine Dobutamine	6 × body weight (in kg) is the mg dose added to make 100 mL	Then 1 mL/hr delivers 1 μg/kg/min

Cardiac Rhythm Disturbances

Life-threatening cardiac rhythm disturbances in infants and children are more often the result than the cause of acute emergencies.

The electrocardiogram should be monitored in any child who has sustained, or is at risk for, a cardiac or pulmonary arrest. One limitation of electrocardiographic monitoring is that it gives no information about the effectiveness of myocardial contractility or adequacy of tissue perfusion. Management decisions must therefore always be based on clinical evaluation of the patient in correlation with information derived from the electrocardiogram.

The Normal Heart Rate

The normal heart rate in children is related to age and is influenced by level of activity and pathologic conditions such as fever, blood loss, etc. Table 1 is a composite of several studies[27-30] and shows the wide variation in the normal heart rate and its gradual decrease with age. It should be appreciated that a febrile infant with a normal cardiovascular state can achieve heart rates close to 200 beats/min. The differentiation of sinus tachycardia in a sick infant, from paroxysmal supraventricular tachycardia as a cause of vascular collapse, can be problematic and is discussed below.

Abnormal Rhythms

In infants and children, arrhythmias should be treated as an emergency only if:

- They compromise cardiac output or
- They have the potential for degenerating into a rhythm that compromises cardiac output.

Since cardiac output (CO) is the product of stroke volume (SV) and heart rate (HR), both very rapid rates and very slow rates may adversely effect cardiac output. Very rapid rates compromise diastolic filling and preclude adequate stroke volume, and very slow rates will not eject sufficient CO even though the stroke volume is increased. Rhythm disturbances, such as premature ventricular contractions, may require cardiac evaluation but do not usually require emergency treatment in children.

When rapid rates produce cardiovascular instability, they should be treated by the most rapid and effective method — synchronized cardioversion. In the non-emergency situation, there are other methods of management, but a discussion of these is beyond the purpose of this chapter.

The slow rhythms associated with an acute cardio-pulmonary emergency in children usually result from atrioventricular block or suppression of normal impulse generation caused by a combination of acidosis and hypoxemia. Initial therapy consists of proper ventilation and oxygenation; if needed, medications such as atropine and sympathomimetics are useful.

Supraventricular Tachycardia (SVT)

This rapid regular rhythm is often paroxysmal and, though better tolerated in older children, can cause cardiovascular collapse with clinical evidence of shock in infants. The heart rate varies with age; in infants it is usually around 240 beats/min, but can be as high as 300 beats/min. The rhythm is usually regular since associated atrioventricular block is rare. QRS duration is normal in over 90% of children; a wide QRS resulting from aberrant conduction is infrequently seen.[33]

In severely ill infants it may be difficult to distinguish sinus tachycardia (ST) secondary to an underlying illness (most commonly sepsis or hypovolemia) from supraventricular tachycardia (SVT) with secondary cardiogenic shock. The following may be helpful in the differentiation:

Heart rate: In ST, usually < 200 beats/min; in SVT, more likely > 230 beats/min.

ECG: P waves may be difficult to see in both at rates > 200 /min. In ST, rate may vary from beat to beat. In SVT there is no beat-to-beat variation; termination is abrupt.

Chest X-Ray: In SVT sufficient to cause cardiovascular instability, heart size may be enlarged. In ST, depending on the cause, it is often normal.

Synchronized cardioversion (0.5–1.0 J/kg) is the treatment of choice for patients with SVT who have cardiovascular instability. If SVT persists, the dose is increased to 2.0 J/kg. If conversion still does not occur, the diagnosis may not be correct; the child may have ST.

In nonemergency situations various techniques and medications are used, but a discussion of these is beyond the scope of this chapter. Verapamil has been associated with irreversible cardiovascular collapse in infants and should therefore be used with caution, if at all, in this age group.[34,35]

Ventricular Tachycardia (VT)

Heart rate may vary from close to normal to above 400 beats/min. Slow rates may be well tolerated, but rapid rates compromise cardiac output and may degenerate into ventricular fibrillation. The majority of children with VT have underlying structural heart disease or a prolonged QT interval. Other causes include hypoxia, acidosis, electrolyte imbalance, and insults caused by medications and poisons, especially the tricyclic anti-depressants. It may be difficult to differentiate SVT from VT; fortunately, aberrant conduction is present in only 10% of children with SVT.

In the presence of cardiovascular instability with clinical evidence of low cardiac output, synchronized cardioversion (0.5–1.0 J/kg) is the treatment of choice. A lidocaine bolus (1.0 mg/kg) prior to cardioversion results in a higher success rate; infusion therapy with lidocaine

20–50 μg/kg/min will help maintain the rhythm. If lidocaine is unsuccessful, bretylium is the next agent of choice. If initial cardioversion is unsuccessful, the electric dose should be increased to 2.0 J/kg.

Bradycardias

Sinus bradycardia, sinus node arrest with a slow junctional or ventricular escape, and various degrees of atrioventricular block are the most common terminal rhythms in children with cardiopulmonary arrest.[36] In the context of cardiopulmonary resuscitation, it is not important to diagnose the exact rhythm.

Every slow rhythm associated with evidence of a poor cardiac output is first treated by ensuring good ventilation and oxygenation and by external chest compressions. Medications, especially epinephrine, can then be used (see above).

Ventricular Fibrillation (VF)

VF is an uncommon terminal event in the pediatric age group (9%)[37] and is especially rare in infants. Defibrillation should be attempted only if VF is demonstrated by ECG monitoring.

Electromechanical Dissociation (EMD)

Underlying causes of EMD must be sought and corrected. These include hypoxemia, severe acidosis, tension pneumothorax, and hypovolemia. EMD is treated with ALS support using the same approach used for asystole.

Defibrillation and Synchronized Cardioversion

The ideal paddle size for the pediatric patient is not currently known. The largest electrode size that allows good chest contact over its entire area and which allows the two electrodes to be well separated, is preferred. Among currently available electrode paddles, the 4.5-cm diameter is adequate for infants, and the 8.0-cm and 13-cm paddles for older children.

The optimal energy dose for defibrillation has not been conclusively established for infants and children. The controversy over a relationship between patient weight and optimal energy dose is recognized. Nevertheless, the available data in the pediatric age group suggest that a dose of 2 J/kg be used initially. If defibrillation is not successful, the dose should be doubled and repeated twice, if necessary. If VF continues, attention should be turned to adequacy of ventilation, oxygenation, correction of acidosis, and hypothermia before another attempt is made.

Pharmacologic Management of Ventricular Arrhythmias

Lidocaine

Lidocaine should be administered to the child with ventricular tachycardia, ventricular fibrillation, or to the hemodynamically unstable child with ventricular couplets. Its use in a hemodynamically stable child with frequent PVC's is controversial, but probably unnecessary. A constant infusion should be used in ventricular tachycardia or ventricular fibrillation that reverts after a lidocaine bolus.

Dose: 1 mg/kg IV, ET, or via intraosseous route. Another dose can be given in 10–15 minutes, but if this is required, a continuous infusion of 120 mg lidocaine in 100 mL of D5W at a rate of 20–50 μg/kg/min (1–2.5 mL/kg/hr) should be used. To assure adequate plasma concentrations, the patient should receive a 1 mg/kg bolus of lidocaine at the time the infusion is begun. In the presence of shock or known liver disease, the infusion should be started at 1 mL/kg/hr to prevent toxicity from impaired lidocaine clearance.

Bretylium Tosylate

There is currently no published information on the use of bretylium in pediatric patients. The benefits of bretylium in adults suggest that it would also be useful in children in the treatment of ventricular fibrillation and tachycardia resistant to defibrillation (or cardioversion and lidocaine).

Dose: 5 mg/kg by rapid intravenous infusion followed by another attempt at electrical defibrillation. If ventricular fibrillation persists despite this dose and countershock, the dose can be increased to 10 mg/kg and the countershock repeated.

Bretylium may also be helpful in refractory or recurrent ventricular tachycardia. It should be administered in a dose of 5 mg/kg over 8–10 minutes since, in the conscious patient, nausea and vomiting may follow more rapid administration. If necessary, this dose may be repeated in 20 minutes.

Postresuscitation Care

Principles of Care

Any infant or child who has suffered a respiratory or cardiac arrest, no matter how good the initial response to resuscitation, should have repeated and regular cardiopulmonary assessments and should be transferred to a pediatric intensive care unit for further observation and care.

General postresuscitation care prior to and during transport includes the following:

1. Humidified oxygen at the highest attainable concentration should be provided until objective

assessment by an arterial blood gas indicates that less oxygen is needed.

2. Regular and repeated cardiopulmonary assessments including a) continuous ECG monitoring of heart rate and rhythm, b) blood pressure recording, directly by intraarterial cannula or indirectly by a Doppler measuring device or sphygmomanometer, every 5 minutes until stable and every 15 minutes thereafter, c) evaluation of peripheral circulation and end-organ perfusion, including skin temperature, capillary refill, quality of distal pulses, level of consciousness, and urine output (the latter can best be monitored if an indwelling Foley catheter has been inserted), d) evaluation of ventilation by observing chest motion, use of accessory muscles, nasal flaring, auscultation of lung fields, and evaluation of arterial blood gases. In addition, continuous noninvasive monitoring of oxygenation is helpful in preventing episodes of hypoxemia, e) serial neurologic exams.

3. Optimally, there should be two well-secured, functioning intravenous lines. The following are guidelines for maintenance fluids:

   < 10 kg: an infusion of D10W with ¼% NS at a rate of 4 mL/kg/hr.

   10–20 kg: an infusion of D5W with ¼% NS at a rate of 40 mL/hr + (2 mL/kg/hr for kg > 10); e.g., maintenance rate for a 15-kg child is 40 + (2 × 5) = 50 mL/hr.

   > 20 kg: an infusion of D5W in ¼% NS at a rate of 40 + 1 mL/kg/hr; e.g., maintenance rate for a 30-kg child is 40 + 30 = 70 mL/hr.

4. Blood studies are determined by specific circumstances but may include arterial blood gases, electrolytes, calcium, glucose, and hematocrit. Arterial blood gas analysis, after at least a 15-minute period of equilibration on the ventilating system to be used during transport, should be repeated just prior to transport.

5. A nasogastric tube to gravity drainage is useful to keep the stomach decompressed, especially in patients receiving positive-pressure ventilation. This step is almost always indicated in critically ill children, especially if they are obtunded.

6. A search should be instituted for the precipitating cause of the arrest, and if appropriate, therapy (e.g., antibiotics) should be started.

7. Careful attention should be given to preserving body temperature. This is especially, but not exclusively, important in infants. The method is determined, in part, by need for exposure for monitoring and therapy. Prior to transport, overhead heating units can be used for infants and heating lamps for children. During transport, portable incubators are useful for infants; older children should be covered, including the head, which represents a relatively large portion of the body surface.

Pediatric Transport System[39]

The goals of postresuscitation care and transport are to avoid secondary organ injury and have the patient arrive in the best possible physiologic state. The airway should be secured and ventilation carefully assessed. Frequent examination of peripheral perfusion and organ function is essential to making an early diagnosis of organ dysfunction and thus permitting early therapy. Finally, a system establishing good communication between the referring and accepting hospitals can improve patient outcome.

Every pediatric tertiary care facility should be part of an organized pediatric transport system. Such a system is usually regionalized, with central control at a pediatric tertiary care facility, under the direction of a physician trained in pediatric emergency or critical care, and should be capable of rapidly delivering advanced pediatric care at the referring hospital and of maintaining that level of care during transport. Transportation of a critically ill infant or child is best performed by a team experienced in pediatric transport and care, even if this causes a delay in the referring institution awaiting arrival of this team. Part of the responsibility of both the referring facility and the tertiary care unit is to establish well-defined protocols dealing with specific clinical situations. Protocols for transporting pediatric patients directly to hospitals and facilities equipped to handle their critical care needs should be included in EMS protocols so as to avoid a secondary transport.[40,41]

Critical to the success of a transport system is early communication between the referring and the tertiary care facilities. When contacting a tertiary care facility, the following information should be transmitted:

- The child's name, age, and weight.
- A description of the child's current illness and significant past medical history, including medications.
- The child's present clinical state, including measured heart rate, respiratory rate, blood pressure, and temperature, as well as assessment of capillary refill and distal pulses.
- Laboratory data, especially a recent arterial blood gas.
- The number of intravenous lines, infusion rate, and medications given.
- Ventilator settings.

A transport medical record should include a legible copy of the history, physical findings, laboratory data, medications, response to therapy, current clinical findings, name and telephone number of the referring and family physicians, and the names and telephone numbers of family member(s) who were notified of the transfer. Vital sign flow sheets, nurse's notes, and a copy of all x-rays should accompany the patient.

References

1. Gillis J, Dickson D, Rieder M, et al: Results of inpatient pediatric resuscitation. *Crit Care Med* 14:469, 1986.
2. Friesen RM, Duncan P, Tweed WA, et al: Appraisal of pediatric cardiopulmonary resuscitation. *Can Med Assoc J* 126:1055, 1982.
3. O'Rourke PP: Outcome of children who are apneic and pulseless in the emergency room. *Crit Care Med* 14:466, 1986.
4. Downes JJ, Fulgencio T, Raphaely RC: Acute respiratory failure in infants and children. *Pediatr Clin North Am* 19:423, 1972.
5. Crone RK: Acute circulatory failure in children. *Pediatr Clin North Am* 27:525, 1980.
6. Perkin RM, Levin DL: Shock in the pediatric patient, Part I. *J Pediatr* 101:319, 1982.
7. Perkin RM, Levin DL: Shock in the pediatric patient, Part II. *J Pediatr* 101:319, 1982.
8. Ellner JJ: Septic shock. *Pediatr Clin North Am* 30:365, 1983.
9. Plum F, Posner JB: *The Diagnosis of Stupor and Coma,* 3 ed, Philadelphia, Davis, 1980.
10. Eckenhoff JE: Some anatomic considerations of the infant larynx influencing endotracheal anesthesia. *Anesthesiology* 12:401, 1951.
11. Sellick BA: Cricoid pressure to control regurgitation of stomach contents during induction of anesthesia, preliminary communication. *Lancet* 2:404, 1961.
12. Rosetti VA, Thompson BM, Aprahamian C, et al: Difficulty and delay in intravascular access in pediatric arrests, abstracted. *Ann Emerg Med* 13:406, 1984.
13. Rosetti VA, Thompson BM, Miller J, et al: Intraosseous infusion: An alternative route of pediatric vascular access. *Ann Emerg Med* 14:885, 1985.
14. Meola F: Bone marrow infusions as a routine procedure in children. *J Pediatr* 25:13, 1944.
15. Heinild S, Sondergaard T, Tudvad F: Bone marrow infusion in childhood: Experiences from 1,000 infusions. *J Pediatr* 30:400, 1947.
16. Berg RA: Emergency infusion of catecholamines into bone marrow. *Am J Dis Child* 138:810, 1984.
17. Kanter RK, Zimmerman JJ, Strauss RN, et al: Pediatric emergency intravenous access: Evaluation of a protocol. *Am J Dis Child* 140:132, 1986.
18. Simmons MA, Levine RL, Lubchenco LO, et al: Warning, serious sequelae of temporal artery catheterization. *J Pediatr* 92:284, 1978.
19. Bull MJ, Schreiner RL, Garg BP, et al: Neurologic complications following temporal artery catheterizations. *J Pediatr* 96:1071, 1980.
20. Miyasaka K, Edmonds JF, Conn AW: Complications of radial artery lines in the pediatric patient. *Can Aneasth Soc J* 23:9, 1976.
21. Ward JT, Jr: Endotracheal drug therapy. *Am J Emerg Med* 1:71, 1983.
22. Roberts JR, Greenburg MI, Knaub MA, et al: Blood levels following intravenous and endotracheal epinephrine administration. *JACEP* 8:53, 1979.
23. Roberts JR, Greenburg MI, Knaub MA, et al: Comparison of the pharmacological effects of epinephrine administered by the intravenous and endotracheal routes. *JACEP* 7:260, 1978.
24. Cohen RD, Simpson BR, Goodwin FJ, et al: The early effects of infusion of sodium bicarbonate and sodium lactate on intracellular hydrogen ion activity in dogs. *Clin Sci* 33:233, 1967.
25. Clancy RL, Cingolani HE, Taylor RR, et al: Influence of sodium bicarbonate on myocardial performance. *Am J Physiol* 212:917, 1967.
26. Graf H, Leach W, Arieff AI: Evidence for a detrimental effect of bicarbonate therapy in hypoxic lactic acidosis. *Science* 227:754, 1985.
27. Alimurung MM, Lester GJ, Nadas AS, et al: The unipolar precordial and extremity electrocardiogram in normal infants and children. *Circulation* 4:420, 1951.
28. Ziegler RF: *Electrocardiographic Studies in Normal Infants and Children.* Charles C. Thomas, Springfield, Ill 1951.
29. Furman RA, Halloran WR: Electrocardiogram in first two months of life. *J Pediatr* 39:307, 1951.
30. Tudbury PB, Atkinson DW: The electrocardiogram of 100 normal infants and young children. *J Pediatr* 34:466, 1950.
31. Olley PH: Cardiac arrhythmias, in Keith JD, Rowe RD, Vlad P, (eds): *Heart Disease in Infancy and Childhood, ed 3.* New York, Macmillan Publishing Co, Inc, 1978, pp 279-280.
32. Gikony BM, Dunnigan A, Benson DW Jr: Cardiovascular collapse in infants: association with paroxysmal atrial tachycardia. *Pediatrics.* 76:922, 1985.
33. Garson A Jr: Supraventricular tachycardia, in Gillette PC, Garson A Jr. (eds): *Pediatric Cardiac Dysrhythmias,* New York, Grune and Stratton, 1981.
34. Radford D: Side effects of verapamil in infants. *Arch Dis Child* 58:465, 1983.
35. Epstein ML, Kiel EA, Victorica BE: Cardiac decompensation following verapamil therapy in infants with supraventricular tachycardia. *Pediatrics* 75:737, 1985.
36. Walsh CK, Krongrad E: Terminal cardiac electrical activity in pediatric patients. *Am J Cardiol* 51:557, 1983.
37. Eisenberg M, Bergner L, Hallstrom A: Epidemiology of cardiac arrest and resuscitation in children. *Ann Emerg Med* 12:672, 1983.
38. Chameides L, Brown GE, Raye JR, et al: Guidelines for defibrillation in infants and children: Report of the American Heart Association Target Activity Group: Cardiopulmonary resuscitation in the young. *Circulation* 56 (suppl):502A, 1977.
39. Guidelines for air and ground transportation of pediatric patients. American Academy of Pediatrics Committee on Hospital Care. *Pediatrics* 78:943, 1986.
40. Boyd D: Comprehensive regional trauma and emergency medical delivery systems: A goal of the 1980's. *Crit Care Q* 5:11, 1982.
41. Haller JA, Shorter N, Miller D, et al: Organization and function of a regional pediatric trauma center: Does a system of management improve outcome? *J Trauma* 23:691, 1983.

Medicolegal Aspects of Cardiopulmonary Resuscitation (CPR) and Emergency Cardiac Care (ECC)

Chapter 19

Just as the preferred approach to the problem of sudden death is prevention, the preferred approach to potential liability in CPR and ECC is prevention. This implies a definition of foreseeable problem areas and appropriate strategies to deal with identified points of legal vulnerability. The touchstone for prevention of legal liability in CPR and ECC, as in other forms of medical care delivery, is good quality medical care.

In considering the quality of ECC it is important to emphasize that the provider is not obliged to render the best possible care to the patient. Rather, the provider must provide care appropriate to the patient's condition and desires. Increasing attention is focused on patients' rights, and an awareness and respect for them is part of the obligation of care providers. The physician's decision to withhold or withdraw life-sustaining care should not be arbitrary but should reflect the best possible assessment of the condition of the patient (diagnostic certainty), the patient's prognosis to the extent that this can be determined (including appropriate protection of the patient's life and well-being while diagnosis and prognosis remain in doubt), the desires of the patient, and the availability of certain medical care capabilities.

The preceding chapters of this text rely on the "Standards and Guidelines for Cardiopulmonary Resuscitation (CPR) and Emergency Cardiac Care (ECC)" that were published in the *Journal of the American Medical Association (JAMA)* in June 1986. Accordingly, they represent the "standard of care" for a wide range of cardiovascular emergencies, and emergency cardiac care provided according to these standards would be generally accepted as beyond reproach. With such an objective "standard of care" available care providers can take steps to bring their practice within these standards and guidelines, and in doing so, they should decrease liability risk significantly. In addition to "standard of care" issues, however, are issues of decision making, including whether to provide or withhold CPR or ECC, when to discontinue BLS, and whether to suspend or continue life support. These issues have become increasingly important and will be addressed in this chapter in addition to general concepts of legal liability and some pertinent recent case law.

General Concepts of Legal Liability

The physician's duty to his patient is generally considered by the courts as contractual in nature. It is established when the physician–patient relationship is established. The contract is implied since no actual terms of agreement are usually expressed. The physician's duty begins when the patient presents him- or herself for medical care and the physician undertakes to provide that care. In certain circumstances, such as in an emergency facility which holds itself out as such, as discussed below, the physician responsible may not have the option to refuse to undertake the care of the patient.

While the basis of the physician–patient relationship may be considered contractual, the legal action is usually based on the claim that the physician failed to exercise "reasonable care" in his treatment of the patient and that the physician's failure was the direct cause of the patient's injury. The duty to exercise reasonable care is imposed by the law on every man with regard to his dealings with every other man. When failure to exercise reasonable care results in injury, the injured party has a legal right to an action for recovery or compensation. In legal parlance, this is known as a "tort" — a civil wrong based on the violation of the duty to exercise reasonable care, a violation resulting in the injury of another.

Ingredients of a Malpractice Action

There are four elements that must be established if a malpractice claim is to be successful. The plaintiff, i.e., the patient or his or her representative making the claim against the physician, must establish

1. that a duty to provide care existed on the part of the physician, i.e., that a physician–patient relationship existed;
2. that a breach of the duty to provide reasonable care was committed, i.e., that the physician was negligent;
3. that the patient suffered an injury;
4. that there was a cause-and-effect relationship between the breach of medical practice or duty and the injury that the patient sustained, i.e., that the physician's negligence was the proximate cause of the patient's injury.

The Physician–Patient Relationship and the Duty of Care

The physician–patient relationship establishes the duty to provide care conforming to accepted standards of medical practice and can be established in a number of ways. It is most frequently instituted when a physician accepts an individual as a patient. When a patient seeks medical care at a hospital emergency facility, the duty to perform in the best interest of the patient may be established by the patient arriving at the emergency facility and indicating one way or another that he is seeking care. The duty to perform in the patient's best interests may be established even when the patient is unconscious. For example, the arrival of a cardiac arrest victim at an emergency department will establish a duty to perform in the best interest of the patient because the law considers that, were the patient able to communicate, he would request appropriate medical care.

On the other hand, no duty is usually owed by a physician confronted by an unknown person who has collapsed on the street. While a moral and ethical obligation to care for the collapsed individual may exist, a legal obligation usually does not. However, once emergency care is initiated by a physician passerby, the duty to perform reasonably and not to abandon is established.

Negligence and the Standard of Care

How are the patient, the physician, and the court to establish the kind of care that the patient should have received in order to decide whether or not the care provided by the physician (or the nurse, or the paraprofessional, or the hospital) was adequate or negligent? The courts have defined the physician's duty to the patient in rather specific terms:

The physician is required to possess that degree of knowledge and skill, and to exercise that degree of care, judgment, and skill which other physicians of good standing of the same school or system of practice usually exercise in the same or similar localities under like or similar circumstances.[1,2]

The physician's performance is measured against the medical knowledge and professional performance of the average reputable physician in his community, not against that of the most skillful physician. This standard of conduct can usually be defined only through the use of expert testimony and the opinions of the defendant's colleagues unless the physician's performance was so obviously negligent as to be recognized as such by the common knowledge of the layperson. Usually, the physician's peers by their testimony ("the expert witness") inform the judge or jury what constitutes the usual performance of a physician under the same or similar circumstances. In the last analysis, therefore, the physician is judged to a large extent by his colleagues through their testimony, although the judge or the jury has the final say in deciding whether or not the physician's performance measured up to the standard offered by the medical experts.

Increasingly, the standard of care for the physician is based on a nationwide standard rather than on a local standard. This is particularly the rule for medical specialists. The reference in the definition above to "the same or similar localities" is generally left out when the legal duty of the medical specialist is stated. When criteria for performance are widely promulgated on a national basis, as they are in the area of CPR and ECC, it is very likely that the standard against which performance will be judged by the court will be a national standard.

The heart of the legal duty imposed on the physician is expressed by the following portions of the quotation above: "The physician is required . . . to exercise that degree of care, judgment, and skill which other physicians . . . usually exercise . . . under like or similar circumstances."[1,2] The physician is not required to effect a cure nor is he obligated to obtain a good result in every instance. The failure to effect a cure or obtain a good result does not, of itself, infer negligence. The physician promises, by implication, only that he will use that degree of skill, knowledge, and care which would be used by the average reputable physician and will exert his best judgment in an effort to bring about a good result. The legal duty is measured by the degree of skill and care which would have been exercised by the average physician under the same or similar circumstances.

The fact that the physician's peers will ultimately pass judgment on the appropriateness of his or her treatment should a law suit ensue dramatizes the importance of judicious use of consultants by the physician who is managing difficult, complex, and potentially controversial cases.

It is important to emphasize that there are certain capabilities which the physician staffing an emergency room is expected to have, one of which is the ability to mobilize a resuscitation effort. The emergency room physician will be judged according to the way a physician staffing an emergency room would be expected to perform. There are objective expressions of training and performance, listed by specialty groups like the American College of Emergency Physicians, which can be used to help establish a "standard of care" within such an emergency facility. It may be particularly important that the physician be aware that he or she is likely to be judged according to the average performance of the expert in the field of therapy which the doctor undertook to apply, rather than the performance of a physician in his or her own specialty. Thus, if the general practitioner treats fractures, he may be expected to treat fractures to the standard of the average orthopedic surgeon. And when a general practitioner is performing as the emergency facility physician, he will generally be expected to provide care to the standard of the average emergency care physician.

Injury and Causation

The patient claiming that malpractice was committed must show that injury occurred, whether physical, emotional, or both. However negligent the physician, the litigation cannot be sustained without evidence of injury. Further, the injury must be shown to be the direct result of the substandard care of the physician. This means that it must be shown that the injury would not have occurred unless the doctor either failed to act or acted improperly.

Great Danger and Due Diligence

When the danger of serious injury or death is great, the physician's obligation to exercise diligence in his effort to protect the patient must be proportionately high. When cardiac arrest or any other serious cardiac or pulmonary problem is present or suspected, the risk to the patient of death or brain damage is high and reasonable steps to protect the patient from such foreseeable consequences must be taken.

Brain Death

Criteria for the definition of brain death were first developed by an ad hoc committee of the Harvard Medical School. Since then, brain death statutes have been passed in Kansas,[8] then in other states. The brain death criteria developed by the ad hoc committee of the Harvard Medical School were recognized by the Massachusetts Court in the Golston case and by other courts as a medically and legally acceptable definition of death.[9] In fact, in every case in which the definition of death was made according to such criteria was challenged, the courts, in Curran's words, "have uniformly upheld the physician's actions as medically proper, ethically justified and legally sound."[10] Approaches to severe brain damage which fell short of those strict criteria continued to be dealt with by the physician, family, and/or prognosis committee, but rarely by the court, up to the time of the Quinlan decision.[11]

Decision-Making in CPR and ECC

Successful resuscitation is generally thought to require the reestablishment of effective cardiovascular functions and complete neurological recovery. The fact that serious brain damage is the consequence of resuscitation efforts in some cases has led to efforts to predict the likelihood of full neurologic recovery. This practice has influenced and continues to influence decision-making in CPR, including the decision whether or not to initiate CPR and whether or not to discontinue CPR. Accordingly, the legal implications of making such decisions on this basis need to be considered.

The Question of Brain Recoverability

As alluded to above, the decision to initiate resuscitation for the cardiac arrest victim is based on the fundamental presumption that the brain may still be viable even though the heart has stopped. The accepted medical standard assumes that when the possibility exists that the brain is viable, and there are no compelling medical or legal reasons to act otherwise, resuscitation should be initiated.[13-15] As a result of that presumption and the implementation of resuscitation, many patients who would have been declared dead in the traditional sense have survived. The fact that there are a number of people alive with residual brain damage, some mild, some severe, is equally true, but the number of individuals with severe neurological sequelae represents a small percentage of total resuscitative attempts. Under most circumstances it is not possible to determine the likelihood of brain recovery at the time the decision to initiate or withhold resuscitation needs to be made.[14,15] Furthermore, there are undoubtedly patients who might have recovered completely but who are now dead because CPR was not provided in a timely manner, or was improperly or ineffectively performed, implying the necessity for clear guidelines in both decision-making and in the quality of performance in the area of resuscitation.

The extent to which improper decision-making, including improper omission or termination of CPR and inappropriate maintenance or suspension of life support, affects outcome is a question that continues to be among the most significant in this area. All too often, the conscientious physician finds that guidelines may be very difficult to apply to the circumstances of a particular patient. Thus, a reappraisal of medical and legal concepts that bear on decisions to provide or withhold resuscitation, the cessation of resuscitative efforts, the standard of care in resuscitation, and associated practices is timely.

There are several sets of circumstances that are both frequent and recurrent and, accordingly, will continue to present the CPR–ECC care provider with difficult medical, ethical, and legal decisions.

Initiating CPR: To Start or Not to Start

The current standard of care as is applied to resuscitative efforts requires that resuscitation be implemented by a responsible person or agency when two conditions are fulfilled: 1) when there is the possibility that the brain is viable, and 2) when there is no legally or medically legitimate reason to withhold it.[13-15] It is clear that persistent, severe brain damage is the more dreaded outcome than death for both care provider and, in most cases, family and loved ones. The *possibility* of brain recovery implies as well the possibility of permanent brain damage. Since accurate prognostication of postresuscitation brain status is not possible at present, resuscitation efforts should be implemented promptly when the two conditions above are present.

Consider one important situation in which the decision to initiate or withhold CPR must be made over and over again: the cardiac arrest victim arrives at the emergency facility in a condition that was once referred to as "Dead On Arrival".

Dead on Arrival

Resuscitation of the out-of-hospital cardiac arrest victim has met with increasing success undoubtedly because of broad-based improvement in emergency medical services along with the education and training of laypersons and first responders.[16,17] Still too frequently, however, a cardiac arrest victim is rushed to the emergency facility without benefit of resuscitation efforts. Prior to the time resuscitation became a standard procedure, this patient would qualify as "Dead on Arrival", or "DOA".

Although it is usually impossible to determine accurately the duration of complete cessation of cardiovascular function because of the lack of competent and reliable observers at the scene, efforts to do so are often made. For the responsible physician to make a decision not to initiate CPR in this setting, however, he must be confident at the least 1) of the ability of the observer to recognize cardiac arrest, 2) of the reliability of that observer in documenting the time elapsed, 3) that the observer is acting in good faith, and 4) that no independent influences such as drugs or cold are operative.

The argument that the patient could have collapsed, due to a cardiac or noncardiac cause, and continued to have cardiac activity at a level sufficient to sustain the brain until the victim was rushed through the door of the emergency facility may be an insurmountable one. Armed with the knowledge that weak or slow pulses may be missed by inexperienced observers, a plaintiff's attorney may inquire as to the person on whom the physician should reasonably rely as his witness to the onset and progression of the process of brain death. And does the care and interest of the family, however positive and legitimate, render them sufficiently expert at recognizing cardiac arrest so that the physician can rely on them? The same questions can be asked about a friend, neighbor, or policeman, unless that person had received special training in recognition of cardiac arrest as part of a resuscitation course. And even then, should the physician rely on the expertise of a person claiming to be practiced in the recognition of cardiac arrest who is either unable or unwilling to provide CPR? In short, the physician or other responsible care provider is usually obliged to initiate resuscitative measures and may be held liable if he elects not to do so on an arbitrary basis. One justifiable basis for withholding resuscitation would be, for example, the certain knowledge that the patient would have qualified for a "Do No Resuscitate" designation, discussed below.

For the emergency medical technicians (EMT's) and the paramedics who staff mobile emergency units, there are comparable areas of vulnerability. When these medical care personnel respond to the cardiac arrest victim in the field, they often find themselves in the same predicament as the emergency department physician, attempting to determine how long circulatory arrest has

been present. The history provided by witnesses is generally not a reliable basis for withholding resuscitation in such settings. Furthermore, the number of case reports of complete recovery after extended periods of unsupported cardiac arrest, particularly as a result of cold water immersion, is growing.[18-20] When brain viability is in doubt, the EMT or paramedic should initiate CPR.

Manifestations of Brain Damage as a Basis for Witholding CPR

Is the suspicion of irreversible brain damage or "brain death" a valid basis for withholding CPR? The absence of a pupillary response to light is not a reliable sign of brain death since certain disease states and certain drugs can render the pupil nonreactive, as do some cataract operations. Perhaps more importantly, initially unreactive pupils may become reactive in the course of resuscitation, demonstrating the unreliability of this sign as a prognosticator of brain nonrecoverability.

The use of a single observation of a "flat" electroencephalogram (EEG) to document irreversible brain damage is unacceptable for a number of reasons: 1) The duration over which electrocerebral silence by EEG should exist before it can be assumed that all possibility of resuscitation is past remains to be defined.[21] 2) To take the 10–20 minutes to perform the EEG is to assure brain death since resuscitative efforts must be withheld during this procedure. 3) Drugs may affect the EEG independently, resulting in a "flat" response. 4) A single flat EEG does not meet the current legal or medical "brain death" standards.[7]

"Boxcars" in the fundi have been recognized as indicators of cessation of cerebral perfusion and therefore indicators of brain death. But the acceptability of this sign, assuming its validity, depends on the reliability of the observer. Since there is no permanent record, how many observers should verify it? For how long should fundi be explored while the brain remains hypoxic? One is left with the reality that there are no practically useful, reliable signs of brain death which can be applied in a timely manner to the cardiac arrest victim with the exception of decapitation, rigor mortis, and perhaps established dependent lividity.

Case law supports the medical priority for supporting cardiovascular and ventilatory function before attempting to assess brain status. In the case of *Dubry vs. Gardena Medical Center*, neurologic experts found that generalized irreversible brain damage had occurred and, based on this finding, recommended that life support be withheld.[22] But the court, on expert testimony, found this unacceptable because support of cardiovascular and respiratory function, both of which were severely impaired, was not performed prior to neurological evaluation. Furthermore, misdiagnosis of irreversible cessation of all brain function has been reported in the case of brain contusion in association with reduced cerebral function due to hypovolemia. Vigorous treatment of hypovolemic shock resulted in recovery despite that misdiagnosis.[23] In short, therefore, since it is usually not possible to predict nonrecoverability of a brain acutely insulted by cardiac arrest, and since attempts to do so increase anoxia time and the likelihood of further permanent brain damage, the responsible physician, nurse, or paramedic is usually obligated to commence CPR. Evaluation of brain status and the difficult decisions which may be forthcoming in this regard should be deferred until the issue of cardiovascular responsiveness, as discussed below, is determined. The designation DOA is in large measure an anachronism and an invitation to legal as well as medical sanctions.

Termination of CPR: When to Stop

A number of criteria for deciding to discontinue CPR have been offered. Clearly, the physician has the primary responsibility for this decision. It has been recommended that the nonphysician continue basic life support as long as it is needed or until the rescuer is exhausted or relieved by a physician, another rescuer, or a rescue team.[13,14] The often-discussed liability risk of the layman functioning in good faith in this capacity has been shown not to be supported by facts.[24] With increasing frequency the lay rescuer or other first responder who provides manual support is relieved by a rescue team capable of providing advanced cardiac life support (ACLS) with definitive drug and electrical therapy. The decision to terminate ACLS at this level also must be made with increasing frequency. Practical, workable guidelines for terminating ongoing resuscitative efforts have not been available.

The duration of resuscitation has been considered as a possible criteria for the decision to terminate.[25] It is well known that the longer resuscitative efforts continue to be unsuccessful, the less likely it is that the victim will recover fully. On the other hand, it is also well known that complete recovery has followed resuscitative efforts lasting two or three hours or more.[20,26] Thus, duration of resuscitative effort as the sole criteria for a decision to terminate CPR is arbitrary and unacceptable.[27] Suspicion of permanent brain damage has been based on estimates of duration of unattended cardiac arrest, lack of pupillary response to light, and lack of any neurologic signs of life. These criteria, too, are unreliable for reasons previously discussed. The concern for guidelines for the cessation of CPR has been strengthened by the reality that litigation is more likely to follow when the patient survives with permanent brain damage than when the patient dies. And the troubling awareness on the part of the physician that the risk of permanent brain damage increases with the duration of the resuscitative effort also favors the decision to terminate.

An additional difficulty arises when a physician makes the decision to terminate resuscitation contrary to the feelings of trained paramedical personnel who initiated resuscitative efforts, a circumstance which at times belies the shared medical and legal responsibilities of the emergency facility physician and the out-of-hospital emergency team. But what medically and legally sound guidelines can be used to decide on termination of CPR?

Cardiovascular Unresponsiveness as a Basis for the Termination of CPR

It is well known that the heart tolerates hypoxemia far better than the brain, so that in many circumstances cardiovascular function may be reestablished while the brain may not recover. Since CPR is initiated because both brain and heart may recover, and since there is presently no reliable means of defining "brain death" during resuscitation, the decision to discontinue resuscitative efforts should be based on cardiovascular unresponsiveness. The major thrusts of resuscitation include the reestablishment of circulation and oxygenation of brain, heart, and other organs, correction of metabolic disturbances such as hypoxemia and acidosis, stimulation of electrical activity in a depressed heart or suppression of excessive electrical activity in a heart which is electrically hyperexcitable, and application of appropriate electrical therapy such as defibrillation. In the critically important though infrequent circumstances in which cardiovascular collapse occurs as the result of a readily reversible process such as cardiac tamponade, therapy must be directed toward that cause. The use of therapeutic modalities in appropriate combination and sequence, from administration of basic life support through the application of ACLS, will often result in the establishment of effective cardiovascular activity. When these techniques have been properly applied, and the cardiovascular system fails to respond, the cardiovascular system can be said to be unresponsive to standard resuscitative therapy. Accordingly, the decision to terminate a resuscitative effort that was initiated because of the possibility of brain and heart viability may be reasonably based on the determination that death in traditional terms has supervened, i.e., cardiac death as defined by cardiovascular unresponsiveness to acceptable resuscitative techniques.[14,15] At this point, the issue of brain viability becomes, at least for the present, an academic concern.

Proof of the medical and legal validity of the definition of death by "cardiovascular unresponsiveness" in a particular case may depend on the care provider's ability to demonstrate that therapeutic techniques appropriate to test the "unresponsiveness" of the cardiovascular system were employed, should the question arise subsequently. The possibility that the question may arise in litigation underscores the importance of adequate documentation.

Withholding Resuscitation and "Do Not Resuscitate" Orders

Prior to the Saikewicz case, considered below, it was held by many within the medical, religious, philosophical, and legal communities that resuscitation was a form of medical therapy which, as with most other forms of therapy, was indicated in some situations but not in others. This conviction was clearly enunciated at the National Conferences on CPR and ECC in 1974 and 1979.[13,14] When there is doubt, however, resuscitation should be instituted.[13,15] One of the situations in which it is usually not indicated is in the care of the terminally ill patient for whom no further therapy for the underlying disease process remains available and death appears imminent.[28] In examining this issue, it is worth considering the history of "Do Not Resuscitate" orders.

Time is a critical ingredient in successful resuscitation efforts. The vital importance of prompt support for the cardiac arrest victim was recognized from the inception of resuscitation programs. Accordingly, mechanisms were established by which individuals competent in resuscitation would respond immediately to a signal that indicated an arrest had occurred, and the cardiac arrest team was born. It was not too long before CPR was performed almost reflexly, so much so that a mechanism had to be developed to prevent resuscitative efforts in patients who were hopelessly ill. "Do Not Resuscitate" (DNR) or "Care and Comfort Only" orders were invoked. But resuscitation had become so automatic that withholding it appeared to some to be an interference with patients' rights. The fear of liability for withholding CPR then developed in some areas and resulted in the elimination of DNR from the order sheet. Such orders were then passed on by word of mouth to the nurses so that the patient for whom resuscitation had no long-term justification might be permitted to die peacefully, if not occultly. In a number of areas, however, this procedure ultimately led to revolt among nurses who refused to follow unwritten orders with "life-and-death" implications.

But the central issues remain, i.e., that the purpose of CPR is the prevention of sudden, unexpected death and that CPR is not indicated in certain cases such as terminal, irreversible illness where death is not unexpected. Credible medical support for this view has been offered.[13-15,28] It has even been suggested that resuscitation in some circumstances may represent a violation of an individual's right to die with dignity.[13]

But as discussed later in this chapter, recent case law dealing with decision-making in cases in which life-saving and life-supporting therapy is to be withheld has created widespread uncertainty and controversy. The Massachusetts Supreme Judicial Court in the Saikewicz case argued strongly that in some circumstances the court and the court alone should make decisions for the incompetent.[29] Speculation as to whether this statement applied to all incompetents or only to special classes was rampant in Massachusetts. Heated debate among physicians, attorneys, and other commentators resulted.[30-33] A subsequent Massachusetts case held in favor of the validity of DNR orders in appropriate cases and provided a special insight into the courts' view of justifiable "prolongation of life":[34]

It is apparent . . . that, when the court spoke of life prolonging treatments, it referred to treatments administered for the purpose, and with some reasonable expectation, of effecting a permanent or temporary cure of or relief from the illness or condition being treated. 'Prolongation of life', as used in the Saikewicz case, does not mean a mere suspension of the act of dying, but contemplates, at the very least, a remission of symptoms enabling a return toward a normal, functioning, integrated existence.

The implication that "prolongation of life" may be inappropriate and unjustified, or perhaps at times cruel in so far as it results in a ". . . suspension of the act of dying" is unmistakable. This case is discussed in more detail below.

When the decision not to provide CPR is made in the case of a hospitalized patient, this intent should be expressed clearly on the physician's order sheet for the benefit of nursing and other personnel who may be called on to initiate or participate in CPR. The patient's family should understand and agree with the decision although the family's opinion need not be controlling. Physicians and the entire medical team should be in general agreement with the decision. In questionable circumstances, it may be advisable to support the DNR decision with a confirmatory written opinion from appropriate qualified consultants.

Indications for DNR Orders

In what kind of circumstances may CPR not be medically indicated? Rabkin and colleagues in discussing orders not to resuscitate, referred to an "irreversibly, irreparably ill patient whose death was imminent."[28] Those authors went on to define "irreversible" in the sense that no known therapeutic measures could be effective in reversing the course of the illness. They employed "irreparable" to characterize the physiologic status of the patient in whom the process of the illness had progressed beyond the capacity of existing knowledge and technique to stem it. And they defined death as "imminent" when, in the ordinary course of events, it would probably occur within a period not exceeding two weeks. Rabkin, et al., echoed the recommendations of the Medicolegal Panel of the National Conference on Cardiopulmonary Resuscitation (CPR) and Emergency Cardiac Care (ECC), suggesting that a note summarizing the patient's condition and the basis for the decision to withhold CPR be written in the patient's chart and the order written on the physician's order sheet.[13]

It may appear at first blush that the burden placed on the physician and the medical community at large, i.e., to distinguish consistently between "life and death" therapy that is indicated and that which is not, is excessive. Yet the responsibility is very likely no different than it was before the Saikewicz decision and other such decisions considered below. The physician has always borne the responsibility of his or her decision-making. In causing questions to be brought unnecessarily to the court, the physician is abdicating an authority and a responsibility that is appropriately, and legally, his or her own.

Discontinuation of Life Support Systems

The decision to discontinue life support in most cases revolves around a determination of brain viability and, particularly, the extent that such a determination reliably supports a diagnosis of "brain death". The concept of brain death has been accepted by both medicine and law.[8-10,35,36] The strict definitions of brain death, such as that of the Harvard Ad Hoc Committee, require total absence of responsiveness, reflexes, and EEG activity over a 24-hour period in the absence of certain drugs or other conditions such as extreme cold, which could independently affect these parameters of brain viability.[7] It has been claimed that there is no case in which a patient who satisfied these criteria subsequently recovered brain function.

Brain death legislation has been enacted in more than half the states in the USA since 1970. Efforts to develop a uniform brain death act applicable to all jurisdictions are ongoing. Where brain death is recognized by statute, the express statutory criteria must be met. If they are, death may be pronounced and support mechanisms withdrawn. Where there are not statutory criteria, strict standards such as those developed by the Harvard committee may be applied based on the broad acceptance of such criteria in both the medical and legal communities. When such standards are met, death may be diagnosed with confidence.

Far more problematic are those cases in which the patient may have a severe central nervous system deficit and little or no chance of recovery, but the strict criteria for brain death are not satisfied. Diagnostic criteria for brain death which are less stringent but which may prove useful in improving our capability for recognizing those in whom brain damage is irreparable have been offered, but as yet these standards are not generally accepted.[37]

Because certain recent appellate court opinions have dealt specifically with the issue of suspension of life support, this issue will be discussed in relation to those cases.

Recent Case Law

Some recent cases have dealt directly with certain of the most critical aspects of CPR–ECC, addressing such questions as who will be the decision-maker for suspension of life support and the circumstances in which withholding resuscitative efforts may be justified. While some of these questions have been discussed earlier in this chapter, the pronouncements of the courts as they have evolved over the past several years have sometimes seemed confusing. And yet, the appellate decisions discussed have reflected a continuity and consistency of thought and approach that should be instructive for us in our efforts to determine both the physician's and the patient's rights and obligations.

One of the most pressing problems in the eyes of some courts has been the pursuit of a mechanism by which the incompetent patient can be assured to the extent possible the same rights as the competent patient. Consider, first, some cases that bear on the courts' view of the rights of the competent patient, particularly in the matter of refusal of care which could be life-saving or life-prolonging. We may then consider how the courts have attempted to deal with critical decision-making for the incompetent individual.

The Competent Patient

An example of the attitude of the court towards decisions by competent patients is demonstrated by a recent Massachusetts case, Lane vs. Candura.[38] Mrs. Candura was a 77-year-old widow who had developed gangrenous changes in her right foot and lower leg. Her physicians recommended amputation without delay, indicting she would very likely die without it, but the patient refused. The patient's daughter went to the probate court to seek to be named temporary guardian for her mother for the purpose of consenting to the operation. The daughter, Mrs. Lane, was appointed guardian for the purpose of providing consent for her mother who had been found by the probate court on the weight of the testimony provided by a psychiatrist to be incompetent. On appeal, Mrs. Candura was found to be competent to make the decision herself and the court upheld her right to refuse the surgery. Additional history involved in the case included the fact that Mrs. Candura's husband had died in 1976 and she had been depressed and unhappy since his death. She had lived in her home until 1977 but had not been able to live there alone since part of her right foot had been amputated. It appeared that the probate court had based its opinion on the psychiatrist's opinion that her refusal of therapy, knowing that she would otherwise die shortly, was evidence of incompetency. The appellate court determined that Mrs. Candura's basis for refusing therapy was that she had been unhappy since her husband's death, that she did not wish to burden her children, that she did not believe that the operation would cure her, that she did not wish to live as an invalid, that she did not wish to live in a nursing home, and that she did not fear death, but welcomed it. The court concluded that, while Mrs. Candura was not entirely mentally clear at all times, she was aware of the nature of her decision and of the consequence of her refusal of therapy and was competent to make this choice. The court stated:

> Mrs. Candura's decision may be regarded by most as unfortunate, but on the record in this case it is not the uninformed decision of a person incapable of appreciating the nature and consequences of her act. We cannot anticipate whether she will reconsider and will consent to the operation but we are all of the opinion that the operation may be not forced on her against her will.[38]

Thus, the court distinguished between dementia and competence, indicating that, although Mrs. Candura may be incapable of naming presidents back to Grover Cleveland or subtracting 7 from 100 and then serially, she did know that if she agreed to operation she would be alive with one leg and that if she refused operation, she would die. By so limiting its test of competence to a test of the patient's understanding of the outcome of her decision, the court provided us with a guideline for determining competence for the purpose of therapeutic choice.

Another case demonstrating the court's respect for the competent patient's right to determine whether or not he or she is to receive a certain form of therapy is *Satz vs. Permutter*.[39] This case involved a 73-year-old man with amyotrophic lateral sclerosis who was virtually totally paralyzed by the disease and required respirator support for adequate ventilation of his lungs. The disease process had not affected his intellectual function and, as a competent patient in October 1978, he requested that the respirator be disconnected. His relatives approved of his decision but the hospital refused to cooperate. The state attorney apparently indicated that anyone assisting Mr. Satz would be prosecuted criminally. The case was taken to court and the court affirmed the patient's right to have the respirator disconnected. The Florida Supreme Court indicated that Mr. Satz was a competent adult with no minor dependents. They observed that he had a terminal illness and that he had, as well, a constitutional right to refuse or discontinue extraordinary medical therapy where all affected family members consented. The court did indicate that it limited its ruling to nearly identical cases and planned to proceed on a cautious, case-by-case basis. The respirator was disconnected, and Mr. Satz died shortly thereafter.

These two cases indicate the consistent interest of the courts in sustaining the rights of the individual to either refuse a form of therapy or have it discontinued even if a fatal outcome should invariably follow. The process by which the right of an individual patient to have his or her

wishes carried out very likely should be dictated by the facts of the case. It is likely, for example, that when a respirator-dependent competent individual like Mr. Satz requests that his respirator be discontinued, steps should be taken to assure that, should any civil or criminal question arise after the patient's death, adequate evidence to justify the action should be available to satisfy the inquiry. In such cases, discretion would seem to indicate that the wiser recourse at the present time would be to request a ruling from the court.

As indicated previously, cases involving brain death justify suspension of life support since brain death is generally acceptable as a legal definition of death in this country. A recent Colorado case reaffirmed this position.[40] It involved a 17-month-old child who was hospitalized after extensive head trauma inflicted by the mother. Examination by a neurologist revealed no clinical evidence of central nervous system function. Three flat EEGs were recorded. The court agreed that brain death was present according to current medical criteria and ordered discontinuance of life support. Thus, when brain death can be diagnosed by such accepted medical standards as the Harvard criteria, death in a legal and medical sense is defined and life support should be discontinued.

The Incompetent Patient

Critical decision-making for incompetent patients may be considered in two categories: 1) Those who were once competent and, therefore, may have provided a credible indication of the medical decision which they would make in a given set of circumstances; 2) Those who were incompetent since birth. This division permits us to consider decision-making for incompent patients in light of the desire of the courts to have the patient be the decision-maker, i.e., to permit incompetent individuals to receive or reject medical care in the same manner in which the competent patient is permitted to do so, at least to the extent that this is possible. One way in which the courts have tried to preserve the right of incompetent patients to therapeutic self-determination has been to indicate that credible expressions of choice made before the patient became incompetent *may* continue to be controlling in the period of incompetency. Two such cases are considered immediately below. When no such credible indication is available or discoverable, it would appear that the decision-making process should be comparable to that employed in the case of patients incompetent from birth. One approach that appears to be gaining favor is the appointment by a competent person of an individual who would stand in the patient's stead should incompetency occur and make medical decisions with the same force as the individual by whom he had been appointed.

The Case of Karen Quinlan

Karen Quinlan was a 21-year-old female who suffered several periods of apnea after which she remained in a vegetative state.[11] The father sought to be appointed guardian for the purpose of discontinuing what he considered to be "extraordinary" procedures on behalf of his daughter. The Superior Court in New Jersey had denied authorization for the suspension of life support, but the New Jersey Supreme Judicial Court indicated that Karen Quinlan had a right to "permit noncognitive vegetative existence to terminate by natural forces" as a "valuable incident of her right to privacy which could be asserted on her behalf by her guardian". Karen Quinlan's neurologic status at the time included the fact that she was comatose although she moved at times, her pupils reacted to light and sound, and she reacted to noxious stimuli. In addition, she blinked her eyes, grimaced, made chewing motions, and occasionally made stereo-typed cries. Brain stem function was preserved to the extent that she continued with respiration after the mechanical ventilator was discontinued. Clearly then, Karen Quinlan did not fulfill criteria for brain death. Thus, in granting Karen Quinlan's father's request to be appointed guardian for the purpose of discontinuing life support measures, the court was saying in effect that this person who failed to meet brain death criteria could be permitted to die. The New Jersey court advised that an ethics committee from the hospital be consulted in the course of the final decision-making process.

The decision to suspend life support in the case of Karen Quinlan was, at the direction of the court, to depend on the diagnosis and prognosis as determined by the managing physician and the desires of the family as expressed through her guardian, her father, with the advice of an ethics committee appointed within the hospital. It is noteworthy that the court itself did not make the decision to discontinue life support, that Karen Quinlan by current standards was not dead according to brain death criteria, that the decision ultimately was made according to rather conventional standards, that is by consensus of treating physician and family with consultation in this case with an ethics committee.

It is of particular interest that the court took notice of expressions made by Karen Quinlan while she was competent that indicated she would not want to continue life if she had to be maintained by a life-support system. While this evidence was not controlling in the courts decision, it is a clear indication of the extent of the court's commitment to the principle of therapeutic self-determination.

In re Eichner: The Case of Brother Fox

An approach to the termination of life support mechanisms was offered by a New York State appellate court[46] only to be rejected by the highest court of the state.[47]

Brother Fox was an 83-year-old member of a religious community who suffered a cardiac arrest during a hernia repair. Cardiovascular function was restored but Brother Fox remained comatose and in a chronic vegetative state. Medical experts indicated that there was virtually no chance of recovery. The court, in commenting on the medical record, stated that there was a "reasonable degree of medical certainty that his cerebral function had been irrevocably destroyed."[46] Brother Fox's relatives as well as other colleagues in the religious community in which he lived agreed that a request should be submitted to the court for permission to suspend life support in the case of Brother Fox. The lower court gave permission for the discontinuation of life support and the district attorney appealed. Pending appeal, Brother Fox died. The appeals court heard the case in spite of Brother Fox's death because it recognized the need for judicial precedent on the issue of termination of such treatment. The court at the appellate level indicated that the lower court was justified in permitting discontinuation of life support because 1) The competent adult had a right to refuse therapy even if the outcome would almost certainly be fatal. 2) The court cannot interfere with the competent decision. 3) The same standard had to be applied to the incompetent as was applied to the competent patient. The court concluded that a mechanism had to be made available by which incompetents could have this right exercised. In defining such a mechanism, the court indicated that there had to be clear and convincing evidence in the form of certification by the treating physician with the approval of a designated hospital committee that to a reasonable degree of medical certainty the patient's cognitive function would not return. In addition, in the absence of any evidence of an express wish on the part of the patient, there could be reliance on the "substituted judgment" of a person close to the patient as to what that patient would have chosen in terms of the continuation of suspension of life support. Notice was given to the attorney general and the district attorney and a guardian *ad litem* was to be appointed. In addition, the court indicated that an order from the court must be obtained if immunity from civil and criminal prosecution was to be secured. Then, should all agree, the life-support mechanism could be suspended and any and all individuals involved would be immune from both criminal and civil liability. The case was appealed to the highest court in the State of New York, the Court of Appeals.

The New York State Court of Appeals dealt with the matter far more simply and directly than did the lower court.[47] The Court of Appeals found that Brother Fox's personal desire was that he not be provided an extraordinary treatment should he be in a situation similar to that of Karen Quinlan. The court found that this fact was undisputed and, accordingly, that the hospital could not continue to maintain the respirator contrary to the expressed will of Brother Fox. On the issue of the certainty and seriousness of Brother Fox's wishes, the court stated the following:

> In this case the proof was compelling. There was no suggestion that the witnesses who testified for the petitioner had any other motive but to see that Brother Fox's stated wishes were respected. The finding that he carefully reflected on the subject, expressed his views, and concluded not to have his life prolonged by medical means if there was no hope of recovery is supported by his religious beliefs and is not inconsistent with his life of unselfish religious devotion.[47]

The court refused to impose a higher burden of proof than that there be "clear and convincing evidence" of Brother Fox's refusal, rejecting the request by the district attorney for evidence "beyond a reasonable doubt". The court saw no need to invoke such doctrines as substituted judgment or constitutional right of privacy but based its position on the common-law right of a competent individual to refuse medical therapy which survives the incompetency of the individual if the evidence of the refusal is "clear and convincing".

While the New York Court of Appeals rejected the complicated judicial review process offered by the lower court, the court did indicate its willingness to hear cases when uncertainties exist as to the patient's wishes, concluding that "Responsible parties who wish to comply with the law . . . need not act at their peril."[47]

It is particularly noteworthy in the Eichner case that the court based its decision on the oral testimony from Brother Fox's colleagues in the religious community that Brother Fox had made clear on more than one occasion that he would not wish to live in a condition requiring extraordinary care in the form of life-support mechanisms such as a mechanical ventilator. Brother Fox apparently reaffirmed this preference not long before the surgical procedure during which he suffered cardiac arrest. The court relied on testimony to this effect even though the testimony was based on Brother Fox's oral expression. Thus, the court looked back at Brother Fox's expressions while competent as to whether he would choose to continue to live in a vegetative state on a life support system and found that Brother Fox would have elected to be permitted to die, as it appeared Karen Quinlan would have done as well. In the Fox case, however, the court was prepared to permit Brother Fox's choice while competent to be controlling.

Joseph Saikewicz

Sometime after the Quinlan case, an important and highly controversial opinion was written in the state of Massachusetts involving an incompetent named Joseph Saikewicz.[29] Mr. Saikewicz was a 67-year-old man who had been severely retarded from birth and had lived most of his life in the Belchertown State School as a ward of the state of Massachusetts. He had never learned to speak but communicated through grunts and gestures. He was found to have acute myeloblastic monocytic leukemia in April 1976. Since Mr. Saikewicz was a ward of the state, the superintendent of the institution petitioned the probate court for the appointment of a guardian to assist the court in making the necessary decisions concerning his medical care. Because he would be unable to comprehend the reasons for his treatment and because the treatment would very likely require restraining Saikewicz, and because of the well-recognized side effects of the chemotherapy which included pain, anemia, hair loss, bladder irritation, and bone marrow depression as well as the poor prognosis even with therapy, the court entered an order that chemotherapy be withheld.

An appeal was taken immediately and the Massachusetts Supreme Judicial Court affirmed the decision on July 9, 1976. Saikewicz died quietly of pneumonia in September 1976 and the court issued its full opinion more than fourteen months after Saikewicz' death, in November 1977.

Certain comments in the Saikewicz opinion led many physicians and commentators to believe that the court intended to get actively involved in the business of medical practice, for example:

> Rather, such questions of life and death seem to us to require the process of detached but dispassionate investigation and decision that forms the ideal on which the judicial branch of government was created. Achieving this ideal is our responsibility and that of the lower court and is not to be entrusted to any other group purporting to represent the morality and conscience of our society no matter how highly motivated or impressively constituted.[41]

The latter reference, of course, was unmistakably directed toward the medical profession. The Massachusetts court specifically rejected the mechanism for decision-making offered by the New Jersey Supreme Judicial Court in the Quinlan case, stating:

> We take a dim view of any attempt to shift the ultimate decision-making responsibility away from the duly established courts of proper jurisdiction to any committee, panel or group, ad hoc or permanent. Thus, we reject the approach adopted by the New Jersey Supreme Court in the Quinlan case of entrusting the decision whether to continue artificial life support to the patient's guardian, family, attending doctor, and hospital "ethics committee."[41]

Did the Massachusetts court mean that the court must be petitioned in all cases in which the question of suspending artificial life support arose? That is unlikely, since brain death is a legally accepted basis for defining death in the state of Massachusetts.[9] But how should one deal with cases of severe brain damage without reasonable hope for improvement which do not fulfill brain criteria? The broad applicability of the language of the Massachusetts court created great anxiety and speculation in this whole area, including the basis for decisions to initiate and to withhold resuscitative efforts.[30,33,42] The question of "Do Not Resuscitate" orders was broadly argued and, in some quarters, legal advice was that such orders could no longer be written and that resuscitative efforts ought to be mobilized even in the case of, for example, the incompetent severely brain-damaged, multiple-stroke victim unless the court had permitted withholding of resuscitative efforts in that specific case.

At issue in the Saikewicz case was whether to provide or withhold a therapy which a competent patient in the circumstances of Joseph Saikewicz could in fact accept or reject, i.e., a genuine therapeutic option. The question in the case of Mr. Saikewicz was who should decide whether he, Joseph Saikewicz, should be treated? The Massachusetts court invoked a mechanism referred to as the "substituted judgement" theory by which the court attempted to determine what Joseph Saikewicz would decide were he competent. The Massachusetts court came to the same conclusion as the probate court 14 months earlier. But the concept of "substituted judge-ment" and the absence of guidelines by which the physician could decide whether or not the court had to be petitioned remained subjects of intense concern and debate.

The Case of John Storar

In a case that was considered by the New York Court of Appeals along with the case of Brother Fox, the court indicated that in circumstances in which it is impossible to know the desires of a patient, e.g., the patient's incompetency existed since birth, a parent could not refuse life-saving blood transfusions.[47] This case in-volved a 52-year-old resident of a state facility, John Storar, who had a mental age of 18 months. His mother, a 77-year-old widow, lived nearby and visited Mr. Storar almost daily.

Cancer of Mr. Storar's urinary bladder was found in July 1979 and the mother was appointed guardian for the purpose of consenting to radiation therapy. By March 1980 the malignancy had metastasized to his lungs and elsewhere and bleeding from his urinary bladder was difficult to control, so much so that blood transfusions were begun in May with his mother's consent. His condition was considered terminal and inoperable at the time. He was described by physicians as experiencing intense pain and discomfort, a pain described as "strangling" in nature due to the frequent contractions of his bladder in an attempt to expel the cancerous mass. In June his mother requested that transfusions be discontinued because she believed they caused him unnecessary suffering and increased the bleeding from his bladder, which appeared to cause him pain and frighten him. The director of the facility brought a petition before the court for authorization of further blood transfusions, which was opposed by the mother. There was agreement that Mr. Storar would probably bleed to death without the transfusions but would die within six months even if they were continued. Mr. Storar was receiving sedation and pain medication on a regular basis. Mrs. Storar testified that, because the transfusions obviously caused distress, she believed her son would want to have them stopped. The lower court held that Mrs. Storar was in the best position to understand her son's needs and discomfort and that Mr. Storar's right to refuse therapy could be exercised on his behalf by his mother.

The New York Court of Appeals reversed the decision on the grounds that there was in fact no way to determine what Mr. Storar himself would decide under the circum-stances. The court went on to argue that since Mr. Storar was mentally an infant he had to be granted the rights of an infant. The court went on to say that parents cannot refuse blood transfusions which would be life-saving for their children even on religious grounds. The court concluded that Mrs. Storar could not refuse to have blood transfusions administered to her son.

There are clear similarities between the Storar case and the Saikewicz case including the fact that both were severely retarded and incompetent since birth. The Massachusetts court made it clear in the Saikewicz case that in certain circumstances the court alone would decide when a treatment which represented a reason-able therapeutic option and was life-prolonging could be withheld. They employed the "substituted judgement" theory, in an attempt to best identify the decision that Mr. Saikewicz would have made were he competent. The New York Court of Appeals indicated that there was in fact no realistic way to determine what Mr. Storar would have chosen to do since he had never been competent. The New York court relied on common law, which required that a parent or guardian act only for the benefit of the child or ward. The court would not permit Mr. Storar to bleed to death for lack of blood transfusions based on the mother's refusal of consent.

It may be argued, particularly in comparison to the Saikewicz case, that the Storar opinion is regressive. While many commentators criticized the Saikewicz opin-ion, few criticized the decision not to treat Mr. Saikewicz. It may be argued that the outcome might well have differed had the thinking of the Storar court been applied to Saikewicz. Mr. Saikewicz, like Storar, was incompetent since birth and according to the Storar opinion, perhaps should have been treated as an infant. One right of the infant which the court properly insisted on protecting was the right to receive life-saving and life-prolonging therapy. In the case of Mr. Saikewicz, this may well have included antileukemic agents which, among a number of other untoward side effects, predictably depressed bone-marrow red blood cell production, causing anemia which could require transfusion therapy. Mr. Saikewicz would have had to have been restrained since he would have been unable to understand why needles had to be pushed into his flesh and left there for prolonged periods of time (one of the arguments, incidentally, used to support the decision not to treat Saikewicz). In addition to the similarity of the cases in terms of lifelong incompetence and the likelihood of the need for blood transfusions, the prognosis for life in each case was the same, about six months. Mr. Saikewicz had no pain or discomfort, was not treated (granted, the court was persuaded that treatment may or may not have pro-longed his life, but predictably would cause unpleasant side affects in addition to the transfusion requirement), and died quietly of pneumonia several months later. Mr. Storar's condition, on the other hand, was characterized by pain and fear (in addition to his inability to understand that the transfusions were "good" for him), a virtual guarantee of progression of the malignant process as long as he lived, a high likelihood of more diffuse and more severe pain along with the progressive malaise of terminal malignancy, all of which were sustained by transfusion therapy.

Further, it may be argued that the Storar court's rejection of the substituted judgement theory, while logical, begged the question as to how the lifelong incompetent will be guaranteed in a timely way his right to refuse treatment. This question, in turn, may be seen to revolve around the manner in which the incompetent experiences his existence, rather than either his insuffi-ciency of cognitive capability or the manner in which a certain competent decision-maker might perceive the incompetent's existence. The very lack of cognitive capabilities perhaps dramatizes the extent to which sensory function — particularly the avoidance of pain — must dominate the existence of the incompetent. To defer, if not to deny, the incompetent's right to refuse therapy might then be considered a particularly harsh injustice.

But with regard to the likely impact of providing or withholding therapy, the Storar and the Saikewicz cases differ greatly. In the matter of Mr. Storar, there was an immediate need for transfusion therapy, else Mr. Storar would die. Mr. Saikewicz, on the other hand, had no immediate need for any form of therapy which was withheld. And in both cases, there was time, relative to prognosis for life, to go to court.

And while the Quinlan, Saikewicz, Eichner, Candura, and Perlmutter cases were "right to refuse treatment" cases, Storar is clearly an "obligation to treat" case. The previous cases all focused on the right of the patient, whether competent or incompetent, to refuse life-saving and life-prolonging therapy under most circumstances. The Storar opinion comes down squarely on the side of providing life-saving therapy for the lifelong incompetent, at least in some instances: "A court should not in the circumstances of this case allow an incompetent patient to bleed to death because someone, even someone as close as a parent or sibling, feels that this is best for one with an incurable disease."[47]

Thus, the Storar opinion shifted the emphasis from the right to refuse treatment to the obligation to treat the life-long incompetent in at least certain circumstances. In rejecting the substituted judgement theory and failing (or refusing) to offer an alternative rationale for deciding to withhold treatment, the court would seem to be indicat-ing that treatment should be provided unless there is sufficient reason to withhold it and that when a substan-tial question exists, it should be submitted to the court for disposition. Thus, the Storar case is, in this respect, reminiscent of some of the strong language of the Saikewicz case regarding the role of the court in such decision-making, although it falls short of the infamous language that caused such a vigorous response from the medical community and played a major part in stimulat-ing subsequent litigation (see discussion of the Saike-wicz opinion). Yet, with this renewed emphasis to treat, Storar may well increase recourse to the courts.

There are, then, a number of positive points in the Storar opinion: 1) The court reduced the complexity of the legal basis for affirming the right of a lifelong incompetent to receive certain life-prolonging and life-saving therapy despite the wishes of parent or guardian by basing it on a common law principle. 2) The court expressed its view that the substituted judgement theory was inapplicable to the lifelong incompetent. 3) The court's approach may well tend to minimize arbitrary decisions to withhold from the lifelong incompetent indicated life-saving therapy. 4) The opinion places the burden on the family, guardian, and physician to assure that, when there is effective and indicated life-saving therapy available, such treatment is provided. 5) The opinion restricts the right to withhold such treatment by implying that any exception to the treatment rule (with-holding indicated therapy which may be lifesaving from a person who was never competent or from a person whose wishes while competent are undiscoverable) remains the prerogative of the court.

The Courts on DNR: Shirley Dinnerstein

One of the cases that helped to clarify the Saikewicz case, especially on the issue of "Do Not Resuscitate" (DNR) orders, was that involving Shirley Dinnerstein.[43] Mrs. Dinnerstein was a 67-year-old woman with Alz-heimer's disease, a chronic disorder of the nervous system characterized by progressive deterioration of memory and intellectual function to the point of severe dementia. Her symptoms had begun in 1972. The diagnosis was made in 1975, and she was placed in a nursing home. She was completely disoriented and suffered psychotic outbursts from time to time, had no control of bodily function, and required intensive nursing care. In 1978 she had a stroke that resulted in total left-sided paralysis. In the time of the hearing at the probate court, she was confined to bed, was unable to speak, move,[3] or swallow, had a nasogastric feeding tube in place, and her condition was described as hopeless. The recommendation of her physician was that, should cardiac arrest occur, resuscitative efforts should be withheld and Mrs. Dinnerstein should be permitted to die. The family concurred. The hospital, however, was not willing to accept this plan and it was for this reason that the case came to the probate court and, eventually, to the appellate court in Massachusetts. The uncertainty that had followed in the wake of the Saikewicz case was clearly responsible for the arrival of Dinnerstein in court.

The following clarifying statements were made in the text of the opinion of the appellate court:

It must be borne in mind that the Saikewicz case, while discussing incidentally the doctor's duty to administer treatment, was primarily concerned with the patient's right to refuse treatment and the manner in which the exercise of that right may be secured to persons unable to make the decision for themselves.[42]

And later in the opinion:

It is apparent . . . that, when the court spoke of life-prolonging treatments, it referred to treatments administered for the purpose, and with some reasonable expectation of effecting a permanent or temporary cure of or relief from the illness or condition being treated.[43]

And, as quoted earlier,

Prolongation of life, as used in the Saikewicz case, does not mean a mere suspension of the act of dying, but contemplates, at the very least, a remission of symptoms enabling a return towards a normal functioning, integrated existence.[43]

Thus in the Dinnerstein case, the Massachusetts appellate court affirmed the appropriateness of withholding certain forms of life-prolonging and life-saving therapy, including resuscitative efforts. It also specifically condoned the use of DNR orders in certain circumstances. Although the Massachusetts Supreme Judicial Court endorsed the Dinnerstein opinion in a later opinion of its own (in the case of Earle Spring) a number of other questions still remained as part of the fallout of Saikewicz.

Discontinuation of Feeding

Incompetent Patients

Increasingly, courts are being asked to consider whether nasogastric feeding and other comparable methods for sustaining life may be discontinued. In the Conroy case, the New Jersey Supreme Court permitted withdrawal of life-supporting feeding from an elderly nursing home patient. According to the Conroy case,[48] it would appear that such life support could be withdrawn or withheld from an incompetent, elderly nursing home patient if 1) the patient had no more than one year to live, 2) the patient had clearly expressed this desire through a "living will" or oral directive to family, friends, or physician, or 3) the patient had established a durable power of attorney or proxy to decide on the patient's behalf. Other criteria were offered if the latter criteria could not be met. Importantly, however, the ruling appeared to reject the tradition of shared decision-making by physicians and families of incompetent patients. Instead, the court required the State Ombudsman to investigate cases like that of Claire Conroy as possible cases of elder abuse. Questions as to whether or not such administrative review will safeguard incompetent patients have been raised.[49]

Much discussion has followed from this and similar decisions in other jurisdictions and it is likely that a considerable experience with case law or statutory clarification will be necessary before clear guidelines for providing adequate protection for patients are established.

Competent Patients

A California Court of Appeals has recently found no valid state interest in overriding a competent patient's right to refuse any medical treatment, including nutrition and hydration, even if the patient is not comatose, terminally ill, or in a vegetative state, and who may be expressing a wish to die. The case is that of Elizabeth Bouviae, a 28-year-old woman who had suffered with severe cerebral palsy since birth. Her disease had progressed to the point that she was quadriplegic, completely bedridden, and, except for a few fingers of one hand and some slight head and facial movements, immobile. She also suffered from degenerative and crippling arthritis and was in constant pain. She was physically helpless and totally dependent on others for all of her needs. She was unable to stand or sit upright in either a bed or a wheelchair. She had a surgically implanted chest tube and received automatic injections of morphine which relieved some, but not all, of her physical pain and discomfort. Despite her debilitating condition, she was intelligent, earned a college degree, and remained "very mentally competent".

A three-judge Appeals Court unanimously reversed the lower court, declaring that, on the contrary, "a desire to terminate one's life is probably the ultimate exercise of one's right of privacy," and, therefore, "we find no substantial evidence to support the (lower) court's decision." "This matter," the court recognized, "constitutes a perfect paradigm of the axiom: 'Justice delayed is justice denied.'" "Her mental and emotional feelings are equally entitled to respect. She has been subjected to the forced intrusion of an artificial mechanism into her body against her will. She has a right to refuse the increased dehumanizing aspect of her condition created by the insertion of a permanent tube through her nose and into her stomach . . . [She] sought to enforce only a right which was exclusively hers and over which neither the medical profession nor the judiciary have any veto power."

In a separate but concurring opinion, a judge affirmed the decision described above but went on to indicate that Ms. Bouviae should be accorded additional considerations, as follows:

> Elizabeth apparently has made a conscious and informed choice that she prefers death to continued existence in her helpless and, to her, intolerable condition. I believe she has an absolute right to effectuate that decision. This state and the medical profession, instead of frustrating her desire, should be attempting to relieve her suffering by permitting and, in fact, assisting her to die with ease and dignity. The fact that she is forced to suffer the ordeal of self-starvation to achieve her objective is in itself inhumane.

> The right to die is an integral part of our right to control our own destinies so long as the rights of others are not affected. That right should, in my opinion, include the ability to enlist assistance from others, including the medical profession, in making death as painless and quick as possible.

> . . . Whatever choice Elizabeth Bouviae may ultimately make, I can only hope that her courage, persistence and example will cause our society to deal realistically with the plight of those unfortunate individuals to whom death beckons as a welcome respite from suffering.

> If there is ever a time when we ought to be able to get the 'government off our backs' it is as we face death — either by choice or otherwise.

This opinion not only reaffirms strongly the court's view that the patient be the decision-maker virtually without regard to the outcome, but it raises the issue of physician assistance in the process of dying, a subject that continues to gain support both here and abroad. In such vigorous support of the patient as ultimate decision-maker, the importance of prospective decision-making, particularly among patients at high-risk of becoming incompetent, as a critically important means of assuming that the patient's rights are respected even after they are incompetent, is reaffirmed.

Conclusions

1. With regard to the "standard of care" performance in CPR and ECC, a National Conference on Cardiopulmonary Resuscitation and Emergency Cardiac Care was held in Washington in 1973. Standards for CPR and ECC were developed and subsequently published.[13] These standards were updated by national conferences in 1979 and 1985.[14] Based on these standards, the American Heart Association has continued to develop teaching and testing materials applicable at every level of ECC. These materials provide a definition of the current standard of care at virtually every level of performance in CPR and ECC.

2. A responsible physician or other responsible medical or paramedical person has a duty to provide CPR to the cardiac arrest victim as a form of routine and ordinary care unless there is a medically or legally justifiable reason to withhold that care.

3. Resuscitation may be withheld if there is a medically or legally justifiable reason to do so. "Do Not Resuscitate" orders or their equivalent (e.g., "Care and Comfort Only") should be written in such cases. As with other forms of therapy, the locus of decision-making as to whether CPR represents a reasonable therapeutic option is initially with the physician. If he determines it is not, the question need not be presented to the patient in most cases although, for practical purposes, an understanding by the patient and family of diagnostic and prognostic realities and their therapeutic implications is desirable.

4. Termination of CPR should be based on cardiovascular unresponsiveness to competently delivered BLS and ACLS unless there is another medically or legally justifiable reason to terminate.

5. Life support mechanisms and efforts can and should be suspended when the patient's status meets brain death criteria.

6. Life support mechanisms and life-prolonging therapy and efforts may be suspended in appropriate circumstances without recourse to the court.

7. In circumstances which are less well defined or in which there is a disagreement among physicians or between physicians and family, or substantial questions persist, recourse to the court may be advisable before termination of life support mechanisms or life-prolonging therapy.

8. In the case of a life-long incompetent, there is judicial opinion to suggest that life-prolonging and life-saving therapy which represents a reasonable therapeutic option should be continued unless its termination is authorized by the court.

References

1. Derr vs Bonney, 231 P 2d 637, 1951.
2. Lane vs Calvert, 138 A 2d 902, 1958.
3. Zoll PM, Linenthal AJ, Gibson W, et al: Termination of ventricular fibrillation in man by externally applied electric countershock. *N Engl J Med* 254:727-732, 1956.
4. Safar P: Mouth-to-mouth airway. *Anesthesiology* 18:904-906, 1957.
5. Elam JO, Green DG, Brown ES, et al: Oxygen and carbon dioxide exchange and energy cost of expired air resuscitation. *JAMA* 167:328-334, 1958.
6. Kouwenhover WB, Jude JR,Knickerbocker GG: Closed-chest cardiac massage. *JAMA* 173:1064-1067, 1960.
7. A definition of irreversible coma: Report of the Ad Hoc Committee of the Harvard Medical School to Examine the Definition of Brain Death. *JAMA* 205:337-340, 1968.
8. Kansas Session Laws of 1970, chap 378.
9. Commonwealth vs Golston, 336 NE 2d 744, 1977.
10. Curran WJ: Setting the medicolegal issues concerning brain-death statutes: Matters of legal ethics and judicial precedent. *N Engl J Med* 299:31-32, 1978.
11. In the matter of Karen Quinlan, 70 NJ 10, 355 A 2d 647, 1976.
12. Kuller L: Sudden death in arteriosclerotic heart disease: The case for preventive medicine. *Am J Cardiol* 24:617-628, 1969.
13. Standards for Cardiopulmonary Resuscitation (CPR) and Emergency Cardiac Care (ECC). *JAMA* 227(suppl):833-868, 1974.
14. Standards and Guidelines for Cardiopulmonary Resuscitation (CPR) and Emergency Cardiac Care (ECC). *JAMA* 244(suppl):453-509, 1980.
15. McIntyre KM: Medicolegal aspects of cardiopulmonary resuscitation (CPR) and emergency cardiac care (ECC). *JAMA* 244:511-512, 1980.
16. Thompson RG, Hallstrom AP, Cobb LA: Beneficial effect of bystander-initiated CPR in out-of-hospital ventricular fibrillation, abstracted. *Circulation* 56(suppl 3):111-114, 1977.
17. Lund I, Skulberg A: Cardiopulmonary resuscitation by lay people. *Lancet* 2:702-704, 1976.
18. Seibke H, Rod T, Breivik H, et al: Survival after 40 minutes; Submersion without cerebral sequelae. *Lancet* 1:1275-1277, 1975.
19. De Villota ED, Barat G, Peral P, et al: Recovery from profound hypothermia with cardiac arrest after immersion. *Br Med J* 4:394-395, 1973.
20. Sims JK, Penick M: How much CPR is enough CPR? *JACEP* 7:218-220, 1978.
21. Silverman D, Saunders MG, Schwab RS, et al: Cerebral death and the electroencephalogram. Report of the Ad Hoc Committee of the American Electroencephalographic Society on EEG Criteria for determination of cerebral death. *JAMA* 209:1505-1510, 1969.
22. Dubry vs Gardena Medical Center, California Superior Ct, Los Angeles Co, Docket No. SWC1098, 1972.
23. Grenvik A, Powner DJ, Synder JV, et al: Cessation of therapy in terminal illness and brain death. *Crit Care Med* 6:284-291, 1978.
24. McIntyre KM, Hampton AG: Status of liability risk for out-of-hospital (OH) cardiopulmonary resuscitation (CPR). *Circulation* 54(suppl 2):II-224, 1976.
25. Eliastam M. Duralde T, Martinez F, et al: Cardiac arrest in the emergency medical service system: Guidelines for resuscitation. *JACEP* 6:525-529, 1977.
26. Sandoe E, Flensted-Jensen E, Dupont B: Long-term prognosis in patients resuscitated from cardiac arrest. *Isr J Med Sci* 5:769-771, 1969.
27. Lambrew C: Medical control, editorial. *JACEP* 6:66-67, 1977.
28. Rabkin MT, Gilerman G, Rice NR: Orders not to resuscitate. *N Engl J Med* 295:364-366, 1976.
29. Superintendent of Belchertown State School vs Saikewicz, 370 NE 2d 417, 1977, p 433.
30. Relman AS: The Saikewicz decision: Judges as physicians. *N Engl J Med* 298:508-509, 1978.
31. Baron CH: Assuring "detached by patient investigation and decision": The role of guardians ad litem in Saikewicz-type cases. *Am J Legal Med* 4:111-130, 1978.
32. Buchanan A: Medical paternalism or legal imperialism: Not the only alternative for handling Saikewicz cases. *Am J Legal Med* 5:97-117, 1979.
33. Annas GJ: Reconciling Quinlan and Saikewicz: Decision making for the terminally ill and incompetent. *Am J Legal Med* 4:367-396, 1979.
34. In the matter Shirley Dinnerstein, Mass Adv Sheets, 1978.
35. Veith FJ, Fein JM, Tendler MD, et al: Brain death: I. A status report of medical and ethical considerations. *JAMA* 238:1651-1655, 1744-1748, 1977.
36. Black PM: Brain Death. *N Engl J Med* 299:338-344, 393-401, 1978.
37. An appraisal of the criteral of cerebral death: A summary statement. A collaborative study. *JAMA* 237:982-986, 1977.
38. Lane vs Candura, 376 NE 2d 1232, 1978.
39. Satz vs Perlmutter, 379 So 2d 359, 1980.
40. Lovato vs District Court, Colorado Superior Ct, Colorado, Docket No. 79SA407, October 15, 1979.
41. Superintendent of Belchertown State School vs Saikewicz, 370 NE 2d 417, 1977, pp 434,435.
42. Curran WJ: Law-medicine notes. The Saikewicz decision. *N Engl J Med* 298:499-500, 1978.
43. In re Dinnerstein, 380 NE 2d 134, 1978, pp 137,138.
44. In re Spring, 399 NE 2d 493, 1979.
45. In re Spring, 405 NE 2d 115, 1980.
46. Eichner vs. Dillon, 426 NYS 2d 517, 1980.
47. New York State Court of Appeals opinions concerning: In the matter of John Storar, in the matter of Father Philip K. Eichner. *NY Law J* 185(63):1, 4-6, 1981.
48. In the matter of Clair C. Conroy, 486A 2d 1209 (N.J. 1985).
49. Lo, B, Dornbrand, L. The case of Clair Conroy: Will administrative review safeguard incompetent patients? *Ann Intern Med* 104:869-873, 1986.
50. Case of Elizabeth Bouviae. California.

Automated External Defibrillation

Chapter 20

Importance of Automated External Defibrillation

The AHA adds this chapter to the latest edition of the *Textbook of Advanced Cardiac Life Support* because of greater awareness of the importance of early defibrillation and growing availability and use of automated external defibrillators (AEDs).[1–11] Every person trained in ACLS must be familiar with AEDs and know how to interact with emergency personnel equipped with these devices.

Defibrillation was once a skill reserved for emergency care providers trained in all aspects of ACLS, but it is now often performed by lesser-trained, BLS personnel.[5–7] The availability of AEDs has sparked this extension of defibrillation capability.[2] AEDs eliminate the need for training in rhythm recognition and make early defibrillation by minimally trained personnel practical and achievable.[1–11] AEDs were originally conceived as devices that would be used by emergency personnel and by family members and associates of people at high risk of sudden cardiac death.[12] Now, the range of personnel who may be trained in the use of these devices is much broader.[13] Providers of ACLS, both in-hospital and prehospital, should be able to use AEDs and know the protocols for AED use because they may need to use these devices and because they will be called on with increasing frequency to interact with medical personnel or community members who also can use these devices.

Principle of Early Defibrillation

The principle of early defibrillation states that all BLS personnel must be trained to operate, equipped with, and permitted to operate a defibrillator if in their professional activities they are expected to respond to people in cardiac arrest. This concept has now achieved wide acceptance.[6,8,10,11,14–17] BLS personnel include all first-responding emergency personnel, whether in-hospital or out-of-hospital (e.g., EMTs, non-EMT first-responders, firefighters, volunteer emergency personnel, physicians, nurses, and paramedics). As a result of the AHA's 1985 Standards and Guidelines Conference, early defibrillation has become the standard of care for patients with either prehospital or in-hospital cardiac arrest,[18] except in sparsely populated and remote settings where the frequency of cardiac arrest is low and rescuer response times are excessively long.[19–21]

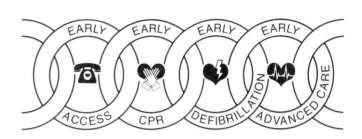

Figure 1. The emergency cardiac care systems concept is displayed schematically by the "chain of survival" metaphor.

ECC Systems Concept

The AHA has adopted and supported the ECC systems concept for years.[1,18] The phrase "chain of survival"[22] provides a useful metaphor for the elements of the ECC systems concept (Figure 1). The ECC systems concept summarizes the present understanding of the best approach to the treatment of persons with sudden cardiac death. The four links in this chain are early access to the EMS system, early CPR, early defibrillation, and early advanced cardiac care. Epidemiological and clinical research have established that effective ECC, whether prehospital or in-hospital, depends on strong links that are closely interconnected.[23–25] To achieve maximum effectiveness, each link must receive special attention. Through the education and training in its BLS program, the AHA strengthens the first two elements: early access and early CPR.[10,11] Through ACLS training, the fourth link, early advanced cardiac care, is established. Now, this educational material for automated defibrillation training strengthens the third component, early defibrillation. When the entire ECC system is brought together effectively, the potential for incremental improvement in survival from cardiac arrest is immense, as displayed in Figure 2.

Rationale for Early Defibrillation

A simple rationale supports early defibrillation:
- The most frequent initial rhythm in sudden cardiac arrest is ventricular fibrillation.
- The most effective treatment for ventricular fibrillation is electrical defibrillation.
- The probability of successful defibrillation diminishes rapidly over time.
- Ventricular fibrillation tends to convert to asystole within a few minutes.

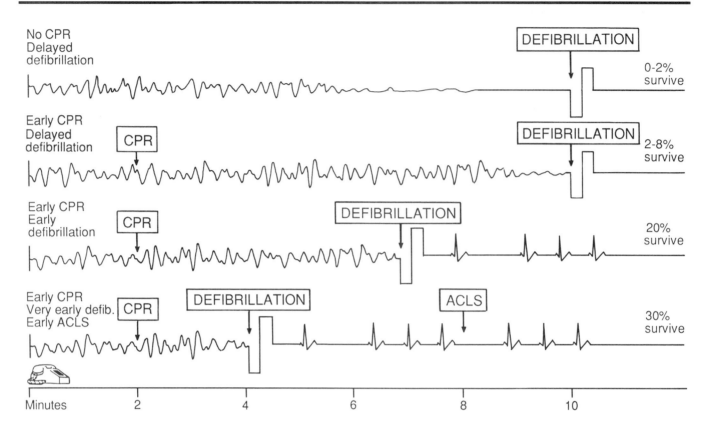

No CPR
Delayed
defibrillation

DEFIBRILLATION

0-2%
survive

Early CPR
Delayed
defibrillation

CPR

DEFIBRILLATION

2-8%
survive

Early CPR
Early
defibrillation

CPR

DEFIBRILLATION

20%
survive

Early CPR
Very early defib.
Early ACLS

CPR

DEFIBRILLATION

ACLS

30%
survive

Minutes   2   4   6   8   10

Figure 2. **Survival rates are estimates of probability of survival to hospital discharge for patients with witnessed collapse and with ventricular fibrillation as initial rhythm. Estimates are based on a large number of published studies, which are collectively reviewed in References 26 and 27.**

Many adult patients in ventricular fibrillation can survive neurologically intact even if defibrillation is performed as late as 6–10 minutes after the arrest.[23,28–31] CPR performed during this period of waiting for the defibrillator appears to extend the existence of ventricular fibrillation and to contribute to preservation of heart and brain function.[30–32] The use of basic CPR, however, cannot convert hearts in ventricular fibrillation to a normal rhythm.

The speed with which defibrillation is performed is a major determinant of the success of resuscitation attempts. Nearly all neurologically intact survivors, who in some studies number more than 90%, were patients with a ventricular tachyarrhythmia that had been treated by emergency personnel.[23,28–31] It appears from studies in which Holter monitors were used that ventricular tachycardia is the initial rhythm disturbance[30] in approximately 85% of persons with sudden, out-of-hospital, nontraumatic cardiac arrest. Ventricular tachycardia, however, is frequently short lived and converts rapidly to ventricular fibrillation, from which the only hope for successful resuscitation lies in early defibrillation. Furthermore, the proportion of patients with ventricular fibrillation also declines with each passing minute as more and more of these patients deteriorate

into asystole, from which successful resuscitation is extremely unlikely. The remaining nonventricular fibrillation patients have a low probability of survival with current resuscitation techniques. By 4–8 minutes after the attack, approximately 50% of patients are still in ventricular fibrillation.[10,11,24,25,28]

Survival rates from cardiac arrest can be remarkably high if the event is witnessed. For example, when people in supervised cardiac rehabilitation programs suffer a witnessed cardiac arrest, defibrillation is usually performed within minutes; in four studies of cardiac arrest in this setting, 90 of 101 victims (89%) were resuscitated.[33–36] This is the highest survival rate reported for a defined out-of-hospital population.

Improved survival rates of patients with cardiac arrest have been reported from communities that had no prehospital ACLS services but added early defibrillation programs. The most impressive results were reported from King County, Washington, where the survival rate of patients with ventricular fibrillation improved from 7% to 26%,[37] and from rural Iowa, where the survival rate for ventricular fibrillation rose from 3% to 19%.[38] More modest results have been observed in rural communities of southeastern Minnesota,[39] northeastern Minnesota,[40] and Wisconsin[41] (Table 1).

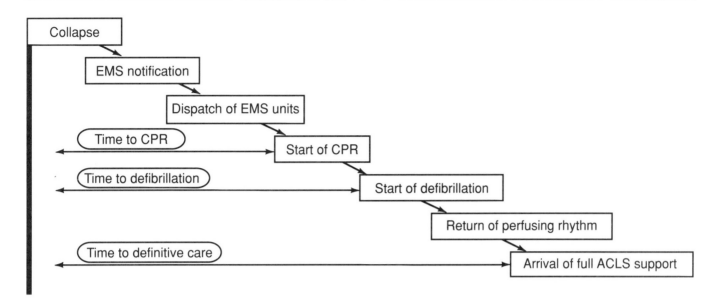

Figure 3. Sequence of events and key intervals that occur with cardiac arrest, based on Reference 27.

Table 1. Effectiveness of Early Defibrillation Programs[17]

Location	Before early defibrillation	After early defibrillation	Odds ratio for improved survival
King County, Washington	7	26 (10/38)	3.7
Iowa	3 (1/31)	19 (12/64)	6.3
SE Minnesota	4 (1/27)	17 (6/36)	4.3
NE Minnesota	2 (3/118)	10 (8/81)	5.0
Wisconsin	4 (32/893)	11 (33/304)	2.8

Values are percent surviving and, in parentheses, how many patients had ventricular fibrillation.

Table 2. Range of Survival Rate to Hospital Discharge for All Cardiac Arrests and Ventricular Fibrillation by System Type: Data From 29 Locations[26]

System type	Survival: All rhythms (%)	Weighted average (%)	Survival: Ventricular fibrillation (%)	Weighted average (%)
EMT only	2–9	5	3–20	12
EMT-D	4–19	10	6–26	16
Paramedics	7–18	10	13–30	17
EMT/paramedic	4–26	17	23–33	26
EMT-D/paramedic	13–18	17	27–29	29

A major determinant in these studies was time. It is clear that the earlier defibrillation occurs, the better the prognosis. Emergency personnel have only a few minutes after the collapse of a person to reestablish a sustained perfusing rhythm (Figure 2). The use of CPR can sustain a patient for a short period of time but cannot directly restore an organized rhythm. Restoration of an adequate perfusing rhythm requires defibrillation and advanced cardiac care, which must be administered within a few minutes of the initial arrest. Table 2 compares the differences in survival observed in different types of EMS systems. These systems differ in how well they strengthen the chain of survival. Figure 3 displays the sequence of events that must occur to ensure a successful resuscitation from cardiac arrest. The use of AEDs increases the range of personnel who can use a defibrillator and thus shortens the time between collapse and defibrillation. This exciting prospect accounts for the addition of this material to the ACLS training curriculum.

Overview of Automated External Defibrillators

Types of Automated External Defibrillators

The generic term "automated external defibrillators" refers to external defibrillators that incorporate a rhythm analysis system. Some devices are considered "fully" automated, whereas others are "semiautomated" or "shock-advisory" defibrillators.[42] All AEDs are attached to the patient by two adhesive pads and connecting cables,[43] as shown in Figure 4. These adhesive pads have two functions — to record the rhythm and to deliver the electric shock. A fully automated defibrillator requires only that the operator attach the defibrillatory pads and turn on the device. The device then analyzes the rhythm; if ventricular fibrillation (or ventricular tachycardia above a preset rate) is present, the device will charge its capacitors and deliver a shock.

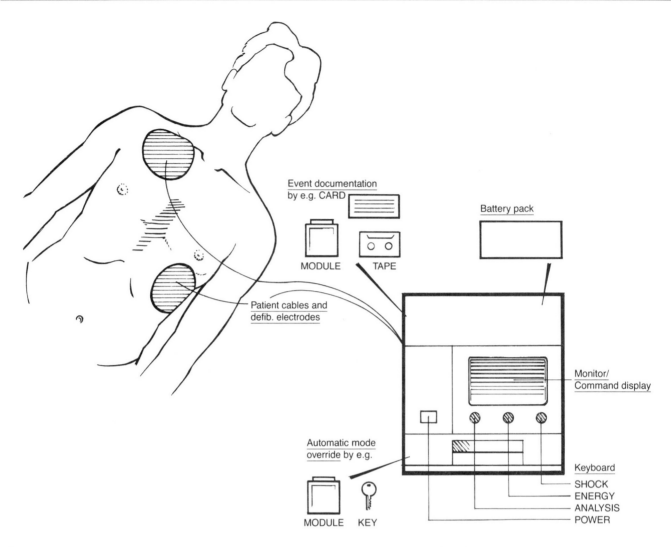

Figure 4. Schematic drawing of automated external defibrillator and its attachments to patient.

Semiautomated or shock-advisory devices require additional operator steps, including pressing an "analyze" control to initiate rhythm analysis and pressing a "shock" control to deliver the shock. The shock control is pressed only when the device identifies ventricular fibrillation and "advises" the operator to press the shock control.

Fully automated defibrillators were developed with simple requirements for use by inexperienced operators. Primarily, this user group has comprised family members of high-risk patients and emergency personnel who are rarely called on to treat patients in cardiac arrest.

Shock-advisory AEDs may be safer because they never enter the analysis mode unless activated by the operator and they leave the final decision of whether to deliver the shock to the operator. This increase in safety is more theoretical than real because clinical experience suggests the devices are equally safe with or without a human operator to push the final shock button.[42]

Automated Analysis of Cardiac Rhythms

Unlike many other devices and approaches in emergency medicine, AEDs have been extensively tested, both in vitro against libraries of recorded cardiac rhythms[44] and clinically in numerous field trials.[39,45–52] The accuracy of the devices in rhythm analysis has been high. The rare errors noted with AEDs in field trials have been almost solely errors of omission where the device failed to recognize certain varieties of ventricular fibrillation or tachycardia.

The presently available AEDs are highly sophisticated, microprocessor-based devices that analyze multiple features of the surface ECG signal, including frequency, amplitude, and some integration of frequency and amplitude such as slope or wave morphology (Figure 5). A variety of filters check for QRS-like signals, radio transmission, or 60-cycle interference as well as for loose electrodes and poor electrode contact. Some

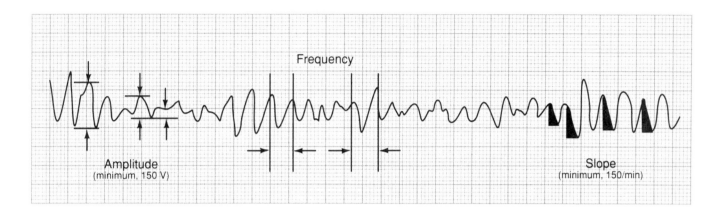

Figure 5. Features of surface electrocardiogram analyzed by automated external defibrillators.

devices are programmed to detect spontaneous patient movements, continued heartbeat and blood flow, or movement of the patient by others.

AEDs take multiple "looks" at the patient's rhythm, each look lasting a few seconds. If several of these analyses confirm the presence of a rhythm for which a shock is indicated and the other checks are consistent with a nonperfusing cardiac status, the fully automated defibrillator will charge and deliver a shock to the patient. The semiautomated devices will signal the operator that a shock is advised. It does this after charging the capacitors, which does not occur until appropriate ventricular fibrillation or tachycardia has been identified. Once the capacitors are charged, a shock is advised. The operator can then push a shock button, and the shock is delivered.

Inappropriate Shocks

Extensive clinical experience has revealed that AEDs are not misled by patient movements (e.g., seizures and agonal respirations), by the patient being moved by others, or by artifactual signals.[45–52] Although the occurrence of inappropriate shocks in such circumstances has not been reported, AEDs should be placed in the analysis mode only when all movement, particularly the movement of patient transport, has ceased. The only major errors reported in clinical trials have been occasional failures to deliver shocks to rhythms that may benefit from electrical therapy, such as extremely fine or coarse ventricular fibrillation.

Ventricular Tachycardia

Although not designed to deliver synchronized shocks, all AEDs will shock monomorphic and polymorphic ventricular tachycardia if the rate is more than preset values. All rescuers who operate AEDs are trained to attach the device only to unconscious patients who are pulseless and apneic. With this approach, the operator serves as a second verification system to confirm that the patient has suffered a cardiac arrest. In an apneic, pulseless patient, electrical shocks are indicated whether the rhythm is supraventricular tachycardia, ventricular tachycardia, or ventricular fibrillation. There have been no reports of shocks delivered to conscious patients with perfusing ventricular or supraventricular dysrhythmias — a testament to good training and good patient-assessment skills of rescuers.

Interruption of CPR

Emergency personnel must not touch the patient while the AED analyzes the rhythm, charges the capacitors, and delivers the shocks. Chest compression and ventilation must cease while the device is operating; this permits accurate analysis of the cardiac rhythm and prevents accidental shocks to the rescuers. Movements induced by CPR can cause the AED to stop its analysis. The time between activating the rhythm analysis system, which is when CPR must stop, and the delivery of a shock averages 10–15 seconds.

This time without CPR that occurs with the use of AEDs is a recognized exception to the AHA guidelines, which recommend that CPR not be stopped for more than 5 seconds. With the use of AEDs, the negative effects of temporarily stopping CPR are outweighed by the positive effects of delivering an early defibrillatory shock. For patients in refractory ventricular fibrillation after the first shock, CPR may have to be interrupted for even longer periods of time to deliver the recommended three sequential shocks. Consequently, the standards for CPR and ECC accept a period of a maximum of 90 seconds for diagnosing ventricular fibrillation and delivering three shocks.[18,p2942]

Advantages and Disadvantages of Automated External Defibrillators

The major distinction between an automated and a conventional defibrillator is that a person must interpret the cardiac rhythm when a conventional defibrillator is used, but an electrical device interprets the rhythm when an AED is used.

Initial Training and Continuing Education

Conventional defibrillators require regular training and continuing education in rhythm recognition and device operation. The only psychomotor skills required by an AED user involve recognition of a cardiac arrest, proper attachment of the device, and adherence to the memorized treatment sequence. Learning to use and operate an AED is easier than learning to perform CPR.[53] Many of the advantages of AEDs stem from brief, convenient training sessions and continuing education.[54] In systems in which compensation must be provided for the initial training time and skills review classes, the use of AEDs offers considerable financial savings.[55] In systems in which the anticipated number of cardiac arrests is low, skills maintenance is a major concern.[19,20] AEDs offer considerable advantages in these situations because little continuing education is needed.

Speed of Operation

In clinical trials, emergency personnel using an AED deliver the first shock an average of 1 minute sooner than personnel using conventional defibrillators.[48,49]

Rhythm Detection

Two field studies have compared the rhythm detection ability of AEDs with that of emergency personnel.[48,49] Although AEDs have not achieved 100% accuracy in rhythm detection, they perform as well as EMTs who use conventional defibrillators.[48,49] The errors of AEDs have generally been limited to identification of very fine or very coarse ventricular fibrillation. Presently available AEDs have responded appropriately to perfusing rhythms and to cardiac arrest rhythms for which shocks are not indicated.

Remote Defibrillation Through Adhesive Pads

Another advantage of AEDs stems from the use of the adhesive defibrillatory pads attached to the patient by connecting cables.[56] This approach permits remote, "hands-off" defibrillation, which is a safer method from the operator's perspective, particularly in the close confines of aeromedical and ground transport vehicles.

Adhesive defibrillatory pads may also offer consistently better paddle placement during a lengthy resuscitation attempt. Although some conventional defibrillators have adapters that permit operation through remote adhesive pads, they are not widely used. All AEDs, however, have adhesive monitor-defibrillatory pads. With adhesive pads, the operator cannot bear down with the heavy pressure that is required to use the paddles of conventional defibrillators. This pressure is recommended to lower the transthoracic resistance by improving contact between the electrodes and the skin, decreasing the intrathoracic volume, and bringing the paddles closer to each other. The adhesive pads offer comparable low impedance, however, due to their larger pad surface area.[57]

Rhythm Monitoring

In clinical settings that require frequent rhythm monitoring, the liquid crystal rhythm displays of some AEDs are less suitable than the bright cathode-ray displays of conventional defibrillators.

Use of Automated External Defibrillators During Resuscitation Attempts

Operational Steps

All AEDs can be operated by following four simple steps:
1. Turn on the power.
2. Attach the device.
3. Initiate analysis of the rhythm.
4. Deliver the shock, if indicated.

Different brands and models of AEDs have a variety of features and controls and may differ in characteristics such as paper strip recorders, rhythm display methods, energy levels, and messages to the operator. Operators can orient themselves best by understanding how each brand and model approaches the previously mentioned four steps.

Standard Operational Procedures

Compared with the Megacode resuscitation procedures for ACLS, resuscitation attempts in which AEDs are used are relatively simple because there are fewer therapeutic options when only automated defibrillation and basic CPR can be implemented.

Most response teams, including those in-hospital, in medical clinics, or out-of-hospital, consist of at least two persons. One team member operates the defibrillator, and one member begins BLS. No other activities, including setting up oxygen delivery systems, suction equipment, intravenous lines, or mechanical CPR devices, should take precedence over or delay rhythm analysis and defibrillation. Instead, these interventions should proceed simultaneously if possible. The rescuer responsible for defibrillation concentrates on operating the defibrillator, while other rescuers attend to airway management, ventilations, and chest compressions.

The rescuer places the AED close to the supine patient's left ear and performs the defibrillation protocols from the patient's left side. This position provides better access to the defibrillator controls and easier placement of the defibrillatory pads and allows the other rescuer room to perform CPR. However, this position may not be possible in all clinical settings.

Depending on the manufacturer, the AED is turned on by pressing a power switch or by lifting the monitor screen to the "up" position. This activates the voice-ECG tape recorder and permits environmental sounds and operator statements to be recorded along with the patient's cardiac rhythm.

The adhesive defibrillatory pads are opened quickly and attached first to the defibrillatory cables and then to the patient's chest. The pads are placed in a modified lead II position (upper-right sternal border and lower-left ribs over the apex of the heart). When the pads are attached, CPR should be stopped, and the analysis control should be pressed. All contact with the patient during analysis must be avoided. Assessment of the rhythms takes from 5 to 15 seconds, depending on the brand of the AED. If ventricular fibrillation is present, the device will announce that a shock is indicated by a written message, a visual alarm, or, often, a voice-synthesized statement.

The rescuer must always state loudly a "clear-the-patient" message, such as "I'm clear. You're clear. Everybody clear" or simply "Clear," before pressing the shock control. In most devices, pressing the analyze button initiates charging of the capacitors if a treatable rhythm is detected. The device shows that charging has started with a tone, a voice-synthesized message, or a light indicator. Shock delivery should produce a sudden contraction of the patient's musculature like that seen with the use of a conventional defibrillator. After the first shock is delivered, CPR is not restarted; instead, the analyze control is pressed immediately to start another rhythm analysis cycle. If ventricular fibrillation persists, the device will indicate this, and the "charging" and "shock indicated" sequence is repeated for the second and third shocks. The goal is to analyze quickly for any persisting rhythm treatable by electrical shocks (Figure 6).

Age and Weight Guidelines

Cardiac arrest in the pediatric age group is seldom caused by ventricular fibrillation. Defibrillation, therefore, is of minor importance in pediatric resuscitation and certainly should not take priority over airway clearance and maintenance. It is recommended that presently available AEDs not be used in pediatric cardiac arrest; they are not capable of the lower energy settings required for pediatric defibrillation. The recommended maximum energy level for defibrillatory shocks in children is 4 J/kg. AEDs now have a minimum energy level of 200 J, which is high for patients weighing less than 50 kg (110 lb). Most experienced EMS systems recommend the following approach, which is also recommended by the AHA: Attach AEDs only to patients in cardiac arrest who weigh more than 90 lb.

Persistent Ventricular Fibrillation and No Available ACLS

The energy levels of the second and third shocks can range from 200 to 360 J. The guidelines for CPR and ECC recommend the use of 200–300 J for the second shock and an energy level "not to exceed 360 J" for a third shock if the first two shocks fail to defibrillate. Some AEDs are programmed to automatically increase the energy level to 360 J on the third shock. Others allow the operator to either remain at 200 J or increase the energy level for subsequent shocks. Neither approach has been established as superior. Some evidence suggests that lower energy shocks have a greater likelihood of leaving the patient in persistent ventricular fibrillation, whereas higher energy shocks may more frequently leave the patient in asystole.[58]

If no pulse returns after these three shocks, rescuers with AEDs but without immediate ACLS backup should not press the analysis button but should instead resume CPR for 60 seconds. They should then deliver additional rounds of three "stacked" defibrillatory shocks after the appropriate analysis period if ventricular fibrillation continues. Presently available AEDs will return to a sequence of 200-, 200-, and 360-J shocks at this point, although programmable modules allow a variety of protocols, depending on local practice. If the patient must be transported by the AED response team, then standing orders and guidelines will vary depending on local protocols.

AEDs can be left attached to the patient during transport in moving vehicles. However, AEDs should never be placed in the analyze mode in such circumstances because the movement of the transport vehicle can interfere with rhythm assessment. If a patient requires rhythm analysis and treatment during transport, then the vehicle must be brought to a complete stop. CPR should be administered during transport when indicated.

Ventricular Fibrillation and Pulseless Ventricular Tachycardia

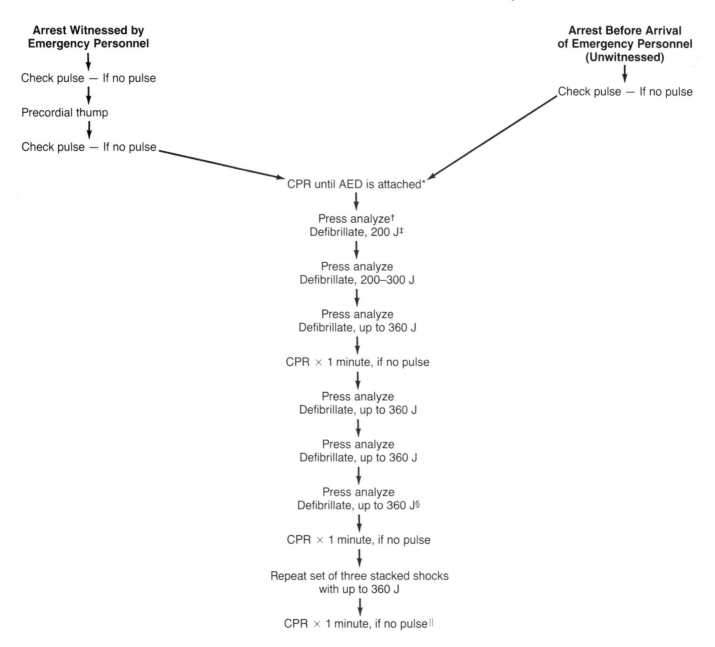

Arrest Witnessed by Emergency Personnel

Check pulse — If no pulse

Precordial thump

Check pulse — If no pulse

Arrest Before Arrival of Emergency Personnel (Unwitnessed)

Check pulse — If no pulse

CPR until AED is attached*

Press analyze†
Defibrillate, 200 J‡

Press analyze
Defibrillate, 200–300 J

Press analyze
Defibrillate, up to 360 J

CPR × 1 minute, if no pulse

Press analyze
Defibrillate, up to 360 J

Press analyze
Defibrillate, up to 360 J

Press analyze
Defibrillate, up to 360 J§

CPR × 1 minute, if no pulse

Repeat set of three stacked shocks with up to 360 J

CPR × 1 minute, if no pulse‖

*The single rescuer with an AED should verify unresponsiveness, open the airway (A), give two respirations (B), and check the pulse (C). If a full cardiac arrest is confirmed, the rescuer should attach the AED and proceed with the algorithm.
†If "no shock indicated" appears, check pulse, repeat 1 minute of CPR, and then reanalyze. After three "no shock indicated" messages are received, repeat analyze period every 1–2 minutes.
‡Pulse check is not required after shocks 1, 2, 4, and 5 unless the "no shock indicated" message appears.
§If ventricular fibrillation recurs after transiently converting (rather than persists without ever converting), restart the treatment algorithm from the top.
‖In the unlikely event that ventricular fibrillation persists after nine shocks, then repeat sets of three stacked shocks, with 1 minute of CPR between each set.

Figure 6.   Recommended treatment algorithm for ventricular fibrillation and pulseless ventricular tachycardia when ACLS cannot be provided and an automated external defibrillator and a trained provider are present.

Recurrent Ventricular Fibrillation — Refibrillation With No Available ACLS

If the patient regains a perfusing rhythm after receiving shocks and at some later time refibrillates, the rescuer using an AED should restart the treatment sequence from the beginning.[53] Whenever the "no shock indicated" message is received, the rescuer should check for a pulse and, if there is none, resume CPR. Three "no shock indicated" messages indicate that there is a low probability that the rhythm present can be successfully shocked. Therefore, the rhythm analysis time periods should be repeated only at 1–3-minute intervals.

Single Rescuer With an Automated External Defibrillator

In some situations, a single rescuer equipped with or with immediate access to an AED may have to respond to a person in cardiac arrest. Traditional BLS guidelines recommended that whenever the rescuer is alone, "CPR should be performed for about 1 minute and then help should be summoned."[18,p2919] The purpose of this 1 minute of CPR was to provide circulation of oxygenated blood before efforts to activate the EMS system. Activation of the EMS system, in turn, aims to get a defibrillator to the patient as fast as possible. Because defibrillation, in the form of the AED, is already available, the minute of CPR and the immediate activation of the EMS system becomes of less importance. The need for rapid identification and defibrillation of shockable rhythms dictates attachment of the AED and analysis of the rhythm before 1 minute of CPR. A full cardiac arrest with an unobstructed airway must be confirmed. The prescribed period of CPR by the lone rescuer, however, can be omitted. Consequently, the rescue sequence becomes verify unresponsiveness, open the airway, give two respirations, and check the pulse. If no pulse, attach the AED and proceed with the algorithm for ventricular fibrillation and pulseless ventricular tachycardia (Figure 6). Activation of the EMS system should occur whenever the "no shock indicated" message is displayed or when someone else arrives on the scene.

No Pulse Checks Between Shocks

The ACLS Subcommittee Task Force on Early Defibrillation recommended that there be no pulse check between the stacked shocks, that is, after shocks 1, 2, 4, and 5. The conventional ACLS ventricular fibrillation protocols require a pulse check after these shocks because the leads may have become dislodged, an artifact may be producing "false" ventricular fibrillation, or an unrecognized perfusing rhythm may have returned. These sources of error do not occur with the use of AEDs; they have sensors to detect loose electrodes,

artifactual rhythms, and regular rhythms associated with return of palpable pulse. Mandating a pulse check between shocks for AEDs will delay rapid identification of persistent ventricular fibrillation, interfere with the assessment capabilities of the devices, and increase the possibility of operator errors.

Summary of Standard Operational Procedures

The rescuer using an AED in the absence of ACLS can memorize an easy treatment sequence:
1. Attach AEDs only to people in apparent cardiac arrest.
2. Always shock in sets of three.
3. Every time the chest is touched after the first assessment, it should be to perform CPR for 1 minute.
4. Continue to shock until the "no shock" indicated message is received.

Coordination of ACLS-Trained Provider With Personnel Using Automated External Defibrillators

With the increasing availability of AEDs, ACLS-trained emergency personnel will interact more frequently with AED-trained personnel. The following guidelines are suggested for this interface between ACLS personnel and personnel using AEDs.
1. ACLS-trained (and authorized) providers always have authority over the scene.
2. On arrival, ACLS-trained providers should ask for a quick report from the automated defibrillation providers and direct them to proceed with their protocols. This is particularly applicable when ACLS-trained providers are unfamiliar with the operation of the AED.
3. ACLS-trained providers should use the AED for additional shocks and rhythm monitoring. They can direct the providers to operate the AED. To save time, avoid disorganization, and allow a coordinated transfer of care, ACLS providers should not remove the AED and attach a separate conventional defibrillator, unless the AED in use lacks a rhythm display screen. Most AEDs have the capacity for "manual override" by ACLS-trained providers, should that be necessary. The method and ease for manual override will vary among models.

4. ACLS-trained providers should consider the shocks delivered by the AED operators as part of their ACLS protocols. For example, if the patient remains in ventricular fibrillation after three shocks by the AED, then the ACLS personnel should enter the ACLS ventricular fibrillation treatment sequence at the point at which the first three shocks have been delivered. Consequently, ACLS providers should move immediately to establish intravenous line access, administer epinephrine, and perform endotracheal intubation.

5. In most circumstances, the AED should be removed and a conventional defibrillator attached only when the patient has regained a spontaneous rhythm or is ready for transport to another location or when the ACLS provider has reason to believe the AED is malfunctioning. Some models of AEDs lack a rhythm display monitor; thus, ACLS personnel will want to attach a conventional defibrillator when clinically convenient.

Postresuscitation Care

Once an automated external defibrillation provider team completes its protocol, several things could happen. Patients could display a maximal response to resuscitation (see Chapter 14) and be awake, responsive, and breathing spontaneously; a palpable pulse may be restored with a variety of hemodynamic profiles and thus a variety of neurological and respiratory responses; cardiac arrest may persist without a rhythm that will respond to shocks; or a pulseless ventricular tachycardia or fibrillation may remain. In each event, patient care remains paramount. If the patient regains a pulse, the resuscitation team will continue to provide supportive care with one or a combination of the following.

- Proper airway control and ventilatory management
- Supplemental oxygen, if available
- Appropriate airway clearance if vomiting occurs
- Continued monitoring of vital signs
- Physical stabilization and transport
- Continued support while awaiting the arrival of the ACLS team

Training

Sources of Information

The AHA training materials on AEDs are provided in the *Instructor's Manual for Advanced Cardiac Life Support* and the *Supplement to the Instructor's Manual for Advanced Cardiac Life Support*. These sources also include information for the electrical therapy lecture and the electrical therapy teaching station in the ACLS provider's course.

The instructor's manual and supplement include a detailed instructor's curriculum and instructor's guidelines for a separate provider's course on AEDs. The AHA does not intend to approve, control, or directly supervise such courses because EMS agencies of most states already provide these functions. Instead, this material is intended to provide a standardized, national curriculum and course content that can be adapted for local use. It is hoped that the AHA-approved algorithms and recommendations for the proper use of AEDs will lead to greater national uniformity in the use of these devices.

General Points About Training

Because of the intrinsic simplicity of AEDs, a markedly expanded range of individuals can now be trained to provide early defibrillation. Individuals who may want training in the use of AEDs include general hospital floor nurses, general office nurses, oral surgeons, dentists, physician assistants, nurse practitioners, security and law enforcement personnel, ship and airplane crews, supervisory personnel at senior citizen centers and exercise facilities, and the entire range of professional prehospital providers, including first-responders, firefighters, and EMTs. In addition, physicians who are not involved in daily emergency care but nevertheless perceive themselves at risk of encountering a patient in cardiac arrest may be interested in learning to use AEDs.

Maintenance of Skills

Survey results and experience in rural communities have demonstrated that depending on the rate of cardiac arrest in a community, an emergency responder may go several years without treating a patient in cardiac arrest.[19,21] Therefore, every program director must determine how to ensure correct performance when such an event occurs. Principles of adult education suggest that frequent practice of a psychomotor skill such as operating an AED in a simulated cardiac arrest offers the best skill maintenance.

Practice Frequency

The frequency and content of these practice sessions have been established by several successful programs.[6,19,37] At the present time, most systems permit a maximum of 90 days between practice drills and have found this to be satisfactory. Note that this is a **maximum** interval between drills. Many emergency personnel and systems drill as often as once a month.

The most successful long-term skill maintenance occurs when individual rescuers voluntarily take a few minutes to perform a quick check of the equipment on a frequent and regular basis. This check includes a visual inspection of the defibrillator components and controls and a mental review of the steps to be followed and the controls to be operated in the event of a cardiac arrest.

Session Content

The practice sessions can be as elaborate as interest and time allow and can include more advanced discussions of ECC. The following is recommended as a minimum content of a 30–60-minute practice session that should occur at least once every 90 days.
- Performance review of recent patients
- Review of equipment operation and maintenance
- Review of standing orders
- Discussion of treatment possibilities
- Scenario practice of field protocols with a training manikin, a defibrillator, and a rhythm simulator; this practice should simulate actual cardiac arrests and include entrance to the scene, two-person response teams, ongoing CPR, a variety of initial rhythms, and a variety of postshock responses
- An objective skills test, with a skills checklist (see the supplement to the instructor's manual)

Medical Control

In emergencies, critical medical procedures must be performed by the first trained personnel who respond. Within the constraints of state law, health providers can perform some medical procedures in emergencies but only with the medical authorization of a physician. The authorizing physician assumes medical control and takes legal responsibility for the performance of the emergency care providers. The authorizing physician issues standing orders, which are in effect direct orders to perform specified tasks for a patient. The emergency rescuer must always operate under the authority of the medical license of the medical director and the enabling administrative codes of the state.

Successful Completion of Course

The AHA does **not** provide medical control for interventions taught in BLS or ACLS classes. "Successful completion" of an AHA course, including any automated external defibrillation provider's course that follows AHA recommendations, means only that a certain level of cognitive and performance standards has been met. Successful completion does not warrant performance, nor does it qualify or authorize a person to perform any procedure on a patient. Licensure and certification is a function of the appropriate state legislative or local health or EMS authority. Such licensure and certification may or may not be related to successful completion of a course following ACLS guidelines. The primary objectives of any automated defibrillation provider's course that follows AHA recommendations are educational.

Case-by-Case Review

Every event in which an AED is used (or could have been used) must be reviewed by the medical director or designated representative. This means that every incident in which CPR is performed must have a medical review to establish whether the patient was treated in accordance with professional standards and local standing orders. In each review, whether ventricular fibrillation and other rhythms were treated appropriately with shocks and with BLS must be considered. Other dimensions of performance that can be evaluated include command of the scene, safety, efficiency, speed, professionalism, ability to troubleshoot, completeness of patient care, and interactions with other professionals and bystanders.[59]

Methods of Case-by-Case Review

The three ways in which the case-by-case review is performed are by a written report, by review of the recordings made by the voice-ECG tape recorders attached to AEDs, and by solid-state memory modules and magnetic tape recordings that store information about each use of the device. The latter two methods are innovative approaches to event documentation, record-keeping, and data management that have been recently developed and incorporated into AEDs.[59] Case reviews that use all three approaches appear to offer the most complete information. Particular requirements or constraints in some systems, however, may dictate various combinations of these approaches rather than all three. Future innovations in event documentation, such as digital voice recordings, annotated rhythm strips, and other microprocessor-based approaches, offer even more options.

Quality Assurance

Quality assurance refers to both the microperformance, that is, the performance of personnel involved in the treatment of individual patients, and the macroperformance, that is, the overall effectiveness of a system that uses AEDs. Quality assurance requires establishment of a system's performance goals, a review to determine whether those goals are being met, and feedback to move the system closer to unmet goals.[54] Review of the treatment of an individual patient in cardiac arrest can lead to identification of a problem in a system's training program.

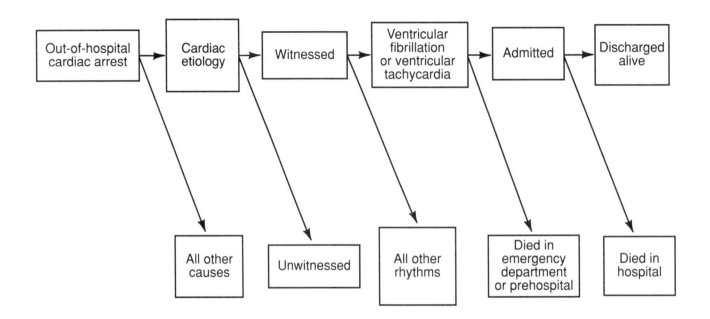

Figure 7. Recommended uniform data reporting approach for out-of-hospital cardiac arrest, based upon data from Reference 27.

Organized collection and review of patient data can identify systemwide problems and allow assessment of each link in the chain of survival for the adult victim of sudden cardiac death. Figure 7 presents the recommended minimum data that a system should obtain on cardiac arrest patients. Adult victims of witnessed cardiac arrest of presumed heart etiology and caused by ventricular fibrillation appear to be the best group on which to focus. The lower-than-expected hospital discharge rates of this group may be explained by long ambulance response times, delayed EMS activation, infrequent witnessed arrests, rare bystander CPR, or slow on-scene performance. Each of these problems can be addressed with a specific programwide effort. Continued systematic and uniform data collection will determine whether the new efforts succeed.

References

1. Atkins JM: Emergency medical service systems in acute cardiac care: State of the art. *Circulation* 1986;74(suppl IV):IV-4–IV-8
2. Cummins RO, Eisenberg MS, Stults KR: Automatic external defibrillators: Clinical issues for cardiology. *Circulation* 1986;73:381–385
3. White RD: EMT-defibrillation: Time for controlled implementation of effective treatment. *American Heart Association Emergency Cardiac Care National Faculty Newsletter* 1986;8:1–3
4. Atkins JM, Murphy D, Allison EJ Jr, Graves JR: Toward earlier defibrillation. *Emerg Med Serv* 1986;11:70
5. Eisenberg MS, Cummins RO: Defibrillation performed by the emergency medical technician. *Circulation* 1986;74(suppl IV):IV-9–IV-12
6. Cummins RO: EMT defibrillation: National guidelines for implementation. *Am J Emerg Med* 1987;5:254–257
7. Ruskin JN: Automatic external defibrillators and sudden cardiac death (editorial). *N Engl J Med* 1988;319:713–715
8. Cummins RO, Eisenberg MS: EMT defibrillation: A proven concept. *American Heart Association Emergency Cardiac Care National Faculty Newsletter* 1984;1:1–3.
9. Cummins RO, Eisenberg MS, Moore JE, Hearne TR, Andresen E, Wendt R, Litwin PE, Graves JR, Hallstrom AP, Pierce J: Automatic external defibrillators: Clinical, training, psychological, and public health issues. *Ann Emerg Med* 1985;14:755–760
10. Newman MM: National EMT-D study. *J Emerg Med Serv* 1986;11:70–72
11. Newman MM: The survival advantage: Early defibrillation programs in the fire service. *J Emerg Med Serv* 1987;12:40–46
12. Cummins RO, Eisenberg MS, Bergner L, Hallstrom AP, Hearne T, Murray JA: Automatic external defibrillation: Evaluations of its role in the home and in emergency medical services. *Ann Emerg Med* 1984;13:798–801
13. Jacobs L: Medical, legal and social implications of automatic external defibrillators (editorial). *Ann Emerg Med* 1986;15:863-864
14. ACT (Advanced Coronary Treatment Foundation): EMT defibrillation — ACT Foundation issues policy statement. *J Emerg Med Serv* 1983;8:37
15. American College of Emergency Physicians EMS Committee: Prehospital defibrillation by basic-level emergency medical technicians. *Ann Emerg Med* 1984;13:974
16. Paris PM: EMT-defibrillation: A recipe for saving lives. *Am J Emerg Med* 1988;6:282–287
17. Cummins RO: From concept to standard-of-care? Review of the clinical experience with automated external defibrillators. *Ann Emerg Med* 1989;18:1269–1275
18. American Heart Association: Standards and guidelines for cardiopulmonary resuscitation (CPR) and emergency cardiac care (ECC). *JAMA* 1980;244:453–508
19. Stults KR, Brown DD: Special considerations for defibrillation performed by emergency medical technicians in small communities. *Circulation* 1986;74(suppl IV):IV-13–IV-17
20. Ornato JP, McNeill SE, Craren EJ, Nelson NM: Limitations on effectiveness of rapid defibrillation by emergency medical technicians in a rural setting. *Ann Emerg Med* 1984;13:1096–1099
21. Cummins RO, Eisenberg MS, Graves JR, Damon SK: EMT-defibrillation: Is it right for you? *Emerg Med Serv* 1985;10:60–64

22. Newman MM: The Chain of Survival concept takes hold. *J Emerg Med Serv* 1989;14:11–13

23. Eisenberg MS, Bergner L, Hallstrom AP: Paramedic programs and out-of-hospital cardiac arrest: I. Factors associated with successful resuscitation. *Am J Public Health* 1979;69:31–38

24. Eisenberg MS, Bergner L, Hallstrom AP: Paramedic programs and out-of-hospital cardiac arrest: II. Impact on community mortality. *Am J Public Health* 1979;69:39–42

25. Eisenberg MS, Copass MK, Hallstrom AP, Cobb LA, Bergner L: Management of out-of-hospital cardiac arrest: Failure of basic emergency medical technician services. *JAMA* 1980;2243:1049–1051

26. Eisenberg MS, Horwood BT, Cummins RO, Reynolds-Haertle R, Hearne TR: Cardiac arrest and resuscitation: A tale of 29 cities. *Ann Emerg Med* 1990;19:179–186

27. Eisenberg MS, Cummins RO, Damon S, Larsen MP, Hearne TR: Survival rates from out-of-hospital cardiac arrest: Recommendations for uniform definitions and data to report. *Ann Emerg Med* 1990;20 (in press)

28. Eisenberg MS, Hallstrom AP, Copass MK, Bergner L, Short F, Pierce J: Treatment of ventricular fibrillation: Emergency medical technician defibrillation and paramedic services. *JAMA* 1984;251:1723–1726

29. Weaver WD, Copass MK, Bufi D, Ray R, Hallstrom AP, Cobb LA: Improved neurologic recovery and survival after early defibrillation. *Circulation* 1984;69:943–948

30. Cobb LA, Werner JA, Trobaugh GB: Sudden cardiac death: I. A decade's experience with out-of-hospital resuscitation. *Mod Concepts Cardiovasc Dis* 1980;49:31–36

31. Cobb LA, Hallstrom AP: Community-based cardiopulmonary resuscitation: What have we learned? *Ann NY Acad Sci* 1982;382:330–342

32. Bayes de Luna A, Coumel P, Leclercq JF: Ambulatory sudden cardiac death: Mechanisms of production of fatal arrhythmia on the basis of data from 157 cases. *Am Heart J* 1989;117:151–159

33. Fletcher GF, Cantwell JD: Ventricular fibrillation in a medically supervised cardiac exercise program: Clinical, angiographic, and surgical correlations. *JAMA* 1977;238:2627–2629

34. Haskell WL: Cardiovascular complications during exercise training of cardiac patients. *Circulation* 1978;57:920–924

35. Hossack KF, Hartwig R: Cardiac arrest associates with supervised cardiac rehabilitation. *J Cardiac Rehab* 1982;2:402–408

36. Van Camp SP, Peterson RA: Cardiovascular complications of outpatient cardiac rehabilitation programs. *JAMA* 1986;256:1160–1163

37. Eisenberg MS, Copass MK, Hallstrom AP, Blake B, Bergner L, Short FA, Cobb LA: Treatment of out-of-hospital cardiac arrests with rapid defibrillation by emergency medical technicians. *N Engl J Med* 1980;302:1379–1383

38. Stults KR, Brown DD, Schug VL, Bean JA: Prehospital defibrillation performed by emergency medical technicians in rural communities. *N Engl J Med* 1984;310:219–223

39. Vukov LF, White RD, Bachman JW, O'Brien PC: New perspectives on rural EMT defibrillation. *Ann Emerg Med* 1988;17:318–321

40. Bachman JW, McDonald GS, O'Brien PC: A study of out-of-hospital cardiac arrests in northeastern Minnesota. *JAMA* 1986;256:477–483

41. Olson DW, Larochelle J, Fark D, Aprahamian C, Aufderheide TP, Mateer JR, Hargarten KM, Stueven HA: EMT-defibrillation: The Wisconsin experience. *Ann Emerg Med* 1989;18:806–811

42. Stults KR, Cummins RO: Fully automatic vs shock advisory defibrillators — What are the issues? *J Emerg Med Serv* 1987;12:71–73

43. Stults KR, Brown DD, Cooley F, Kerber RE: Self-adhesive monitor defibrillation pads improve prehospital defibrillation success. *Ann Emerg Med* 1987;16:872–877

44. Cummins RO, Stults KR, Haggar B, Kerber RE, Schaeffer S, Brown DD: A new rhythm library for testing automatic external defibrillators: Performance of three devices. *J Am Coll Cardiol* 1988;11:597–602

45. Diack AW, Welborn WS, Rullman RG, Walter CW, Wayne MA: An automatic cardiac resuscitator for emergency treatment of cardiac arrest. *Med Instrum* 1979;13:78–83

46. Jaggarao NS, Heber M, Grainger R, Vincent R, Chamberlain DA: Use of an automated external defibrillator-pacemaker by ambulance staff. *Lancet* 1982;2:73–75

47. Cummins RO, Eisenberg M, Bergner L, Murray JA: Sensitivity, accuracy and safety of an automatic external defibrillator: Report of a field evaluation. *Lancet* 1984;2:318–320

48. Stults KR, Brown DD, Kerber RE: Efficacy of an automated external defibrillator in the management of out-of-hospital cardiac arrest: Validation of the diagnostic algorithm and initial clinical experience in a rural environment. *Circulation* 1986;73:701–709

49. Cummins RO, Eisenberg MS, Litwin PE, Graves JR, Hearne TR, Hallstrom AP: Automatic external defibrillators used by emergency medical technicians: A controlled clinical trial. *JAMA* 1987;257:1605–1610

50. Gray AJ, Redmond AD, Martin MA: Use of the automatic external defibrillator-pacemaker by ambulance personnel: The Stockport experience. *Br Med J* 1987;294:1133–1135

51. Weaver WD, Hill D, Fahrenbruch CE, Copass MK, Martin JS, Cobb LA, Hallstom AP: Use of the automatic external defibrillator in the management of out-of-hospital cardiac arrest. *N Engl J Med* 1988;319:661–666

52. Jakobsson J, Nyquist O, Rehnqvist N: Effects of early defibrillation of out-of-hospital cardiac arrest patients by ambulance personnel. *Eur Heart J* 1987;8:1189–1194

53. Stults KR, Brown DD: Refibrillation managed by EMT-D's: Incidence and outcome without paramedic backup. *Am J Emerg Med* 1986;4:491–495

54. Bradley K, Sokolow AE,Wright KJ, McCullough WJ: A comparison of an innovative four-hour EMT-D course with a "standard" ten-hour course. *Ann Emerg Med* 1988;17:613–619

55. Ornato JP, Craren EJ, Gonzalez ER, Garnett AR, McClung BK, Newman MM: Cost-effectiveness of defibrillation by emergency medical technicians. *Am J Emerg Med* 1988; 6:108–112

56. Kerber RE, Martins JB, Kelly KJ, Ferguson DW, Kouba C, Jensen SR, Newman B, Parke JD, Kieso R, Melton J: Self-adhesive preapplied electrode pads for defibrillation and cardioversion. *J Am Coll Cardiol* 1984;3:815-820

57. Wilson RF, Sirna S, White CW, Kerber RE: Defibrillation of high risk patients during coronary angiography using self-adhesive preapplied electrode pads. *Am J Cardiol* 1987;60:380–382

58. Weaver WD, Cobb LA, Copass MK, Hallstrom AP: Ventricular defibrillation — A comparative trial using 185-J and 320-J shocks. *N Engl J Med* 1982;307:1101–1106

59. Cummins RO, Austin D Jr, Graves JR, Hambly C: An innovative approach to medical control: Semiautomatic defibrillators with solid-state memory for recording cardiac arrest events. *Ann Emerg Med* 1988;17:818–824